LESSONS LEARNED

LESSONS LEARNED

Stories from the Oncology Unit

David M. Mastrianni, MD

ISBN-13: 9781975657789
ISBN-10: 1975657780

" Cancer sucks." These two words are embossed on a small metal pin given to me by a patient. I could never wear it, so for years it sat on my desk as a bleak reminder of the sadness often shared by patients and their families in our oncology unit. Yet every day, laughter and the sounds of daily life could be heard in the exam rooms and treatment area. As a family member once said, "I used to think heroes were those who do something extraordinary. But now I know that heroes are also those people who keep doing the ordinary in extraordinarily difficult circumstances." These are stories of our heroes.

Someday, this pin will be wrong. Soon, it may be less true. A transformation in cancer treatment is underway in which molecularly targeted therapies are replacing chemotherapy. This change is the result of years of investment in basic science to understand the workings of normal tissues and thus cancer. It is the culmination of many events, some obvious and others seemingly small, which have occurred in labs and clinics across the world. It is the work of thousands of scientists, physicians, nurses, technicians, administrators, investors, executives, politicians, families, and patients. For those with cancer, this era is bringing new hope mixed with the enduring struggle to make sense of the human condition. These are also stories of this transformation.

This book tells the stories of twenty-one (fictional) patients seen during a typical day in our medical oncology practice in Saratoga Springs, New York. Some patients are undergoing traditional chemotherapy while others receive new targeted treatments. Some have dealt with their cancers for years and are witness to both sides of this transition. All of them have lives outside of their cancers. Each hour of this imaginary day contains three patient visits which can be read and understood independently. Each hour begins with an interlude containing the ongoing story of a (fictional) patient treated in the 1980s during my training at the Beth Israel Hospital/Harvard Medical School. Her story illustrates how far we have come but must be read serially.

Contained within these stories are nonfictional essays on the history of cancer medicine. For many years, I have been privileged to teach medical students from Albany Medical College. These essays grew from discussions with these remarkable students, which often included our physicians, nursing staff, and colleagues in the pharmaceutical industry. I have learned much from these students, including that our medical future is in good hands. Although the direct purpose of this work is to (hopefully) interest students in oncology, I have tried to use vocabulary which will allow patients, families, and others in the world of cancer medicine to read these essays without a medical dictionary. For those searching for a specific cancer or topic, the diagnosis of each patient and the subject matter of the essays appear in the table of contents.

A few disclaimers are required. No one should make any medical decisions based on these stories. The science, medicine, and surgery are often simplified. Cancer treatments are changing rapidly, and the specific therapies will soon be out of date. I believe the recent history of the development of cancer treatments is accurate since it occurred during my career. These brief essays do not provide a comprehensive accounting, and omit many key figures. To place these essays in broader context, I have relied heavily on the work of many skilled historians and fully anticipate I have misinterpreted some of their writings. Any errors are mine.

The settings are real. Saratoga Springs is a charming town of thirty thousand in upstate New York. It was originally known for its mineral springs, gambling, and as the home of the longest running Thoroughbred racetrack in the country. As described at points in this book, the City endured despair from the 1940s through the 1970s and has been reborn in the last quarter century. It is worth a visit. The major academic medical centers visited by these patients are national treasures, driving this transformation in cancer care. Our small office and local community hospital typify the delivery of much of the medical care in our nation. The diverse staffs in these varied settings are fictional, but their dedication is not. That the transformation of oncology has reached from large centers to local hospitals is a tribute to these people and our often maligned but truly remarkable medical system.

The patients are entirely fictional. Even when a specific name, title, or job is applied, any resemblance to an actual person is coincidental. The vignettes and comments have come from real people, although any identifying characteristics were removed. Despite this necessary editing, I hope the courage and expressions of our humanity which occur every day in oncology units have been left unaltered.

David M. Mastrianni, MD
Saratoga Springs, New York

Notes for the general reader

A few notes may be helpful to the general reader, starting with a short course in oncology.

Cancer is the uncontrolled growth of cells which can invade normal tissue. Many patients are surprised to learn that cancer develops in series of steps which damage once normal cells and cause them to become increasingly abnormal. This process can take years. Most normal cells which are damaged will not become cancers—they will either be repaired, commit suicide, or be destroyed or held dormant by the immune system. When deranged cells successfully escape these checks and become cancers, we name them after their site of origin. For example, the breast duct cells which undergo this process become a breast cancer. Over time, these cells may spread to other areas of the body, the process called metastasis. When cancer cells metastasize, we still name them after their origin. In the example of breast cancer, spread to the liver is described as "breast cancer metastatic to the liver." Usually, the cancer cells which have metastasized will have some of the features of the original cancer and the tissue from which it originated.

The past fifty years have seen remarkable advances in our understanding of cancer development based on knowledge of normal cellular growth—including the role of DNA, RNA, proteins, tissue development and structure, and the immune system. All of these components can be deranged in cancers. For simplicity, most of the scientific discussion in this work describes abnormalities in DNA (mutations) which then lead to abnormal proteins which cause the cancers. There are many different combinations of DNA abnormalities which lead to different cancers and thus offer the possibility of specific treatments. Derangements in the immune system which aid in cancer growth and immunotherapy are also discussed. The amazingly complex interplay of all the other components of normal growth is not reviewed. Breakdowns in these systems also contribute to cancer and will occupy scientists for years to come.

A brief review of the structure and nomenclature of DNA is useful. DNA is made of two strings which are wound together in the famous "double helix" then further folded for storage. Each string is a series of "nucleotide bases" (adenine, thymine, guanine, and cytosine) which pair with a base on the other string (adenine and thymine form a pair, guanine and cytosine form a pair). The sequence of the bases makes the DNA code which is translated into RNA and then into the proteins which perform the functions of life. Groups of DNA bases are called a gene if they produce RNA which in turn produces a protein. Human cells have roughly six billion base pairs of DNA, referring to a base on one strand and its opposite base on the other strand. Our DNA is broken up into forty-six chromosomes, each containing fifty million to three hundred million base pairs. Only about 2 percent of our DNA is used in genes; the rest is empty space which may serve other functions. A typical gene is a few thousand base pairs grouped in multiple short stretches (called exons) separated by stretches of other DNA (called introns). Humans have an estimated twenty-one thousand genes. The names of genes are written in italics while their corresponding proteins are not. Thus, the *BRCA* gene produces a BRCA protein. Mutations are damage to the DNA and can lead to the production of abnormal proteins. A common theme in cancer is that genes needed for normal growth proteins are damaged, resulting in abnormal cell growth. The resulting unstable cell acquires further damage to multiple critical genes which can lead to cancer.

The standard treatments for cancer have been surgery, radiation, and chemotherapy. Surgery to remove the primary site of the cancer is usually the first treatment. Modern surgery began in the middle of the nineteenth century with the introduction of anesthesia and antisepsis. Amazingly complex cancer operations are now routine. Radiation is used to destroy cancer in a specific area of the body. It was introduced in the 1950s and has also undergone remarkable advances. For most cancers, the combination of surgery and radiation means the primary sites are effectively treated. Thus, it is the metastasis or spread of cancer throughout the body which poses the greatest threat to patients. The main treatment for cancer spread throughout the body has been chemotherapy. Following a rocky start after World War II, chemotherapy was successfully used to cure some lymphomas and leukemia. In the 1970s and 1980s, chemotherapy improved the survival rates after surgery in some situations, most notably for women after breast cancer surgery. The use of chemotherapy markedly expanded in the 1990s after the development of modern antinausea medications. In attempts to improve results, multiple combinations, maintenance treatments, and high-dose chemotherapy were all tried with limited success. By the end of the twentieth century, most of the benefits of chemotherapy were maximized—the limit was reached. Unfortunately, these relatively nonspecific poisons simply do not help all patients.

The remarkable advances in our understanding of cancer have led to new treatments which are replacing chemotherapy. One approach is to target the abnormal proteins produced by mutated genes, called "targeted therapy." The best example is the rare disease chronic myelogenous leukemia (CML), where a single specific abnormality has led to a targeted treatment which cures this previously often fatal cancer. For patients with more complex cancers, finding combinations of mutations unique to their cancer can also lead to specific treatments, called "personalized and precision medicine." A second modern approach has been to unleash the immune system to destroy cancers. Both of these approaches are changing oncology care and signal the start of an exciting new chapter in cancer medicine. These treatments come to us from the amazing combination of our academic institutions, pharmaceutical companies, and the biotech industry. The cost is staggering. How we will pay for this science and medicine and allocate rewards are unresolved issues.

A few other practical notes might also be useful to the general reader.

Whether they are old or new, most medications have two names: the generic name and at least one brand name (capitalized). These multiple names are a long-standing source of consternation to physicians, nurses, and pharmacists and discouraging for patients trying to understand their medications. In medical literature, medications are written using generic names. In medical conversation, generic and brand names are often mixed. That pattern is followed here—the patient stories and titles use the mixed names as we would in daily life while the formal essays use the generic versions. If the reader is unsure of the proper pairing, the index may be helpful.

The training programs for oncology professionals are often unfamiliar to people outside medicine. Physicians attend medical or osteopathic school for four years. Residency follows medical school and includes the first year called an internship. For many cancer surgeons, a surgical residency of five years continues with several additional years in a specific training program. Radiation oncologists undergo four to five years of residency training and may also have additional subspecialty programs. For oncologists, a general medical residency of three years is followed by a fellowship of three years. Thus, all these physicians can expect a decade of training after college. Oncology nurses typically spend several years after nursing school to become certified. Those who become Nurse Practitioners spend an additional three to five years of training.

Terminology in cancer medicine is notoriously confusing, generally due to the complex nature of these illnesses. The common use of two specific words warrants comment. "Tumor" can refer to a mass of cancerous cells ("the tumor in the breast") but is often also used to mean all the cancer in the body ("your tumor is resistant to the treatment"). This use is a common source of confusion for patients. More destructive is the use of the word "failed." When a treatment fails to work, we often state that the patient failed the treatment ("she failed multiple treatments for breast cancer"). We should abandon this pejorative use of that word.

Table of Contents

October 30, 2017
Saratoga Springs, New York

Carol Feinman 1: Breast cancer (Boston, 1988)

Carol Feinman was twenty-seven on that beautiful fall day in 1988 when she found her breast cancer. As she walked across Boston Common and rubbed an itch, there it was—a small pebble in the upper outer part of her left breast. Carol always remembered that she had just reached the "Make Way for Ducklings" sculpture, Robert McCloskey's recently installed depiction of a larger-than-life mother duck named Mrs. Mallard leading her eight ducklings. As usual, it was crowded with children.

Carol's childhood had been in nearby Brookline with her mother Betty, older sister Rose, and younger brother Steven. When she was seven, Carol's father was killed in an auto accident. Richard had been a highly successful banker, fondly remembered as an intelligent and warm man who deeply loved his family. Since he had the rare foresight to be well insured, Carol's family was financially secure. The loss of their father had bound the girls tightly to their mother, a proud woman who never remarried or even dated another man and still lived in their family home. Rose was a married lawyer in her early thirties who lived in the Boston suburb of Newton with her two young girls, Cynthia and Alisa, while Carol enjoyed single life in the City's downtown. Steven, always more independent, was a film producer in New York City.

Cancer was familiar to Carol's family. Betty, now sixty, had been diagnosed with breast cancer at age forty, four years after Richard's death. Knowing that she had to raise the children alone and fearing another cancer if any tissue was left behind, she had insisted on the removal of both her breasts. At the urging of her surgeon, her ovaries were also taken. Betty had been free of cancer ever since. Her older sister Christine had not been so fortunate. Shortly after Betty's surgery,

Christine developed ovarian cancer and rapidly died. As a teenager, Rose witnessed her aunt's suffering and the haunting images, while Carol, being four years younger, was always partially shielded by the family.

WHY OUR FAMILY? BEFORE GENETIC TESTING.

For many years it has been understood that women in some families develop breast and ovarian cancer at young ages. Even in eras when discussions of cancer were taboo, these families were often aware of the danger and known to their doctors. Major medical institutions collected blood and tissue samples from these families in hopes that researchers might someday unlock their dangerous secret. When advances in technology in the 1970s allowed the study of DNA, scientists began searching for the genes responsible for these so-called "familial breast and ovarian cancers." During the 1980s a highly publicized race to discover these genes began, but it was not until the mid-1990s that scientists identified the two genes responsible for most of these familial breast and ovary cancers. The genes were named *BRCA-1* and *BRCA-2* (BR for breast and CA for cancer). The discovery of these genes was the lead story on the evening news since it promised the opportunity for genetic testing and even treatment. Women who carry mutations in the either the *BRCA-1* or *BRCA-2* genes are at very high risk: 65–80 percent will develop breast cancer and 20–40 percent ovarian cancer.

Inherited *BRCA* gene mutations cause only about 5 percent of breast cancers, so most women with breast cancer do not have this problem. Typically, families with a *BRCA* mutation have women who develop breast and ovary cancer at young ages in several generations. The discovery of the *BRCA* genes allowed the women with cancer in these families to be tested to see if they carried a mutation—there are over three thousand different ones. If a specific family mutation was found, the women who did not yet have cancer could be tested to see if they were carriers. If they were carriers, they could be watched closely or even have their breasts and ovaries removed before cancer developed. If they were not carriers, their risk would be the same as the general population of women. Some specific mutations are found in ethnic groups. For example, three mutations are common in Ashkenazi Jewish families (those from eastern Europe). These mutations first appeared by some accident thousands of years ago and were concentrated in Jewish families by the powerful forces of religion and history which caused them to marry and reproduce within their faith.

Scientists later discovered that the *BRCA* genes repair damage to the DNA in the cells of the breast and ovary. Since DNA damage occurs regularly in all cells from exposure to toxins or radiation and during normal functioning, repair is important to prevent damage which might lead to cancer. Being born with a *BRCA* gene mutation means that breast and ovary cells will not properly repair the damage done to their DNA, hence the cancer risk.

Although the Feinman women could not know about *BRCA* genes, they knew that within their family there was genetic cancer time bomb waiting to explode. Carol and Rose had reacted to this potential terror in very different ways. Rose managed the uncertainty by planning every part of her life. She found her husband in college, a reliable man who idolized her and willingly allowed her to set the agenda. She had her two daughters early, becoming pregnant as she finished law school. Betty cared for the young girls as Rose developed her law practice.

Carol chose a different path. She graduated from Boston University with a degree in English and no clear destination. She had dated several men of varied personalities but had not felt a sense of commitment despite pressure from Rose and her mother. Her work in product evaluation was lighthearted; surveying women about tampons hardly met their expectations. Unlike them, Carol had a free spirit. Despite their differences, Carol was bound to her mother and sister. Although she admired her brother and shared his easy, ironic view of life, Carol also knew that she could not escape the tight links of genetics and life which bound the Feinman women.

Even with the history of cancer in her family, Carol did not initially think of her lump as serious. Somehow, she just felt it was a nothing. She did not tell her mother or sister but did call her doctor on Monday morning. Dr. Carl was a portly, middle-aged man known for embracing alternative treatments for many ailments. Carol found his emphasis on a healthy lifestyle despite his body shape and his distrust of many medical technologies fit in well with her optimistic view of the world. Dr. Carl saw her that afternoon and immediately recognized that the hard mass in Carol's breast needed traditional medical attention. Even as he scheduled a mammogram, ultrasound, and a visit to a surgeon for the next day, Carol felt no fear and was confident as she called her boss to ask for time off.

"I'm sorry, Roger," she said. "My doctor wants me to have a few tests tomorrow. It is nothing serious, but since the Miller report is pretty well done, I thought it would be good to get them done."

Since her graduation from BU six years ago, Carol had worked for a market research firm in downtown Boston which specialized in evaluating women's products. She enjoyed the job and its periods of intense activity punctuated by quieter times, a pattern that seemed a natural extension of collegiate life. Carol's team of three women about her age was led by Roger, a gay man about ten years older. Carol felt somewhat guilty that she was not more forthcoming and not exactly sure why she could not confide in him about this matter. Roger insisted that Carol should take the rest of the week off since their current project was complete and she had been working extra hours.

Carol reported to the impressively decorated main lobby of the Beth Israel Hospital the next morning. A donor list that recorded the history of the Jewish community in Boston adorned the wall.

"Can I help you dear?" asked the older, almost elderly woman behind the desk.

"I need to go for a mammogram," Carol replied.

"Well, dear, take the main elevator to the second floor and go out straight ahead. You will see the signs. You look too young and healthy to be there, though."

Thanks, thought Carol, surprised that this woman, who was just trying to be helpful and probably had both limited vision and no medical training, could somehow make her feel foolish and out of place. The receptionist at the mammogram suite was welcoming and the waiting room warmly colored and comfortable. In the dressing room, Carol removed her top and bra, put on her gown and then entered the mammogram room.

Mammograms are low-dose x-rays of the breast. To have the mammogram, Carol stood at the machine with her breasts pressed between two plates. It was relatively painless. She was somewhat surprised since she had heard older women complain of the dreaded the squeezing of their breasts each year. She remembered the comment that it was probably a man who designed the equipment and the suggestion that he should have his testicles put into the machine. Although the image was amusing, she concluded it might have been a bit harsh.

When the mammogram image is viewed on the x-ray film (or now the computer), the normal breast tissue looks like thin white strands on the black background. Some breast cancers appear as dense white growths which distort the normal structure of the breast tissue, while others produce small calcium specks called microcalcifications. The radiologist's challenge is to distinguish normal tissue and calcifications from cancer. Carol's mammogram was normal. Young women like Carol often have dense breast tissue which appears white and makes it difficult to see cancerous changes. Modern radiologists can use MRIs to see cancers within this dense tissue, but at the time of Carol's diagnosis, the only other available procedure was the ultrasound. She immediately went into the next room where she lay on the exam table as the ultrasound technician applied lubricant and moved the probe over her breast. The technician was a young woman about Carol's age; professional looking and trained to be pleasant but non-committal. As she watched the image of her breast on the screen, Carol began to have her first sense of unease. It was then that she also first noticed the faintly mechanical smell of the jelly lubricant used to allow the probe to glide over her breast. It was a smell which would later make her nauseous whenever she needed that test. More remarkably, Carol later found that this smell could even faintly appear on its own at stressful times to make her queasy.

"It wasn't how I expected to have my first ultrasound," she recalled. "I kept thinking she should be checking my baby as the man of my dreams, or at least my mother's dreams, sat nearby."

The ultrasound showed the small lump was solid and looked cancerous. The technician's face was impressively impassive, but Carol's unease grew with her lack of reassurance. She began to wish she had brought her mother or sister. Immediately after the ultrasound, she dressed and went down the hall to meet the surgeon, Dr. Scanlon. As she sat in his waiting room completing forms and was again forced to write about her mother and aunt, the reality of her situation began to cause a slow rise of panic. The room became warm and the faint smell of the ultrasound jelly still on her skin began to exert its powerfully nauseating effect. When she was brought into the exam room and again placed into a gown, her anxiety and confusion were obvious. Dr. Scanlon was in his mid-fifties, a tall, gaunt man with long, thin fingers and an air of no-nonsense professionalism and experience which was immediately comforting to Carol. After a brief examination, he sat with her and insisted she drink a glass of cold water. The sharpness of the water and his direct clarity briefly cut away her confused panic.

"Carol, you have a lump in your breast which may or may not be cancer. It must be biopsied, and I will do that tomorrow morning at eight. You are not to eat or drink after midnight tonight. The nurse will provide you with all the instructions."

Carol was surprised at how few questions she had. In fact, her only real question was how she would explain this to her mother and sister during their planned dinner at Betty's that evening. The nurse had no answer for this dilemma but gave Carol the instruction sheet and sent her home. As she showered, Carol carefully avoided touching the lump in her breast out of fear that she would feel it grow. She also desperately wanted the last traces of the ultrasound jelly off her breast since even the faint smell of it made her sick. Carol was relieved to find a large bath sponge worked perfectly to clean her breast without allowing her to feel what she was washing. Drying required bunching a large towel then dabbing it gently while sipping a glass of chilled white wine. As she dressed, Carol rehearsed how she would present this to Rose and Betty. She decided she would wait until after dinner and break the news over coffee.

"Don't worry," she would say. "I have a tiny lump in my breast. You know Dr. Carl is very careful and made me have an ultrasound. They're doing a biopsy just as a precaution. Dr. Scanlon didn't think it was anything. I'll be fine . . . No, you don't need to come."

As she walked up the stairs to Betty's brownstone in the cool autumn air, she practiced one more time. She rang the bell and Betty opened the door to reveal the scene of the familiar entrance hall followed immediately by the wonderful smells she always associated with her childhood. She could see Rose sitting in the formal room off to the left. The sudden contrast of her day with the comfort of her childhood home took her by surprise and brought her confused panic rushing back. She again faintly smelled the ultrasound jelly as her composure crumbled.

"What's wrong?" asked Betty after one look at Carol's face.

"I found a lump and think I have breast cancer. I have a biopsy tomorrow."

"What? Why didn't you tell me?" asked Rose, rising quickly and striding to the door as if in a courtroom. "I'll call my surgeon friend at Massachusetts General for another opinion. We need another opinion. You can't have surgery tomorrow without it. Besides I am in court. Who will take care of you?"

"I'll take care of her," said Betty. "You go to court."

"I can't go to court knowing she is in surgery. And I want to know about the surgeon operating on my sister."

"I'm sure they have fine surgeons at Beth Israel," said Betty.

"That's not the point. This is serious and we should have an opinion from somebody we know."

"Could I come in?" asked Carol, her returning composure accompanied by a profound sense of fatigue. Her faint look brought the discussion to a temporary halt until they had her settled on the sofa. When she recovered, Carol revised her story.

"I found the lump by accident and called Dr. Carl. He had me have a mammogram and ultrasound and then meet with Dr. Scanlon—all this afternoon. It happened so fast that I didn't have time to call you. I like Dr. Scanlon. He said he wasn't sure if this was cancer or not, but that it should be biopsied. He can do it tomorrow. I can't eat after midnight and have to be at the hospital at six-thirty in the morning. You don't need to miss work, Rose. I'll be fine if Mom can take me. I don't need another opinion now; it's just a biopsy."

Dinner was unusually quiet as they processed the day's events. For her part, Carol was both relieved that she delivered the news and so tired she could barely eat and certainly not think or converse. While she would later understand that the fatigue produced by medical visits and procedures could be overwhelming, tonight was her first experience with that mind-numbing exhaustion. Opposite her at the table, Rose's thoughts were moving at the speed of light. She had already planned how she would rearrange her schedule for the day and upcoming week. Some part of her mind had known this day would come for either herself or Carol and she was ready for action. She knew after this biopsy would come more surgery and maybe chemotherapy or radiation. Even if Carol was not yet thinking ahead, Rose was determined to be prepared. Betty quietly served the meal, a warm vegetable soup followed by a roast. It was a dish from Carol's childhood, and Betty was content to see that it met Carol's needs in an unplanned but special way.

The pattern of the relationship between the three women had emerged years ago, during the time of Christine's ovarian cancer. She had been a quiet, delicate woman in her forties when the swelling in her abdomen developed. Like many women with ovarian cancer, her early symptoms were subtle, only mild bloating and vague nausea. Eventually, they became more noticeable, and she entered the hospital with an intestinal blockage. Modern CT scans were not yet available, and an initial exploratory surgery found widespread cancer throughout her abdominal cavity. In Christine's time, there were no effective chemotherapy treatments, and women with ovarian cancer often suffered repeated intestinal blockages and fluid build-up in the abdomen. Hospice programs did not exist, so the period leading to death was often included repeated hospitalizations, attempts at surgery, tubes and drains, vomiting, pain, and malnutrition.

Christine's husband Samuel was a wonderful man who loved her dearly but was constitutionally unable to provide her with intimate personal care. He grew weak at the sight or smell of vomit, urine caused palpitations and, when she required a colostomy, changing the bag nearly produced a seizure. Yet, Samuel would sit with Christine for endless hours, talking, reading, and even singing. Since they had no children, it fell to Betty to provide for her physical needs, which she did with graceful competence. At the start of the illness, each morning Betty prepared breakfast for Rose, Carol, and Steven, sent them off to school, and then walked the two blocks to Christine's home. Betty bathed, dressed, and fed her sister before moving her to the living room where she would sit with Samuel. Betty returned in the afternoon to help Christine into bed for her nap and prepared dinner for Samuel to feed her. Betty returned a third time each evening and readied Christine for the night. Visits to the emergency room and admissions to the hospital punctuated the routine. Over nine months, Christine came to need more and more of Betty, who never complained and faced each visit with a resigned stoicism despite her own recent cancer.

During Christine's illness, fourteen-year-old Rose assumed an adult role in their family. Since by nature she was an organized child who had always acted beyond her years, Betty's increasing distraction allowed her to assert her leadership. She began by organizing ten-year-old Carol and seven-year-old Steven each morning and assuming the responsibility of preparing breakfast and walking them both to school. As Christine declined, Rose took over the afternoon and evening responsibilities of homework, studying, and bedtime. Rose never had an interest in cooking, although she quickly learned how to order out when Betty was with Christine in the emergency ward. On most evenings, Betty would be home to prepare dinner and take report from Rose about Carol and Steven. Even in this early time, Rose and Betty worried together about Carol, whose approach to school and life was relaxed, almost flippant.

"I know she can do the work, mother," said Rose one evening as Betty sliced vegetables at the counter. "But she simply is not serious about it. I have tried to explain it to her, but she will not listen."

"I know, Rose. She has always been a little different. But she is a smart girl, and we must be patient with her."

Christine's illness started the pattern that replayed over the ensuing years and which Rose referred to as "waiting for Carol." The older sister tried to make plans and decisions for her sister while Carol refused to go along fully and occasionally resisted but never broke free. Betty usually agreed with Rose yet supported Carol in a less judgmental fashion. Steven, being male and independent, could do as he wished with only an occasional ineffective attempt by Rose to induce guilt.

After telling Rose and Betty of her impending biopsy, Carol stayed the night with her mother. They arrived at the Beth Israel Hospital at six-thirty the next morning, Rose followed shortly afterward.

"You didn't need to . . .," began Carol, giving up once she saw the look on Rose's face.

Carol was met by Dr. Scanlon in the operating room. After the anesthesia was given, he cut into her breast and removed the one-inch hard tumor. A pathologist took a preliminary look at the tissue under the microscopic and reported that it was cancer.

Today, Carol would not have had a surgical biopsy, but rather a "core needle" done by a radiologist using local anesthetic in a mammogram or ultrasound room. This simpler test would make the diagnosis and Carol would then meet with a surgeon to discuss her options. In the 1980s, this technology was only recently introduced, and most surgeons still did biopsies in the operating room. Even this was a significant advance for women. Shortly before Carol's time, when women went to the operating room for a biopsy and cancer was found, the surgeon would commonly remove the breast. The woman awoke in the recovery room unsure of whether she still had her breast, a nightmarish moment described by many as one of the most terrifyingly of their lives and often revisited in dreams for years. Thankfully, this "one-step" procedure ended as women objected and the option of limited surgery and radiation became available.

In the recovery room with the three of them, Dr. Scanlon spoke slowly and carefully.

"This was a cancer, Carol. Today I removed what I could easily take out. Next week you will need more surgery. At that time, I will either remove the entire breast with a mastectomy or just remove more tissue from the area around where the cancer grew. With either surgery, I will also remove the lymph nodes under the arm. If you choose not to have the whole breast removed, you will need radiation treatments. Today is Wednesday. On Friday, you will meet with the radiation oncologist, Dr. Morris, to discuss that option. If you decide to have the mastectomy, you may have reconstructive surgery and meet a plastic surgeon. On Monday, you will meet with me to tell me your decision, and I will schedule your next surgery."

Then he was gone. It was Rose who spoke first. From this initial meeting, she did not like Dr. Scanlon. Although she would later admire his dedication to Carol, she hated his spare style that never offered a single extra word or explanation. Rose described him as the perfect witness, stating only the facts and never speculating. Worse yet, although he was respectful to Betty, he never acknowledged Rose's needs and always spoke directly to Carol.

"How does he know that it's cancer already? The written pathology report isn't even out. Now we really need another opinion. I'll set it up at Mass General," she said emphatically, her pace only a little less rapid than the night before. Carol lay back on the recovery room stretcher, numb and tired.

"Rose, let's worry about that later. I want to go home."

"You'll stay with me," said Betty.

"No. I can go home. I want my own bed."

"Don't be silly, Carol," said Rose. "You need Mom tonight."

This time Carol successfully resisted. Betty brought her home, stayed with her for a few hours, and then left her alone in her bed. Carol thought briefly about calling some of her close friends to update them, but her second experience with post-procedure fatigue made even this simple act overwhelming. Carol did not remember any specific dreams that night. When she awoke early the next morning in her room with the sun coming through the windows as it always had, it seemed an ordinary day. It took her a moment to remember what had happened. Carol often recalled that morning's brief interval between when she awoke and when she remembered as the last moment when she had possession of her old life, free of cancer. As she began to move, the mild soreness in her breast and the tugging of the dressing made her surgery undeniable. As she bathed carefully to avoid wetting the bandage, her discomfort was partially offset by her relief that she no longer had to worry about accidentally touching the hard lump in her breast. Her breakfast routine and coffee were comforting, but as she finished cleaning up the small kitchen area, Carol faced a day with no definition. Her breast began to ache, and she was unsure what to do. Fortunately, Betty arrived and settled Carol into her most comfortable chair in her small living room, carefully arranged pillows to support her arm away from her breast, and gave her one of her forgotten pain pills.

As Carol was beginning to relax, the phone rang. She elected not to answer it, and the message machine played her taped greeting.

"This is Carol. I cannot take your call, but I'm sure it is very important to me, so please leave a message . . ."

"Carol this is Roger calling to check and be sure you were all right. Give us a call if you need anything. The ladies also want you to know that they will be going to the Black Rose on Friday night and would love to see you there. I cannot imagine why you all would go to such a dreadful place, but there it is. Anyway, love you, so let me know, dear."

"He sounds delightful," said Betty.

"He is."

"Why haven't we met him?"

"Do you mean why haven't I brought him home for you and Rose to get your hopes up?"

"Well . . . yes, dear."

"Roger is gay, mother."

"And there is no hope of converting him?" asked Betty, partially seriously.

"No, mother," Carol answered. And not just because he is gay, she thought, but because by next week I might not have any breasts. It was the first time she had thought seriously about her options. She could undergo a mastectomy as Betty had chosen almost twenty years earlier. The other choice was to remove more tissue near where the cancer had been and an extra rim of normal surrounding tissue, followed by radiation treatments to the breast to kill any isolated cancer cells which might remain. This procedure was commonly called "lumpectomy" or "partial mastectomy" and radiation.

MODERN SURGERY: SAVING WOMEN THEN SAVING BREASTS. For women with breast cancer in the 1980s, the choice to try and save their breast was relatively new. Since about 1850, mastectomy had been the main treatment for breast cancer.[1] Before that time, there had been no useful treatment. Early surgeons found removing just the cancerous lump was futile because the tumors grew back at the site of the surgery. Since they did not have anesthesia, removing the whole breast was horribly painful. Saint Agatha, the patron saint of women with breast disease, was tortured in the third century by having her breasts amputated. Her suffering is depicted in graphic art showing her carrying her breasts or being healed by Saint Peter. While these iconic renditions carried many religious messages, they were also a clear warning to surgeons not to perform mastectomies. A few surgeons did very rapid breast amputations with barbaric looking instruments; usually their patients died of infection since the need for sterile conditions was also not understood. Until the middle of the 1800s, therefore, breast cancer could not be treated, and women died with disfiguring foul tumors which eroded their breasts and spread through their bodies.

Two discoveries in the mid-1800s changed surgery forever: the discovery of anesthesia by Boston dentist William Mortin in 1846 and the promotion of antisepsis to prevent infection by Joseph Lister in 1867.[2] Mortin was a dentist who administered a gas he called "Letheon" to his patients to produce anesthesia. Interestingly, Morton patented his recipe and operated in secrecy. Fortunately, surgeon Henry Jacob Bigelow at the Massachusetts General Hospital in Boston smelled the ether in Letheon and publicized it in the *Boston Medical and Surgical Journal* (later to become the *New England Journal of Medicine*, the premier medical journal in the United States). Prior to ether anesthesia, the skill of the surgeon was usually measured by the speed of the operation. With ether, operations could be done carefully without immediate pain. Unfortunately, most serious operations risked death from infection. Surgeons often did not wash their hands and operated while wearing old heavy coats which were rarely cleaned and often covered with old blood and body fragments. They performed surgery in dirty rooms or "operating theaters" with a variety of notoriously unkempt students and observers. Thus, the second key for safe surgery was the discovery of germs (or at least cleanliness). In 1867, Joseph Lister published a series of articles in the *Lancet*, now the premier British medical journal, which described the use of carbolic acid to produce antisepsis and prevent infection.[3] At the time, Lister's work was very controversial. Many surgeons and physicians refused to believe they could be the guilty parties in transmitting these infections, instead blaming airborne substances called "miasmata," a medical term historically meaning "bad air." This resistance in the profession was not new. A classic example is the story of Dr. Ignaz Semmelweis, a physician who worked in a Vienna obstetrical clinic in the 1840s. Semmelweis found that women who gave birth attended by physicians died of an infection at a much higher rate than those attended by midwives. Semmelweis concluded that this was because many of the physicians attended their patients after visiting the morgue and participating in autopsies. His insistence upon strict hand washing and cleaning of instruments reduced the infection rate. Semmelweis encountered so much opposition that he reportedly quit and ended up in a lunatic asylum.[4] Despite these battles, the combination of anesthesia and antisepsis started the era of modern surgery. For women with breast cancer, the ability of surgeons to do mastectomies meant some were cured.

Once mastectomies became possible, a debate began over how much tissue to remove. Some surgeons argued that only the breast itself needed to be removed, while others felt that more extensive surgery was required.[5] The latter group was led by two famous surgeons, William Halsted from Johns Hopkins and William Handley of London. The debate revolved around the scientific understanding of breast cancer. While it was well known to surgeons of the day that breast cancer was fatal because it spread to other parts of the body, it was not clear whether it spread widely through the blood stream or the lymph system. If the cancer had spread through the blood stream before it was removed, then doing more extensive surgery on the breast would probably not be helpful. The woman's fate was already decided when the surgeon operated. Expressed more roughly, the surgeon who did the more extensive surgery was "closing the door when the horse was already out of the barn." If the breast cancer spread primarily through the lymph system, more surgery to remove the lymph nodes and channels could be useful.

The lymph system was (and still is) less well understood than the blood system. Lymph channels are found throughout the tissues of the body and serve as "storm drains" to collect the fluid that leaks from the blood vessels into our tissues (among other functions). The lymph fluid travels through the small channels into larger lymph channels and lymph nodes until it finally reaches the largest lymph channel, called the thoracic duct, in the chest. Here the fluid is put back into the circulation. Hanley and Halsted reasoned that if breast cancers first spread into the lymph system before they go into the blood stream, it might be possible to "catch them" before they spread by removing all the lymph tissue. Hanley did careful dissections of mastectomy specimens and found that the cancers from these women had spread extensively into the lymph channels. He deduced that the cancers spread through the lymph system and, if he could remove that system, he could remove the cancer. Halsted agreed, and these two surgeons pioneered a more extensive "radical mastectomy" which included removal of all the lymph tissue under the arm, the muscle under the breast, and even some lymph tissue from within the chest. They became known for their brilliant surgical techniques, and the radical mastectomy became the standard surgery for breast cancer by the time of Halsted's death in 1922. Although cure rates were still low, their surgery saved the lives of some women with breast cancer, and, for others, removed the visible cancer for a time.

Since the radical mastectomy was partially successful, surgeons including Halsted, Handley, and his son Richard Handley, then advocated the "extended radical mastectomy," an extreme surgery which reached its peak in the 1930s and 1940s. This operation left women "skeletonized"—missing all the tissue except a thin tight layer of skin covering their ribs. Often women lost much of their arm strength and developed terrible lymphedema, swelling of the arm which occurred from the buildup of lymph fluid which could no longer escape from the tissue since all the lymph channels were gone. Although this operation could reduce the rates of recurrence of the cancer in the areas the surgeons removed, it did not improve the cure rate.[6]

Why did these more extensive surgeries fail to increase the cure rate? The answer is that most breast cancers spread through the blood system independently from their spread into the lymph system. The conceptual mistake that Hanley and Halsted made resulted from the fact that the women diagnosed with breast cancer in their era usually had very large tumors which often occupied the entire breast and therefore filled all the lymph channels. When Hanley did his dissections, these large cancers made the lymph system look like the primary means of spread. We now understand that almost all breast cancers spread (metastasize) via the blood system. By the time of surgery, either spread has already taken place through the blood system or not. The cancer must be removed, but also taking extra tissue surrounding the breast and lymph system cannot prevent those metastases that have already happened. While a few early surgeons had indeed argued that this was the case and only limited procedures were needed, the preponderance of advanced cases and the enthusiasm for trying more extensive surgery carried the day.

In the 1960s, Halsted's radical mastectomy was replaced with the "modified radical mastectomy" which removed the whole breast but left the muscle underneath. By the late 1970s, the modified radical mastectomy had become the most popular breast cancer operation in the United States. About that time, an even more radical concept developed. Since the spread of the cancer cells through the blood would ultimately determine if it was lethal, why remove the whole breast? Advances in radiation treatments had made it possible to focus the radiation beam on the breast and spare other tissues, so it seemed reasonable to remove just the cancer and use radiation treatments to kill any cancer cells which were nearby in the breast. The ideas of Hanley and Halsted were challenged by surgeons like Bernard Fisher in the United States and Umberto Veronesi in Italy. Around the world, a series of clinical trials took place in which women with small breast cancers agreed to undergo the proverbial coin flip and have either a mastectomy or lumpectomy and radiation. These studies all gave very similar results: survival from breast cancer was equal with either treatment. Since more women were having mammograms, cancers were discovered at the smaller sizes that made choosing "breast conservation" (treatment with lumpectomy and radiation) possible. In 1990, the National Cancer Institute endorsed breast conservation as the preferred treatment for women with early stage breast cancer.[7]

Breast conservation was not universally accepted. In the United States, surgeons on the East and West Coast tended to offer their patients this treatment, while surgeons in the middle of the country clung to recommending mastectomies. In part, this difference was due to the more conservative medical, and probably non-medical, culture in the heartland. Having easier access to radiation facilities in cities on the coasts also played a role. But much of the resistance to lumpectomy and radiation came from a harsh reality: even though survival with either treatment was the same, women who had lumpectomy and radiation instead of mastectomy did have a higher risk of the cancer returning in the spared breast. If this were the case, how could survival be the same? The answer was that those cancers which returned in the spared breast were the aggressive cancers which had already spread throughout the body. Still, depending on how this was presented and her own personality, an individual woman could see this set of facts as either supporting her decision to save her breast ("my survival is no different") or have mastectomy ("I don't want to have a higher risk of it coming back in the breast").

Carol understood her choices. She also instinctively realized that her mother's decisive action with her own breast cancer twenty years earlier set the standard for her family. Carol knew that both Betty and Rose would want her to undergo a mastectomy of the left breast and would probably feel better if she underwent removal of both breasts. Since facing Betty and Rose together was formidable, she decided to test out her mother alone. The room was peaceful and the morning sunlight highlighted the bright cubist prints of Picasso and Juan Gris on her walls as she spoke.

"I'll be glad to meet the radiation doctor tomorrow . . . Dr. Morris," she started.

"Yes, dear," replied Betty, hoping to avoid a discussion.

"Mother, I would like to try and save my breasts if he thinks it's possible to treat me with radiation. I don't want to have mastectomies and lose my breasts. I know that's what you did, but I think I might rather try a different treatment."

"Let's hear what he says," replied Betty, trying to delay a serious discussion. Betty knew that her own decision to undergo bilateral mastectomies had been the correct one. Treatment with lumpectomy and radiation was not yet offered, but she would have refused in any event. She had the three children to raise alone and wanted all her breast tissue gone. Betty could have later undergone breast reconstruction, but with her responsibilities she did not wish to spend the time or effort. Her parent's history also helped make her decision. Once they had recognized the impending Nazi takeover in Germany, they had abandoned everything to come to the U.S. Although her parents lost their fortune, they avoided the holocaust—a decision Betty admired and one that vindicated decisive action. Betty hoped Carol would undergo the same procedure but, in her heart, she was afraid that Carol was different. Her naturally optimistic temperament was not shaped by the sacrifices of World War II, and she had not yet met a man she loved. Betty quietly despaired that Carol did not have the strength to choose correctly.

The next afternoon, Rose joined them for their appointment in Radiation Oncology. Meeting Dr. Morris was very different from her visits with other physicians. His office was in the basement of the hospital, chosen for most radiation oncology units to reduce the cost of installing the heavy shielding needed to protect the outside world. The waiting room for patients undergoing treatment contained only a few people, a testament to the careful attention paid to running the treatment schedule on time. A separate waiting room for consultations was nice, almost richly appointed. Carol again completed the obligatory questionnaire. This time the forms did not produce the same sense of panic, and she wondered whether her relative calmness was because she now knew her diagnosis or because she was with Rose and Betty. They were promptly escorted into Dr. Morris' office by an attractive young Asian woman who introduced herself as Asa, "Dr. Morris' nurse." The elegant office was windowless but impressive as mementos of trips around the world and photographs with various dignitaries attested to an accomplished life. The man himself was in his mid-fifties, elegant, poised, and dressed in finely cut clothing. He examined Carol in an adjoining room and, once she had dressed, sat with the three of them and Asa.

Dr. Richard Morris' presentation was a tour de force. He summarized Carol's history, acknowledged Betty's life accomplishments despite her cancer, and complimented Rose's intellect. As he succinctly reviewed the history of breast cancer treatment, his enthusiasm for radiation became obvious. He explained the physics and recent clinical trials as Asa nodded and supplemented the presentation with some professionally produced diagrams and well-timed knowing smiles. He ended by answering a few questions then gracefully exiting the stage, allowing Asa more time with the patient and family.

Rose and Betty were both impressed. Rose likened his presentation to that of a brilliant trial lawyer. Yet they were still convinced that Carol should undergo mastectomies of both her breasts. At Betty's home that evening, the three of them ate quietly in an unspoken agreement not to discuss the issue until dinner finished. Over coffee, Rose opened the discussion.

"I can't see you doing anything but mastectomies like Mom," said Rose. "Even Dr. Morris said if you do the lumpectomy and radiation, you'll have a higher risk of a recurrence of the cancer. And we'll still have to worry about another new cancer."

"But the chance of beating the cancer is the same," said Carol. "Dr. Morris and Dr. Scanlon both agreed about that. And that's what is most important."

"Yes, but why worry about the possibility of having to do this again?" asked Rose.

"Well, it's just a chance I guess you have to take," replied Carol. The discussion was now heading into a tense territory. She knew she would opt for lumpectomy and radiation, but did not want to challenge the decision her mother had made years ago. It was a bit ironic, she thought. I am the one with cancer, yet I need to be careful what I say. Rose was oblivious to Carol's dilemma and pushed on.

"I don't see why you have to take any chances," she restated.

"There's more to it, Rose," Carol replied.

In fact, Carol had made her decision years before Dr. Morris spoke, at the time of Betty's mastectomies. Carol had been eleven and remembered how upset she had been when her mother returned home looking pale and drawn. In an era when cancer, and particularly breast cancer, was not discussed openly, Betty had never hidden her scars from either Rose or Carol. Although Betty never spoke of her loss, Carol had been silently horrified by her appearance. Later, as a teenager, Carol intellectually understood her mother had no choice, yet somehow vaguely mourned for her. It was in college that the strength of her feelings had become apparent in, of all places, a Russian literature class. They had been reading Alexandr Solzhenitsyn, a Russian writer whose works documented the oppression inside the Soviet Union at the height of the Cold War. Carol had found his description of life in a Soviet penal colony in *A Day in Life of Ivan Denisovich* compelling. She had also chosen to read one of his less well-known books, *Cancer Ward*, a description of patients in a Soviet hospital undergoing treatments for cancer.

In that work, a young woman with breast cancer waited in the ward for days to undergo her mastectomy for breast cancer. The night before the surgery she asked a fellow patient if he would place his hand on her soon to be amputated breast. She wanted him to remember how it felt before it was lost forever.

Carol was surprised how this scene crystallized her feelings about Betty's surgery and how, even as a college student, she felt like crying for her mother. For a normally lighthearted woman, it had been a striking feeling. But when she tried to discuss it with Rose, she again ran into the fierce determination that characterized her sister.

"Of course she was upset," said Rose sharply. "Do you think that she had a choice? Come on, Carol, Daddy was dead, and she had us. And don't talk to her about this. It's over. She has moved on and is happy. The best thing you can do is honor her sacrifice and get on with your life."

Carol was also surprised how this scene forced her as a college student to think about the possibility that she too might someday develop breast cancer. Carol understood how Solzhenitsyn's character felt. While Rose was organizing her future, Carol was also planning for this decision.

"I do not want to lose my breasts. I appreciate what you are trying to do, Rose, but it is wrong for me. I understand why you wanted mastectomies, mother, but I do not. I am too young to just give them up."

Betty and Rose were not pleased.

"I still don't understand why you would leave anymore to worry about," tried Rose again. "You never know when the rest will go bad."

"And if something else happens, then I will have the mastectomy. But until then, I want to try to keep my breasts."

"And I don't understand," said Betty. "You will be a beautiful woman even without breasts. Any man would be lucky to have you. Please, dear, don't do this. It's too risky." In a final plea, she added, "Look at me. Haven't I had a good life? And you could have reconstruction."

Carol was silent for a moment as she tried to compose her thoughts. A part of her was so upset that she wanted to tell Betty the truth: Carol could not face the disfigurement and loss she had seen her mother undergo. But Carol paused, afraid of wounding her mother. For once, she was thankful when Rose, with her continued irritating determination, spoke before Carol's silence was noticeable.

"We can't be worrying about this, Carol," said Rose. "Don't be crazy."

"Too bad, Rose, you'll just have to suffer because it's my decision and I've made it."

Carol had never so directly disagreed with them about such a substantial decision. Selecting her college, majoring in English instead of a useful subject, leaving various favored boyfriends, and her choice of work had each brought some disapproval. Rose and Betty had always found a way to excuse her indiscretions. But this was different. Carol was opposing them in a way they could never understand. For Rose and Betty, this was a challenge to both the authority they saw in their mother-sister and sister-sister bond and their own decisions in life. They could not accept Carol's plan and, in unspoken agreement, knew that if circumstances changed they would take control.

8:00 Harold Crimons: Small cell lung cancer

Early appointments are given to reliable patients. The staff knows that having that first patient arrive even fifteen minutes late starts the day off badly and begins a ripple effect which will inconvenience many people who will express their irritation directly to them. Harold Crimons was a good starter because he always arrived ten minutes early.

The door to the exam room was open. Harold, an outwardly healthy, good looking man in his mid-fifties, sat in a chair sipping his coffee and reading the *New York Post*. He wore comfortable jeans, a polo shirt, and a Yankees cap. He had already given the medical assistant who checked him in the prescriptions he needed to be refilled and, in a characteristic display of courtesy, had his cell phone turned off.

"Good morning, Mr. Crimons. How are you?" asked Dr. John Matthews as he walked in.

"Getting my gossip," Harold replied as he waved his *Post*, then folded the paper quickly and moved to the exam table in a practiced sequence. Today would start his second round of a new chemotherapy for recurrent high-grade neuroendocrine small cell lung cancer.

Harold was the quintessential Saratoga boy. His father Dan had been a groundskeeper at the famous Saratoga Race Track while mother Peg worked in the cafeteria at Division Street Elementary School. During a childhood shared with his younger sister Colleen, Harold was a mild-mannered, well-liked Yankees fan. After graduating from Saratoga High School, relieved that the Vietnam War had ended, he worked a series of construction jobs. At twenty-three, Harold married his high school sweetheart. Five years later, his life "took a bad turn" when she ran off with another man. His thirties brought a "rough patch" of depression and alcoholism, a time during which Harold's Yankees also collapsed following their 1981 World Series loss to the traitorous Dodgers. With the help of his parents, Harold eventually stopped drinking and rebuilt his life. Although never remarried, he had a network of close friends, work as a middle school janitor, and a small home a few miles outside town. Dan and Peg, both still healthy despite being in their late eighties, were nearby while Colleen lived in town with her husband and two children. Harold's middle years had been good ones, filled with the routines of the school year, his friends and family, Yankees baseball, and life in Saratoga Springs. As he often said, Harold was a happy man.

Harold's only remaining curse from his early years was smoking. He was never quite sure why he had started in high school, but his addiction had been immediate and profound. The stranglehold that cigarettes held on him began with his very first successful deep inhalation. In his late thirties, he had tried to quit a few times without success. His doctor told him that nicotine was like a key that fit into a lock in his brain. The better the key fit, the stronger the addiction. Harold remembered thinking his brain must be filled with locks just waiting for that key, because, man, did it fit nicely with his morning coffee, breaks during the day, and after dinner—to the tune of three packs per day.

THE TOBACCO INDUSTRY: THE HISTORY OF A KILLER.
Tobacco is the leading cause of cancer death worldwide.[8]

Almost all smokers start before they finish high school, a perverse tribute to the tobacco industry. The history of this lethal product begins with the tobacco plant *Nicotiana*, probably first grown in South America and used by Native Americans across the adjoining continents. Early European explorers found tobacco smoke a part of many native spiritual and healing rituals and came to appreciate that it produced feelings of both stimulation and relaxation. New World settlers, particularly in the Virginia area, soon learned to grow and export tobacco to Europe, where it was rapidly incorporated into daily life and spread throughout the world.[9] There was even hope tobacco might ward off the plague.[10] By 1604 King James felt the need to publicly deplore the excessive use of tobacco, although his words clearly had little effect as by 1670 it is reported that half of the men in England smoked, primarily using clay pipes. A series of European wars were effective mechanisms for spreading tobacco addiction deeper into that continent.[11] Supplying this worldwide craving led to the growth of tobacco farming in the colonies which, in turn, stimulated the development of the Southern plantation economy and culture, including slavery.

In the early United States, the average man chewed and spat out his tobacco—brands like the famous Bull Durham. Cigarettes were rolled by hand, and the supply was limited. Cigar smoking was the province of the powerful men in business and politics. Pipe smoking was common but never gained the tremendous popularity it had in England. Chew was so popular in the mid-1800s that when the famous writer Charles Dickens toured the United States, he reported the young nation's Capital City of Washington was covered with tobacco stained saliva.[12]

The twentieth century brought advances that allowed cigarettes to replace chewed tobacco. Machines to roll cigarettes tremendously increased production and matches, the underappreciated but critical partner of the cigarette, became available. Equally importantly, aggressive businessmen fashioned small companies into the beginnings of a powerful industry which controlled the entire process of manufacturing, developed modern marketing, and reached monopoly status with the formation of the American Tobacco Company.[13] Although this company, like the Rockefeller's Standard Oil, was broken up using the

Sherman Anti-Trust Act, the industry remained a powerful force which acted in a coordinated fashion to expand the market for cigarettes.

As smoking became more widespread in the early 1900s, there was opposition from some portions of society, including the people associated with the Temperance movement. Smoking was criticized on moral and health grounds, and there were attempts to limit the sale of cigarettes. Remarkably, it was World War I which legitimized smoking when supplying soldiers with cigarettes to ease terror or boredom became a patriotic act. Beginning in 1918 the War Department took responsibility for issuing Camels, Chesterfields, and Lucky Strikes to the troops. When the Great War ended, the smoking debate resumed, but the ranks of smokers were reinforced by the returning troops and women who were beginning to insist on their right to smoke. The cigarette industry had developed effective ad campaigns which targeted all parts of society, including women and children, and made smoking an integral part of modern American culture. The sheer numbers of smokers and the failure of Prohibition made it virtually impossible to imagine ending the sales of cigarettes.[14]

World War II massively increased smoking in the United States as again the War Department issued cigarettes with C-rations to help the GIs cope. The health risks of smoking were not understood. Even if they had been known, for many soldiers the benefits outweighed the risks. One soldier who fought as a tank gunner in the Battle of the Bulge and was diagnosed in the 1980s with terminal lung cancer expressed his feelings.

"The Germans were attacking us with everything they had, and we were taking a terrible beating. Every day we would drive past wrecks of our tanks, some still smoking, and I would think of those guys being burned alive. The more I saw, the harder it got for me to get into my tank. I kept waiting for my turn to be cooked. They only thing that got me into that damn tank each day was those cigarettes. They saved my life then. So, you tell me now they have killed me, and I say they were worth it . . . Every damn one."[15]

When the GIs returned home from World War II, they exposed their wives and girlfriends to smoking. Unlike at the end of World War I when there had been significant social obstacles to women smokers, the combination of increased women's rights in the 1920s and 1930s and the successful advertising by the industry set the stage for a rapid expansion of smoking by women. In addition, during World War II women had taken over many of the traditionally male roles vacated by the men who were off fighting. They had worked in factories like "Rosie the Riveter," run businesses, and managed family finances. While these women did not need cigarettes to climb into a tank for combat, smoking was an accepted part of their new modern lives.

The massive increase in cigarette smoking did not cause any immediate change in the health of the nation. There were several reasons why the bad effects of cigarettes were not immediately appreciated. Life expectancy rates had just begun to rise to the point where smoking could exert an effect. Before this time, so many people died of infectious diseases, accidents, or general poor health and nutrition that it was hard to see an effect from cigarettes. Secondly, it takes about ten or fifteen years of widespread smoking to produce increased rates of heart or lung disease or cancer. This delay is called the latency period, and it made understanding the relationship between smoking and these serious illnesses more difficult. In addition, physicians and scientists needed to learn how to understand the effects of smoking. Methods to collect data, analyze statistics, and correlate these with lab findings needed developing. Doctors were familiar with infections and injuries, but a complex situation where many different people were exposed to various levels of a mix of toxic chemicals and in which only some would become sick years later was much harder to comprehend.

The lack of knowledge about lung cancer in the medical profession is seen in the 1950 edition of the *Merck Manual*, a widely-used resource text for physicians of the era. This book had over fifteen hundred pages, of which only three were devoted to cancers in the lung and stated the "cause of primary pulmonary carcinoma is almost completely unknown. The only recognized etiology is that of certain radioactive ores . . . Tobacco, oils, fumes, tarred roads, and other possible irritants have been suspected but proof of their effects is lacking."[16] The *Merck Manual* did comment on the rise in lung cancer diagnoses, but it took a diverse group of scientists in Europe and the United States years of work to clearly identify smoking as the main cause of lung cancer. The stakes in this research were high, and a well-organized and ruthless tobacco industry attempted to block every effort to link smoking to diseases. They advertised physician smokers, promoted "less irritating" smokes, and issued statements about their concern for the health of the American public. In a brilliant marketing strategy, the tobacco industry also pledged to study the causes of lung cancer by forming its own research group, the Tobacco Research Counsel. This group recruited skeptical scientists with their own agendas to create a scientific smoke screen using debates about the meaning of proof, discussions of other potential contributing factors, and the promise of endlessly more basic science research.

Despite the industry's efforts, by the late 1950s the scientific data regarding the bad health effects of cigarettes were clear to most reasonable physicians and scientists. In men who were smokers, lung cancer rates rose so sharply after World War II they could not be ignored. Since rates of smoking among women rose later, the rise in lung cancer rates in women also occurred later. For women, a perverse milestone was reached in the 1990s when lung cancer caused by cigarettes killed more women than breast cancer (which is not caused by smoking). In 1964, the Surgeon General's Advisory Committee issued their famous report declaring cigarettes caused lung cancer.[17] Over the next fifteen years, smoking rates among men declined from a high of nearly 60 percent down to about 30 percent while women's rates went from about 35 percent to about 25 percent. This progress did not come easily as the tobacco industry fought the scientific demonstrations of the harms of cigarettes with its own pseudo-research and waged sophisticated advertising campaigns to lure women, children, and minorities to smoking. They vigorously opposed any legislative or legal efforts to limit the use of their products. The combination of addiction and advertising made smoking in homes, clubs, workplaces, and even confined spaces like airplanes, part of our culture. The tobacco industry was tremendously profitable and, although there was competition in the marketplace for individual brands, it was united in its actions to preserve the industry.[18]

In the 1960s and 70s, public health advocates and some lawyers challenged the tobacco industry in a series of political and legal proceedings which they generally lost and in which their few victories were ineffective. When restrictions on cigarette advertisements on television began in 1971, the industry easily converted to print advertising, selling branded merchandise, and sponsoring public and sporting events. A baseball fan in 1976 watching the Yankee's Chris Chambliss hit his famous walk-off home run on the first pitch of the ninth inning to beat the Kansas City Royals and win the American League Championship Series would have their view of Yankee Stadium dominated by a Marlboro billboard. When warnings were required on cigarette packaging, the industry made sure they were bland and timid by flexing its tremendous financial and political muscle throughout the government. Throughout this period, the industry successfully argued smoking was an individual American's choice. Even while they made this argument, the cigarette manufacturers understood the power of nicotine and the need for new young recruits. Since the most smokers are hooked before they are eighteen, the industry promoted cigarettes to children with cartoon advertisements like the famous 1980s' "Joe Camel" series. They also modified the production process to raise nicotine levels while offering filtered low tar brands which seemed safer but were not.

It took until the 1980s and 1990s for the tide to turn against the tobacco industry. Authoritative public figures like Surgeon General C. Everett Koop ensured the ill effects of smoking were undeniable. The addictive effects of nicotine were documented, and cigarette smoke formally classified as a carcinogen. In 1994, the leaders of the largest tobacco companies were called before Congress where they all testified that smoking was not addictive and faced public ridicule. Shortly thereafter, in a series of events worthy of a John Grisham novel, internal company documents stolen from lawyers representing the tobacco companies were made public which showed the industry's manipulation of nicotine levels to recruit and retain more smokers. These events gave additional ammunition to those trying to restrain smoking. The effects of secondhand smoke also became an important public issue in the fight against cigarettes as non-smokers were mobilized to protest the habit. Even more importantly, the cost of smoking to the health care system and the States became greater and more obvious. Many State Attorneys General began to use new legal tools to seek money from the industry.[19]

By the late 1990s, the pressure on the tobacco industry had mounted, and court cases which they had previously won now seemed threatening. Public opinion had turned against smoking in general. Americans at least partially held the industry responsible for smoking related illnesses, although smokers themselves were often still blamed for their diseases. Public health advocates had successfully raised issues of secondhand smoking and advertising to children. Some leaders within the industry recognized the need to stabilize the external environment to secure their ability to continue to do business. A complex series of legal cases and political negotiations culminated in the 1998 Master Settlement Agreement. In this uniquely American compromise, the industry agreed to pay over $200 billion to States over the next four decades, fund an independent national foundation to combat smoking, and agreed to some additional restrictions on advertising. In return, they were freed from further legal challenge from the States and now had a secure business environment. The initial versions of the Agreement were much harsher on the industry, and the final Agreement showed the political power the industry still retained. The Agreement was a bitter disappointment to many public health advocates as it made the States directly invested in the survival of the industry if they wanted to continue to be paid.[20]

About 20 percent of Americans still smoke. It is the leading single preventable cause of death and disease in our country. Eliminating smoking would probably correct the health care financial crisis. Nor has the industry given up recruiting new smokers using the same old tactics—recent advertisements for "American Spirit" cigarettes promote "100 percent additive-free natural tobacco." Sadly, the same story of tobacco is now being replayed throughout the developing world as our companies export cigarettes to impoverished countries. The same successful advertising strategies, arguments about "freedom of choice," and desire to enhance our manufacturing exports combine to allow the tobacco industry to poison smokers, particularly children, around the world.

Harold understood the dangers of smoking. His parents and sister begged him to stop. As his niece and nephew grew older, they tormented him with the relentless and loving indignation of children. His physicians frequently discussed his options. He watched as smoking was completely banned from the workplace, airplanes, restaurants and nightclubs, and even many outdoor areas. He suffered the righteous verbal assaults of ex-smokers, increasingly graphic public service announcements, and the marked rise in cigarette prices. Yet, he had no choice. Harold knew in his heart that his addiction was so strong that he would never overcome it. By his forties, he had stopped trying and simply hoped he would be spared.

Sadly, Harold developed lung cancer. Since cancers are named by the organ in which they arise, Harold's cancer had started in his lung before it spread (or metastasized) to other areas of his body. Even when they have spread, cancers are still named by their site of origin. Thus, lung cancer in the liver is called "lung cancer metastatic to the liver." Since the lung has several different types of cells which can become cancerous, there are several types of lung cancer. Harold's cancer developed from the small "neuroendocrine cells" which produce hormones which help regulate the functioning of the other cells in the lung. Hence, his cancer was called neuroendocrine small cell lung cancer.

MAKING A CANCER: MULTI-STEP CARCINOGENESIS.

Patients often describe cancers as a "bolt of lightning," coming out of nowhere. Yet scientists have learned that most develop over a period of many years in a process called "multi-step carcinogenesis."[21]

Cancers start from normal tissues, a basic concept which eluded many early scientists and physicians. "Morbid growth" is the term which best characterizes the understanding of cancer in the early nineteenth century. In 1838 German scientist Johannes Muller reported that cancers form from cells which resemble the tissues from which they arise, yet his definition was not immediately accepted. Even Muller's famous student Dr. Rudolph Virchow, a prominent German physician known as "Hippocrates with the microscope," believed that all cancers started from connective tissue.[22] It was not until the twentieth century that it was generally understood that cancers result from uncontrolled cellular growth leading to the invasion of normal tissue and metastasis (spread) to other parts of the body.

The sequence of changes from normal tissue to cancer are visible under the microscope. When benign growths are examined microscopically, increased numbers of normal appearing cells are seen, called "hyperplasia" (hyper meaning excess, plasia meaning growth). In most cases, the excess of normal cells does not lead to cancer. For example, "hyperplastic polyps" removed at the time of colonoscopy are usually not of concern. When the appearance of the cells becomes abnormal, "dysplasia" (dys meaning bad, plasia meaning growth) is diagnosed.

Most growths with dysplasia will not progress to cancer, but their risk of becoming cancer is higher. As dysplastic cells multiply, they may form growths called "adenomas" (adeno meaning glands) which can become cancerous over the years. "Tubular adenomas" found in the colon are removed at colonoscopy because they "might become cancer." When cells become very abnormal but do not invade the neighboring tissue, they are "non-invasive cancers," sometimes named "pre-cancers." Actual cancers appear under the microscope as highly abnormal cells which invade normal tissue and may spread to other areas (metastasis). Once cancers have formed, the degree to which the cancer cells have microscopic features of the normal tissues from which they evolved is described by pathologists as "differentiation." Cancers which are "well differentiated" look more like the normal tissue while "poorly differentiated" cancers are more abnormal. The time it takes for normal cells to pass through these stages and become cancerous is usually measured in years, as seen when the exposure of GIs to smoking in World War II led to an increase in lung cancer about a decade later.

Breathtaking advances over the past fifty years have given us an understanding of this complex series of events on a molecular level. One key concept is that damage to cellular DNA accumulates during each step—a process of increasing "genetic instability" in which damage begets more damage. Normally, our DNA is under constant attack from external agents such as chemicals or radiation and internal errors inherent in the replication process. Fortunately, our cells have many different DNA repair mechanisms. Some patients are born with the first step in genetic instability because they have defects in DNA repair mechanisms. An example is the *BRCA* mutations which may lead to breast or ovarian cancer. As cancers develop, the pattern of damage to various critical genes will determine their appearance and behavior. In a typical cancer, many genes are altered, some "drive" the process while others are less important "passengers." Most cancers probably require mutations in five or six critical driver genes.[23] Given that a human cell has twenty-one thousand genes and a cancer may have hundreds or thousands of mutations, sorting out the important damage is a challenge.[24] Factors which promote cell division and activity, such as inflammation or hormonal stimulation, may increase the likelihood of cancer, but determining exactly what caused the damage may be impossible (without invoking either a higher power or chance).

Cancers continue to evolve as they grow and spread. Within a cancer, there will be differences among the individual cells and their environment which can become magnified over time, called "tumor heterogeneity." These differences among the various cancer cells may determine which spread, where they go, or how well treatments work. Over time, most cancers become more aggressive and less like normal tissue. As treatments are given, the hardiest cancer cells survive, and resistance to chemotherapy develops—Darwin's "survival of the fittest" is often used as an imperfect analogy. The hope is that if the underlying molecular events can be understood, possibly they can be reversed.

When Harold finished high school, the normal neuroendocrine cells in his lungs produced small amounts of various hormones. As Harold began working, each morning started with coffee from the local Stewart's Shop and the deeply satisfying inhalation of several hundred toxic chemicals which penetrated the cells of his lungs and damaged their important machinery—including the DNA. The code for the proteins of the cell is in the DNA, the beautiful double helix described in 1953 by James Watson and Francs Crick in one of the most important achievements of the twentieth century. This structure must be maintained in perfect form. The toxic chemicals in Harold's smoke chipped and smashed his DNA in an act of cellular vandalism.

When DNA damage occurs in an important gene, it can lead to abnormal growth of the cell. As that cell divides, the damaged or mutated DNA can be passed down to daughter cells which can then get further mutations. If enough critical genes are damaged, the cell can grow out of control and become cancerous. Fortunately, the cell has many repair mechanisms. Each day they would repair the damage done by Harold's smoking before the cell divided so that the mutations would not be passed along to the daughter cells. The normal cell also has "check-point genes" which halt cell division until the repair work is done. If the cell cannot be repaired, there are genes which cause the cell to commit suicide, called "apoptosis" by scientists. During Harold's start of work life and marriage, his cells managed to repair themselves each day and continue their normal jobs. Some could not repair themselves and were killed by their own suicide genes so they would not reproduce.

As Harold's smoke assaulted his DNA, it also carried chemicals like nicotine which stimulated the growth of some cells in his lung. Nicotine itself does not cause cell damage or lung cancer, but the more rapid growth of the cells meant less time to repair the daily damage. About the time his wife left him, the first irreparable genetic damage was done. A damaged gene caused his neuroendocrine cells to release more gastrin releasing peptide (abbreviated GRP), a substance that caused all the nearby cells to divide and grow a little faster. If Harold had stopped smoking when his marriage dissolved, it is possible that this extra growth would have ended, but in his rough patch, he smoked even more. The nicotine in the cigarettes and the extra GRP together caused the cells to grow too rapidly for the repair mechanisms to undo all the daily damage to the DNA caused by the smoke. Something had to give. In his thirties, Harold's smoking caused a second mutation, this time in the gene that produced a protein called c-kit. The rushed repair process failed, and this defect was also passed along to daughter cells. The mutated *C-KIT* gene in Harold's neuroendocrine cells further sped up the cell growth and division.

In Harold's forties, serious trouble occurred. As he was watching his beloved Yankees win the Divisional Series from the Twins in 2009, some of the genes responsible for the repair mechanisms were mutated.

This terrible blow to the cells did not mean they were cancerous, but they were now unstable and vulnerable. If Harold had quit smoking, he still might have escaped lung cancer but would have always been at very high risk. He was blissfully unaware of these events and rejoiced as his Yankees won their twenty-seventh World Championship by beating the Philadelphia Phillies.

For a while, nothing happened. Harold certainly did not notice any dramatic changes in his body, although he did have a vague sense of the passage of time as George Steinbrenner, the longtime Yankee owner, and Bob Sheppard, the longtime voice of the team, both died in 2010. Eventually, however, further damage occurred in two more critical genes in his neuroendocrine cells. The first caused the *C-MYC* gene to become duplicated, pushing the unstable cells into division even more rapidly. The second was a mutation in the Retinoblastoma gene (*RB*) which is responsible for slowing the cell cycle, giving further speed to the growth of his neuroendocrine cells. His neuroendocrine cells were not yet cancerous, but they were close.

The 2014 season was the last for famed Yankee shortstop Derek Jeter. As Harold read about Jeter's plans in the *Post* and inhaled from his cigarette, the chemical benzopyrene reached one of these stimulated cells and caused a mutation in the *TP53* gene which was overlooked by the increasingly disorganized repair equipment. Since the *TP53* gene was supposed to stop cell division and signal the cell to commit suicide if it was growing out of control, that final safety check was now gone. In early 2015, damage to one more gene called telomerase made the neuroendocrine cells immortal and, although he was still unaware of it, Harold had lung cancer.

As his Yankees 2015 season ended with a loss to Houston in a one-game playoff, the cancer in Harold's lung had reached a diameter of about a millimeter or one-twentieth of an inch. Although tiny, the growth rate was rapid, doubling in size every forty-five days, compared with one hundred eighty days or even longer for other cancers. Even worse, Harold's cancer invaded the lung tissue by overcoming the normal stop signals that cells get when they are crowded by other cells (called "contact inhibition" by scientists). They produced enzymes to dissolve the barriers of fibrous tissue which separate our cells and structures. Harold's cancer cells also started making their own blood vessels to supply nutrition and oxygen in a process called "angiogenesis" (angio meaning blood vessel and genesis meaning creation). Normally angiogenesis occurs during wound repair as a beautiful but carefully choreographed ballet involving many different cells. The cancer cells pervert this wonderful dance to make shoddy blood vessels to aid their growth. This poor blood vessel construction explains why many cancers bleed and how the invading cancer cells get access to the blood system to spread. In lung cancer, the combination of invasion and angiogenesis is particularly deadly since the cancer cells will have very easy access to the lung's normal arteries, a highway system to travel to other areas.

Over the winter of 2015, Harold's cancer cells begin the dreaded process of metastasis. In one part of his growing mass of cancer cells, a particularly aggressive group formed. They made powerful enzymes to break down the fibrous tissue barrier, slipped into the ragged new blood vessels, then poured out into the circulation like millions of demented attackers in a horrible video game. As Harold started thinking about spring training, his organs were showered with millions of cancers cells searching for new places to colonize and grow. When the right seed found the right soil, a colony was established. In Harold, the cancer cells from his lung found the right soil in the bones of his spine and ribs, and there began to grow. A series of small steps had led to widespread cancer.

The summer of 2016 in upstate New York was beautiful, the sunlight contrasting the intense greens of the Adirondack Mountains with the shimmering blue lakes. In Saratoga Springs, the eagerly awaited summer season began. June brought the arrival of the thoroughbred race horses to the Oklahoma practice track. July opened with the Saratoga Performing Arts Center's Jazz festival and continued with pop stars, the New York City Ballet, and the Philadelphia Orchestra. The City's Victorian main street Broadway became filled with diners and tourists. The climax began in late July with Opening Day at the Track, starting six weeks of racing which peaked in mid-August with the famed Travers. Harold's work at the middle school was quiet, time off was easy to arrange, and he enjoyed it all with friends and family. And, of course, a few day trips to Yankee Stadium.

As summer ended and Saratoga became quiet, the cancer cells in Harold's bones had grown to the point that he felt a dull aching in his lower back and right arm. With the excitement of the start of school followed by the disappointment of the Yankees' 2016 season, it barely registered. By October, though, the aching became a steady pain, and his co-workers noticed he was moving slowly. Since he was normally a strong man and hard worker, at first they teased him.

"Harold, man, you are leaning on the broom pretty heavily. You look like one of them Yankees that couldn't even win one from Detroit," joked Roger, a long-time co-worker.

"Keep this up, and you'll be out like A-Rod. Hey Roger, let's call Joe Girardi and get a real janitor here," joined in Frank, another old timer.

Gradually, though, his friends became concerned and recruited the school nurse to examine him.

"Harold," she said. "You have strained your back and look pale. I want you to see your doctor right away. You need some x-rays and medication."

Harold saw the Physician Assistant in his primary care office the following Monday. She examined him, ordered x-rays of his spine, and prescribed rest and a muscle relaxant. He called work and took the rest of the week off. At home, Harold tried the medication but found it made him even more tired. He had trouble keeping track of the days and forgot to have the x-rays done. Movement became harder and harder until, at the end of the week, he collapsed onto his sofa.

Dan did not know Harold had taken the week off from work but was surprised that he had not heard from him. He called Sunday evening and when there was no answer, spoke with Colleen.

"Do you know where Harold is?" he asked. "I haven't heard from him this week."

"No, Dad. I spoke with him last week, and he didn't mention anything about going anywhere."

"It's not like him not to call."

"Let me check with Roger and see if he knows where he might be."

When Colleen found out that Harold had missed work, she drove her father to his house where they discovered him on the couch and called 9-1-1. Over the radio to the Emergency Room, Harold was described by the EMTs as a "mid-fifties-year-old-man found unresponsive by his family" with a mildly low blood pressure and rapid heart rate, normal blood oxygen, glucose, and EKG. They reported Harold moved all his extremities and was moaning, but would not respond to any of their commands. One of the EMTs knew Harold well and, although he had not seen him in a few months, assured his colleagues that he was not a drinker or drug user.

In the Emergency Room, the reason for Harold's confusion became clear. His sodium level was dangerously low. A chest x-ray showed a large mass in the right lung and a CT scan done immediately afterward showed this growth was about four inches in size and looked cancerous. There were several spots in his liver and many in his bones, including his spine, right arm, and ribs. A CT scan of the brain showed no cancer. The conclusion was that Harold appeared to have lung cancer which had spread to the bones and was causing the pain. The cancer cells were also secreting hormones into his bloodstream, including one called antidiuretic hormone (ADH) which caused Harold's kidneys to retain water. This lowered his sodium, a condition called "hyponatremia" (hypo meaning low and natremia meaning sodium in the serum). The extra water and low sodium caused swelling in Harold's brain and confusion. If his case were an exam question for a medical student, the correct answer would be that this was metastatic neuroendocrine (small cell) lung cancer.

Harold could not appreciate the spacious room and flat screen televisions in the new emergency ward which allowed his sister and parents to sit comfortably as they anxiously waited. At midnight the ER physician, Dr. Gary Newcomb, earnest but hurried, came in and spoke rapidly.

"The CT scan shows a large mass in his lungs which looks like cancer. It has spread to the liver and bones. His sodium is low, and that is making him confused. We'll admit him to the hospital to correct that and have the oncologists see him."

"But... don't we need a biopsy?" asked Colleen. Peg started crying while Dan held her hand.

"Yes. You can talk to the oncologists about that tomorrow," said Dr. Newcomb as he left the room to speak to the admitting hospital physician, Dr. Cindy Alison.

"Gary here. Got another smoker with cancer all through him. Sodium is 110, so he's out of it. Doesn't need the unit, though. Good luck."

Harold was moved to a private room on the cardiology ward so the rhythm of his heart could be monitored while his sodium was corrected. Peg and Dan were exhausted, and Colleen sent them home. She reviewed the history with Dr. Alison, a compassionate woman in her early thirties.

"I am sorry that your brother is so sick," Dr. Alison said, sitting next to Colleen by the bedside as Harold lay quietly moaning. "We will be correcting his sodium slowly over the next few days, and hopefully he will wake up. The oncologist will come by tomorrow, and we can decide about doing a biopsy."

"It looks bad, doesn't it?"

"Well, I'm not an oncologist, and sometimes these cancers can be treated. But it has spread throughout his body, so it doesn't look good. You should go home. He doesn't need you tonight, but he will over the next few days."

Monday was brutal. As the intravenous fluid and medications slowly corrected Harold's sodium level, more of his brain functioned and registered the terrible pain in his back and right arm. Any movement caused Harold to shriek like a wounded animal. The only thing that gave relief was morphine, which in turn made him more sedated. He could not eat and lay in bed, soiling himself despite the efforts of the aides who cared for him. Several of them knew Harold and were upset to see him in this state. Patty, a long-time nursing aide, was particularly sad.

"He was in my class at high school, such a nice guy. I never did see what he saw in that Marilyn he married. Serves her right for leaving him, though. She ended up with that loser Joe what's-his-name, a miserable drunk if there ever was one."

"Sounds like you had a sweet spot for him," said Cindy, another aide, as they worked to finish gently washing Harold and making up his bed.

"I was too stupid to look for a nice guy like him then," said Patty. "But it breaks my heart to see him like this. I hope they can do something."

Dr. Matthews consulted that evening after Colleen and Dan had returned. Harold was quiet.

"Mr. Crimons, this is Dr. Matthews. Can you hear me?"

"Yes," said Harold in a surprisingly clear voice. Colleen and Dan looked up hopefully.

"Do you know where you are, Mr. Crimons?"

"Oh, God, stop it it's killing me," he screamed.

"Where does it seem to hurt him most when you move him?" Dr. Matthews asked Patty.

"His right arm . . . here, and his low back." Cindy nodded agreement.

"That makes sense, that is where the scans show the worst of his problem."

"He's a great guy, doc," Patty added.

Dr. Matthews sat with Colleen and Dan.

"Mr. Crimons, your son is very popular around here," he began. "He sounds like a good man."

"We love him," said Colleen, as her father's eyes filled.

"What have the other doctors and nurses told you?"

"Well, we know he has lung cancer which has spread to his bones and liver, but we're not sure what will happen now."

"That seems to be true. We would like to get a biopsy to tell us the type of cancer, but first we need to get him more comfortable and more alert. We will adjust some of his medications and give him radiation to his arm and back. Radiation is a beam aimed at a specific part of the body. It will not treat the cancer outside that area, but it could help his pain in those areas.

"Can he stand radiation?" asked Colleen.

"Yes. The main side effect will be the pain of moving him downstairs for the treatment. If you speak to people who have had radiation, always ask where the beam was aimed. Obviously, if it is aimed at a place like the mouth, you can have bad side effects. On the low back and arm, it should not cause any major problems. Hopefully, he will get more alert and comfortable over the next few days. When we can make sure he can stay still, we will do a biopsy of the liver. The doctors will use a thin needle which usually does not cause much pain. Then, depending upon the result and how he is, we can talk about chemotherapy."

"Is there any hope?" asked Dan. "What can I tell his mother?"

"If this is the type of lung cancer we think it is, we will be able to treat him. We will not be able to cure him, but it is possible that he will feel better for some time, months or a year or two. I do not know how you will tell his mother this, but it is where he stands."

That evening Dr. Matthews spoke with Dr. Stephen Chris, the radiation oncologist. They decided to begin radiation treatment. Dr. Chris was a cheerful, young looking man in his mid-thirties who, except for his tie, could have just come from a college campus. Harold's parents immediately warmed to him.

"Dr. Matthews tells me your son is a favorite around here. Well, we can kill the cancer where we can aim the beam, and I think we can help his pain. Then you and Dr. Matthews can get going on some treatment for the rest of his body."

Harold was heavily medicated when the nurses moved him carefully onto the stretcher for the ride downstairs to the Radiation Oncology Center. He was wheeled through massive lead doors into the large room which contained the linear accelerator and gently transferred onto the table in the center. Around him was some of the most impressive looking machinery in the hospital, including the large mechanical arm weighing over a ton which would move around him to deliver the beam of radiation which would pass through his body in a fraction of a second.

RADIATION: HISTORY OF THE BEAM.

Radiation is an integral part of cancer treatment. For newly diagnosed patients with cancer, almost one third will receive radiation as part of their initial treatment plan.[25] When cancers recur, radiation treatments can control the disease at specific sites, often relieving pain or other symptoms. Most radiations treatments are from an "external beam" which is carefully aimed into the body.

In 1895 Wilhelm Roentgen found that x-rays would pass through objects that light could not and took a picture of the bones of his wife Bertha's left hand. Roentgen's discovery began when he observed that phosphorescent screens in his lab would light up when a power source was turned on. After he had determined the cause was not any known form of energy, he named the energy "x-ray." Within weeks of the reports of his discovery, the use of x-rays in medical diagnosis spread across the world with a speed which seems improbable in a pre-internet era. Only a year later Dr. Emil Grubbe noted that x-rays damaged the skin of his own hands and used them on a woman with an ulcerating breast cancer with some success, beginning the modern era of radiation treatment. Understanding of x-rays and radioactivity increased dramatically with the work of Antoine Becquerel, Marie Curie, and Pierre Curie, who shared the 1903 Nobel Prize (the first awarded to a woman).[26]

Radiation is energy packed into bundles called photons or into particles (electrons, protons, and neutrons). The main problem early physicians and scientists faced as they tried to harness photons to destroy cancer cells was obtaining enough energy in a beam. Early x-ray machines produced enough energy to take a picture, but not enough to treat a cancer unless it was on the surface of the body, as with Dr. Grubbe's patient. To treat tumors inside the body, the first therapists used radioactive pellets of radium which they implanted inside the tumor. This technique is called brachytherapy and is still used today for some cancers, particularly cervical and prostate cancer. Brachytherapy is limited since it requires access to the tumor, a way to hold the pellets in place, and does not treat nearby lymph nodes or other areas. In the 1950s and 1960s, methods for producing powerful beams of energy which could reach deep into the body were developed, called external beam radiation. The first machines typically used radioactive Cobalt to make the energy. These were eventually replaced by linear accelerators (also called linacs), which produced intense beams of photons using electricity and did not need radioactive materials on site (although some of the parts of the machines do become radioactive with use). The first of these accelerators for medical use opened in 1953 at Hammersmith Hospital in London. In 1957, Dr. Henry Kaplan of Stanford famously treated and cured a young child with a retinoblastoma of the eye.[27] Reports like these encouraged the use of external beam radiation for a variety of different cancers and the technology rapidly spread.

Controlling and aiming the beam to administer the proper dose is a tremendous challenge. The anatomy of the area and the tumor to be treated are identified. The dose to kill the specific type of cancer and the tolerance of the normal structures must be known. Since the beam deposits its energy in a predictable shape, the amount released into both the cancer and the nearby healthy tissue are calculated. The beam is aimed at the tumor from different directions to avoid giving a high total dose to the same area of skin or other healthy structures. The beams can also be modified by partially blocking them with shields. Treatments are given each day since more frequent and smaller doses allow the normal tissues more time to heal and therefore do less damage. When linacs first became widely available, treatments were planned by radiation oncologists and physicists using x-rays and tedious calculations while the beams were shaped using lead blocks. The development of advanced computer systems with CT scans to plan and control the beams and the ability to shape the beams using movable fingers built into the machines tremendously advanced the field of radiation oncology.[28]

When the beam bombards the cancer cell with photons, the energy damages the DNA. The highest energy photons energize electrons which slice the DNA directly while lower energy photons strike water atoms nearby and produce "free radicals," molecules which can further cut the DNA. The cancer cells die as their DNA is ripped and shredded by each daily dose. In an ironic twist, those cells which had become cancerous since they started with damaged DNA repair mechanisms may be more vulnerable to the radiation.

By Thursday, Harold's sodium level was in the low end of the normal range. He was aware of his surroundings, recognized his family, could eat and drink, but was easily confused. Movement still caused terrible pain in his arm and back, but the medications kept it under control when he lay quietly. Using the CT scan, a needle was inserted into his liver to obtain a piece of the cancer.

On Friday, Dr. Matthews received a call from the pathologist.

"It certainly is a malignancy. I've sent off special stains which should be back on Monday, but it looks like small cell lung cancer."

DISEASES: WHAT'S IN A NAME?

In the pre-molecular era, physicians divided lung cancer into two groups: "small cell lung cancers" and "non-small cell lung cancers" (everything else). The small cell cancers grew and spread rapidly, but shrank with chemotherapy. The non-small cell cancers were less rapidly growing, but more resistant to the drugs. As our understanding of lung cancers has improved, these categories were divided into further subtypes.

Small cell lung cancer has had different names. When the GI smokers from the World Wars started to die of lung cancers in the 1950s, this type was named "oat cell cancer" because the cells looked like oats under the microscope. Later, as fewer pathologists knew what oats looked like, the name changed to small cell lung cancer because the cells were small compared with other lung cancers. Finally, when the function of the cells was discovered, the name "high-grade neuro-endocrine carcinoma" was introduced, although many practicing physicians still cling to small cell.

Descriptive titles like oat cell cancer came from an era in medicine when diseases were often named after their appearance, an early patient, a historical feature of the condition, or most commonly, the physician or pathologist who discovered the condition. Perhaps the best-known example of a medical eponym (person, place or thing after which an item is named) is Alzheimer's disease. This dementia is named after Dr. Alois Alzheimer, a brilliant cigar smoking pathologist who described the microscopic features of the disease in 1906 and had the historical fortune of having his boss name it after him in a classic textbook. In the cancer world, the best-known condition named after a physician is Hodgkin's lymphoma, named after Thomas Hodgkin who described abnormalities of the lymph system in 1832. These unique descriptions of diseases often make them more memorable and give physicians and patients a convenient way to label the illness while honoring medical history. They also have served to make generations of physicians who could quote the eponym seem more learned in the eyes of their students and patients.

These eponyms occasionally have memorialized evil. An example is the rare inflammation of the blood vessels called Wegener's Granulomatosis, acknowledging its original description in 1936 by Dr. Friedrich Wegener. Countless physicians, medical students, patients, and their families have referred to the condition by this name. In 2006, Drs. Woywodt and Matteson reported in the journal *Rheumatology* that Wegener had been an early supporter of the Nazi party. Their research uncovered that Wegener had later worked near the Jewish ghetto of Lodz, Poland, in a medical office linked to some of the chilling medical tortures inflicted upon prisoners. Although they could not show Wegener himself carried out any of these atrocities, Woywodt and Matteson called for renaming the condition "ANCA-associated granulomatous vasculitis."[29] Perhaps justice might be served if the condition was renamed after Dr. George Livchitz, a physician in the Jewish Defense Committee, executed in 1944 after trying to resist the deportations to Auschwitz.[30]

The era of colorful and occasionally upsetting nomenclature in medicine is ending. The World Health Organization (WHO) has developed International Classification of Diseases (ICD) system to give diseases standardized names and codes. The first of these systems, called ICD-6, was published in 1948 and successive editions have increased the number of codes. The ICD-9 system had approximately thirteen thousand disease codes and three thousand procedure codes while the newer ICD-10 has sixty-eight thousand disease codes and eighty-seven thousand procedure codes.[31] Oat cell or small cell lung cancer is now defined as "poorly differentiated neuroendocrine tumor" of the lung and listed as code 209.30 in the ICD9 coding system and C7A.1 in the ICD10 coding system. On the positive side, the ICD system uniformly reports diseases, allowing data to be stored and compared across the globe. The WHO website displays the health of the world graphically using this data. On the negative side, the codes are cumbersome and often do not capture medically useful information, particularly rapidly changing molecular or genetic data.

The codes are here to stay. Payments in many countries, including the United States, require the proper ICD code for each interaction and bill. Given the complexity of ICD system, armies of trained medical coders are needed for billing. Since huge amounts of money are involved, coders and providers in these countries spend more time defining patients' illnesses using multiple codes. Auditors are hired by the insurers to review the coders. A whole industry has formed to use, teach, and police the billing aspects of the ICD system. Since billions are spent on medical care according to this system, the gradual loss of medical history which many find lamentable will be unstoppable.

After Monday's results had confirmed the diagnosis, Dr. Matthews met with Dan and Colleen. Harold was clearly better, but still on heavy doses of morphine for pain and sedatives to calm him before his radiation treatment.

Dr. Matthews spoke to Harold.

"Mr. Crimons, you might not remember, but last week we did a biopsy of your liver and found you have cancer. We want to give you some treatment tomorrow. Hopefully, it will make you feel better."

"I have cancer?" he replied in a puzzled voice.

"Remember, we told you," said Colleen.

"Oh. Okay. That must be what hurts so much." said Harold. "I guess I don't have much choice. Cancer is not good." He put his head back and drifted off again.

Dr. Matthews outlined the treatment for Colleen and Dan in more detail.

"He will receive three days of chemotherapy every three weeks. There will be two medications, called carboplatin and etoposide. Don't worry about remembering the names; the nurses will give you handouts with information. On the first day, he will get both medications, and it will take about three hours. On the second and third day, he will get only one medication, and it will take about an hour. He will get medications to prevent nausea or vomiting. I do not think he will feel much. Normally these treatments are done in the outpatient unit and patients go home each day, but he needs to be here in the hospital. We call these three days of treatments a cycle. After three cycles or nine weeks, we will do another set of scans to see if they are working, but we hope to see improvement in a few weeks."

The chemotherapy medications would stay in Harold's blood for only a few hours, but their effects on the DNA of his cells could linger for days or weeks. The image of DNA in the beautiful double helix we often see is rare, most of our DNA is kept tightly wound up for storage. When DNA is reproduced or access to the code is needed, like in active cancer cells, it is unwound. Harold's chemotherapy drugs interfered with this process. The carboplatin links onto the DNA, impairing its flexibility. The etoposide complements the carboplatin by poisoning the enzyme topoisomerase 2 which helps uncoil the DNA. When cancer cells are rapidly dividing, and these chemicals disrupt their DNA, they die. Unfortunately, these chemicals also have effects on rapidly dividing normal cells such as those of the bone marrow and lining of the mouth or intestinal tract, producing side effects of low blood counts, mouth sores, or diarrhea.

Harold did not feel anything as the chemotherapy entered his body. Kim Johnson, the oncology nurse, had given him anti-nausea medications and a mild sedative. Dan and Peg had come for the treatment, but Harold had slept, so Kim used the time to talk with them about discharge.

"Harold is still easily confused and will need some help with his medications for the next few weeks. These narcotics could really cause trouble if he takes too much of them or if he forgets. We need to lock them up and give Harold only what he should be taking each day. He can do simple things, but I think he will need help when he bathes or showers. Even though the discharge planner is getting you equipment, Harold is a big man, and I don't think you should help him by yourself, Mr. Crimons. If he fell on you, it would not be pretty. The discharge planner is also working on getting some aides."

Peg nodded and said, "Colleen called one of Harold's buddies, Roger, who will be over each morning to help us get him up and showered. Her husband will come at night to help us get him in bed."

"We will keep the medicines and Colleen will help us set them out," added Dan.

"You are very well organized. I wish all our patients had families like you. He's lucky to have you."

"I hope you get to meet him when he is better," said Peg, her eyes starting to well up again. "He really is a good son, and funny, too."

Following his treatment, Harold improved enough to be discharged. His sodium level remained normal, his pain was controlled with oral narcotics, and he began to eat. Since he was still unsteady on his feet and a bit confused, each morning Roger got Harold up and showered then stayed for Peg's breakfast. Colleen and her family often joined them for dinner so her husband Bill could help Harold get ready for bed.

Colleen, Dan, and Peg all brought Harold for his first visit to the outpatient oncology unit. He had was walking with much less pain, using a wheeled walker. Dr. Matthews reviewed the plans.

"It's nice to see you so much better," he said to Harold. "You have put together a good team here. We would like to give you another three-day chemotherapy treatment. You did very well with it in the hospital, and I think you will do well as an outpatient, too."

"Did I have chemo in the hospital?" asked Harold.

"Remember? We told you," said Colleen.

"I guess."

"You probably do not remember much from the hospital, Mr. Clements," said Dr. Matthews. "You were very sick there."

Karen Lange, the senior nurse on the unit, brought Harold to his chair in the large, windowed treatment area with a pretty view of the countryside. In her forties, Karen had been raised in Boston and practiced there for ten years before moving to upstate New York. Since Harold was wearing his Yankees cap and 2009 Championship jacket, Karen stopped near Rebecca Lotito, another of the nurses who was working on the computer.

"You'll need to take off your jacket before the treatment," Karen told Harold. "And you might as well take off the cap, too."

Harold looked puzzled. "Do you do something with my head?"

"No, this unit is part of the Red Sox nation. You can't wear that silly hat in here."

"Don't listen to her, Mr. Crimons," responded Rebecca in a Brooklyn accent. "She's just mad that you obviously know something about baseball. Come on in and bring all those Yankees fans with you."

Colleen and Dan laughed, while Harold looked puzzled.

The third nurse in the area, Beth Franklin, entered the discussion. "I can't stand any more of this baseball stuff. Sports, sports, sports. And anyway, don't you people know it's almost winter. How can you think about baseball?"

"Baseball is a metaphor for life," answered a man receiving treatment. "I should know, I'm from Cleveland. A lifetime of the Indians has taught me that."

"I think you'll fit in here, Harold," said Colleen.

Harold tolerated his treatments well and continued to improve. After the third cycle, he could walk without pain, his narcotic use was minimal, and his mind was clear. Although his mother refused to let him go home yet, Harold came by himself to his next visit.

"You look very good. I am glad you have made so much improvement," said Dr. Matthews.

"I feel good, doc. I am going to move back to my own home soon, probably after Christmas."

"Good. Now is a good time for us to get a CT scan to compare with the one you had in the hospital. I expect we are going to see a significant improvement."

"What happens with my treatments then?" asked Harold.

"If the scans look good, I would like to do three more treatments for a total of six, then another scan. When we see that you have made the maximal improvement, we will stop and take a break."

"What are my chances?" asked Harold.

Dr. Matthews gestured for Harold to sit in a chair and joined him.

"You were so sick in the hospital that we could not talk to you in detail about your cancer. Your small cell lung cancer cannot be cured. After we have finished our treatments, the cancer may stay away for a while, possibly several months to a year, but then it will come back, and you will need more treatments. Usually, the treatments do not work as well the second or third time, but we will try to keep them going as long as we can."

"What happens when they stop working?"

"Then we do our best to keep you comfortable."

"So, I die, then . . ."

Dr. Matthews nodded. "Yes."

They sat in silence for a moment.

"My parents and Colleen know this?" Harold asked.

"I told them in the hospital when we had to make decisions about your treatment."

Harold sat quietly for another moment, rotating his Yankees hat in his hands.

"Well, I feel good today, so we'll go with that for now." He put his hat on, rose, and moved out the door.

SMALL CELL LUNG CANCER: THE PROMISE AND LIMITS OF CHEMOTHERAPY.

Small cell lung cancer is an example of how the promise of chemotherapy turned to frustration with its limits. For the rare patient in whom this cancer is found as a tiny growth, cure is possible with a combination of surgery, radiation, and chemotherapy. For most patients, the cancer is widespread when discovered. For them chemotherapy produces shrinkage, sometimes so dramatic the cancer appears completely gone. Yet despite this tremendous effectiveness, chemotherapy has not produced cures.

When the GIs from World War II began to develop lung cancers from their tobacco addiction, it rapidly became clear surgery was rarely successful. This is still the case today; lung cancers are usually widespread when they are detected. To deal with the mounting numbers of men with inoperable or metastatic cancers, VA doctors in the 1960s used the first chemical treatments including, ironically enough, derivatives of mustard gas used in the World Wars (particularly World War I). These first clinical trials produced very few durable successes, but they did show that the lung cancer most likely to respond was oat cell lung cancer—now called neuroendocrine small cell lung cancer.[32]

There were reasons to hope these chemicals might work. After a difficult start, the use of combination chemotherapy treatments in the 1960s produced cures for Hodgkin's and other lymphomas. In general, scientific optimism was high following the success of the space program and the July 1969 Apollo lunar landing. In his January 1971 State of the Union address, President Nixon declared his intention to seek funds to cure cancer. The "War on Cancer" was formally declared later that year when Nixon signed the National Cancer Act. Over the next few years, the National Cancer Institute was reorganized, cancer centers were designated across the country, and the specialty of medical oncology drew physician-scientists to the challenge. Scientists discovered more chemotherapy drugs and developed scientific and mathematical models of cancer. Investigators tested concepts like the Goldie-Coldman hypothesis, which predicted that using multiple different agents is a more effective way to kill cancer cells. It seemed that researchers only needed to find the proper drugs and use them in the correct manner to cure many cancers.

The treatment of small cell lung cancer is a good example of the excitement, progress, and ultimate disappointment of this era. When combination chemotherapy for small cell lung cancer was first used, it often dramatically shrank tumors. While these responses were encouraging, the cancers would always regrow. In attempts to produce cures, physicians tried combining many drugs in complex treatment schemes like those used for lymphomas. These produced no cures, but often more side effects. Physicians tried maintenance drugs for longer periods, but again there was no long-term success. Finally, in the 1980s the ultimate in chemotherapy was attempted: combinations to kill most of the cancer cells followed by "high-dose chemotherapy with bone marrow transplantation" to eliminate any surviving cancer cells. In these high-dose procedures, patients were given about six to ten times the standard amounts of chemotherapy, a dose that would destroy the patient's bone marrow and be fatal. Before the chemotherapy was given, some bone marrow was removed from the person, frozen, and then given back after the drugs were gone from their system. Patients were hospitalized for several weeks and suffered terrible side effects from the treatments, which require impressively skilled physicians and nurses. Yet even these huge blasts of chemotherapy could not eliminate the cancer cells.[33]

Why doesn't chemotherapy finish the job for most cancers? Why can it kill 99 percent of cancer cells in some patients, but not the last few? One answer may lie in the "cancer stem cell." These parent cells may not be dividing rapidly and thus escape chemotherapy, but can produce progeny which divide rapidly. Cancer stem cells may hide in protected areas of the lung, sheltered from the chemotherapy. They may have evolved specific mechanisms to resist the drugs. Whatever the reason, the era of chemotherapy made it clear that once many cancers are widespread, other approaches would be needed to cure.

Harold returned with Colleen to review the results of his CT scan. The news was good.

"Your CT scan is much better. The lung tumor is almost gone, and the spots we could see in the liver are now gone," said Dr. Matthews.

"What about the bones?" asked Colleen.

"For the bones, it's harder to tell. It takes a long time for them to heal. The CT scan is also not the best test for them, but we do not see anything new, and I believe they are also getting better since your pain is so much better," he replied.

"So, we keep going," said Harold.

"Yes, we should keep going and recheck after three more treatments." Then, after a pause, Dr. Matthews asked, "Are your parents okay? I expected to see them here today."

Harold nodded. "They are fine, but this is hard on them. I wanted to prepare them for the results."

Christmas was happy in the Crimons' home. Although Harold had never been religious, he always enjoyed hearing his mother read the Bible passages announcing the birth of Jesus on Christmas Eve. This year as she reached the birth, Peg stopped.

"And thank you, God, for giving us our son back. For this year, Harold has been reborn to us."

The New Year of 2017 revealed the funny Harold Clements his mother had promised. One day he marched into the chemotherapy area wearing a Yankee shirt and large plastic ears, pointed to Karen and announced,

"Look what you've done to me. You didn't tell me about this."

A silence fell over the treatment area. Karen looked up from her work, studied him carefully and spoke with her best Boston accent.

"We only see this reaction in Yankees fans. But we know the cure. A Red Sox cap will shrink those ears back to normal in no time."

"That treatment is worse than any disease," Harold replied to generalized laughter.

"Maybe not if you're from Cleveland," replied Harold's treatment buddy, the Indian fan.

For many fellow patients, Harold was a large, reassuring figure who set a relaxed tone in the treatment area with his omnipresent *New York Post* and Stewart's coffee. After his sixth session in March, his CT scan showed no signs of cancer in the lungs or liver and the bones were healing.

"Your CT scan looks very good. We should stop now and take a break," said Dr. Matthews.

"I can take more if I need to . . ."

"I know you can. You have been very determined, but the studies show us that there is no benefit to continuing beyond this point. We know that at some time in the future you will need more chemo. This is a good time to rest so you can take more when you need it."

"Well, having the summer off would be nice," Harold agreed.

"Good," said Dr. Matthews. "Let's plan a CT scan in three months. That will be June. If that one is good, we can do the one after that in September."

Harold stopped to visit "my nurses" on the way out.

"I am free for three months," he told them. "No more chemo for now."

"Then stand over here," replied Karen. "Dr. Matthews can tell you you're done, but we still need to end your treatments."

Harold stood still as the nurses gathered around him and sprayed him with their automatic turbo bubble maker, a ritual that ended a course of therapy. Suitably blessed, he left the office.

When Harold returned in June, his CT scan remained unchanged, and he enjoyed another summer in the town he loved. In September, Harold's CT scan again showed cancer in his liver. The spots were very small, and unlike the first time, he felt well. Harold was alone to receive the news.

"You have three choices," said Dr. Matthews. "One choice is not to take any further treatment. If you do not take more treatment, you will probably feel good for several months before you get sick again. You can then join the hospice program, and we will try to make you as comfortable as possible. This choice is the best for those people who had a tough time with chemo. The second choice is to try a different chemotherapy. You know what these treatments are like. We may soon have some immune treatments available as well. The final choice is to visit a major cancer center like Memorial Sloan Kettering in New York or Dana Farber in Boston. They might have a clinical trial of new medicines, particularly these new immune treatments."

"I don't want to leave here."

"If you do enter a clinical trial in Boston or New York, we will still take care of you. They might not let us give all the treatments, but we would help however they let us," offered Dr. Matthews.

"I understand the score, doc. I am not putting myself and my family through travel back and forth to New York and all that." His eyes were moist, but his voice determined. As he left, Harold stopped by the chemotherapy nurses station and found Karen.

"I'm coming back to you, " he said.

"I'm sorry, Yankee. We'll take care of you again."

As he left, Karen caught Rebecca's eye.

"Shit," she swore softly. "I didn't want him back yet."

Rebecca nodded, the Red Sox and Yankee nurse agreeing on this call.

Today Dr. Matthews finished examining Harold and sat down on the stool.

"You look good," he said. "How are you managing with the new chemotherapy treatments?"

"I'm okay, doc." He took off his Yankees cap, reached into his pocket and pulled out a ball of plastic with elastic straps. "Except for these damn ears." He put them on and headed into the back for more.

"My father used to sing 'When Irish Eyes Are Smiling' to me when I was sick," said Kelly Mulvaney, a forty-two-year-old Irish woman with red hair and a pretty, modestly freckled face. "Most of the time it was for colds or silly stuff. But when I was about fifteen I was in bed for three weeks with mono. Every evening he would come upstairs into my room to check on me. He would stand there, so large in his police uniform that he seemed like a mountain, and sing in that deep beautiful voice."

She paused.

"At first they told me I had 'kissing disease' and I was so scared."

"Because you were sick?" asked Dr. Matthews.

"No, I remember being sick, but that's not what scared me. Joe O'Neil, a neighbor boy, and I had kissed about two months earlier in the woods behind the house, and I knew if my father found out he would kill us. I thought I would have to tell the doctor."

"And did you?" asked Dr. Matthews, drawn into the story.

"No. Thank God one of my older cousins, Gracie, came over to visit. She had had mono a year or two before and explained it to me. I was so thankful I didn't have to tell anyone about Joe. He and I still laugh about it when we meet at reunions."

She wrinkled her lip, a habit when she was thinking.

"Do you think that was it?" she asked.

Dr. Matthews laughed. "Do I think kissing Joe gave you mono which then gave you Hodgkin's lymphoma?"

She nodded. It was a good question.

Kelly was treated for Hodgkin's disease ten years earlier. She was thirty-two, a stay-at-home mom with two children. John Jr., known as Jack, was nine and Mary was seven. Kelly had developed a harsh cough, and after a course of antibiotics did not help, her primary physician sent her for a chest x-ray which hinted at swollen lymph nodes in her chest. A CT scan was scheduled a week later. During that time, Kelly's cough improved, and she even debated canceling the scan but, being dutiful, went ahead. Dr. Oakley called that evening while Kelly and John had been watching *Jeopardy* and the children played. For some reason, it always stuck her mind that only a few days earlier they had watched the first three-way tie in the history of the show.

"Kelly, you have some enlarged lymph nodes in the center of your chest. I don't know if they are due to an infection or something more serious, but you need to see the lung specialist, Dr. Martin. I spoke with him, and he will see you tomorrow at four o'clock. Call our office tomorrow, and the staff will give you instructions."

"Is this serious?" was all that she could say as Alex Trebek carried on until John turned down the volume.

"I don't know. Hopefully, this is an inflammatory condition or the result of an infection. The radiologists did not see anything in the lungs themselves. Dr. Martin is an expert, and he will tell you what he thinks about it."

"What is it?" asked John after she hung up.

"I'm not sure," Kelly answered. "Dr. Oakley said I have swollen lymph nodes in my chest and he wants me to see a lung specialist at four tomorrow. He said it might just be infection—"

"Mom! Jack took my Claire! Make him give her back," came the distressed cry of an exhausted Mary.

"John, Junior, you give your sister back that doll. Then both of you, pick up those toys and get ready for bath."

Once the evening fighting over the toys started, Kelly knew that her own issues needed to be deferred until after the highly-ritualized bedtime sequence of events. A brief toy pickup was followed by the bath, pajamas, and then story in bed. Any deviation risked the dreaded outcome of an awake and partially invigorated but very needy young child. After the four hundredth reading of *Dinosaurs Before Dark* for Jack and a chapter in a *Junie B. Jones* book for Mary, the children were kissed, and the lights were out. Kelly and John sat in the living room.

"Did the doctor say anything else?" John asked.

"Not really," she replied. "He said it might be infection or inflammation. He didn't mention cancer or anything like that . . ."

"I bet he's just being cautious. And your cough seems better these past few days," John added.

"Yeah, it's not gone, but I feel pretty good."

A night with the internet ended that feeling. A search of "enlarged lung lymph nodes" led to a long list of sites dealing with lung cancer, some with lymphoma, a few about sarcoidosis, and many detailing horror stories of surgeries gone wrong and misdiagnoses. After two hours of reading, she sat awake in bed while John snored next to her. Fortunately, the day ahead was a busy one as she had volunteered to help in Mary's classroom. When school was over, Kelly settled Jack and Mary with the sitter before she and John headed to her appointment.

Kelly was easily the healthiest looking patient in the pulmonary office. Most of the others were older; some were in wheelchairs and on oxygen with labored breathing. Dr. Martin was a warm man in his late fifties who examined Kelly and discussed her situation.

"You do have some swollen lymph nodes the middle of your chest. It is possible they could be from an infection, but they are a bit large for most routine infections, and you have not been exposed to anything unusual. The most likely possibility is that these nodes are a condition called sarcoidosis. That is a benign, usually very manageable condition that often does not need treatment. The most serious thing they could be is a cancer. A lymphoma would be the most likely cancer, and those are very treatable. Lung cancer is possible, although that is not likely since you are not a smoker and we do not see any other spots in your lungs. Whatever they are, we need to get a biopsy of them to know what to do."

"How?" asked John.

"I will start with the easiest test called a bronchoscopy. This is a scope which I pass into the breathing tubes of the lung. If that does not give us an answer, then we will have our thoracic surgeon do a mediastinoscopy. That is a surgical procedure where he will make an incision at the top of the breastbone and insert a scope to do the biopsy. The ladies out front will set you up with everything and give you instructions."

Kelly had very little memory of the bronchoscopy. Dr. Martin had seen some narrowing of the main air passages in the lung, but nothing to biopsy. In the recovery room afterward, he explained to Kelly and John that they needed to proceed with the mediastinoscopy the following afternoon.

The staff prepared Kelly for the procedure, but not for Dr. Ben Joe. The next day as she lay on the hospital gurney, a self-assured Hispanic man in surgical garb entered.

"Miss Kelly Mulvaney. I'm Dr. Joe. First, I sing for you. 'Old Danny Boy, the old piano's calling.' You look surprised. I'm no good? Okay, then I cut your throat. But just a little and only because Dr. Martin tells me to." He smiled. "I cut in just the right place, about this much." He held up his finger and thumb about two inches apart. "I take out a few of the lymph nodes. You go home and this fellow over here," he pointed to John, "he takes care of you. Very good, no?"

Kelly burst into laughter.

"Don't worry," he said as he patted her arm, "everything will be fine."

The biopsy went well. Kelly woke in the recovery room and found John sitting beside her. Dr. Joe came to check on her.

"You have a beautiful neck," he said. "My scars, they always heal well but this man," he pointed to John, "he still must buy you a nice necklace to cover the thin line."

Kelly smiled, and he went on.

"I got a good sample for Dr. Martin, very nice lymph nodes. Now you wait. It's very hard, but that is what you must do. But I will tell you something," he paused as they both looked at him. "I believe in the end you will be fine."

Kelly and John returned to a quiet house as the children had stayed with neighbors after school and for dinner. They had been uncertain how to prepare them for Kelly's procedure. They debated telling them the doctor needed to make a small cut in her neck see what was inside, but were unsure how that would be understood. They finally settled on saying that the doctors were going do a test on Mom and figured they would explain later. They were pleased when Kelly was able to hide the bandage under a high-necked shirt. The children were so excited about the disruption to their routine that they did not notice Mom's mildly pale appearance and her early trip into bed.

The next morning, Kelly supervised the usual routine of breakfast and putting the children on the bus while John went to work. Although her neck was mildly sore, Kelly otherwise felt well. Since she had not known what to expect following the biopsy, she had left the day open and now did not know what to do with herself. In anticipation of surgery, she had cleaned the house, done the laundry, and baked cookies, so she had no chores. She lacked the focus to start any new projects, the television didn't hold her interest, and she wasn't sure what to tell her friends. My neck was cut by a crazy surgeon. I feel okay but am scared to death somehow didn't seem appropriate. Nor did she particularly feel like discussing the various possible results. In the end, she found herself sitting in the study with a cup of tea looking through her old yearbooks. The pictures from high school of her and Joe O'Neil brought a smile. The youthful, enthusiastic writing of her friends spoke of the endless possibilities of her life ("you are the best and the smartest" and "you can do anything!"). In her college yearbook, she and John were featured in pictures together at a school dance and football game. Her formal photo gave her the look of a serious student and listed her major (history), activities (newspaper editor) and plans (teaching). His picture was wilder, but she was still struck by how handsome he looked. It was a pleasant way to pass the morning. After lunch, she fell asleep on the living room couch.

The slam of the door ended her vaguely enjoyable dream. Jack and Mary came tearing into the living room, full of energy after school.

"Mommy, where are you?"

As Kelly sat up, the children suddenly stopped short a few feet in front of her. Jack's mouth fell open while Mary froze, eyes wide and terrified. Jack reacted first.

"What's that?" he pointed to her bandage, now visible over her unbuttoned her shirt. For a moment, Kelly wasn't sure what he meant until her hand involuntarily touched the dressing, and she realized what had happened.

"It's a special Band-Aid," Kelly responded. "I have a little cut underneath where the doctor had to check me yesterday. But it's almost all better now."

"Will I get a boppy when I go to the doctor?" asked Jack.

"A what?"

"A boppy," insisted Jack.

"Where did you learn that?" asked Kelly.

"I heard Dad talking about it to Mr. Newton."

"No," Kelly said. "You won't need a biopsy."

"Can I have some cookies?" he asked, turning toward the kitchen.

"Go ahead, but only two," she answered.

Kelly turned back to Mary, who still stood frozen.

"It's okay, honey," she said and reached out for her. Mary ran into her arms and hugged her tightly. Kelly could feel her little heart beating rapidly as she trembled.

"Your cookies are awesome, Mom," came the boy's voice from the kitchen. "Can I have one more?"

Mary stayed near Kelly as she prepared dinner. When John returned home from work, he noticed her quiet determination not to leave the kitchen. He understood when Kelly caught his eye and pointed to her bandage. During dinner, the always more vocal Jack described his day while Mary ate little and sat quietly. Afterward, as *Jeopardy* played, she leaned on Kelly, twirling her hair and holding Claire. She said almost nothing during bath and book.

"Are you worried about Mommy, honey?" asked Kelly, stroking her hair as she lay in bed. Mary nodded.

"It's okay. Everything is going to be fine. You understand?"

Mary nodded again, but still did not look convinced.

The routine of the week initially kept Kelly's mind off the waiting for the results, but as the visit approached she felt a sense of dread. Her cough worsened again, and with each episode Mary froze, her eyes wide and scared. Although Kelly outwardly remained calm, by the time of their drive to Dr. Martin's office, she was anxious. John sensed her nervousness and tried to reassure her. After checking in, they waited quietly in the exam room. They could faintly hear Dr. Martin's muffled voice in the room next door. Although they could not make out any of the words, they knew when he finished. In the silence that followed, Kelly began to hear her heart beat as John held her hand.

"That crazy surgeon was right," she said. "This is very hard."

"It will be okay. He said that, too," answered John.

"Can you believe a guy who sings like that, though?" she joked weakly.

"Well, I believe it, no matter what."

Dr. Martin entered the room, said hello, then moved right to the point.

"Kelly, we did not get an answer from your biopsy. Dr. Joe removed several swollen lymph glands, and they have been studied by the pathologists here and at an outside lab. They cannot say for sure what is wrong. The lymph nodes show only inflammation."

"Isn't that good news?" asked John, puzzled.

"It is good news in the sense that we did not find lung cancer. If this were a lung cancer, I would have expected to find cancer cells in the lymph nodes. If it was the condition sarcoidosis, we should have seen that, too. Lymphomas can fool us, and that is what I am concerned you have in the deeper lymph nodes."

"What do we do now?" asked Kelly, stunned.

"We need to do another biopsy," said Dr. Martin. "This time the surgeon will make an incision lower down in your chest and try to take some of the deeper lymph nodes. It is a slightly more complex procedure. Usually, you go home the same day, but sometimes the surgeon needs to put a chest tube into the space, and you stay overnight. Although Dr. Joe is an excellent surgeon, I want you to go to a hospital with specialized pathologists who can look at the lymph nodes immediately. That way we know we will get a sample which gives us an answer. I have spoken to Dr. Mark Robinson, a thoracic surgeon at the Brigham and Women's Hospital and Dana Farber in Boston. He will meet you next week, and you will have the surgery the following morning."

Kelly and John returned home to relieve Kate, the sitter. As usual, Jack had his car collection out to impress his tall blonde love. Mary usually painted with Kate, but today there was no easel, and she sat quietly on the couch holding Claire. As they hugged, Kelly could tell she was checking her neck for a bandage.

After the bedtime routine, Kelly and John sat in the family room.

"I'm scared," she said. "I don't think Dr. Martin would send me to Boston if he did not think it was cancer."

"We don't know that," began John, but stopped when he saw her look of disbelief. "Okay, let me try again. It sounds like he thinks you have lymphoma, but that if we find it, you can be treated."

"Treated doesn't mean cured."

"Don't think that way, honey."

"Don't tell me how to think, John," she snapped. "This waiting, not knowing, is driving me crazy. Plus, what do I tell people? What about the children? What do I tell them? You see how Mary is. What if something happens to me?"

"Jesus, I don't know Kelly. What do you want me to say?" he snapped back.

"I don't know," she said forcefully, then started to cry.

John moved to hug her as she sobbed.

"It's going to be all right, Kelly."

She pulled away.

"You're not the doctor, John. And even they don't know. So stop patronizing me."

He looked stunned, and his face reddened.

"Well, for Christ's sake, Kelly, tell me what you want."

Kelly sat for a minute with her head down, then looked up.

"I'm sorry," she said. "I didn't mean to snap at you. I mean, I guess I did mean to snap at you. John, I'm scared. Something bad is inside me, and the doctors don't know what it is. I'm worried when they find out it will mean that I'll die and you and the kids will be without me."

"You don't know—," he started until she held up her hand to silence him.

"I know that you mean well when you tell me that everything is going to be all right. But you don't know that, and it's not what I need to hear. I need you to tell me that you understand why I'm scared. That nobody knows what is going on. All our lives together you have protected me and tried to make everything all right for me, but you can't fix this now. I can accept that, but don't pretend it will all be okay."

"All right. But listen to me. I do believe it, Kelly. I believe you're going to be all right."

Kelly and John made the trip to Boston together. Fortunately, they had close neighbors with children who would gladly look after Jack and Mary. They were reluctant to rely on their families. Kelly's father had died a few years ago and her mother, although only a few hours away and theoretically willing to come, would not be able to keep pace. John's parents were both still living but spent their winters in Florida. The chaos that their return would have caused was not worth the effort.

The first issue was what to tell the children. John argued that they try to keep it a secret.

"Look, Mary was scared when she saw your band aid. This one will be lower down, and she won't have to see it. We can tell them we are going to visit friends in Boston."

"I don't think that will work, John. They will hear from someone that I need another boppy."

"A what? What's a boppy?" he asked. Kelly relayed Jack's story.

He laughed. "I guess you're right. They hear a lot."

Kelly bit her lip. "The question is what exactly do we say? We don't want to scare them, but we want them to understand. Who would know?"

"Dr. Anthony will have an opinion," offered John. Kelly nodded.

Dr. Benjamin Anthony, the family pediatrician, was a tall, upright man in his late sixties who habitually wore a bow tie and could have walked off a Norman Rockwell painting. Despite his years of practice, he was still fascinated by children and both awed them and comforted their parents.

"I am sorry to learn of this, but your children are fortunate to have two wonderful parents. For children of the ages of Mary and Jack, you must tell them the truth when you know the facts, but do not share your anxieties over all the possibilities. Explain what is happening simply. Tell them they may hear things from other people and if they have any questions they must not keep them inside but come to you."

"What words should I use to explain things like a biopsy?"

"You might as well use the medical terms since that is what they will hear. You should explain them as simply as you can and then answer in more detail as they ask. You can be surprised what they focus on. Sometimes a little thing you would never think of is what they will ask about. They are often worried that something will happen to them as well as you. You can reassure them by explaining any changes in their daily routine. Remember that they have great imaginations and what they do not understand can be worse than what they do know. The main thing is to just be yourself and be with them."

She tried that night while John was at the office, finishing work in anticipation of their trip. After bath and pajamas but before books, Kelly gathered Jack and Mary with her on the sofa.

"I want to talk with you for a few minutes about next week. Mommy and Daddy are going away for a few days, and you will be staying with the Newtons. They will get you on the bus for school, and you will sleep at their house."

"Why Mommy?" asked Mary.

"Mommy needs another biopsy from the doctors in Boston."

Mary looked alarmed, "No, Mommy. I don't want you to go."

"She has to go," said John. "She has cancer. That's where they cure it."

Kelly sat upright quickly. "Where did you hear that?" she asked.

John looked at her proudly. "I heard it from the message machine. And I know about Boston because they talk about it when we watch the Red Sox. Are you going to be like the bald women they had on TV?"

Mary started to sob. "Where's my Claire?" she wailed, her nose immediately running.

"Sometimes they have the kids on TV, too," continued Jack. "Do you think we will be on TV?"

"Where's Claire?" cried Mary, sobbing uncontrollably now.

Shit, thought Kelly, what have I done? Overwhelmed, she wanted to cry, too. Then the memory of being sick as a child flashed by and she heard her father singing. Calm down; you can do this, she thought. She first brought Mary to bed and sat with her, stroking her hair. Mary sucked her left thumb while cradling Claire and twirling her hair with her right index finger. It would have been difficult for her to look more vulnerable.

"Are you scared, honey?"

Mary just looked at her.

"It's okay, honey. Mommy will be fine. The doctors just need to check me so they can fix my cough."

Mary lay still.

"Do you know what my Daddy used to do for me when I was scared?"

Mary shook her head.

"He would sing to me, like this,

> 'When Irish eyes are smiling,
> Sure, 'tis like the morn in Spring.
> In the lilt of Irish laughter
> You can hear the angels sing.
> When Irish hearts are happy,
> All the world seems bright and gay.
> And when Irish eyes are smiling,
> Sure, they steal your heart away.' "

Mary relaxed a little and closed her eyes.

"That will be our song, too," said Kelly. "And whenever we are nervous, we will sing it to ourselves or each other, okay?"

As Mary nodded, Kelly dimmed the light and lay beside her until she fell asleep.

But the night wasn't over. In the next room, Jack sat on his bed with his thirty or forty small stuff animals arrayed around him. Kelly sat next to him.

"What are they all doing?" she asked.

"Well, you see," began John. Kelly knew she was in for a long, convoluted explanation. "It starts over here with Uncle Pickle (the blue bear). He is the leader. Next to him is Squirrel. He is the assistant . . ."

Ten minutes later, when the story finished, and Jack's eyes were finally starting to get heavy, Kelly spoke.

"Are you worried about Mommy and Daddy going to Boston?"

"Yes," he nodded.

"What are you worried about?"

"How will I sleep at the Newton's?"

"They have an extra bed in Charlie's room. Mrs. Newton said you can sleep there."

He looked at her. "I can't sleep without Uncle Pickle."

"Honey, you can bring Uncle Pickle to the Newton's."

He looked at her again. "But Charlie will see him."

Then Kelly understood. Nine-year-old-boys needed their Uncle Pickle but did not want their friends to see Uncle Pickle.

"Let me talk to Mrs. Newton. I won't mention Uncle Pickle, but I'll see what we can do, okay?"

He nodded, rolled over, and fell asleep.

The few days before the trip to Boston were busy. John had to work long hours. Kelly had to be sure the insurance approval was in place, collect her records, and prepare the house. The children's clothing, schoolwork, and activities had to be arranged at the Newton's. And most importantly for two boys, Uncle Pickle had to be introduced to Fuzzy, a larger and slightly worn brown bear belonging to Charlie.

The Longwood Brookline area of Boston is a center of American medicine, containing the Brigham and Women's Hospital, Dana Farber Cancer Institute, Children's Hospital, Beth Israel/Deaconess, and Harvard Medical School. After a four-hour drive from Saratoga Springs, Kelly and John arrived at the Brigham and Women's Hospital and found a small city within the complex. In the main wide corridors streams of fast-moving, white-clad young doctors, nurses, and students, admixed with an occasional senior physician, swirled around slow-moving clumps of patients and families. Kelly found the atmosphere electric. Even the signs in elevators announcing lectures added to the intellectual energy which powered the place. After a walk, short elevator ride, and another impressive corridor, they turned into a quieter hallway belonging to the thoracic surgery department. Portraits of past surgeons and modern photos of "The Best of Boston" left no doubt that here they practiced serious medicine.

Dr. Mark Robinson was a pleasant and obviously brilliant man in his late thirties with wire-rimmed glasses who reminded John of a young

Terry Francona, the Red Sox manager. He reviewed Kelly's history and briefly explained the procedure he would perform the next morning. He would make an incision to the left of Kelly's breastbone and remove a portion of cartilage to expose the lymph nodes while avoiding the important blood vessels just above the heart. If the pathologist felt they had a diagnostic sample, Dr. Robinson would stop, and she would go home. If not, he would enter the deeper space near the lung to get more tissue. In this case, Kelly would need to stay in the hospital for several days with a chest tube to suck the air out from around the lung. Kelly's surgery was called a "Chamberlain procedure" after the famous surgeon who developed it in the late 1950s. Although Dr. J Maxwell Chamberlain was a larger-than-life thoracic surgeon, he had trained at the rival Massachusetts General Hospital, and thus his portrait was not found in this office. Chamberlain tragically died in 1968 in an automobile accident as he drove from New York to Boston, yet his legacy was still acknowledged in the instruction sheet for the procedure which bore his name. After the visit, Kelly and John checked into their hotel and called the children. Predictably, Jack answered first.

"Guess what, Mom? We had hot dogs tonight! Mrs. Newton is awesome!"

"Did you have a good day at school?" asked Kelly.

"Yeah. We had a fire drill, and the fireman came and everything. Oh, I gotta go, Charlie and I are playing. Bye."

Mary's voice was quieter but she, too, seemed content. Kelly thanked Cindy Newton.

"They are good kids, Kelly. Don't worry about them. Just take care of yourself and don't hurry back."

The biopsy went well. Dr. Robinson made the incision and removed several lymph nodes. The pathologist stationed in the operating room froze a portion, examined it under the microscope, and assured him that it would provide an answer after the final processing. Since he did not need to go deeper, Kelly was discharged to the hotel that evening. The phone call that night was brief as Jack remained excited and Mary was content to hear her voice. She and John returned to the hospital the next morning for a brief check with the resident physician and then left for home.

A week later Kelly and John again were in Dr. Martin's office. Although Kelly was coughing more, she was less anxious. By now she was confident she had lymphoma and spent time on the internet in a focused search. Kelly understood that if this was lymphoma, it might be either Hodgkin's lymphoma or non-Hodgkin's lymphoma. She hoped for Hodgkin's lymphoma since that seemed to have a higher cure rate, but she felt either type was manageable. Her studies made her confident that she could participate in any upcoming decisions. In some strange way, she was vaguely reminded of her college days. All in all, she thought, I'm ready for the exam.

Surprisingly, it was John who became more anxious. His hours in the Brigham surgical waiting room had been sobering as he watched other family members wait for news of their loved ones. After Kelly was in the operating room, John tried to walk off his nervous energy. Wandering randomly, he crossed from the Brigham and Women's Hospital into the Dana Farber Cancer Institute through an elevated causeway. John found himself in a quiet hallway where small groups of young scientists walked passed, some speaking foreign languages and others unintelligible English. The walk was calming until he rode the elevator down to the main lobby. There he saw patients heading for various parts of the hospital, many obviously bald and wearing masks, some in wheelchairs looking like they were not doing well. All with cancer, he thought. Once he and Kelly returned home, John had to answer questions from several friends and coworkers who shared stories of their own, a few even with terrible endings. Cancer talk was replacing sports in his life, and he did not like it.

Dr. Martin walked in and gently went right to the point.

"Dr. Robinson called this morning. You have Hodgkin's lymphoma, Kelly."

"Good," she replied forcefully as John and Dr. Martin exchanged surprised glances. "Now we have an answer and can go forward. What is next and what are my chances?"

"What's next is you see Dr. Matthews, our oncologist. He will do some additional tests and then treat you with chemotherapy. You might also need some radiation treatments. It will probably take about six to nine months. It is a hard road, but you can do it. Your chances of being cured are very high. There are no guarantees, but we certainly hope you will return to near normal."

"Do I need to go back to Boston?" Kelly asked.

"No. Dr. Robinson spoke with his lymphoma team, and they say the treatment is the same here. The person he spoke to knew Dr. Matthews since he had worked there many years ago."

She looked at John and wrinkled her lip, then turned to Dr. Martin.

"That's good. Thank you for figuring this out. You and your staff have been great. We are ready to get started. Okay, John? Are you ready to go?"

"I guess so," he looked a bit dazed.

"She is ready." Dr. Martin smiled and patted John on the shoulder.

That night Kelly returned to the internet and continued her study of Hodgkin's lymphoma. She was intently focused when John entered the study. For a moment, he saw the serious student he met those years ago.

He whistled softly.

"You remind me of the beautiful girl I met in college, studying away."

She looked up, pursed her lips, and signaled for him to get lost, just like she did in college when she would be studying and he wanted to go out. That had been their pattern. Kelly was the serious student while John, a popular and handsome lacrosse player, did only what was required. After they married, it was his career that had directed their lives. John used his sports contacts to obtain a position in an advertising firm. When the company opened a new office in Saratoga Springs, John became the head of sales. His success and their decision to move had cost Kelly her own less lucrative first job as a junior news writer for a small paper. Unlike John, she found the transition from the orderly world of college academics into the work environment challenging. When she became pregnant, Kelly had put her career dreams aside with mixed feelings. Her energy had gone into the children and volunteer work, but now this once serious student had reason to study.

"This is my disease, John," she said, "and I'm going to learn all I can about it."

THOMAS HODGKIN AND THE START OF MODERN MEDICINE. The question "How was Hodgkin's lymphoma discovered?" is the correct response to the *Medical Jeopardy* answer that "in 1832 a physician at the famous Guy's Hospital in London wrote 'On some Morbid Appearances of the Absorbant Glands and Spleen.' " Like so much in science and medicine, the truth is much more complicated. For Thomas Hodgkin lived and described his lymphoma at a time we now identify as the start of modern medicine.[36]

Thomas Hodgkin was born in England in 1798 into a world in turmoil. Europe was transforming as the Industrial Revolution gained speed, fueled by rapid population growth. Established governments with aristocratic and religious leadership struggled with the demands of the common man to have access to traditional institutions. Britain had been stung by the loss of its American colonies. In France, the brilliant ideals of the revolution had turned to slaughter and then Napoleonic hero worship. A long period of War between these two great powers was beginning across the continent and on the seas. From an intellectual viewpoint, the early nineteenth century saw human reason begin to challenge the Word of God as defined by the Church. The Age of Science was beginning. During this time of upheaval, fortunate individuals could have profound influence while the unfortunate could suffer greatly.[37]

Medicine in the early 1800s was also changing. At the start of the century, medical treatments were largely useless and surgery brutal. In Hodgkin's England, the highest level of practitioners, at least as defined by social status, were physicians who obtained a university medical degree. University medical education combined the study of Greek and Latin with philosophy and the traditional practices of ancient medicine, but very little practical training. Graduates could then obtain additional training in surgery or medicine if they desired at hospitals. Although some physicians performed surgery, many did not and used bleedings, purgings, blisterings, and the various compounded remedies of the day to treat illnesses. A university degree from Oxford or Cambridge could allow entry into the Royal College of Physicians, which controlled and limited physician practice in the London area, probably to the public's benefit.[38] Surgeons were the next level of practitioners. They trained at hospital medical schools where they followed surgeons on rounds and into the operating room. Surgeons practiced their art without anesthesia or an understanding of antisepsis. Patients in need of an operation were strapped down, and the skill of the surgeon could be in large part measured by the speed of the operation. Apothecaries were the lowest social tier of practitioners but provided the majority of care to the public. Their training typically included several years in an apprenticeship in retail settings working long hours preparing and dispensing various remedies combined with some time at hospitals.

From this bleak point, the start of the nineteenth century saw some important advances in medicine. For non-surgical practitioners, France and the "Paris School" of physicians began the serious study of the diagnosis and pathology of illness. Historian Roy Porter notes that these advances largely took place in hospitals where many of the famous physicians were themselves Napoleon-like figures. One famous example was Rene-Theophile-Hyacinthe Laennec, who studied heart sounds by placing his ear on the chest of his patients. When he encountered a young woman whose heart he wished to hear but whose sex and age precluded such an "intimate" approach, he invented the listening tube we now call the stethoscope.[39] Although Laennec and others like him improved the understanding of diseases, medical treatments were still usually futile and remained so through much of the century. Surgeons in the first half of the century were also very limited by the lack of anesthesia and antisepsis, but the slaughter on the battlefields and in the seas provided ample opportunities to practice rapid amputations and wound care. Trauma in the work place and daily life provided the opportunity to set fractures, although any open fractures which exposed the bones would usually result in infection requiring amputation.[40] While bladder stones could be removed to relieve obstruction in painful operations, surgeries involving the abdomen and chest were still generally avoided. A few surgeons in America had begun to operate on the female organs, their relative aggressiveness attributed to both lack of medical regulation and the availability of slaves who had little opportunity to resist any "treatment."[41] Fortunately, by the second half of the century, the introduction of anesthesia and the understanding of the need for cleanliness started the modern "age of surgery."

During this time of change in both the world and medicine, Thomas Hodgkin was raised in England by a devoutly Quaker family. Hodgkin's faith, which had a profound influence on his life, had begun in the mid-1600s when George Fox taught that it was possible for a person to have a direct relationship with God and therefore not need the Church of England (or other formal religions). The name Quaker, which came from Fox's suggestion that a hostile magistrate tremble before the word of God, was initially insulting but gradually became an accepted way to refer to members, also formally known as the Religious Society of Friends. Early Quakers adopted plain dress and language, refused to take oaths, serve in wars, or pay taxes which would be used to support the Church of England. Quakers also gave women a substantial role and supported the education of girls. For their beliefs, early Quakers were severely persecuted by the government, but by the time of Hodgkin's birth tensions had eased. The Toleration Acts gave religious dissenters more protection and the faith had both diminished in size and became less demonstrative. Some Quakers succeeded in business where they were regarded as honest and hard-working, yet considerable prejudice remained. Quakers were not admitted to many parts of society while many higher educational institutions such as Oxford and Cambridge Universities required students to take an oath to the Church of England. Thus, most educated their children privately. Hodgkin's father was a well-known teacher of penmanship, mathematics, and Greek who studied Latin.[42] Hodgkin himself had beautiful penmanship as a youth which, perhaps predictably as a physician, later became almost illegible.[43]

In addition to calligraphy, Hodgkin's parents instilled in him a strong belief in hard work, an appreciation for intellectual endeavors, and a desire to serve. He expressed an early interest in science and through his family's connections with other Quakers with similar interests, was exposed to botany, chemistry, electricity, and geology. The early 1800s were an exciting time for scientific study as new theories and experimentation challenged centuries old dogma, usually religiously based. In geology, evidence began to support theories that the earth was both changing and much older than had been calculated by biblical scholars, revolutionary ideas proposed in 1830 by Charles Lyell in his famous work *Principles of Geology*. As a young man, Hodgkin himself was a contributor to geologic science in a period textbook.[44] These advances in science often caused tension with established religious beliefs. Charles Darwin famously visited the Galapagos Islands in 1835 and developed his theory of evolution, but was afraid to have it published until 1859 for fear of reprisal from the Church and the damage it might cause his reputation. Hodgkin had several Quaker role models who managed to balance their quest for scientific study with a strong faith, and he appears to have been able to reconcile these parts of his life.

Hodgkin's entry into medicine began when he served as secretary to William Allen, a Quaker with a broad range of scientific and philanthropic interests who owned Allen & Hanbury's, a London apothecary which was also a remarkable place of scientific and intellectual discourse. In an interesting historical twist, Allen had been tutored by Hodgkin's father. Although their short relationship ended with Hodgkin's disappointment at being denied an apprenticeship, the work introduced him to Guy's Hospital, where he studied before obtaining his medical degree at the University of Edinburgh in Scotland.[45] Hodgkin wrote his thesis on the role of the lymphatics in the body and, although many of his theories were wrong, his approach was scientific. Following graduation, he spent time in France with Rene-Theophile-Hyacinthe Laennec and learned the use of the newly devised stethoscope to hear heart and lung sounds.

In 1826, Hodgkin returned to Guy's Hospital as "Inspector of the Dead" and "Curator of the Museum of Morbid Anatomy." Since this position allowed him to both treat patients and perform autopsies, Hodgkin linked the clinical care of the patient with the science of pathology. Over the next decade, he made key contributions including organizing the pathology lab, developing a comprehensive teaching program, introducing the stethoscope from France, and producing a large two volume lecture series. Hodgkin performed numerous autopsies and wrote reports for treating physicians, making valuable contributions in describing many medical conditions, including perforation of the appendix and valvular heart abnormalities. It was a risky job and Hodgkin, like many other physicians, nearly died from an infection he acquired while cutting himself doing an autopsy. At Guy's, Hodgkin formed a famous trio with well-known physicians Thomas Addison (famous for Addison's disease, a deficiency in the functioning of the adrenal glands which affected President Kennedy) and Richard Bright (well known for his description of kidney diseases). Hodgkin also collaborated with Joseph Jackson Lister to describe the appearance of various cells under the microscope. Hodgkin's Lister, a wine merchant and developer of optics for the microscope, was also the father of Joseph Lister, the man soon to revolutionize surgery with his theory of antisepsis.[46] Hodgkin is described as a passionate man who had a formidable intellect and a stern and rather unbending personality. Since he had fallen in love with his first cousin, a match forbidden by his faith, and did not marry another woman until much later in life and never had children, his personal life left him free to devote himself to his professional activities.[47]

In addition to his medical life, Hodgkin was also a prominent social reformer. He had a special concern for native peoples who were displaced by the British empire, opposed slavery, and was an active supporter of Liberia as a state for freed slaves. Hodgkin was particularly invested in the protection of "Indians" in North America and was a key member of the Aborigines Protective Society which challenged the policies of the government and Hudson Bay Trading Company. Hodgkin championed the Medical Preservation of Health (promoting healthy lifestyles), female education, and humane treatment of the mentally ill. In advocating these causes, Hodgkin combined his Quaker beliefs with his powerful intellect and strong personality, a combination which certainly made him enemies.[48]

Hodgkin's medical career at Guy's Hospital ended in 1837 when he was turned down for the second-in-command position of Assistant Physician which he coveted and certainly deserved. Hodgkin's vocal views about the Hudson Bay Company and its treatment of the "Indians" of North America were a direct challenge to the Treasurer of Guy's Hospital, Benjamin Harrison, who was on the Board of the Company. Harrison had been the driving force behind the formation of the medical school at Guy's Hospital and was a formidable opponent. Harrison was infuriated by Hodgkin's liberal ideas, could not tolerate his sternly rigid personality, and was probably prejudiced against his Quaker faith.[49] At the end of their confrontation, Hodgkin resigned from Guy's. Harrison, in an act of revenge, had much of Hodgkin's work either buried or expunged, and it has been only in modern times that his legacy at Guy's has been fully acknowledged.[50]

Hodgkin's somewhat inglorious end at Guy's cut short his academic medical career (although he briefly did similar work at the rival St. Thomas Hospital), but did not end his contributions to medical science or social causes. Following his departure, Hodgkin remained active as a physician at the London Cutaneous Infirmary where he worked with patients exposed to toxic substances from the developing industrial revolution and continued to speak out about the need for preventative medicine. He published lectures on pathology, which included brilliant descriptions of many organ systems. Hodgkin debated the origin of diseases such as tuberculosis with colleagues such as his former teacher Laennec and discussed the structure of medical education. He was a founding member of the Syrian Medical Aid Association, a group which sought to bring practicing physicians to underserved regions and continued to advocate for slaves and oppressed native peoples. Hodgkin died while on a journey in Jaffe (in modern day Israel) in 1866 after a fascinating, multifaceted life.[51]

This history leads to the irony of the naming of Hodgkin's lymphoma. In 1832, in the middle of his brilliant and expansive career, Hodgkin lectured on six autopsy cases having unusual lymph nodes which he described from their "gross" or visual appearance without the use of the microscope.[52] Often swollen lymph nodes associated with death in Hodgkin's era were the result of tuberculosis, yet these nodes seemed different. Hodgkin did not understand they were cancerous in the modern use of the term and later pathologists arguably determined that only three of the six cases were true "Hodgkin's lymphoma." After his lecture, Hodgkin learned that a Dr. Malpighi had earlier reported a similar case and, in keeping with his scientific honesty, he made note of this in his written report. Hodgkin's work sat quietly until thirty years later when Sir Samuel Wilks, a prominent physician at Guy's Hospital, published a report of cases with similar unusual lymph node enlargement.[53][54] Wilks was alerted by Dr. Richard Bright to Hodgkin's earlier report and his work in the Guy's Hospital Museum.[55] Although he was probably disappointed at not being the first to report the condition, Wilks graciously named the condition Hodgkin's disease in a paper published in 1865, the year before Hodgkin's death.[56] Thus, Thomas Hodgkin, the brilliant Quaker physician who made many contributions to medicine and was an activist social reformer with a broad reaching agenda, ended up being a historical figure whose name is frequently repeated two hundred years later. His enduring fame was not for the breadth of his work but for a brief lecture and description of some peculiar lymph nodes.

Kelly and John met Dr. Matthews two days later. He ordered a PET scan and bone marrow biopsy to look for signs of the lymphoma elsewhere in her body.

"If the lymphoma is only in the chest, which is what we expect, then you will be treated with six months of chemotherapy followed by radiation to the chest," he told Kelly.

"Is that the chemotherapy called ABVD?" she asked. John looked surprised.

"Yes. Good. You've been doing your homework," Dr. Matthews replied. "The letters stand for the four medications which make up the treatments. This chemotherapy is given by vein one day every two weeks for six months. Have you read about side effects?"

Kelly nodded.

"Okay. Well, remember, everyone is different. Our nurses do a teaching program where they tell you about the side effects that we think are most important because they are either serious or most common. They have written some information which they will give you as well." He looked at John. "You should come to this meeting with the nurses; it is very important that you understand the treatments."

Dr. Matthews paused for a minute. "Here is the quick version. On the day of your chemotherapy, I will check you over. Then you will go in back to the chemotherapy area for your treatments, which take about three hours and are hopefully boring. Occasionally a person has an allergic reaction to the medications, but those are pretty rare. For the next few days, you could feel nausea. Vomiting is unusual with the medications we have now, and we can adjust them if needed. For the rest of that week, you are likely to be tired. One week after your treatment, we will see you and check your blood counts. Low white blood counts are what we worry most about. If you get an infection with a low white blood count, you might not be able to fight it and can get very ill. If you get a fever during this time, you will need antibiotics and probably need to be in the hospital. By the end of the second week, you will feel better and then you are back to do it again. After the second treatment, you will lose your hair."

He paused and when Kelly nodded with clear eyes and no tears, continued.

"Usually, what you experience after the first treatment is what you will feel after that, but by the fourth month you will be really tired of it all. Most people do many of the things they want to but are exhausted by the end. We will be checking your kidney, liver, heart, and lung function with various tests to be sure we do not do any damage. There are other different side effects which the nurses will discuss. Most people get some but not all of them, and they slowly go away when the treatment is over. It takes a good nine to twelve months to recover. We advise patients not to become pregnant during these treatments, as the chemo can damage the baby."

"Will I need a catheter for the chemo?" asked Kelly.

"Yes, but not now. These medications are given into a vein, and it is important that they do not get into the tissue under the skin because they can cause a burn. I noticed you have very good veins, so at the start that will not be a problem. Later, however, the medications can scar the veins, making it more difficult to use them. Because of this many patients have a port placed. That is a quarter sized device put in under the skin on the chest with a catheter which goes into the vein behind the collarbone. You can shower or swim with it. When the nurse needs to get access to the vein, he or she just put the needle into the device. They can draw blood or give medications into the vein. Since you know where they are aiming the needle, you can numb it with cream ahead of time."

He paused. "Having the port put in is a day procedure, and Dr. Joe can do it for you."

Kelly smiled at the mention of his name.

Dr. Mathews continued. "I would like to wait until you have had several treatments and the lymph nodes are back to normal size in your chest. I do not want them pressing on the veins when that port is in because it might raise the risk of a blood clot involving the catheter."

On the way out, Dr. Matthews showed them the treatment area, a large room with windows and a panoramic view of the country-side. Several patients were finishing their infusions and the late afternoon sun filled the area, giving it a peaceful look. A sign on the wall which read "no children beyond this point" caught Kelly's eye and Dr. Matthews saw her read it.

"What do your children know?" he asked.

"Not much yet," Kelly replied. "We will tell them this weekend. Any advice?"

"Tell them the truth. You are getting medicines to get rid of your lymphoma, and you will be fine once it is over. If you want, you can bring them here to see the place and meet us once you get started. For some kids that is helpful, but not all. As you know, they are all different."

At home, Kelly's cough had worsened, and she was noticing some shortness of breath when she walked up the stairs. Mary was increasingly clingy, and even Jack seemed to be watching her more closely. Kelly and John gathered them on the couch that night and explained.

"The doctors in Boston found out why Mommy is coughing so much," she told them. "I am going to get some medicines to fix it and then I will be better."

"Will they taste bad?" asked Jack.

"Some," said Kelly. "The medicines are called chemotherapy. Some will be pills, and some will be shots. Mommy will have to go to the doctor's office to get the shots, and I will lose my hair. But when I'm all better, it will grow back."

"Can you make a wig with your hair?" asked Jack.

"No, honey. I will buy a wig to wear until it grows back." She turned to Mary. "Will you help me pick out my wig, Mary? I could use your help."

Mary nodded and clung tighter as Kelly stroked her hair.

CURING WITH CHEMOTHERAPY: THE LUNATIC FRINGE, LASKER PRIZE, AND HEROIC CHILDREN.

The 1960s saw the first cures for many patients with widespread Hodgkin's disease using chemotherapy. This remarkable breakthrough raised hopes that the other widespread cancers could be cured with the proper drugs and started the "age of chemotherapy."

Chemotherapy treatments began in the 1940s and 1950s as scientists studied treatments for acute leukemias, rapidly growing cancers of the white blood cells which are quickly fatal. Although it is surprisingly difficult to grow leukemic cells from a person in the lab, when it is successfully done these cells can be studied. Growth rates and sensitivities to drugs can be determined. Leukemic cells growing in the lab can also be transplanted into susceptible mice and treatments tested. One of the most famous scientists of this era, Dr. Howard Skipper in Birmingham, Alabama, was a "mice doctor" who cured some of his rodents of leukemia using combinations of chemotherapy and in so doing established some guiding principles for the use of these drugs.

As these critical laboratory experiments were ongoing, some physicians began to treat acute leukemias and a few other cancers, primarily in children.[57] These early chemotherapy treatments were controversial. Since "Cancer Centers" can now be found in most large cities and some of our most recognizable medical institutions deal exclusively with the treatment of cancer, many are surprised to learn that in this era the specialty of medical oncology did not yet exist. Even more shocking is that many physicians and institutions did not want cancer patients receiving chemotherapy. Some leading institutions like Columbia University and Yale discharged physicians who used these treatments, while even at institutions which allowed this work the criticism was severe. Dr. Vincent DeVita, a pioneer in early chemotherapy treatments, notes they were referred to as the "lunatic fringe" of medicine, their wards "butcher shops" and their treatments "poisons."[58] Of course, there was some truth in these labels. Not only were the early treatments generally ineffective, but the side effects were severe, and management strategies for the complications had to be slowly worked out, often at the expense of patient suffering. The challenge, excitement, hope, and suffering of these early days is poignantly detailed by Siddhartha Mukherjee in the *Emperor of all Maladies*, his remarkable biography of cancer.[59]

Progress in childhood leukemia came slowly but steadily. Each decade saw improvement in survival rates until today more than 80 percent of children are cured. Progress in Hodgkin's lymphoma came more suddenly. In the 1960s individual drugs were identified that worked in Hodgkin's lymphoma and physicians learned from treating childhood leukemia to combine them into combinations. The key was to schedule the drugs to kill the cancer cells but give the normal tissue, particularly the bone marrow, time to recover before the next treatment. The results with programs like MOPP (which are abbreviated using a letter from each of the ingredients: nitrogen mustard, oncovin (vincristine), procarbazine, prednisone) were "startling," in the words of Dr. DeVita.[60] About 60 percent of patients with widespread Hodgkin's lymphoma who previously would have died were cured. Increasingly successful treatments like ABVD (Adriamycin, Bleomycin, Vinblastine, Dacarbazine) followed which cured most patients with advanced Hodgkin's disease. Modern targeted treatments and immune therapies may soon replace these programs, but the treatment of Hodgkin's disease has been one of success stories of the chemotherapy era.

The determination of a handful physicians was critical to the success of chemotherapy in leukemias and lymphomas. In recognition of their efforts, a group of pioneering oncologists received the 1972 Lasker Clinical Medicine Research Award, one of the nation's most prestigious awards referred to as "America's Nobel Prize." They were Joe Burchenal (Memorial Sloan Kettering Cancer Center), Denis Burkitt (Medical Research Council), Paul P. Carbone (NCI), Vincent DeVita (NCI), Isaac Djerassi (Mercy Catholic Medical Center), Emil Frei III (Children's Cancer Research Foundation), Emil J. Freireich (MD Anderson), Roy Hertz (New York Medical College), James Holland (Roswell Park), Edmund Klein (Roswell Park), Min Chiu Li (Nassau Hospital), V. Anomah Ngu (University Centre of Health Sciences), Donald Pinkel (St. Jude Children's Research Hospital), Eugene J. Van Scott (Temple), John L. Ziegler (Uganda Cancer Institute) and C. Gordon Zubrod (NCI/NIH).[61]

Albert and Mary Lasker started the Lasker Awards in the 1940s, and their story illustrates the paradoxical social and political forces which funded early cancer research. Born in 1900 in the small town of Watertown, Wisconsin, Mary Lasker reported a boring childhood. As soon as possible, she left for boarding school in Milwaukee, graduated from Radcliffe as an art history major, and with her first husband owned an art gallery in New York. After this marriage had ended, Mary survived the great depression and developed a successful fabric business which featured her "Hollywood Patterns" decorated with pictures of movie stars. A beautiful and vivacious woman, Mary was socially well-connected. At thirty-nine she married Albert Lasker, the owner of Lord and Thomas Advertising and one of the fathers of modern advertising who promoted "Lucky Strikes" in the days when the link between cigarettes and health problems was not understood.[62] Lasker's highly successful campaigns encouraged vast numbers of men and women to smoke. After their marriage and with her urging, the Laskers used his fortune to promote medical research. Although Albert Lasker died in 1952 of intestinal cancer, Mary lived for over forty more years and used her many political and social connections to advocate for medical and cancer care. She began in the 1940s by revamping the American Cancer Society.[63] Lasker was an early proponent of research funding for chemotherapy and worked to establish the National Cancer Institute. Later, she played an important role lobbying for the National Cancer Act signed by President Nixon in 1971 which led to the "War on Cancer." She organized a group of similarly minded women called "Laskerites" who had tremendous political influence. It is ironic that this determined socialite and philanthropist turned a fortune made in the promotion of smoking into a legacy of progress in medicine, and specifically cancer.[64] For her work, Mary Lasker received the Presidential Medal of Freedom and the Congressional Medal of Honor.

The 1950s and 1960s produced the first cures of leukemia and widespread Hodgkin's lymphoma, political and social elites mobilizing to fund cancer research, and started the era of chemotherapy. The support for medical research, academic infrastructure, and knowledge from this era has led to the modern advances seen today. Often forgotten from this time are the children across the country who participated in this early work. There are no awards for them. Nor are there awards for the parents, siblings, and families who bore witness to these treatments in the hope that they might have their loved one for a few more days or weeks and help the next child to be stricken. For every person who survives today, there is a debt to these young heroes which can never be repaid, but must be acknowledged.

Kelly later described her chemotherapy treatments as a long, dark tunnel. Her world was repeated visits to the office, needle sticks, blood values, nausea, rashes, baldness and, most of all, fatigue. She kept a detailed log of her symptoms and medications as she traveled through the tunnel. These daily, even hourly, events took on tremendous importance as she tried to come to terms with the many toxic effects of the chemicals. Later she hated looking too carefully at the journal but was always glad she had made the effort to keep the record.

Kelly treasured a few memories of her time on chemotherapy, particularly of the people who went through that tunnel with her. John was always present, although for the first time in their lives together, Kelly could see he was befuddled and uncertain. For his part, John watched with admiration as Kelly asserted herself and took control of the decision making. Mary clung to her passionately and was relieved that Kelly's cough improved, even though it meant trading her hair. Jack maintained his young analytic and factual perspective, seemingly content that she was still Mom. Cindy and Mike Newton made the trip with them as well, taking care of the thousands of daily issues which came up: driving, helping with the kids, the yard, and even a car repair when a dashboard light came on, a gift which seemed worth millions at the time.

Some people could not make the trip through the tunnel. Kelly's mother was too terrified to be of any help, and her visits only added to their stress. John's parents had been in senior citizen retirement mode for too long to help with a busy family life. Kelly's Bible study group was also left behind. She had tried to attend a meeting after her diagnosis but found herself the uncomfortable center of prayerful attention. She left, asking for their blessings while pleading fear of infection. Other friends were left behind for a variety of reasons. A few tried to insert themselves into her care by offering advice or alternative treatments. John dealt with them bluntly. A few simply vanished, never quite sure how to acknowledge her illness. Many simply went on with their own busy lives, happy to see her when she was out and offer words of encouragement, but never really understanding.

When her chemotherapy was complete, Kelly had four weeks of daily radiation treatments to her chest. Since the dose of radiation used for lymphoma is low, it produced very few side effects. After her treatment finished, Kelly and John met with Dr. Matthews.

"Your CT scan looks very good," he said. "We will repeat it in four months, then every six months for five years. The odds are that you are cured, but we must watch."

"Thank God it's over," said John, smiling.

"It's true the treatments are over," said Dr. Matthews, "but the recovery is just beginning. Most people get about 85 percent of their energy back over the next three or four months, but that last 15 percent can take six to twelve months or even longer to return. It means that if you have a busy day or two, you will be exhausted. If you wait for that burst of energy in the evening, it won't come. Don't be surprised. This is normal. There is nothing wrong with you. You were treated for nine months and won't get better overnight. Some people get depressed by this, so it is important that you have realistic expectations for yourself."

"Another thing that happens," he continued, "is that everyone else wants this over, too. The people who were being nice to you may stop being nice. Your friends will want you to do normal things. You will look good, and most everyone will forget or not know how tired you are. So, the words 'no' and 'not yet' are important. This is particularly true for patients who finish as we enter the holiday season. You know what it is like to be a mother during the holiday season. You can blame me if you need to and tell people I don't want you doing too much for the next six months."

"She always does a lot during the holidays," agreed John. Kelly nodded.

"Finally," Dr. Matthews continued, "once they have finished treatment, many patients find that they look at some parts of their life differently. When you were diagnosed, everything happened fast, and now you may need time to make sense of it all. We call this re-entry. You have been in a strange world for these past nine months, so don't be surprised if you need time to sort things out. Again, most people do just fine, but some people find this to be an unsettling or even depressing time. Let us know if you are feeling that way."

The rituals of Christmas were particularly vivid that year. The cutting of the tree at Bob's Farm on a clear, cold day produced a smell of pine which was so real and powerful that it seemed as if she had never experienced it before. The sticky sap had a texture she had never felt while the reds and greens of the kissing balls exploded against the whiteness of the snow. The drive home through the countryside was almost new although they had made it many holidays before. Arriving home, the scent of her cookies, the excitement of the children, and John's playfulness seemed too perfect to be real.

Even after the holiday season ended, Kelly did not immediately rejoin her pre-treatment social groups. She intuitively felt Dr. Matthews was right and her world was slightly different. As the winter went on, Kelly regained much of her energy and collected her thoughts. Although she had found the treatments terrible, she realized that as they had been poisoning her, they had also awakened a part of her. Once Kelly had overcome her initial paralyzing fear, she had studied her cancer. She kept returning to that image of herself as a serious student in high school ("you can do anything") and college. She was proud that she had led John and the children through her treatments.

That March, almost a year to the day of the first call about the CT scan, Kelly again reported news to John.

"John, I have been thinking," she began.

"About what?" He held up his *Sports Illustrated*, the March Madness edition with Georgetown's "DeJaun" Summers on the cover. "Can you believe they spelled his name wrong?" He pointed to the title. "See, it should be DeJuan. Either way, though, the Hoyas are not going past Kansas this year."

"I want to go back to school."

"School?" He looked up, surprised, and lowered the magazine. "Are you kidding?"

"I'm serious. I want to go back and get my Master's in Education. I want to teach."

"Where's this coming from?"

"I'm not sure exactly. In some strange way, this cancer made me study, and I liked it . . . I mean, I hated the cancer, but I like learning about it. And I felt like with the kids I could explain things to them, to help them understand. It meant something."

And she did. Kelly returned to school, finished her Master's degree, and took a job editing curriculums. She loved reviewing the material, seeing it presented and interpreted by the students, often thinking of how her children had seen her treatments. John had initially been neutral, but as he saw Kelly recapture her academic life, he became her greatest supporter. The test came two years later when John had the opportunity to move to New Jersey to head a new office. He told Kelly he was declining the offer.

"I don't want the job, Kelly," he said. "We are happy here. The children are doing well in school, you like your work, and all your doctors are here."

"We can all adapt if you want, John. You know that."

"I know that. I don't want it."

"Why not?" she pushed.

"Why not? Because I sat in that damn room in Dana Farber years ago and watched those families wait for the news of whether their loved one was going to live or die. I walked around and saw all those poor bald people fighting for their lives. And I saw you figure all this out and beat this cancer. John and Mary have their mother. You are happy, and so I am. I don't want anything else."

Today, ten years after her treatment, it was Kelly's work that prompted her to ask why she contracted Hodgkin's disease. She had been reviewing a biology class when she came upon a discussion of mononucleosis which mentioned a link to lymphoma. During her illness, she had naturally focused on the diagnosis and treatment of Hodgkin's lymphoma. Now safely cured, this potential cause of lymphoma caught Kelly's eye, and she studied a debate which has gone on for years.

VIRUSES AND LYMPHOMA.

Carcinogens are agents which cause cancer—often classified as chemical, physical, or biologic. Chemical carcinogens are well known to the public. Tobacco is one of our making and the leading cause of cancer death worldwide. Physical carcinogens like radiation are also widely understood. The biologic carcinogens are less commonly recognized. In this group, viral infections such as hepatitis and human papilloma virus are important causes of cancer, particularly in less well-developed areas.[65] The idea that viral infections can lead to cancer has tantalized scientists for years, and Hodgkin's lymphoma has been part of that discussion.

When Thomas Hodgkin described his lymphoma in 1832, the era of modern medicine was just beginning, cancer was not well understood, and swollen glands were thought to result from infection or inflammation. Over the next century, as the modern definition of cancer (uncontrolled cellular growth) emerged, the swollen lymph nodes in patients with Hodgkin's lymphomas came to be understood as part of the cancer. In an interesting twist, several observations suggested an infection might be the cause of the Hodgkin's lymphoma. The lymph node swelling often starts in the neck—mimicking an infection of the mouth, teeth, throat or respiratory system. The lymph node swelling often progresses in an orderly fashion, typically starting from one node group in the neck and proceeding to the next node in what is described in medical texts as "contiguous spread." In addition, Hodgkin's disease generally stays confined to the lymph nodes and spleen for long periods and, unlike other cancers, is usually not immediately invasive into organs. While this ability to predict the spread of Hodgkin's lymphoma later allowed the use of radiation treatments to cure patients with localized disease, it also reminds physicians of an infection. Another similarity is that patients often experience fever and sweats. From the epidemiological viewpoint (the study of diseases in groups), several features of Hodgkin's disease also implied infection might be the cause. The disease occurs in young adults and then again at older ages in what is called a "bimodal distribution." Clusters of cases are found in some neighborhoods and families, and there were suggestions that higher socioeconomic groups were more vulnerable.

When the lymph nodes from Hodgkin's lymphoma were examined using the microscope, pathologists also had the impression that an infection might be involved. The nodes contained many inflammatory cells and often much fibrous tissue, like an infection or inflammation. In fact, the few cancerous cells were not identified for many years. WS Greenfield described these bizarre cells with many nuclei in 1878,[66] but it was not until about 1900 that their identification was credited to the combination of Dorothy Reed and Carl Sternberg, and they were named Reed-Sternberg cells, depriving Greenfield of medical immortality. Regardless of the justness of this allocation of medical fame, the microscopic appearance of an immune reaction also suggested an infectious process.

If an infection was the cause of Hodgkin's lymphoma, what was the agent? Tuberculosis was the first thought of many physicians. In fact, when Sternberg had identified the cancerous cells, many of his cases had both tuberculosis and Hodgkin's disease. In their comprehensive review in the *New England Journal of Medicine* in 1944, Harvard physicians Henry Jackson and Frederick Parker discussed the evidence for an infectious cause of Hodgkin's lymphoma, focusing on the great debate over the role of tuberculosis.[67] In subsequent years, the most likely culprit has been identified as the Epstein-Barr virus (EBV), a virus which infects most humans, who are its only known host. EBV infection usually takes place in childhood and may result in no symptoms or "acute mononucleosis," also known as the "kissing disease" because its transmission is by intimate contact. Mononucleosis (mono) may produce fevers, sore throat, swollen glands and an enlarged spleen. The blood often contains a large number of odd looking lymph cells, called atypical lymphs, which can sometimes be difficult to distinguish from leukemia cells. For most young people, the infection leaves no long-term physical effects. For unclear reasons, some people seem to develop a more long-lasting type of EBV infection which may produce a chronic fatigue syndrome.

EBV infection as a cause of Hodgkin's lymphoma is reasonable since the virus is known to cause Burkitt's lymphoma, a terrifying tumor found in children in parts of Africa. This lymphoma was first described in 1958 by Denis Burkitt, a British surgeon working in Kampala, Uganda, who became aware of rapidly growing cancers of the jaw and abdomen in children from a region he termed the African lymphoma belt. Burkitt's lymphoma has the fastest growth rate of any known cancer—it can grow from a small lump to the size of a baseball overnight. With two physician colleagues, including one described as an expert auto mechanic, Burkitt made a ten thousand mile "tumor safari" in search of cases.[68] In 1961, Burkitt presented his findings in a lecture at Middlesex College in London entitled the "Commonest Children's Cancer in Africa." The speculation was that the cause of this cancer was some agent transmitted by mosquitos. Among those attending Burkitt's lecture was Michael Anthony Epstein, a researcher interested in virology. The duo formed a collaboration in which Burkitt obtained fresh tumor tissue and had it flown to Epstein in England. On late Friday, December 5, 1963, a sample from Uganda reached London (after a detour to Manchester) which Epstein and his associates made into a "cell line"— cells which would continue to grow indefinitely.[69] Most people without lab experience are surprised to learn that growing cancer cells in the lab is a very difficult process and this was a major achievement. The cell line allowed Epstein in 1964 to use the electron microscope to observe viral particles inside the cells, linking a virus with Burkitt's lymphoma. This connection helped establish the concept that viral infections could lead to cancers. The name of the Epstein-Barr virus came from Dr. Epstein and one of his two associates, Yvonne Barr.[70] The third associate, Bert Achong, did not get immortalized in the same fashion, although Dr. Burkitt acknowledged his work when he suggested the virus be named Epstein-Barr-Achong.[71]

After the viral particles in Burkitt's lymphoma were identified, Epstein sent his cell line to the laboratory of Drs. Gertrude and Werner Henle and Volker Diehl at the Children's Hospital of Philadelphia. They made the full connection between EBV, mononucleosis, and Burkitt's lymphoma. Other researchers had demonstrated that antibodies to EBV were found in many people across the world, indicating this infection was a common one. As the Henles and Diehl worked to establish that EBV infection caused infectious mononucleosis, a technician in the lab developed the illness. Her serum showed evidence of EBV and her cells exhibited some of the same chromosomal changes seen in the Burkitt's cell line.[72] Successive years of work using molecular techniques have solidified the theory that EBV causes mononucleosis and can on occasion lead to Burkitt's lymphoma. The pathways by which this happens continue to be studied.

The link between EBV, mononucleosis, and Hodgkin's lymphoma is less direct, but several lines of evidence point to EBV as a cause in many cases. In general, people who have had mononucleosis are found to be at increased risk for Hodgkin's disease. Within the tumor cells of many patients with Hodgkin's lymphoma, EBV can be found while other viruses are absent. The EBV patterns in these cells indicate that the infection took place before the cancer developed. The risk of developing Hodgkin's disease containing the EBV is increased in people with other immune system weakening diseases like HIV infection or autoimmune conditions. In the lab, scientists have identified genes from the virus which may stimulate the Hodgkin's cells (Reed-Sternberg cells) to grow and protect them from death. The evidence is strong, but there are many remaining questions, including why so many people are infected with EBV yet only a few get Hodgkin's disease and why some people with Hodgkin's disease do not have EBV in their cancer cells.

As their yearly visit ended, Dr. Matthews answered Kelly's question.

"Well, I hate to blame some innocent boy who was probably just the envy of all his friends because he got to kiss you because we really don't know. Hodgkin's lymphoma is a mysterious condition. We know it usually occurs in younger people and then again in older people. Sometimes it appears in clusters, but the scientists have debated whether that is just chance or not. In some cases, they have found the Epstein-Barr virus in the cells of the Hodgkin's lymphoma. That is the same virus that causes mono, but it is difficult to tell if the virus is the cause of the lymphoma or just one of several factors. Probably the virus infects cells and then kicks off an immune system reaction and, if you are unlucky and have several other things go wrong that we don't understand, you get the cancer. So, Joe may have been part of the cause, but he was not totally to blame."

She laughed. "Well, it takes two to tango anyway, and it was fun. He was a cutie."

"What happened to him?"

"We dated in high school and went to the prom together, but broke up once we went to college and I met John." She shook her finger at him. "Nothing more than kissing though, not in those days, not with my father."

"Your blood is fine'" reported Dr. Matthews to Mark Luciano, a balding forty-five-year-old Italian-American man who, at five feet seven and over two hundred fifty pounds, occupied most of the exam table. He was wearing a New York Giants sweat suit with a gold chain around his neck and new Nikes. His wife Teresa sat nearby, a thin, attractive, and fashionably dressed woman who could have just left the set of the *Real Housewives of New Jersey*.

"Can I go then?" he asked, smiling.

"After I check you over," said Dr. Matthews. He washed his hands, completed his exam, and gestured to Mark to sit in the chair next to Teresa.

"You are still in remission from your leukemia," he began.

Eleven years ago, Mark Luciano was diagnosed with chronic myelogenous leukemia, known as CML. Mark had felt well, but blood work done by his regular physician showed his white count was 55,000 instead of the normal 7,000. Dr. Matthews did more blood tests and a bone marrow biopsy. For Mark, the whole time was a blur, while Teresa could instantly recall the terror of those days and vividly remembered sitting in the very same exam room when they heard the final reports.

"Mr. Luciano, you do have a form of leukemia called chronic myelogenous leukemia. This is the condition we discussed at our first meeting. It is treatable, and it is important that you understand it," Dr. Matthews had said.

"Oh, my God," gasped Teresa. "What do we do?"

"Shh, let him speak," Mark replied.

Dr. Matthews continued. "Leukemia is a cancer of the white blood cells. When most people hear the word leukemia, they think of acute leukemias which very rapidly make people sick and must be treated with intensive chemotherapy. You do not have that kind of leukemia. You have a chronic leukemia which means that it has been present in your body for some time, several years at least. It will not cause you any problems right away. So, the first message is that we have time to take the proper action. The second message is that scientists have developed a pill that treats this condition. It has few serious side effects and usually works well. We do need to use it, however, because if it is not treated, your chronic myelogenous leukemia will at some point change into acute leukemia."

"Can this pill prevent that?" asked Teresa rapidly.

"Shh, let the man speak," said Mark.

"Does it cure it?" Teresa persisted.

"This pill is only about six or seven years old, so we don't yet know for sure. In most patients, it seems to work so well that after a few years we cannot find the CML, but they keep taking the medication. Some people have been on the medication since the late 1990s when it was first developed, and their leukemia appears gone."

"What if it doesn't work?" she asked.

"Come on, Tee," Mark said. "Don't think like that."

Dr. Matthews answered her. "The pill is called Gleevec, which is the brand name, or imatinib, the chemical name. If it does not work or stops working there are other treatments. In some cases, we can do a bone marrow transplant, but we do not need to consider that now. And we expect more Gleevec-like pills in the next few years."

"When does he start?" asked Teresa.

"We will make arrangements for you to get the pill. It's very expensive, and we need to contact your insurance company and get it ordered, so it usually takes a few days."

"We'll pay if we need to," said Teresa.

"Don't do that yet," replied Dr. Matthews, shaking his head. "The cost is about $3,000 a month, and you will be on it for a long time. It usually works out with your insurance, so let us do the proper paperwork. As I said, we are not in an emergency here, so a few days won't matter."

"As soon as possible," said Teresa sharply.

"Easy, honey," added Mark. As she started to cry, he hugged her.

"I also want you to do one more thing," added Dr. Matthews. "I want to send you to a major cancer center to have you seen by doctors who specialize in this condition. There are several reasons for this. First, it is always useful to have all these tests reviewed, although I am sure they will not find anything different. Secondly, even though we expect you to do well with this Gleevec, it won't hurt you to have a connection to one of these medical centers in case you ever need it. Finally, I suspect you will be getting a lot of advice and information from your family, and this will make it easier on everyone."

Mark laughed. "You got that right. They will all be here this weekend, but some have already called to set me up with doctors in the City and the rest want me to take vitamins or some supplements or other damn thing."

Three years earlier, in mid-2003, Mark and Teresa had moved upstate from Staten Island with their five-year-old twin girls. Teresa's younger brother Thomas, a firefighter and her only sibling, had died when the second World Trade Center Tower collapsed in the September 11, 2001, attack. Brother and sister had been close. Teresa also knew most of Thomas's friends and fellow firefighters, many of who had also died. Their widowed mother, already frail and with early dementia, had been devastated by the death of her son.

The year following the attack had been brutal. The loss of her brother, the seemingly endless series of funerals in their community of firefighters, and the generalized depression and terror the City endured traumatized Teresa. Her mother had never recovered and, until she died about a year later, Teresa had to explain to her, again and again, the reason for Thomas's absence. After the death of her mother, Teresa began to unravel. She could not enter Manhattan. She dreaded driving the New Jersey turnpike or any of the roads which gave a view of the City and the hole left by the loss of the Towers, knowing that void was where her brother was obliterated. When the panic attacks began at night, she would awaken suddenly with terrible images. Over time she had become afraid to leave the house and obsessed over the safety of the twins. Teresa had always been a strong, proud woman and her mental collapse humiliated her. She began medications which made her sluggish and withdrawn. Mark grew increasingly worried. When the opportunity to transfer to the Albany office came, he took it and moved them upstate. A program which had taken firefighters and their families to rest in Saratoga Springs following the attack had given him a peaceful image of the place. He hoped the change in scenery would ease her nerves.

Looking back, the move had paid off. Teresa found Saratoga Springs a pleasant and secure community in which to regain her bearings. Over time, she drove again. She felt safe sending the girls to the small public grade school. The terrifying images of falling buildings and mangled fire trucks faded, and she rarely woke at night. Teresa missed the excitement, shopping, and fashion of the City, but understood that for her the trade was necessary.

Mark was stoic but less sanguine about his deal. He missed his life in the City, sports teams, papers, food, and the immediacy of his large family, which included his parents, three sets of aunts and uncles, a brother, two sisters, and countless cousins.

"They're all dead up here, Ralph," he told his brother six months after the move. "I mean, don't get me wrong, Tee needed this move and thank God she is getting better. The girls love it, but you cannot believe it here. No food, I mean our food. The mozzarella and the bread stink. There's no pork stores. Try to find a diner after midnight, forget it. But there's parking everywhere . . . You never even pay.

And quiet, you wouldn't believe it. Even on the roads. Up here when the light changes they sit like dummies until the guy in front of them moves. Nobody honks, they just sit there. No pro sports, but you want pig races; they got them up here at the County Fair. The twins love the pigs. Ralph, we're raisin farm girls here."

Although Mark's family had initially been horrified by the move, as time went on, they enjoyed their visits. They appreciated the ease of travel and the peace mixed with a taste of excitement during the summer season. But trusting serious medical care to an upstate doctor was another matter entirely, one that would be discussed that weekend. They had arrived loaded with food. Dinner started Sunday at two o'clock with a mixed antipasto, olives, grilled red peppers, sliced tomatoes, mozzarella, and provolone with real bread. Pasta with marinara sauce was followed by a break then sausage, pork, and meatballs accompanied by a salad. When at five o'clock they finally reached the sweats, fruit, and coffee, Mark knew he would have to explain his condition to the family and let the dialog began in earnest. Teresa announced she was going to the basement to check on the twins and their cousins.

"Why are you going, Tee?" asked Mark. "You can't leave me alone."

"Call me when either the Luciano medical conference is over, or you got even one that went to medical school."

Mark told his family of his condition and the treatment.

"You trust this guy?" began Mark's father, Anthony.

"Stop, Daddy," interrupted Samantha, Mark's older sister. "It's not our business who his doctor is—"

"My son is my business until you bury me or he tells me otherwise," said Anthony in a tone which Samantha recognized from her childhood.

"She didn't mean anything by it, Dad," said Ralph. "She just wants Mark to have his privacy."

"Bah," said Anthony. "You think this is the doctor's office where you got to fill out some stupid form to talk to family?"

"It's okay," said Mark, raising his palm to Ralph and Samantha in a gesture to keep the peace. "Yeah, Dad, I trust this guy. But I'm also going to Memorial Sloan Kettering to have them look over everything."

"So maybe you don't trust him," said Anthony.

"He suggested it."

"See, Daddy," began Samantha until Anthony raised his hand.

"So maybe he doesn't trust himself. Mom, where's my cake?"

"You get yours after my poor baby," came the reply as Mark's mother served him first.

Although the Lucianos found Mark's diagnosis a shock, it was not a new event in his body.

❖ ❖ ❖

UNDERSTANDING CHRONIC MYELOGENOUS LEUKEMIA.
The stem cells of the bone marrow produce the red cells, white cells, and platelets which make up the blood. Chronic myelogenous leukemia (CML) develops when the bone marrow stem cells suffer a break in two chromosomes. Why this happens is not known, but one break is in chromosome 9 and the other is in chromosome 22. The broken pieces of each of these chromosomes then move to the opposite chromosome. This produces a longer than normal chromosome 9 with some extra DNA from chromosome 22 and a shorter than normal chromosome 22 with some DNA from chromosome 9. This movement is called a "translocation" by scientists, written t(9;22). On the new longer chromosome 9 the extra DNA does not seem to have much effect, but on the new shorter chromosome 22 there is a problem. Genetic material from an area called the *BCR* (breakpoint cluster region) on chromosome 22 becomes joined to the gene called *ABL* (Abelson murine leukemia) from chromosome 9. A new combination gene forms, called *BCR-ABL*, which produces a protein which is an abnormal variation of an enzyme called a tyrosine kinase. This abnormal enzyme stimulates the CML stem cell to divide faster than normal and produce

excess blood cells, particularly white cells. Although these cells are not entirely normal, most do mature and function adequately.

The difference between the growth rate of a damaged CML stem cell and a normal stem cell is not much, but over a period of years, it slowly allows the progeny of the damaged CML cell to take over the bone marrow. The "leisurely" growth rate of these cells was well worked out by two Japanese investigators from Hiroshima University in the 1970s using an amazing resource: twice yearly blood samples taken from eighty thousand survivors of the atomic bombings in Japan.[73] They found blood samples from one hundred two patients with CML which allowed them to study the growth of the illness over years. On average, it took about eight years for the CML to take over the bone marrow and produce an elevated white blood count.[74] At the start, the person is unaware of the CML, unless the increased white blood cells are detected on routine labs. As the white blood cell count reaches very high levels, the spleen often enlarges, and the person may feel fatigue, prompting a visit to the physician. This early part of the illness is called the "chronic phase" of CML.

The problem with untreated CML is that eventually the condition takes a terrible turn, on average about four to six years after diagnosis.[75] Other mutations occur in the stem cells, and the CML enters "blast crisis." When this happens, the now severely mutated stem cells produce abnormal and immature "blast" cells which fill the bone marrow, resulting in low red blood counts, low platelet counts, and few useful white blood cells—a deadly type of "acute leukemia." The prognosis is grim, even with intensive chemotherapy. The timing of this transformation is variable; some patients live for many years before the blast crisis develops while in others it occurs more rapidly. Before the development of effective treatments, all patients faced the profound terror of waiting for that day.

The first true cure for CML was developed in the 1980s—an allogeneic bone marrow transplantation (bone marrow from another person). In this procedure, the patient is given high-dose chemotherapy to eliminate the CML then receives bone marrow or stem cells from a donor. This is a risky procedure because the high-dose chemotherapy is very toxic and the donor's bone marrow attacks the organs of the recipient in a reaction called "graft-versus-host disease." About one-third of patients die from the procedure, and it is suitable only for young and healthy people. For patients with CML who felt well and had no symptoms, this was a difficult step.

In 2001, the FDA approved a revolutionary new oral treatment named imatinib (Gleevec) for CML. Imatinib blocked the abnormal tyrosine kinase produced by the abnormal t(9;22) and *BCR-ABL* gene, preventing the growth of the CML and allowing the normal stem cells to take over the bone marrow.[76] With the introduction of this drug, the need for allogeneic bone marrow transplantation to treat CML became rare. This previously often fatal leukemia was now treated and hopefully cured with a pill designed to reverse the defect which caused the cancer. The development of imatinib meant the age of "targeted treatment" for cancers had arrived.

The trip to Memorial Sloan Kettering Cancer Center was Teresa's first return to New York since they had moved upstate three years earlier. When they left the City, she had been in regular psychotherapy and on medication. Although it had taken almost a year for the nightmares to fade and another six months for her to be able to leave home without a feeling of dread, for the last year she had not needed any medications and was seeing her therapist only rarely. Mark had hoped she would eventually be able to revisit the City but had feared to make the suggestion. Shortly after their visit with Dr. Matthews, Tee had told Mark she was going to go with him. He was unsure how to answer.

"You don't need to, Tee," he responded. "Ralph can come with me. I promise we will tell you everything."

"That's not it. I'm your wife. He's your brother."

"Honey, you don't need the stress. You are doing great, and we don't want you to get bad again."

"It's been three years, Mark. I'm ready. Besides the two you will probably end up in some restaurant stuffing yourselves and miss the appointment."

A few days later, he approached her again.

"Tee, I've been thinking about this second opinion idea. Why don't we go to Dana Farber in Boston? They've got some good doctors there, and it will be a chance for us to see a different city . . ."

She looked right through him, her jaw tensing and her foot tapping. Mark knew the warning signs.

"Tee?"

"Are you kidding me? Those assholes fly those planes into the buildings, kill all those people, including my only brother, my mother dies, I get depressed so bad you move me upstate and when I finally get over this depression and am feeling good, I find out my husband has some kind of leukemia and now you want me to go to Boston? Boston, of all places? Forget it, okay? I can only take so much."

"Memorial it is."

The trip began with a thirty-mile car ride south from Saratoga Springs to the Albany-Rensselaer train station where they would catch the early morning express for the two-and-a-half-hour journey into Manhattan. Their appointment was in the mid-afternoon, so they had given themselves plenty of time. It was a bitter, gray November day. Mark parked his dark blue Mercedes in the drive and opened the door for Theresa.

"You don't need to . . .," he began.

"Don't start," she shook her head and got into the car.

They rode in silence, and she felt him look over at her as he drove.

"I'm okay," she said. "Remember, this trip is about you and your condition, not me. I don't want you thinking about me. Got it?"

"Got it, Tee," he answered.

She paused and cleared her throat, thinking of the beautiful clear sky on that terrible day. "I'm glad it's a shitty day, though."

"Me, too."

FINDING A MOLECULAR TARGET FOR CANCER TREATMENT. Imatinib revolutionized the treatment of CML and demonstrated that treating cancer treated with "targeted" treatments offered more precision and effectiveness than chemotherapy. The story of imatinib has several chapters; the first is the finding of the target.

Our modern understanding of CML started in 1960 with the discovery of the translocations of chromosome 9 and 22 which triggers the illness by Peter Nowell and William Hungerford. They noticed a small abnormal chromosome (later found to be the small chromosome 22) in the cells of patients with CML and suggested this might be the cause of the disease. Since these scientists were both at the University of Pennsylvania, this short chromosome is named the "Philadelphia Chromosome." These men would later be recognized for their accomplishment with numerous awards, but at the time it was not clear whether this small Philadelphia Chromosome was the cause of the disease or resulted from the illness. Even if the Philadelphia Chromosome was the cause of CML, it was not clear whether this type of genetic damage was applicable to cancers in general or just this uncommon illness.[77]

Time proved the Philadelphia Chromosome was the cause of CML and just the first example of a chromosomal abnormality which produced a cancer. To see genetic abnormalities like the Philadelphia Chromosome, scientists took dividing cells and squashed them (sometimes by dropping them from a height of several feet) to spread out the chromosomes, then stained them using some basic dyes available at the time and looked at them under the microscope. This work is called cytogenetics and, during the 1960s and 1970s, the field expanded greatly. In 1973, a scientist named Janet Rowley stained and photographed some chromosome spreads from patients with CML. She cut out the pictures of the individual chromosomes and laid them out on her dining room table so she could compare and rearrange them. What she found was remarkable: the Philadelphia chromosome was a short version of chromosome 22, and chromosome 9 was longer than normal. Dr. Rowley went on to become a leading figure in leukemia research, but her first paper on a small number of patients was rejected for publication. Only after she expanded her work to include more samples was it finally accepted. Rowley commented that she anxiously waited for it to be published, fearing she would be scooped by someone else—a feeling common even to the greatest scientists in this competitive environment.[78]

Building on Rowley's work, scientists John Groffen and Nora Heisterkamp found the actual *BCR-ABL* gene created by the translocation on chromosome 22. They worked in the late 1970s and early 1980s, an exciting time in molecular biology when "cloning" of DNA became possible. In the broadest sense, cloning refers to the ability of scientists to manipulate DNA by cutting it into specific pieces which are then moved into different combinations, reproduced or amplified, and used to produce new proteins. During this time, the discovery of several key enzymes allowed scientists to work with DNA. "Restriction endonucleases" are enzymes which cut the DNA at a certain code ("endonuclease" meaning cutting the DNA and "restriction" because they cut only at a specific code). These enzymes were found in nature and allowed bacteria to defend their own DNA by cutting up any foreign DNA inserted into them by viruses. In the lab, these enzymes let scientists split the DNA into specific, workable fragments. At the same time, the discovery of other enzymes called "ligases" allowed the pieces of DNA to be sealed together into a longer strand. Enzymes called "polymerases" allowed reproduction of the new strands. The field of molecular biology exploded as scientists could now cut and reassemble DNA into new forms to test and study.

The methods of cutting, moving, sequencing, and studying DNA used in the 1980s seem crude by modern standards, but they were tremendously exciting. Not only were scientists now able to manipulate DNA, but the procedures could be learned with relatively little training and done with simple equipment, much like working on cars in that era. For example, one common procedure called the Southern blot (named after Edward Southern, its inventor) was used to analyze DNA. In this procedure, the DNA was removed from cells and appeared as a visible clump of fine white strands in the bottom of a test tube. The DNA was then cut into pieces using the restriction endonucleases and loaded into one end of an agarose gel, a clear slab of jello-like consistency about six inches long. An electric current spread the DNA fragments out by size in the gel, a process that was made visible using dyes. A few hours later, the spread pieces of DNA were transferred to special paper using absorbent paper towels to suck the solution and DNA out of the agarose, the "blotting" part of the name Southern blot. Once the cut and spread DNA was stuck on this special paper, it could then be analyzed by putting it in a plastic bag with liquid and adding radioactive fragments of a specific piece of DNA called a "probe." The radioactive DNA probe would stick to the DNA fragments on the blot (the paper with the DNA) in a specific pattern and the signals seen using x-ray film and developers. The Southern blot could be washed and probed again and again. Performing the whole process had the same flavor as working in a home shop, garage, or kitchen.

In 1983, Groffen and Heisterkamp used this Southern blot technique to see if the *ABL* gene might be at the breakpoint in the t(9;22) translocation Rowley had identified. Their description of this event, recorded in a commemoration of the 50th anniversary of the discovery of the Philadelphia Chromosome, captures this hands-on sensation.

"The floor on which we worked had a huge darkroom and tanks for the manual developing of x-ray films. You would stand there with the red light on and wait until your eyes adjusted to the gloom. Then you would take the exposed film out of the cassette, attach it to a metal bracket and immerse it in developer. You could monitor a bit what was happening by dipping it out of the tank and seeing black areas emerge. It was always the best part of a day and we usually did this together—you sometimes literally would not know what could develop. The day that we developed Southern blot #57 was a day we will never forget. Seeing an extra band in the lane that contained BamHI-digested DNA of one CML patient was the most exciting moment in our career."[79]

The target for treatment of CML had been found.

The train from Albany-Rensselaer ran south along the Hudson River. The initial portion of the trip took them through the rolling country-side of upstate New York, on that gray day stripped bare and blended with the cold bleakness of the Hudson. Closer to New York City, a growing collection of abandoned and rusted industrial objects added to the dreariness. The journey finished with a depressing view of the gloomy and littered North Side Rail System until they entered the darkness of the tunnel into Penn Station.

During the ride, Teresa and Mark rode in companionable silence that masked swirling emotions. For her part, Teresa found herself anxious about Mark's situation and both excited and nervous about her return to New York City. Despite her protestations, the trip had also become about her condition. Before the attack, Teresa had thought of herself as a strong person. She had been humbled by her breakdown, knew she needed to escape her demons, and had come to enjoy her quiet life in Saratoga. She devoted herself to the twins and their school activities, was well-liked by her neighbors, and made friends easily. Although she knew they would raise the twins Upstate, she had never given up her real identity. With her dress and accent, Teresa would never be mistaken, even at a distance, for a local. In the months leading up to Mark's diagnosis, she had been vaguely thinking about a return to visit the City but had made no definitive plans. Her thoughts were mixed. She wanted to return home but knew that since her brother and mother were gone and their firefighting community forever altered, she would no longer belong. Now Mark's illness had galvanized her desire to return. She needed to go back to complete her recovery.

Mark's thoughts were less complex. He intuitively felt his leukemia would respond to the treatment, so he had relatively little anxiety about the visit to Memorial Sloan Kettering. He was mainly worried about Teresa. Despite his successful business life, Mark always felt his greatest fortune was to have found and married this beautiful, smart, and strong-willed woman. Her breakdown had upset him greatly and, as much as he missed the life of the City, he did not want to take a chance with her health. Still, he reasoned, before this she had always been so strong. Maybe now she was ready. It sure would be nice if they could return together from time to time.

They walked off the train and were immediately surrounded by the City. The speed and numbers of moving people, the sounds and lights, and even the smells quickly overwhelmed any possibility of self-reflection. As they walked through the station to catch a cab, Teresa spoke.

"What did you do to me? I feel like a hick."

Mark laughed. "You'll get it back."

And she did. Even the ride across town in the checker cab with its thick plastic barrier, fare card, meter, and Indian driver playing sports talk radio, all unknown in Saratoga, was both familiar and exciting. The noise and traffic, a few quick lane changes, some horns and a muttered curse from the driver reintroduced her to sensory overload. Teresa knew she was back when her mind began to automatically figure a better route to their destination.

Dr. Dailey was in his mid-thirties, sharply dressed and very blunt.

"You definitely have CML. Before Gleevec the average survival was four years until blast crisis, now we don't know. It seems to have controlled the disease for a long time in some patients, but not all. We will watch your blood with regular blood counts and chemistries every two weeks at the start, repeat the cytogenetic testing and PCR every three months, and do a bone marrow every year. Do not take any other medicines while you are on Gleevec without checking with us."

He handed Mark a printed list of instructions.

"How soon will we know if it is working?" asked Teresa.

"It should start to work very soon, but we may not know for another year or two how well it works."

"But it works for most people," continued Teresa.

"It seems to, but we are not yet sure."

"And if not?" she asked.

"If it does not work, we will put you on the bone marrow transplant list. We would first look for a match from your brother and sisters. If you do not have a match, we will use an unrelated donor."

They were quiet as they checked out and gathered their things. They had stopped in the relative calm of the lobby before they entered the street.

"How are you?" she asked.

"Okay. I know we heard the same thing from Dr. Matthews, but somehow it seemed a little more positive when he said it. This sounded a little more serious."

"It is serious, Mark."

"I know, Tee, I just didn't really want to admit it." For the first time, she saw him look sad and older.

"The pill is going to work, Mark. I know it." She hugged him.

"Well then, we might as well eat. All this medical stuff is making me hungry. There's a good Greek place down the block; then we can get a cab back to the train."

"No," she said. "I want to go to the site. We'll eat someplace there."

He looked at her. "Are you sure?"

"Yes. Let's go."

MOLECULAR SCIENCE: A BRIEF PAUSE FOR THE ANDROMEDA STRAIN.

In 1969, a military satellite which had been collecting microorganisms from the upper atmosphere crashed into the desert outside the small town of Piedmont, Arizona. The team sent to retrieve the satellite and nearly all the inhabitants of Piedmont died horrible deaths. The culprit was an extraterrestrial organism which had contaminated the satellite. The organism was taken to the secret Wildfire Complex, a biologic isolation lab maintained by the U.S. government, where it nearly ran wild and threatened to infect the entire earth. This story, *The Andromeda Strain*, was the bestselling book that started Michael Crichton's career, which later included *ER* and *Jurassic Park*. Although Crichton's lethal organism did not have DNA or RNA, the success of his novel showed the intense public interest in this type of science. It also mirrored the concern many scientists had about the new field of molecular biology.

In the early 1970s, unease began to surface in some members of the scientific community. The identification of the "restriction endonucleases" which could cut DNA made it possible for scientists to make DNA fragments and insert them into viruses which would then infect cells. The scientists could then determine if the cells would then be changed or produce the protein from the DNA fragment. One important virus, called SV40 (Simian Virus), was found to be cut by a restriction endonuclease called EcoRI. This cut area made a perfect place to insert other DNA fragments cut by EcoRI into the virus. Under normal conditions, SV40, a virus collected from monkeys and grown in monkey kidney cells in the lab, was not considered dangerous. In fact, it had contaminated some lots of the polio vaccine which were made using monkey cells in the early 1960s. Many people vaccinated with the polio virus were also infected with SV40. When later studied, these people developed antibodies to SV40 yet did not seem to suffer any obvious bad effects, although it is difficult to be certain.[80] The concern in the early 1970s was that the SV40 virus could become a threat if it were changed or combined with another virus in an experiment. Another area of anxiety was the use of bacteria to reproduce newly constructed DNA fragments. Scientists commonly used strains of the bacteria *E. coli* in the lab. Infecting *E. coli* with a newly fashioned piece of DNA to multiply the DNA was a reasonable expectation. The concern with this procedure was that since *E. coli* is in human intestinal system, it might be possible to unleash a terrible changed *E. coli* which would then produce human illness—our own Andromeda strain.[81]

In 1974, two groups of scientists from Great Britain and the United States issued a call for a voluntary moratorium on experiments using these techniques until they were discussed by the scientific community. Remarkably, this ban was observed by scientists across the world. When one thinks of the pressure that these scientists felt, like Dr. Rowley's anxiety about publishing her work on the CML translocation, this voluntary restraint seems impossible. Today it probably would not happen. In 1975, one of the leaders of the moratorium, Dr. Paul Berg, organized a conference at Asilomar, California. The conference produced a set of guidelines adopted with some modifications by the National Institute of Health and similar governing bodies in other countries.[82 83 84] These actions by the scientific community were particularly remarkable when one remembers the time in which this took place. Distrust of authority was high. The Vietnam War had only recently ended, and Watergate was ongoing. Communication methods were limited. There was no internet or cell phone system, journals were printed and sent by mail, and telegrams were still commonly used. Although we now understand that these initial guidelines were probably too strict and were ultimately relaxed, the story is a remarkable one in the history of the science.

In an added twist to this narrative, Groffen and Heisterkamp had first worked in the Netherlands. The regulations in that country to allow DNA research were not finalized, so they came to the England and then the United States, where they ultimately contributed their important step in understanding CML.[85]

Despite the pause, by the 1980s the widespread use of these techniques caused some to joke that anyone could study DNA in their basement or garage. The age of molecular biology had begun.

The cab left them a few blocks from the site. As they walked the perimeter of the former World Trade Center, Teresa was initially disoriented. Construction barriers and fences lined the sidewalks along the site, shielding the area from view. Overhead the scaffolding and planks formed a dungy tunnel of rough wood on harsh metal bars. For a few moments, she could almost imagine being in any construction site on any block in this ever-changing city. The movement and noise of the traffic and people for whom this was now routine added to the false feeling of normalcy. But unlike most construction sites, this work zone was seemingly endless. When the covering overhead ended, a dusky sky and dark clouds appeared where there should have been buildings. Finally, they reached an opened fenced area where they could stop and see the site below them.

It was still a horrible ragged hole. As they looked down into its exposed layers, the vast panels of illuminated work lights combined with the fading sun allowed them to see that most of the rubble was gone but collapsed rough concrete and metal edges were everywhere. The white construction trailers looked like children's toys, dwarfed by the size of the pit. The red cranes and even brighter red construction barriers lent a sense of emergency even after all these years. On this day, there were large blue coverings over some objects. Together the colors reminded Teresa of the flags handed to grieving families time and time again during those early days. They stood looking together for an unmeasurable few minutes until she turned to him, resolute.

"This is a new day for us, Mark. You're going to start those pills and beat this leukemia. And I'm going to live again. My brother is gone, and Mom is dead. I love our life in Saratoga, but our girls are coming back here to visit next month. They are going to see Times Square, Radio City, and shop at the real Macy's. And when they finally rebuild this place, we're going to see it."

GLEEVEC: TARGETED TREATMENT FOR CANCER.

Once the abnormal *BCR-ABL* gene was identified in patients with CML, the next steps were to understand its function and develop a targeted treatment.

The *ABL* gene had been tested by Groffen and Heisterkamp for involvement in CML because it was one of a relatively new class of genes called oncogenes—normal genes which can cause cancer when damaged or mutated. In CML the combination *BCR-ABL* gene increases the normal activity of *ABL* gene. The proof of the role this oncogene came in 1990 when scientist David Baltimore placed the abnormal *BCR-ABL* gene in mice and found the creatures developed CML.[86] Other scientists studying normal and abnormal *ABL* genes concluded that this gene produced a "tyrosine kinase," a class of enzymes responsible for controlling many cellular activities. This work would ultimately be important for understanding many different cancers.

The final act in the story of Gleevec (imatinib) belongs to a brilliant physician named Brian Drucker. Trained as a medical oncologist at the Dana Farber Cancer Institute, Dr. Drucker studied tyrosine kinase enzymes like that produced by the *BCR-ABL* gene. In years of dedicated work in chemistry labs, other scientists had developed inhibitors of these enzymes.[87] In the medical community, there was little enthusiasm for using these inhibitors to treat cancers. It was generally thought that they would be too toxic and that the cancers would be unlikely to respond since they probably had many different defects. Even worse, CML was a rare disease, and any drugs were unlikely to be profitable. Dr. Drucker thought differently. After moving to the Oregon Health and Science University, he formed a partnership with Nick Lydon from Ciba-Geigy (later Novartis) to study the inhibitor imatinib. Drucker and Lydon, with support from other leading CML physicians, convinced the company to support their studies. The results were amazing: imatinib worked with very little toxicity. The clinical trials started in June 1998 and were reported in December 1999. The FDA approved the medication, brand named Gleevec, for use in May 2001.[88]

For patients with CML, imatinib offered new hope for possibly even normal lives. The discussions of stem cell transplants from other people became rare. And for patients, physicians, and scientists dealing with other cancers, imatinib offered hope that the age of "targeted" treatments for cancer might soon arrive. It was a new day in cancer medicine.

Mark's CML responded rapidly to the treatment. After two months, he was in a "hematologic remission" which meant that his high white count was normal. The CML was still present in his blood and could be found in a small number of the white blood cells using an analysis of the chromosomes called FISH testing, an advanced way of doing the procedure that Dr. Rowley did on her dining room table to find the Philadelphia Chromosome. After a few more months, this testing also became normal, and Mark had what was called a "cytogenetic remission." Dr. Matthews then turned to the most sensitive method of detecting the CML; a test called the polymerase chain reaction (PCR). If this test turned normal, Mark would be in a "molecular remission" with no evidence of CML in his body.

Both Mark and Teresa remembered that Monday appointment. Over the weekend, they had visited Mark's family in Brooklyn and brought the girls to Manhattan for Sunday afternoon tea at the American Girl Doll Store on Fifth Avenue. The twins had been so excited to get dressed up and bring their dolls, Jess and Nicki, whose hair they combed and clothes they repeatedly adjusted during the ride. They looked wide-eyed as they proudly walked up Fifth Avenue holding hands. The store itself was an alternate universe filled with American Girl dolls, clothing, accessories, and even a doll hospital. Mark had been one of the few fathers in this girl's world, which he described later to his brother.

"Ralph, I never saw so many little girls and dolls. The twins loved it, the dining room with all the table settings, the tea, the little cookies, and the waiters and waitresses. It's some operation they have. There's a lot of money in those dolls."

As they made the three-hour drive home north on I-87 that evening, the girls and dolls were fast sleep in the back seat, and Teresa sat reading in the passenger's seat. She caught Mark glance over at her.

"You okay?" she asked.

"Just thinking," he replied.

"Yeah? About what?"

"You and the girls."

After a minute, she looked back at him.

"Would you like to be more specific?"

Another pause as he changed lanes and maneuvered the Mercedes around a truck.

"That was one strange place, that American Girl Doll Store. I mean, outside is Fifth Avenue and the whole world. Inside is this girl's fantasy land, where we're sitting at this table eating hundred dollar cookies served by waiters to dolls. The twins look so excited and cute, and you look so happy and beautiful. And in my mind, I'm hearing the Talking Heads singing 'how did I get here? This is not my beautiful wife.' And I'm thinking about everything that happened to us, to our family, to the City. It all seems to go away at that moment, and it's just us in this crazy place. I know I'm the luckiest man in the world."

The road was straight, and they held hands for a moment.

"No, Mark," she whispered. "You're the best man in the world."

The weekend had been so busy that they had neither the time nor the desire to think about Monday morning's appointment. The glow of the trip was still with them as they pulled into the parking lot. It was only at the entrance of the office that reality intruded. The routine of the noisy elevator, the faint smell of the building, and the ritual of the check-in brought Mark and Teresa back to familiar territory. They again entered exam room number two, into which they always seemed to be placed. Teresa sat in the chair while Mark was weighed and had his blood pressure, pulse, and temperature checked.

Tee caught Mark's eye as John Welt, the medical technician, listened through the stethoscope.

"Bet those hundred dollar cookies look pretty good right now," she said.

"No Talking Heads here," he replied.

Dr. Matthews did not keep them waiting for long. He entered the room, shook hands, and went right to the point.

"Your PCR test now shows a complete molecular remission," he said. "No CML could be found."

"It's gone?" asked Mark.

"As best we can tell."

"Thank God," sighed Teresa as they hugged. "What now?"

"You keep taking the pills. We keep testing your blood every six months. You live your life, and we hope. At this point, we think most people who reach this type of complete molecular remission will remain in remission a long time. We don't know how long, but many or even most may never see the cancer again."

"From your mouth, doc, to God's ears," said Mark. He pointed to Teresa. "I told her this weekend I was the luckiest man in the world."

The PCR test that Dr. Matthew used to track Mark's CML is a variation of the test used to solve crimes, establish paternity, and study a wide variety of diseases. The PCR procedure allows a massive amplification of a small amount of DNA, hence the classic identification of the criminal from a single hair found at the crime scene. PCR works by heating the DNA and causing the double helix to separate into two single strands. The two strands are cooled, then enzymes (which are found in nature to reproduce or repair DNA) are used to reproduce a specific section of each single strand. The specific section to be reproduced is determined ahead of time depending on whether one is looking for CML or trying to identify a killer. These enzymes thus make the two single stranded pieces of DNA into two double stranded pieces of DNA, which can, in turn, be again heated to separate into four single strands. The four single strands are reproduced by the enzymes to become four double strands then heated to become eight singles with the next cycle, then 16, 32, 64, 128, 256, 512, 1024, and so on. Within hours there is a large amount of this specific DNA available for study. In tracking the CML, it is estimated that the PCR test could detect one abnormal cell in 100,000 to 1,000,000.[89] When Mark's PCR test became normal, it was powerful evidence that there were very few of these cells left in his body.

THE BIRTH OF BIOTECH: PCR AND YELLOWSTONE NATIONAL PARK

Scientist Kary Mullis invented the PCR in the 1980s. The test has become one of the most important in medicine and science, earning Mullis a 1993 Noble Prize. The story of the PCR is also an important first chapter in the development of the modern biotech industry and starts in Wyoming's Yellowstone National Park.[90]

Yellowstone National Park offers a lesson in geology which humbles the attentive guest. The oldest rocks in the Park date from the Precambrian era—the era of the Earth's beginning and most of the planet's history which ended 570 million years ago. The next era, the Paleozoic, lasted until 245 million years ago and saw ancient seas flood the region. The Mesozoic era lasted until 66 million years ago and included the famous Jurassic period of the dinosaurs and the start of the formation of the Rocky Mountains. The last 66 million years of the Earth's history is called the Cenozoic era and for Yellowstone was a time of volcanic eruptions, glacier carving, and the building of mountains like the nearby Grand Tetons. For the story of the PCR, however, it is the last 16.5 million years of this geologic history which are critical: the years of the "Yellowstone hotspot."

The Yellowstone hotspot is an area where hot molten rock from deep within the earth erupted through the crust. Although geologists argue about the origin of the hotspot and some of the events of the last 16.5 million years, there is general agreement that three "recent" Yellowstone eruptions have taken place: 2 million, 1.6 million and 600,000 years ago. These eruptions each formed a caldera—a huge hole in the ground. Thus, the Park is a forty-five mile by thirty-mile-wide hole left by the last of these explosions. Thankfully, no eruptions of these type have occurred during recorded history since they are on an almost unimaginable scale of violence. The last eruption 600,000 years ago is estimated to have produced over one thousand times the ash of the Mount St. Helen's explosion and, if it happened today, would probably cover most of the central part of the United States in debris and change our climate.

Beneath Yellowstone today is a collection of molten rock about one hundred twenty-five miles underground which produces the tremendous heat responsible for the eruptions of Old Faithful and the hot springs found throughout the park. The temperature of the water in these hot springs would seem to preclude life, yet over the years some bacteria have evolved which thrive in this environment. They have adapted in part by developing enzymes that are resistant to the heat. One such bacteria, *Thermus aquaticus*, evolved many thousands of years ago, fought for its survival, and then patiently (if one can attribute such feelings to bacteria) awaited its discovery by humans. In 1966, it was found by Thomas Brock, a faculty member at Indiana University, and undergraduate Hudson Freeze as they were studying bacteria from the hot Mushroom Spring in the Lower Geyser Basin. After Brock identified *Thermus aquaticus* and named it, he deposited some of the bacteria in the American Type Culture Collection (ATCC) in Washington, D.C.[91] This private, non-profit organization (now located in Virginia) serves as a repository for microorganisms for researchers across the world. By depositing his new find here, Brock made it available for others to use.

Thermus aquaticus sat on the shelf at ATCC in Washington, D.C. during the turbulent era of the late 1960s and early 1970s. Although insignificant by geologic standards, this period brought great changes in the scientific community. Traditional academic methods of organizing scientific research came under challenge. Part of the pressure was external as increasing sums of money flowed into science from both industry and venture capitalism to develop profitable new products. Within the scientific community, many younger scientists of this era were comfortable challenging established hierarchies—quite a number had opposed the Vietnam War, the government, or their universities. These men, and increasing numbers of women, chafed under the promotion rules, the perception of sexism, and restrictions they saw in university life. Scientific leaders, notably several Nobel Prizes winners, were recruited to Boards of new start-up companies. The result was the emergence of new partnerships between various elements of industry, academics, and individual scientists which led to the new biotechnology industry.

In 1971, biochemist Ronald Cape, physician Peter Farley, and Nobel laureate in physics Donald Glaser formed the first biotech company.[92] Named Cetus, the company recruited talented scientists attracted by its interesting projects and a work environment which emphasized avoiding traditional scientific compartmentalization. The company obtained funding and had success with its initial projects. By the time it went public in 1981, Cetus had three hundred fifty employees, including fifty with MD or PhD degrees.[93] Eventually, the company's research focus turned to interleukin-2 (IL-2), a molecule which stimulated the immune system and which they tested as a cancer treatment.[94] Although IL-2 is still used today to treat some cancers, the company is best remembered for being the birthplace of PCR.

Kary Mullis, a scientist at Cetus, conceived of the PCR reaction in the mid-1980s. By his report, the inspiration came during a drive to his cabin in the mountains.[95] The concept was brilliant, but converting it into reality required tremendous work. One problem was the need to heat the DNA to separate the double strands into two single strands for copying. With each cycle (or doubling of the DNA), the heating to separate the double DNA strands and then cooling to allow copying of the single DNA strands would take place. The difficulty was that heating destroys most enzymes—requiring that a new set of enzymes to reproduce the single strands of DNA be added with each cycle. Adding new enzymes after each cycle was tedious and, to make matters worse, the first enzymes had a high error rate. The solution was the heat resistant enzyme from Brock's *Thermus aquaticus*, called *Taq* polymerase. After all, this organism had learned to survive in extreme heat, so its enzymes would keep working under these conditions. The PCR reaction worked beautifully using this enzyme.[96] The whole process was automated, and Cetus joined with Elmer Perkins to produce the equipment.

Like many great scientific accomplishments, the assignment of profit and fame from the development of the PCR was messy. Shortly after the perfection of the PCR, Mullis left Cetus following a bitter dispute about the publishing of the results—a battle also fueled by the fiery personalities involved. Cetus also had to win a legal patent fight with DuPont, giving the PCR reaction an opportunity to contribute to biotech patent law as well as science. In 1991, after having difficulties with its IL-2 program, a collapsing Cetus sold the rights to PCR to Hoffman-La Roche, then was acquired by Chiron and vanished. The awarding of the 1993 Nobel Prize to Mullis upset many of his former colleagues at Cetus, who felt that their contributions to making the PCR work were not properly acknowledged.[97] Yet despite these battles and its brief existence, Cetus produced the right environment for the right scientists at the right time to produce a critical step for biomedical science. And Yellowstone Park helped.

The brilliant work which led to Gleevec as the modern treatment of CML has allowed many patients to live almost normal lives. It was the rest of Mark's life that now worried Dr. Matthews.

"How has your health been otherwise?" he asked.

"My right knee stinks. It's bone on bone, and Dr. O'Carol wants to replace it if you give the okay."

"Do you have a lot of pain?"

"It's been hurting for years, but these past six months it's killing. I can hardly walk. I want to lose some of this," he grabbed a handful of his ample fat with both hands, "but it's hard to do when you can't exercise."

"How are your heart and your diabetes?"

"Dr. Moon says my heart is fine and my blood pressure and cholesterol are good, thank God."

"But he also says he may need insulin soon," added Teresa.

"From the blood viewpoint, you can have any knee surgery Dr. O'Carol wants to do. Missing a day or two of your medication should not pose a problem," commented Dr. Matthews.

"I told him you would say it's okay."

"Fixing your knee will hopefully help your pain, but you really need to deal with your weight."

"I figure after I get this knee fixed, I can exercise, and I will lose some of this."

Teresa shook her head. "You've haven't exercised since you stopped playing football in high school and you won't give up the food. Every other week, you and your brother, down to Brooklyn to load up that car. Bread, pasta, mozzarella, meats, and the sweets, you name it. And half is gone by the time you even get back here. Probably by the time you cross over the GW knowing you two." She turned to Dr. Matthews. "I think he should go for a gastric bypass."

"Forget it. I'm not doing that surgery." Mark also turned to Dr. Matthews. "She made me go to the info meetings with the other fatties. When I heard what they do to your stomach, I said forget it. Plus, they said you don't always absorb medications well after that surgery. Suppose I don't absorb my Gleevec, then I'm dead from leukemia." He looked over at Teresa. "Is that how you want me? Thin but dead. Some deal."

Teresa turned back to Dr. Matthews. "If he keeps whining about his fat, aching body, I'll kill him before the leukemia ever gets a chance. And is it true about that bypass that he would not absorb the medication?"

Dr. Matthews replied. "There is a possibility of that with the full gastric bypass, but you could probably do the banding or sleeve procedure without the same risk."

"Who wants to live with a plastic cord strangling off your stomach? Not me. I'll exercise this time, you'll see. You won't recognize me in six months."

"Yeah, yeah, we've heard it before. Come on, let's get out of here," said Teresa. "This doctor needs to see other patients, ones he can believe when they speak."

As they left, Mark stopped.

"You like mozzarella, doc?"

"Sure."

"Next week, I'll bring you some bread and mozzarella from Brooklyn. Not the stuff they make up here, but the real stuff." He kissed his fingers and walked out arm-in-arm with Tee.

Carol Feinman 2: Breast cancer (Boston, 1988)

Carol always remembered the worst part of her surgery was not the cut in her breast, but the drain under her arm. That hurt.

She had arrived that morning with Betty and Rose at Beth Israel in control, thankful that she did not sense the oppressive smell of ultrasound jelly. Dr. Scanlon met her in the operating room. She awoke later in the recovery room.

"The surgery went well," he reported. "I removed more tissue from the breast where the cancer was, and it all felt normal. That should heal nicely. As planned, I also removed the lymph nodes from under your arm. I have left a drain in place which will come out in several days. The pathologist's report will take about a week."

"When does she start the radiation?" asked Rose.

"In about a month, when she has healed," replied Dr. Scanlon as he examined Carol's bandages.

"Can she wait that long?" persisted Rose.

He briefly looked up at Rose.

"Yes."

Dr. Scanlon had done a "level one and two axillary lymph node dissection." The axilla is the medical term for the armpit. The lower portion of the axilla near the breast is mainly fatty tissue while the upper portion contains sensitive nerves and blood vessels—as anyone who has had fingers jammed into their armpit understands. There are three levels in the axilla, and by removing only the lower two, Dr. Scanlon avoided damage to the nerves and blood vessels. Within the fatty tissue he removed were Carol's lymph nodes. Most women have about twenty-five pea-sized lymph nodes in their axilla which surgeons usually cannot see or feel unless they are swollen or filled with cancer cells.

Some of Dr. Scanlon's colleagues also removed the highest (third) level of tissue in the axilla to get more lymph nodes out. At the time of Carol's surgery, some surgeons argued taking more nodes helped patients while others felt it only put a woman at more risk for nerve damage and swelling of the arm. In later years, surgeons concluded that removal of only a limited number of lymph nodes should be done to detect cancer cells and determine the risk of spread. More extensive surgery would not improve the cure rate since "the horse was out of the barn." By the 1990s surgeons used dye injected near the tumor to allow them to remove only a select few lymph nodes which drained the area of the cancer, called the "sentinel nodes."

Carol was not aware of this debate, but she knew her underarm hurt. And she hated the sight of the drain sticking out of her body—a clear plastic tube about the diameter of a pencil and a foot long which ended in a pear-sized plastic suction ball collecting blood-tinge fluid. Over Carol's objections, Betty had spent the night sleeping on her couch. While she wanted her mother to feel useful, she worried about subjecting her to memories of her own breast cancer.

Rose had no such scruples. The phone rang at eight the next morning, and Carol overheard her demanding report.

"She's sleeping." Pause.

"Right away. No, she did not have much pain. Of course, she took the pill . . ." Pause.

"No, the drain looks fine." Pause.

"No, stay at work. I'll go home after breakfast and come back this afternoon." Pause.

"Okay. Bye."

After Betty had left, Carol explored her body. The dressing could be pulled back, allowing her to see Dr. Scanlon's work. Her breast was swollen and discolored, about what Carol had expected, but the view of the drain going into her underarm was disgusting. The morning light was coming into her living room, and she smiled ironically as the disassembly of her cubist prints took on a new personal meaning. After a few minutes, Carol realized she was not going to do much that day since the drain hurt when she moved. On impulse, she called work.

"Carlton Associates, Roger Clark speaking," announced the articulate voice.

"Roger, it's Carol."

"Carol, my love, how wonderful to hear you. How are you? We have been dying to know, but did not want to disturb you." She could picture him, meticulously dressed, sitting at his neat desk, fussing with any paper not in perfect order.

"I'm fine."

"Don't lie to me."

"My breast is swollen and bruised, and I have a tube coming out from under my arm," she replied.

"That's better," he said factually, as if he was hearing about the weather. "And the cancer? That better be gone, too. We want you back completely rid of it."

"Well, the surgeon thinks he got it all, but we won't know until we get the pathology reports next week."

"He better have removed it all," Roger continued. "I hope at least he was cute."

"Who?" asked Carol, puzzled for a moment.

"Your surgeon, silly. I could use a nice hot doctor myself."

Carol paused, then burst into laughter at the vision of Roger, gay, black, and thirty-five, making a pass at Dr. Scanlon.

"I love you, Roger, but you are too much for Dr. Scanlon to handle. And Allen would be furious." Allen, a computer scientist at MIT, was Roger's devoted, long-time partner.

"I love you too, dear, but don't think that means you can keep your hot doctor to yourself. Allen will just have to share me." His tone became serious. "Are you eating?" he asked.

"Yes, you sound like my mother. About the eating part, I mean."

"Good, we will be over tomorrow night at six with Thai food."

Carol smiled. Carlton Associates was a Boston market research firm. The projects were interesting; they had just finished an analysis of the use of feminine hygiene products among college students. The other "ladies" on the team were both single and about her age. Mary was a red-headed, Irish Catholic graduate of Boston College with a large family in the area while Sophia was an ethnic-looking, third-generation Italian from the North End who still lived at home with her parents. Roger was the team leader, having been at the firm for more than a decade. They worked well without rivalries and socialized without being intrusive. In short, it was fun, and she looked forward to seeing them for dinner.

The meeting with Dr. Scanlon the next week was a different matter, not fun. He reviewed the pathology reports.

"The was no cancer left in the breast, Carol," he began. "I removed it all with a wide margin. You can start your radiation in three weeks." He turned to look at Rose. "No sooner. Her incision needs to heal." He returned to Carol. "I removed fifteen lymph nodes. The pathologists found two infected with cancer."

"So, thirteen were clear," calculated Rose. "Were the infected nodes the lower ones?"

"Yes."

"What does that mean?" asked Carol.

"It means that you will need chemotherapy. Those treatments have been shown to reduce the risk of a recurrence if the cancer has spread into the lymph nodes."

"Chemotherapy?" asked Betty, puzzled. She looked at Carol. "You need chemotherapy?"

"Yes. She does," said Dr. Scanlon gently.

"When does that start?" asked Carol.

"After the radiation," he replied. "You will meet Dr. Spiegel, the oncologist, to get the details."

At home, Betty was still shaken by the thought of chemotherapy.

"I don't understand why you need the chemotherapy if he got all the cancer," Betty said abruptly as she poured their coffees. "I wish he had done the mastectomy; then you wouldn't need it."

"It would not have mattered, Mom," replied Carol. "Even if I had the mastectomy, I would need to take the chemo. The chemo is in case any cancer got out into the body. It's just insurance. Don't worry; I'll be fine."

"But I never had chemo," said Betty. "And my cancer never came back." She looked so suddenly sad and vulnerable that Carol once again tried to protect her mother.

"It's okay, Mom. They did not do chemotherapy in your day, but now it's routine. It's an advance in medical science. More women are cured of the breast cancer all the time. I promise I'll do fine with it."

Once again Rose seemed oblivious. "Mother, your cancer did not go into the lymph nodes, so there would have been no need for chemo. Since Carol's cancer has already spread into the nodes, it may have spread into her body, and she needs the chemotherapy."

Shit, thought Carol. Did you have to say that? Leave Mom be, Rose. And me, too.

Don't be naïve Carol, thought Rose. Mom knows this is bad news. You might as well face it, too. It's time to get serious here.

They finished their coffees in silence, each exhausted in their own way.

ADJUVANT CHEMOTHERAPY FOR BREAST CANCER?

The success of chemotherapy treatment for Hodgkin's lymphoma in the 1960s had raised hopes that it might cure more common cancers like breast, lung, and colon cancer. Unfortunately, the results with chemotherapy in these other cancers were not as good. It rapidly became clear that once cancers had visibly spread, chemotherapy could produce temporary shrinkage but did not cure. Experiments with various combinations of drugs improved the rates of shrinkage but still could not cure. In frustration, many physicians gave up trying to cure common cancers with chemotherapy.

A different strategy was needed. A few physicians proposed giving chemotherapy immediately after surgery in the hopes that this might cure those patients who had only a small number of cancer cells which were not yet visible. For women with breast cancer, this meant that after mastectomy the chemotherapy would be given to eliminate any cancer cells which might have already escaped the breast. It was called "adjuvant chemotherapy"—meaning "in addition to surgery," and it was controversial. Those women who were cured by the mastectomy would receive the chemotherapy unnecessarily. Some might be harmed or even die from the treatments. For the physicians who had given up on chemotherapy, the idea seemed futile.

Determining if adjuvant chemotherapy worked required randomized clinical trials. In breast cancer, this meant that after mastectomy one-half the women would be given chemotherapy treatment and one-half observed. If the concept were correct, cure rates would be better in the chemotherapy group (also called the treatment arm of the clinical trial). For these clinical trials to produce useful results, many patients would be needed and the effects monitored for long periods of time. Since no single surgeon or hospital would have enough patients, large groups had to be organized. In the United States, one of the first groups to do these types of studies was called the National Surgical Adjuvant Breast and Bowel Project (NSABP).

The start of clinical trials in breast cancer did not go well. The first NSABP study reported in 1968 used a single chemical called thiotepa, which was given for three days after surgery. While this study did show a slightly positive effect of the treatment, it was largely ignored because physicians had not yet learned to accept that progress in many of the common cancers would be incremental—the dramatic cures seen in Hodgkin's lymphoma would not be the norm.[98] In the mid-1970s, two famous clinical changed this attitude. In the United States,

Dr. Bernard Fisher and the NSABP tested a chemotherapy drug called melphalan given by mouth for five days every six weeks for two years following surgery. In Italy, Gianni Bonadonna and Umberto Veronesi tested a combination of the drugs cyclophosphamide, methotrexate, and 5-fluorouracil, given by mouth and vein for two weeks each month over one year, called CMF.[99] They modeled their program after the treatment called MOPP which had successfully cured Hodgkin's lymphoma. Both trials showed that chemotherapy following surgery could modestly improve the cure rate in breast cancer. In a neat bit of international collaboration, the National Cancer Institute promoted and supported both trials. Dr. Fisher became a legend in American oncology for this work and his efforts to promote breast conservation surgery, winning the Lasker Prize in Medicine in 1985. These treatments began an international effort to improve the results of adjuvant chemotherapy which continues today. [100]

Carol was glad to return to work. Roger, Mary, and Sophia were happy to have her back. The firm had been hired to determine the optimal products for vending machines located in the restrooms of nightclubs and bars frequented by college students. It was exactly the kind of project they enjoyed. Together they would design surveys, administer them to their target audience, analyze the results, and present their conclusions. The team would start with some preliminary research and explore their own pre-existing opinions in several days of often hysterical discussions. They always brought their perspectives to projects and this one promised to be even more interesting than usual.

Roger had pulled Carol aside.

"What do you have to do now?" he asked.

"Six weeks of daily radiation to my breast. They say I should be fine to work during that. Then comes chemo. I'm not sure about that. I'll find out next week."

"Do what you need to for your health, Carol. Just let me know what you can and cannot do, and we will work around it. I mean it."

"I know you do, Roger. Thanks. This much is better than thinking about cancer."

"Yes, well, when we get to a discussion about putting edible condoms into the machines, you may reconsider. When do you start that radiation?" he asked.

Carol laughed. "In about three weeks. I get marked for the radiation tomorrow and see the chemo doctor Friday. But don't worry, Roger. I'll be fine to work for the next two months at least. They say the radiation doesn't bother most people much. The chemo might be harder, but we should be well into this project by then, and I hope you won't have to carry me."

Roger looked directly at her. "We don't really care what they put into those vending machines, Carol. We care about you. And we have a deal for you. Sophia, Mary, and I think you have a long road coming up. So if it works for your schedule, we intend to spend a week preparing our project plan and survey offsite."

"Offsite?" said Carol, puzzled. "Where?"

"Well, as it turns out, Allen has been offered the use of a villa in Saint Martin, or Sint Maarten if you are Dutch. Sadly, he cannot use it due to some pressing engagement with a computer. This villa overlooks one of the nicer beaches on the island and has a large veranda suitable for a project meeting space. It somehow seems appropriate that we expose you to some sunshine before your radiation."

The image of the beach was with Carol the next day as she went for her radiation simulation appointment. She was placed on the table under the radiation machine, and temporary magic marker lines were drawn on her chest and breast to allow for the planning of her treatments. Several permanent dot tattoos were then placed, used to aim the beam each time.

As she lay there with her beautiful but wounded breast exposed and the technical talk and marking went on around her, Carol closed her eyes. She had a vision of the hospital stripped bare except for its steel beam frame and floors. It contained only beds and stretchers, no other equipment or staff. In the beds or on the stretches were the naked bodies of the several hundred patients in surgery or on the wards. In the background, their disembodied voices softly spoke or cried or moaned. Carol could not make out distinct sentences. As she concentrated on trying to understand what was being said, she felt unsettled. She was glad when she felt a touch on her arm and opened her eyes. It was Asa, the nurse.

"Hi, Carol. How are you doing?" She smiled warmly.

"Well, it is a little strange here, but I'm okay."

"You think?" Asa laughed. "Millions of dollars and tons of equipment to aim a beam of radiation into this poor bruised breast?" She checked the area, then became more serious. "You won't feel anything the first few weeks, but by the end your skin may be red or burned. We have some creams to help you."

"I have a question for you," said Carol.

"Okay."

"I have the chance to go to Saint Martin for a week with work before I start. Is there any problem with the sun before I get the radiation?"

"It's beautiful there," agreed Asa, "and it would be a nice break before you start. But you are pretty pale and starting radiation with a sunburn on your chest would not be a good idea, so cover up and be careful. But there is no reason I can think of not to go. In fact, it sounds perfect."

Rose wasn't so sanguine.

"Are you crazy? Saint Martin? Suppose you get sick and have to delay your treatment? Then where will you be? You should be resting and getting ready," she said in the stern tone of the reasonable adult addressing a wayward child.

"I'm not going on safari in Africa, Rose. It's a work trip to Saint Martin. I'll be staying in a villa with my team."

"Work? What kind of work will you be doing there? If you need to bond with your team, stay at the Boston Marriott."

Carol laughed. "You sound like the comptroller. I think you're just jealous. Anyway, it's all set. We leave Saturday morning."

Before she left, Carol had a Friday afternoon appointment with Dr. Spiegel, the medical oncologist. She dreaded this visit. Carol had always been mindful of what she put into her body. As a child, she innately favored fresh fruits, vegetables, and nuts over candy while Betty had prepared traditional, but wholesome meals. In college and as an adult, Carol continued a healthy eating pattern. Dr. Carl reinforced her views. Upon learning of Carol's food leanings and her work marketing products to young women, he had given her his old copy of Adelle Davis' book *Let's Eat Right to Stay Fit*. Davis was a pioneering nutritionist famous in the 1960s and early 1970s for advocating natural foods and vitamin supplements while challenging the processed food industry. To his credit, Dr. Carl had shared his belief in Davis' emphasis on natural foods while steering Carol away from some of Davis' more controversial ideas. Carol found the arguments persuasive and incorporated them occasionally into her discussions at work. The concept of putting harsh chemicals into her body was repulsive.

Carol also dreaded this visit because she knew they would discuss the chance of the cancer spreading. She knew that Rose would leave her no place to hide, demanding statistics and facts. Carol loved, respected, and needed her sister, but she also knew that Rose would charge ahead, regardless of how Carol felt. She felt vulnerable and prayed that her sister would be less aggressive and Dr. Spiegel somehow sympathetic.

The oncology unit was depressing. They exited the elevator on the second floor and came immediately to the reception desk. Off to the side was a small waiting area crowded with ill looking people, mostly older, some bald and a few very pale, including two in wheelchairs. It was quiet, and when all eyes turned on her, Carol immediately felt out of place. I'm too healthy to be here, she thought. Just wait until they get finished with you, replied another voice. They found three seats together, and Carol worked on her forms, trying not to look at the other patients. Much to Carol's relief, Rose took the completed papers to the desk and spared her the walk in front of the crowd. She may drive me crazy, but I can always count on her, thought Carol. Thankfully, they were called promptly by Janice, the large and slow moving assistant who brought them into an exam room.

"Sit up there," Janice motioned to the exam table. After Carol sat, Janice leisurely took her blood pressure, pulse, and temperature. After an eternity writing the figures in the chart, she handed Carol a cloth top. "Everything off from the waist up." Then she looked at the chart again. "No, wait, you're seeing Dr. Spiegel. He likes to talk first, so sit here." She pointed to one of the chairs and slowly ambled out.

Rose rolled her eyes. "I hope I never see her in an emergency. At her pace, it's a wonder they ever see a patient."

"I'm sure it's hard working here," offered Carol.

"Some of those people don't look like they have long," answered Rose, "and they might not make it waiting for her to get checked in."

Thanks, Rose, thought Carol. I hope that's not me.

Dr. Roger Spiegel was in his late forties, average height with a bushy Groucho Marx mustache and a manner which immediately put Carol at ease.

"I'm Roger Spiegel, your oncologist. I brought help today. This is Dr. John Matthews, our oncology fellow, and Cathy Johnson, our medical student." Dr. Spiegel reviewed her history and discussed the pathology report, using a diagram of the breast.

"Your type of breast cancer is the most common, called invasive ductal cancer. It starts inside the ducts and then breaks out into the tissue of the breast. Once cancer cells invade the tissue, it possible for them spread to the rest of the body in the blood, called metastases. We will do a CT scan and a bone scan to check for any metastases, but those tests cannot tell us if a few cells got out. We would need to put your whole body under the microscope. When Dr. Scanlon removed the lymph nodes, they were examined under the microscope and cancer was in two of them. This means that there is a chance that some cancer cells spread to the rest of your body. I know you don't want it, but chemotherapy improves the chances that this cancer will be cured, so we just must do it. It's no fun, but you will still have plenty of good days."

"Are there any other choices?" asked Carol.

"Not really," he answered. "You are young. You have to take chemotherapy."

Carol nodded. Dr. Spiegel handed her a chemotherapy calendar. "The standard treatment is called CMF. It is six months long. As you can see, you take Cytoxan pills for fourteen days out of each twenty-eight. On day number one and day number eight you also receive intravenous injections of methotrexate and 5-FU. The pills typically cause mild nausea and fatigue for those first two weeks, and the IV injections can also produce some nausea. There are a lot of medically minor side effects. Fatigue is one. You will probably lose some, maybe even all your hair. Most young women do have their periods stop, go into a temporary early menopause, and have hot flashes. Their periods usually start up again soon afterward, but an occasional woman in your age group does not have her periods return."

"Will she be able to have children later?" asked Rose. Thanks again Rose, thought Carol. Children are about as far away right now as Pluto. I will be bald, vomiting, and have a swollen boob, never mind about that man part of the equation. While Dr. Spiegel answered Rose, Carol caught the eye of Cathy Johnson, the studious looking medical student who seemed about her age. Cathy nodded in sympathy.

"Well, most women under the age of thirty-five will not permanently lose their periods. If a women's periods come back after chemotherapy, she should be able to have children. Many women have had children, and there does not appear to be any higher risk of birth defects."

"That's good," said Betty, speaking for the first time.

"Is this the only chemo treatment?" asked Carol, turning the conversation away from this particularly painful area.

"No. There is another choice. Across the country, doctors are comparing this CMF with a shorter, more intense, three-month treatment called AC, which uses the Adriamycin and Cytoxan, two medicines both given IV every three weeks for four times. Patients sign up for the study, and the treatment is determined by a flip of the coin. That study is being done down the street at the New England Deaconess Hospital. If you were interested in being part of a research study, we could send you there."

"No thanks," responded Carol quickly.

"Is the other treatment better?" asked Rose.

"We don't know. That is why it is a study. It is shorter and might be better or worse or the same."

"When would I start?" asked Carol.

"You can get your tests done now, then have your radiation. We will start the chemotherapy a week or two later."

"I have to be away next week. Can the tests wait until I get back?" Carol asked. Rose looked up sharply, and Dr. Spiegel noted her reaction.

"Yes. Where will you be?"

"Saint Martin."

"Then definitely yes."

Carol turned to Rose and briefly stuck her tongue out. Dr. Spiegel's eyebrows rose, and he laughed, understanding immediately. He turned to Rose and shrugged, hands out and palms up.

"She wins this one, big sister . . . sorry." When he smiled, even Rose had to grin a little.

9:00 Sandra Warren: Breast Cancer

"I'm fine. I'm ready," Sandra Warren announced as Dr. Matthews entered the room. She sat ramrod straight on the exam table, her forty-eight-year-old lean and conditioned body dressed in perfectly fitting Lulu Lemon workout clothes. Her hair looked freshly styled and exactly as it had for her campaign photograph taken six months earlier. Dr. Matthews knew it should match since she had informed him earlier that this human hair wig cost $3,000 at Pieces & Biz in New York City.

"Let me check you over," he replied and began washing his hands, using the time to begin the medical conversation which she despised.

"I heard you had some nausea and vomited once or twice," he tried.

"Yeah. Twice. It was nothing. I felt better after."

"And some mouth sores?"

"They're gone, see," she stated impatiently, opening her mouth to rush the exam.

"Exercising?"

"Did it this morning. Only an hour. Just like you told me."

"Good. Take deep breaths." He listened to her lungs and heart.

She lay back, and he pressed on her flat, hard abdomen.

"My legs are fine," she informed him before he could check them.

"All right," he replied. "This is your last treatment with Adriamycin and Cytoxan. In two weeks, you will start Taxol. That should be easier in terms of the nausea and vomiting—"

"They told me all about it," she interrupted.

"So, you are ready."

"That's what I said." As he raised his hands in mock surrender, she smiled before going to receive her chemotherapy.

Four months ago, highly respected attorney Sandra Warren had been nominated by the Saratoga County Republican Party for election as a judge in the County Family Court. One of two her opponents, longtime Republican insider Phil Johnson, had expected the Republican nomination and was running on the Conservative ticket. The Democrats nominated Kelly Smith, a young liberal lawyer. The district was historically Republican, but since Johnson threatened to split that vote and Smith had an energetic group of women supporting her, the race was closer than usual. The campaign had been in full swing three months ago when Sandra had a routine visit with her longtime gynecologist, Dr. Stacy Gold, a pleasant woman about her age.

After the exam, Dr. Gold asked her about the campaign.

"It's a fight. The Republican Party has never nominated a woman for this position before. It has always been an old boy network for these judgeships. The primary battle was brutal. And now the election will be close since some of the hacks are torn between loyalty to the Party and their hatred of me for knocking out their old boy. So, I make nice in every small town in the County, which covers a lot of territory. But getting the position would mean a great job. With a term of ten years, one reelection and I can reach a nice retirement age."

"How are the girls?" asked Dr. Gold.

"Julie finishes at Colgate this year and is applying to medical school while Sarah is a sophomore at Cornell studying computer science."

"No lawyers?"

"Watching Bill and I took care of that." They both laughed, sharing the moment since neither of Gold's own two college-aged children had shown any interest in following their mother into medicine.

"Well, you seem fine. Do you want your mammogram this year?" asked Dr. Gold.

"Why wouldn't I?" Sandra responded.

"You have no family history of breast cancer and the U.S. Preventative Services Task Force now recommends doing them when you are fifty. And then every other year."

"But we have been doing them every year since I was forty."

"That is true."

"What do you do?"

Dr. Gold smiled. "Like every actively practicing woman doctor over forty I know, counselor, I have my mammogram every year."

"Case closed."

"Good. We have already made a slot for you downstairs on your way out. I know you busy types."

MAMMOGRAM SCREENING FOR BREAST CANCER.

"Give yourself the gift of health. Get a mammogram." In the 1970s and 1980s, it seemed simple. Any doctor or nurse who worked in the years before mammograms remember the repeated heartbreaking stories of women with large cancers which destroyed their breasts and then took their lives. The mammogram was not perfect, but it worked. Breast cancers could be detected when they were smaller and lives saved. The American Cancer Society, radiology groups, and the activists starting the pink revolution joined to promote early detection.

There were some hurdles. Since mammograms embarrassed some women, specialized units with comfortable environments away from sick people were introduced, which later became "Breast Health Centers." The test could still hurt, but having a dedicated staff helped. Another less obvious problem was that the mammogram itself uses radiation which could theoretically cause cancer. Since early mammograms used higher doses of radiation and were not well standardized, they may have had a small risk of causing cancers. More modern mammograms, particularly digital mammograms, produce very little radiation exposure.

As the rates of screening mammograms rose, controversies developed over who should get them, when, and how often. Women have heard many different recommendations, all mixing science, medicine, statistics, emotion, money, and values. Since screening tests like mammograms are done in people without symptoms, the groups making these recommendations study the possible outcomes, which they divide into "true-positive," "false-positive," "true-negative," or "false-negative" results. Studying these different results is important in producing the final decisions about the use of the test, but is a complex undertaking.

A true-positive mammogram would seem to be the ideal goal: the test finds a cancer which is cured. Yet some true-positive mammograms detect cancers which cannot be cured and thus do not improve the survival of the woman. Other true-positives detect cancers that are irrelevant to that specific woman. Obviously, this could occur if she is elderly or has other medical problems limiting her life expectancy. Even if she is younger, mammograms detect some non-invasive breast cancers called ductal carcinoma-in-situ (DCIS)—cancer cells on the inside of the ducts. DCIS may take years to become an invasive cancer, may not progress, or the woman may die of other causes before the transformation occurs. This type of true-positive occurs more in older women. How should these results be factored into the decision to use the test?

The false-positive mammogram is a well-known possibility to women: the worrisome call back for more tests or a biopsy. How do we assign a value to this situation? If the extra mammograms or biopsies were life threatening, the analysis could be more coldly mathematical. But how do you value an afternoon out of work and a bruised breast? How about the anxiety?

The true-negative test is the most common results: a normal mammogram and no cancer. Yet if done in women at very low risk for breast cancer, the test wastefully offers reassurance about something which was not going to happen.

The false-negative mammogram is a devastating result: it provides false reassurance to a woman with cancer. Since mammograms detect only about 70 percent of breast cancers, some women with a negative mammogram are diagnosed with the disease. The false-negative mammogram has led some to add other methods of screening to mammography. MRI of the breast may detect more cancers, but it is a more difficult and costly test which involves the injection of a dye and has a higher false-positive rate. Screening ultrasound of the breast is possible but is a time-consuming test which is hard to standardize.

Over the years, many studies have compared women who undergo regular mammograms with those who do not have the test or do so less frequently. These studies usually report rates of cancer detection, stage, death from breast cancer, and death from all causes. Accurate information is difficult to collect and may change as technology improves, or with the inclusion of different groups of women. In general, the studies have generally shown that for women who are between fifty and seventy doing regular mammograms will save about one woman for every five hundred who participate. Fifty of the women will likely have more tests (false-positives). For women under fifty, it may take about fifteen hundred women to have regular mammograms to save a life. One hundred fifty will have more tests (false-positives). For women over seventy-five, nobody knows. These numbers do not answer questions like how many women will have cancers detected earlier and avoid chemotherapy or how many irrelevant cancers are found. A small army of scientists continue to argue over these numbers, but they are a reasonable starting point.[101]

What you do with these numbers reflects your values. The American Cancer Society, in the front lines of the fight against cancer, tends to support wider use of mammograms, even if it means more expense and trouble. Radiology and surgery professional societies do the same and often face criticism for their financial stake in the test. Activist groups eager to have tools to fight cancer are also usually supportive of more screening.

What about the United States Preventative Service Task Force (USPSTF)?[102] The USPSTF was authorized in 1984 by Congress to evaluate screening tests and preventative medications to determine if they should be part of primary care. Their recommendations are highly influential in determining patterns of care, insurance coverage, and evaluations of doctors and health care systems. The Affordable Care Act (Obama Care) emphasized the importance of the USPSTF recommendations. The USPSTF is composed of sixteen volunteer physicians from a variety of primary care fields who are appointed by the Director of the Agency for Healthcare Research and Quality (AHRQ), part of the Department of Health and Human Services. AHRQ is an organization of three hundred employees with a $500 million budget whose mission is to improve healthcare by promoting patient-centered research, safety, and accessibility.

The USPSTF evaluates an impressive range of subjects including mammograms, PSA testing, colonoscopy, aspirin use, routine physical exams, and counseling strategies for patients of all ages. The physician members of the USPSTF review studies in these various fields and reach conclusions. Their work is supported by the staff of the AHRQ and its experts in "evidence based medicine," who have a culture which influences their view of the data. The difference in recommendations between the USPSTF and the ACS and professional societies reflects their distinct viewpoints.

Which brings us back to mammograms. The USPSTF has recommended that mammograms be done beginning at the age of fifty and then only every two years. From their viewpoint, this strategy maximizes the percentage of positive findings, limits ultimately negative tests, and saves money. It reflects their values. The American Cancer Society recommends that women should have the opportunity to begin yearly mammogram at age forty, certainly begin at age forty-five and consider changing to every two years at fifty-five, continuing for as long as their health is good. This strategy will find more cancers at the cost of more testing—reflecting their values.[103]

For Dr. Gold, whose longstanding practice has about three thousand women between forty and fifty years old, sending them all for mammograms means that one or two more families in the community with school-age children will have mothers. The extra tests and biopsies are annoying, but not deadly. And saving money on mammograms to bet at the Saratoga Race Track seemed like false saving. So she kept ordering them.

The call came late that evening. Sandra had just returned from another indigestible political dinner in nearby Ballston Spa and was getting ready for an evening workout.

"Sandra, it's Stacey Gold. The mammogram you had today shows an area in the right breast which looks suspicious. It is very small, but you need a biopsy. I would like to arrange it immediately."

Shit, she thought, maybe I should have listened to the damn U.S. Preventative whatever. Maybe I can wait. No, take care of it now. She fought back a wave of angst mixed with fear.

"I'd like to think about it," Sandra answered with the instinctive caution of a politician. "You know I'm in the middle of this campaign and any health issues, particularly cancer, will be blood in the water for the political sharks. I might opt to go out of town, probably New York. I do not want anyone to know."

"I will tell the radiologist that you have made other arrangements and they will keep it confidential. You can pick up the mammogram on a disc from our office tomorrow and bring it with you when you go."

Sandra's husband, Bill James, arrived home an hour later. He was a trial lawyer whose face adorned every bus stop in the region, advertising his expertise in injury and disability law. Despite this widespread publicity, Bill James was not classically handsome, and they made a discordant couple. At fifty-two, he was five years older than Sandra. At five feet seven and two hundred and fifteen pounds, Bill was powerful but no match for her on the elliptical trainer. In contrast to her polished presentation, he had the legal persona of a pit bull. Their differences fueled speculation about the stability of their marriage, often manufactured by Sandra's admirers or detractors.

He walked in, his tie loose and jacket over his shoulder, obviously energized.

"We beat the bastards today," he announced, smiling until he saw her sitting on the sofa in unused workout clothes. "What's wrong?"

"Breast cancer," she said.

"Your mother?" he asked, looking concerned. Sandra's mother, a feisty eighty-year-old widow, lived nearby. Sandra was her only child, and her husband had died of heart disease ten years earlier.

"No, Bill. Me."

He sat down.

"What do we know?" he asked. She relayed the conversation.

"So, we don't yet know," he started, stopping when she held up her hand.

"I know. I heard the tone in Dr. Gold's voice."

"Well, we need a surgeon."

"I'm worried about the campaign. You know what it'll be like if they hear I have breast cancer."

"Forget the campaign. You're way better than those other two. And unless you want to make it an issue, no one has to know."

"I'd like to go to New York . . . Sloan Kettering if possible."

"Okay. That's it then . . .," he trailed off.

She looked pensive. "I remember a few years ago the Women's Bar held the annual meeting in Albany. They had two oncologists, a man from Albany Med and a woman televised from New York, talk about breast cancer. I'm pretty sure the woman on the screen was from Sloan Kettering. Anyway, there were about a hundred of us, all women lawyers. Karen Jones introduced the oncologist from Albany Med as the person who had seen the greatest number of the breasts in the room, including hers."

"Nice."

"Well, he took it well for such a nerdy guy. It was the end of the week, and most of us had had a drink or two, so it seemed funny at the time. But now, not so much. The point is, this is a pretty small community, and I don't want this out there."

"I understand. You leave that part to me. I'll make the arrangements and make sure they are kept confidential. You worry about your health. We'll do whatever we need to."

She nodded and hugged him, eyes unusually moist. "Thanks."

He looked hard at her. "Are you kidding?"

The appointment at Memorial Sloan Kettering Cancer Center was the following week. Sandra kept her usual work schedule, including an evening campaign address to a group of senior citizens at the Saratoga Springs Civic Center. Since it was a speech she had given many times, part of her brain was free to wander as she spoke. Sandra usually imagined swimming in an ocean, but that evening was different. She had recently seen a television advertisement for a retirement fund with people who had a number indicating their net worth hovering over their heads. As she was speaking, part of her imagined the audience members with a list of their medical problems floating over their heads. As she looked at them, she could see the names of various cancers. It was an unpleasant vision, but since she had always had the ability to partition her thoughts, it did not influence her presentation.

"Am I nuts?" she asked Bill that night.

"No, only under stress," he replied. "Don't you remember being told in public speaking when you got nervous to imagine the audience naked?"

"Yes."

"Well, this is the same type of thing. Knowing that group, you should be thankful that didn't happen."

The Evelyn H. Lauder Breast Center of Memorial Sloan Kettering Cancer in Manhattan boasted a therapeutic design, natural light, and soothing colors, but Sandra was most impressed that in one day she had another mammogram, ultrasound, breast MRI, and a needle biopsy. The rapid care suited her needs perfectly. Just get the damn thing out and get me back to the campaign, she thought. I do not have time for this.

The next morning, she met an equally well-organized and blunt breast surgeon, Dr. Jenifer Welsh.

"You have breast cancer," said Dr. Welsh. "The good news is that it is small, just over a centimeter in size by the MRI. You have two choices for surgery: either a lumpectomy and sentinel lymph node biopsy followed by radiation or a mastectomy. The only exception to this is if you have a mutation in the *BRCA1* or *2* genes. These are the genes that cause hereditary breast and ovarian cancer. If you have one of these gene mutations, then you should consider bilateral mastectomies. That is not very likely since there is no other cancer in your family, but we will do the test because of your young age. The results take about two weeks to come back. If the test is negative, it's an equal choice. Your choice."

"I understand. No matter what, I want the lumpectomy now," Sandra replied. "I am in the middle of a political campaign, and I can't take time out for a big surgery. If you tell me I need them, I can have the mastectomies later. Right?"

"Absolutely. Good. We will put you on the schedule at the end of next week."

"Will I need chemotherapy?"

"I don't know. That depends on the estrogen receptor and Her-2-neu status of the cancer. We will have those next week when you come back, and you can meet the medical oncologist then."

After they had left the City, the ride was quiet. Sandra turned to Bill.

"What now?" she asked.

"Now you get the damn thing out," he replied.

"No. I mean who do we tell? What about Julie and Sarah? My mother? Your parents? The campaign?"

"One at a time. Let's start with the girls."

Julie was their eldest, a bright, outgoing and no-nonsense biology major at Rutgers who had planned to be a physician since birth. Sarah was a reserved, intellectual young woman with a passion for mathematics which had taken her into theoretical computer science at Cornell. The girls were separated by two years and different in almost every aspect of their lives. Julie had her mother's sense of fashion and poise, while Sarah would wear the same t-shirt for days and ignore everyone while she relentlessly solved a problem. Despite their differences, the girls loved each other and kept in constant communication. Sandra had no doubt Julie would deal with the news calmly and effectively, but she was less certain of Sarah's reaction.

"I'm not sure exactly how to tell them," she began. "Over the phone seems impersonal. I want to be there to tell them, but visiting them is awkward and might give them the wrong impression that I am sick. And do we ask them to keep it a secret?"

"What would you say to them?"

"That I have a small cancer and will have surgery and be fine. Julie will probably know all about it, Sarah has always been harder to read. And I don't want to just drop this on her at the wrong time. You know how she is when she is working on something."

"I think you are underestimating her. They will worry but deal with it. And don't visit or call them, just text them."

"Text them I have cancer?" she interrupted.

"No, honey. Text them that you want them to call us when they have a chance. When they call, you explain it and tell them they need to keep it secret. They can talk to each other for support."

"Okay. I think I will tell my mother later this week. She can keep a secret."

"She's a peach. That leaves my parents," he noted. "What lies, if any, do we tell them?"

She smiled. Bill's parents were both in their mid-eighties. His father had been a well-known lawyer and mother a prominent socialite in Albany. Since his father's retirement fifteen years ago, they spent their summers in Saratoga and their winters in the gated world of Palm Springs. In Florida, their lives became a seemingly endless succession of lunches and dinners at the Club, charity parties, best ball matches, and complaints about the condition of the greens and fairways. Over the past few years, as they had become frailer and their circle of friends dwindled, the complaints had changed from the golf course to the service in the dining room. It was impossible to imagine them keeping a secret or being any help. Mercifully, they had recently completed their fall migration and were safely ensconced in their plush community, a world away from Sandra and the campaign.

"I vote for silence," she responded.

"Agreed. When they come back, we can deal with them, depending upon the circumstances. They probably won't even notice."

Sandra leaned back into the seat and closed her eyes briefly, a moment of fatigue passing over her. Snap out of it, she told herself. When she opened her eyes, she saw Bill looking intently at her.

"Why don't we take a break? We can talk more later," he offered.

"No," she said. "I'd like to think this through before we get home. About the campaign, the question is, do we tell anyone?"

"Not now. I think you should wait until after the surgery and you know what you will be facing, then get together with whoever you want from the campaign to discuss it. Otherwise, you are asking them to keep a secret longer than they need to . . . and you are not sure how big a secret it is. If you don't need chemo, the secret will be fairly easy to keep. If you do, it will be a harder situation, and they will need to understand more."

For the remainder of the week, Sandra was grateful for the distraction of her client's disordered lives. Exercise also worked.

"That help?" Bill asked one evening when he found her drenched in sweat in their basement exercise area.

"I feel good," she replied. "I can't believe I'm sick. It doesn't seem possible."

"I don't think sick is the right word. This is different."

"Yeah . . . You know that if that gene test is positive, I will need to have both breasts removed. And the girls will be in danger, too."

"It's unlikely," he reminded her. "But if it's positive, you will do what you need to do. And so will the girls. Did you text them yet?"

"No, I wanted a little more time. I thought tomorrow."

Sandra and Bill were together when Julie called the next evening.

"Hi, Mom. What's the matter?"

"Why do you ask?" she responded.

"You've never texted to call, so something must be up."

Sandra stuck her tongue out at Bill, who shrugged.

"Well, dear, I did not want to worry you, but I had my regular mammogram, and they found a small breast cancer. I am going to have it removed next week."

After Sandra had answered Julie's questions, Bill explained their decision to keep quiet.

"I understand. I'm glad Mom caught it early."

It was a few minutes later when Sarah called. She also took the news well and strongly approved of the plan to keep everything quiet. When the calls ended, Sandra turned to Bill.

"They both took it well," she said.

"You are their mother. Good genes there."

That night, Sandra awoke at 3:11 a.m. She watched the clock as Bill snored until 3:13 appeared, her special time. Once when Sandra had been a young mother and Bill was away, infant Sarah had been febrile. After an exhausting night, her sick baby finally fell asleep as the clock seemed frozen at 3:13. From then on, Sandra looked for those numbers. When she saw them this night, she sat up, found her slippers with her feet, pulled on her robe, and went downstairs. In the dark study, the modem lights flashed placidly until she sat and moved the mouse to wake up the bright desktop screen.

It's time to face this, Sandra thought. She typed in "breast cancer prognosis." Disturbing cartoons of ugly looking cancers in the breast appeared, drawn in bright colors which emphasized their power. They were shown spreading to the lungs, liver, or bones of bodies drawn in weak, faded colors. From this Sandra learned the staging of breast cancer. Stage I cancers were small and within the breast, usually cured. Stage II and III were larger or involved the lymph nodes, possibly cured. Stage IV meant the cancer had spread to other organs, unlikely to be cured. Sandra also learned that within each stage, some cancers grew rapidly and others that grew slowly, some that responded to chemotherapy while others were resistant. The explanation for this range of behaviors was called the "biology" of the cancer.

Predicting the biology or behavior of a breast cancer is the goal of pathologists who report the microscopic appearance of the cells as high grade (the most aggressive appearing), moderate or low grade (the least aggressive appearing). The 1970s produced tests to determine if breast cancers were stimulated by estrogen, meaning they were less aggressive and treated with anti-estrogen drugs like tamoxifen. In the 1990s, scientists discovered the Her-2-neu receptor on the outside of some aggressive breast cancers which spread rapidly but responded to treatment with the antibody Herceptin (trastuzumab). More recently the expression of various genes has given additional information about the behavior of some cancers. Despite these advances, the behavior of many breast cancers remains hard to predict.

Sandra realized she did not have enough information to learn her prognosis. Even if her cancer was small (which it seemed) and the lymph nodes were clear (which she hoped), she needed the grade, the estrogen and progesterone receptor status, and the Her-2-neu status. She might even need extra gene studies to know what she was facing.

She finished at 4:38 a.m. I won't remember this time, she thought, returning to bed as Bill still snored.

Sandra's information arrived in a phone call a few days later.

"Hello, Sandra. This is Karen James, Dr. Welsh's nurse." Her voice was clear and intelligent. Sandra's first thought was that belonging to Dr. Welsh did not seem to be an appropriate goal for a bright woman.

"You mean you work with Dr. Welsh?" she asked, trying to reframe the relationship.

"Yes, I'm her nurse."

Her nurse? Her belonging? Wait, give up this battle and listen to her, she thought.

"Okay, what's going on?"

"Well, Dr. Welsh asked me to call you and let you know that your *BRCA* genetic test was negative. She said that we expected that, but it's still good news. Dr. Welsh says you should keep the plan for surgery."

"Thank you," replied Sandra gratefully.

"You're welcome. See you next week."

"Wait," she said. "Do you have the other tests on the cancer cells? The estrogen receptor and Her-2 test?"

"Let me see . . .," Sandra could hear her typing. "Yes, they are done. The final report is all available. Do you want me to email it to you?"

Opening the email a few minutes later was surreal. The impressive heading "Department of Pathology" jumped out at her while her name and date of birth seemed to belong to someone else. As she quickly scanned the document, a blur of unfamiliar but ominous phrases rushed together: mammary, high-grade invasive, negative, core biopsy, millimeters, non-amplified.

Stop, she told herself. Handle this like you would a case. She clicked the print icon, waited for the printer to come to life, then exited out of her email account. Once she heard it hum, she stood up, grabbed her Rutgers mug, walked down the hall, and filled it with black coffee. When she returned, she could see the pages had printed. Ignoring them briefly, she cleared her desk, selected the sharpened pencil she would use to mark them, and sipped the hot coffee. Finally, she placed the three sheets across her desk and dispassionately wrote the key words.

"Eight-millimeter core biopsy, high-grade, nuclear grade 3, Bloom and Richardson Grade 9, estrogen receptor negative, progesterone receptor negative, and Her-2-neu non-amplified."

She looked over her notes, sipped her coffee, then briefly stared out the window. Once the part of her brain which had done the translation was finished, another part completed the analysis, referencing her night-time reading and reporting as if to one of her clients.

It is a bad cancer, stated that part of her brain. It better be small and the lymph nodes clear or we are in trouble.

"We will know soon enough," she answered herself aloud and again sipped her coffee.

That evening had been a rare lull in the campaign. Sandra reported the news and studied Bill carefully, looking for his reaction.

"So, it sounds like this is a small but fast-growing cancer. If you take it out now, the odds are it won't have spread anywhere else, right?" he summarized.

"True."

"And they are checking the lymph nodes to help confirm that."

"True."

"Are there any other tests they can do to check the rest of the body. PET scan?" he asked.

"I don't think that would show a few cancer cells," she replied. "If you had a growth somewhere it might show it."

"Sounds like we are still back to get the damn thing out," he nodded. "It scary stuff, but it sounds like you are going to be fine."

I hope, they both thought as they hugged each other.

The next week Sandra went to Memorial Sloan Kettering Breast Center for an injection of radioactive dye into the area of the breast which contained the cancer. The dye would travel to lymph nodes under the arm. The next day, Dr. Welsh would remove both the tumor and the nodes which contained the dye, Sandra's co-called "sentinel nodes."

THE SENTINEL LYMPH NODE BIOPSY: MORE LIMITS ON SURGERY.

The sentinel lymph node biopsy was an important step in the evolution of using less surgery to treat breast cancer. The first theories of how breast cancer spread held that the cancer cells invaded the lymph system then went into the lymph nodes under the arm (called the axillary region or axilla). From the lymph nodes, the cancer cells could "jump out" into the body's circulation. This theory led to the idea that removal of the lymph nodes would be useful to prevent the spread of the cancer. Surgeons therefore combined mastectomies with extensive attempts to remove all the lymph glands under the arms and sometimes the lymph nodes in the chest. Even in the 1980s, when lumpectomy and radiation became an alternative to mastectomy, surgeons still tried to remove many of the lymph nodes under the arm. The average woman has twenty to forty lymph nodes located in three levels of the axilla, with the highest (third) level being in the upper portion near the nerves and blood vessels that go into the arm. For many years, it was the mark of a good surgeon to be able to remove all these lymph nodes. The higher the count, the better the surgeon. A good "level three lymph node dissection" removed most of these nodes and counts of more than twenty lymph nodes in the surgical specimen were considered optimal.

There were problems with the standard lymph node dissection. The removal of so many lymph nodes could result in "lymphedema," the swelling of the arm resulting from an inability of the fluid in the arm tissue to drain into the lymph system. For some women, this condition left them with a swollen arm which was painfully heavy. On occasion, damage to the nerves could lead to severe chronic pain. For the pathologist, having to analyze twenty lymph nodes was no easy task. They would often simply cut the node in half and make a limited inspection of a few slides under the microscope, so a few cancer cells in a node could easily go undetected.

The other problem with the removal of the so many lymph nodes was that it did not help to cure the cancer. The theory was wrong. The ability of cancer cells to invade the lymph system made it more likely they could invade the blood stream and travel, but removing more lymph nodes did not prevent that spread. In the 1980s, surgeons began the use of more limited procedures called "lymph node sampling" or "level one lymph node dissection." Since these removed only the lower lymph node tissue, which usually held about ten nodes, the chances of lymphedema or nerve damage were much less. One important concern about limiting the lymph node dissection was the worry the cancers might skip the lower-level nodes and travel to the upper-level nodes, thus escaping detection. Pathologists meticulously mapped the lymph nodes removed in earlier extensive dissections and found these "skip metastasis" were very unusual, reassuring patients and doctors that if the lower nodes were clear, it was very unlikely the higher nodes would be infected.[104]

After the limited node dissection had become accepted, the next step in further reducing surgery was the sentinel node biopsy. In this procedure, a dye is injected near the cancer. The dye travels to the lymph nodes which collect fluid from that area. The first lymph nodes the dye reaches are called the sentinel nodes—like the military sentinel watching a section of a territory. Removing just these few nodes has less risk of complications and gives the pathologist more time to study each node, increasing the ability to detect even a few cells in the node. The first key question was if the sentinel lymph node biopsy was negative, could doctors and patients be sure the rest of the nodes were clear?

The answer came from a remarkable study. In the 1990s, a group of surgeons did the sentinel node biopsy on women with breast cancer, then immediately followed it with a regular lymph node dissection on the same woman. The results were impressive. If the sentinel node was clear, it meant that there was a 98 percent chance the higher nodes were not involved. The surgeons who did the study proved their point. The women in the study did not get any benefit. They had the dye injection, the sentinel node biopsy, then the limited node dissection. But by agreeing to this extra effort, these women allowed future generations of women to undergo this lesser surgery with confidence—a wonderful gift.[105]

The use of the sentinel node biopsy raised other questions. If the sentinel node was negative, the surgeon could stop. Removing more nodes would not give more information. But what if the node was positive? At the start, surgeons generally accepted that if the sentinel node was positive, they would remove the lower-level lymph nodes. If the sentinel node was found to be positive during the surgery on the preliminary "frozen section" look by the pathologist, the surgeon would do the larger surgery immediately. This meant that the woman would wake from anesthesia not knowing which procedure had been done. A generation earlier, some woman with breast lumps had entered the operating room not knowing if they would wake with only a biopsy or a mastectomy. This was certainly not that terror, but it was still stressful. If the lymph nodes looked clear on the frozen section but were later positive when a full analysis had been done, the woman would have the upsetting prospect of returning to the operating room for more surgery. Could these scenarios be avoided? Could surgeons possibly stop after the sentinel node biopsy, even if it was positive?

Not doing further surgery after a positive sentinel node biopsy was conceptually one of the most difficult steps in the evolution of breast cancer treatment. For many surgeons, it was one thing to leave the rest of the lymph nodes in place when the sentinel lymph node was clear, but leaving the nodes in place when the sentinel nodes contained cancer cells just seemed wrong. The answer came from a randomized study sponsored by the American College of Surgeons in which women with breast cancer underwent a lumpectomy and sentinel lymph node biopsy. If the sentinel node biopsy was positive, they then had either a limited lymph node dissection or no more surgery. Of course, they all then had radiation. The results were striking: there was no benefit to removing the extra lymph nodes even if the sentinel nodes were infected.[106] Why? Probably because the radiation eliminated any cancer cells in the lymph nodes under the arm. Women could now be treated with only removal of the tumor in the breast and a sentinel lymph node biopsy followed by radiation. Breast surgery had gone from its most radical to its most limited.

Following her injection, Sandra and Bill met Dr. Sun Chen, a young, small, and very dynamic Asian medical oncologist who spoke rapidly in clipped but definitive statements.

"Your *BRCA* testing was negative. So, good news. That means Dr. Welsh will do lumpectomy tomorrow. No need for bilateral mastectomy. We have the pathology from your biopsy. Your cancer is triple negative. You're young, so you take chemo. Dose-dense Adriamycin and Cytoxan followed by Taxol. It's eight treatments, one every two weeks, sixteen weeks. I know oncologists in Albany. You get it there. Radiation is after chemo."

"What about the lymph nodes?" asked Sandra.

"They don't change treatment for you. Prognosis only."

"But it's small, and that's intensive chemo," Sandra began.

"Biopsy measures eight millimeters but on MRI one centimeter. It's your best chance to live," responded Dr. Chen. "No question about it. You do it. I tell Dr. Welsh to please put in port, so you ready for chemo."

CHEMOTHERAPY AND BONE MARROW TRANSPLANT FOR BREAST CANCER: TESTING LIMITS.

Chemotherapy given after surgery to eliminate any cancer cells which may have spread elsewhere in the body is called "adjuvant therapy." Although it is now commonly used for many cancers, it was controversial when introduced in the 1960s. One first attempt at adjuvant chemotherapy in breast cancer came in 1968 when women who underwent a mastectomy received either a chemotherapy drug called thiotepa on the day of surgery and for two days following or a placebo. Overall the women given the drug had no marked improvement in cure rate, but later analysis showed that their cancers came back somewhat later and some with more advanced cancers might have benefitted. [107] [108] Although the results of this study were disappointing, there were some important lessons. Chemotherapy had a "biologic but not clinical effect," meaning the treatment did something interesting even if not meaningful for most patients. A second lesson was that the use of chemotherapy following breast cancer surgery would not be as dramatic a success as it was in Hodgkin's lymphoma.

In the mid-1970s, two famous clinical trials which tested adjuvant chemotherapy in women with breast cancer renewed hope. In the United States, Dr. Bernard Fisher and the NSABP tested a chemotherapy drug called melphalan given by mouth for five days every six weeks for two years. In Italy, Gianni Bonadonna and Umberto Veronesi tested a combination of the drugs cyclophosphamide, methotrexate, and 5-fluorouracil, called "CMF," given by mouth and vein for two weeks each month over a one year period. These treatments were given to young (pre-menopausal) women following surgery if cancer was in their lymph nodes. The chemotherapy modestly improved the cure rate and started the use of these adjuvant treatments.[109]

In the 1980s and early 1990s, the use of adjuvant chemotherapy was broadened to include older women and many younger women even when their lymph nodes were not involved. This was a period of intense experimentation in which thousands of women participated in many clinical trials. The CMF program had been one year long, but six months was found to be just as effective.[110] The combination of doxorubicin (brand name Adriamycin) and cyclophosphamide (brand name Cytoxan) in a program of four treatments given once every three weeks further reduced treatment time to three months.[111] This "AC" treatment was harsher in terms of nausea, vomiting, low white blood counts, and hair loss, but it soon became the standard across the country. The idea that more chemotherapy would be better was also proposed, a concept called "dose intensity," and it seemed to work in the laboratory. While some chemotherapy drugs (like doxorubicin) could only be given in slightly higher doses since they would damage the heart or other organs, doses of others (like cyclophosphamide) could be doubled or tripled. A series of clinical trials in patients compared higher doses of chemotherapy with regular or lower dose treatments. Unfortunately, the results with more chemotherapy were not better, although lowering the doses below the standard was worse. It appeared that once a minimum threshold of chemotherapy was reached, using a modestly higher dose did not help.[112]

Since a modest dose increase was not useful, what about a huge increase of seven to ten times the normal chemotherapy dose? There was lab data that this type of increase could maximize the killing of cancer cells. The problem was that it could also kill the patient, usually by destroying their bone marrow cells. The answer was the "autologous bone marrow transplant." In this procedure, bone marrow was removed from a woman and placed in the freezer. She was then given lethal doses of chemotherapy which would destroy her bone marrow. The woman was saved when she received her thawed bone marrow back. The massive doses of chemotherapy would kill any remaining breast cancer cells. In the war on breast cancer, this was the equivalent of dropping the atomic bomb.[113]

Being able to give "high-dose chemotherapy with autologous bone marrow support" or "bone marrow transplant" (BMT) was no easy task. The patient had to survive the chemotherapy, receive her bone marrow back and then wait for it to rebuild (or "engraft"). The initial high-dose chemotherapy could produce nausea, vomiting, allergic reactions, damage to the gastrointestinal tract, heart, lungs, kidneys, and brain. The woman had to be protected from infection until her bone marrow recovered and would need antibiotics, antifungal, and antiviral treatments as well as transfusions of blood and platelets. It was an incredibly complex medical procedure involving physicians, nurses, pharmacists, therapists, laboratory and blood bank personnel.

In the 1990s, major medical centers across the country began BMT programs, recruiting some of their best medical minds to perfect this technology. High-dose chemotherapy was used for other cancers like lymphoma, but very quickly breast cancer became the most common reason for doing the treatment. The treatment was given both to women with widespread breast cancer after it had been shrunk with regular dose treatments (metastatic breast cancer) and to women after surgery who had no obvious metastasis but had many lymph nodes involved (adjuvant treatment for high-risk cancer). These programs reported impressive improvements in the safety with very low deaths rates, although most women would still suffer significant side effects requiring hospitalization for several weeks.[114]

Enthusiasm for the new technology ran high, and dynamic physician leaders promoted their programs. The early results seemed to justify their optimism. When high-dose chemotherapy with bone marrow support was given to women after surgery who had many infected lymph nodes, the results seemed far superior to what was typical. Although true scientific testing was done in the form of a randomized clinical trial, most experts agreed this was the best treatment. The main obstacle was the $100,000 cost, a striking figure at the time, which led to insurance company objections. They argued that there was no proof that this expensive treatment was better than standard chemotherapy. Their intransigence set the stage for a battle which pitted the insurance companies on one side and a combination of hospitals, medical professionals, and breast cancer advocates on the other. In the court of public opinion, the insurance companies lost heavily. The media avidly followed women undergoing the heroic struggles against breast cancer that this technology symbolized. Eventually, the insurance companies lost in courts of law as well and the procedure became standard. By 1995, five thousand eight hundred women with breast cancer had undergone BMT, an impressive feat by a technologically sophisticated medical system.[115]

Unfortunately, BMT for breast cancer did not benefit the vast majority of patients who underwent the procedure. The initial successful reports were not randomized trials which treated women with BMT or standard chemotherapy by "flip of the coin." The key first studies compared the results of BMT with historical results. The randomized studies did not show a clear benefit to the procedure. Patients and many doctors were shocked. Although these randomized studies were not perfect, they spelled the end of BMT for breast cancer. Insurance companies, armed with this data, refused to pay, professional societies agreed, and there was no court in which to challenge these results. Over the course of a year or two, BMT programs across the country closed and many of their highly-trained physicians and staff returned to the world of regular dose chemotherapy. The obvious lesson was that BMT needed careful testing before its promotion in the real world since it resulted in unnecessary suffering. The less obvious lesson was that the premature use of BMT and the forcing of the insurance companies to pay for the procedure resulted in a backlash when the randomized studies did not show any dramatic benefit. All further research into BMT ended and medical science a lost opportunity. It is still possible that BMT was effective for a certain group of women with breast cancer, but we will never know. The baby may have gone out with the bathwater.

As some physicians were giving massive doses of chemotherapy to treat breast cancer, others were taking a different approach by using the new chemotherapy drug paclitaxel (Taxol). Initially found in the bark of the Pacific yew tree, paclitaxel was tested in women with widespread breast cancer. It did not cure but often shrank breast cancer dramatically. Paclitaxel killed cancer cells using an entirely new mechanism of action. While most common chemotherapies affected the DNA, paclitaxel damaged the microtubules, structures important for cell shape and cell division. In the late 1990s, a series of well-done clinical trials showed that adding paclitaxel (Taxol) to doxorubicin (Adriamycin) and cyclophosphamide (Cytoxan) ("AC-T") modestly improved the results for women given chemotherapy after their surgery.[116] It was another step forward.

The addition of paclitaxel (Taxol) to doxorubicin (Adriamycin) and cyclophosphamide (Cytoxan) set the stage for yet another advance termed "dose-dense chemotherapy." The "AC-T" (Adriamycin/Cytoxan followed by Taxol) had been given as a treatment every three weeks for eight times until a group at Memorial Sloan Kettering Cancer Center in New York proposed administering them only two weeks apart. In the laboratory, exposing cancer cells to the chemotherapy drugs more frequently resulted in more "cell kill," but many oncologists were afraid this would be too hard on the patient. Clinical trials proved this dose-dense treatment was more effective than the regular schedule. Although the patients found the treatment difficult, it was over more quickly. This was also another step forward.[117] By the end of the century, the sense was that the traditional chemotherapy programs for breast cancer were optimized. The new tools of molecular biology would be needed to move oncology forward.

Sandra remembered craving coffee the morning of her surgery, but not much else. Dr. Welsh told Bill the procedure went well, a nurse instructed him on her care, and they left the Breast Center late that afternoon. The bandaged wound on her right breast did not hurt, but she felt mild discomfort under her arm when she moved. The port site on the other side of her chest was fine. They returned to the Four Seasons where Bill helped her undress and get ready for bed.

"Not the model you married," she commented as he surveyed her bandages seriously.

"Don't you be running down the model I married, Lady. I was damn lucky to get her," he replied, still looking at the dressings carefully.

"You still think so? Even with all this?" she asked.

"Look," he said, "stop interrupting me while I am trying to be a good nurse and follow all the instructions they gave me." He fiddled with the tape near one bandage.

"There, that's better." He looked satisfied, then turned his attention to her. "Now that you won't bleed to death, do you want me to do the lovey-dovey stuff or tell you I always liked your ass most?" he said, giving her a little pinch.

"Bastard," she laughed.

They drove home the next morning. It was good to be back. The house and the yard looked somehow new, and Sandra found herself almost euphoric. She sent Bill to work the next day and when he returned she was doing campaign paperwork.

"Aren't you sore?" he asked.

"I'm a little sore under my arm and the tape over my chest itches, but I actually feel better, more energetic. Could it be that little cancer was sucking my energy? I really feel different. I didn't realize how tired I was, but now I feel like my old self."

"I guess," he responded, puzzled but pleased. "I wouldn't have thought something so small could do that, but I don't really know."

Sandra was good at compartmentalizing problems. Like Clinton, Bill would say to antagonize her. As she waited for her results, even she found breast cancer intruding into her life. Her morning drive to work on Union Avenue passed by the Saratoga Racetrack, where traffic would often be stopped to allow the Thoroughbreds to cross the street to the Oklahoma practice track. She enjoyed sipping her coffee and watching the beautiful skittish animals and their training riders. On her first morning back, Sandra was annoyed when her gentle reverie was interrupted by a radio advertisement for Mike's Hard Pink Lemonade supporting breast cancer research.

"It's good on so many levels," intoned the announcer, happily ignoring the incongruities.

Pink cigarettes will be next, she thought, the beauty of the horses lost as the moment was gone and her wound began to throb slightly.

A week later, Sandra and Bill returned to Dr. Welsh. She pronounced Sandra healing well, then turned to the pathology report.

"The cancer was one centimeter, under half an inch. The margins were all clear, and the lymph nodes were all clear."

"That's good news," beamed Sandra, relieved.

"Have your chemo, and you'll be fine," answered Dr. Welsh.

They left the office for their next consultation at Pieces & Biz, a New York City Salon specializing in hair for the stars and women undergoing chemotherapy. After they entered the sleek, windowed storefront, stylish mannequins sporting designer wigs of every imaginable style immediately surrounded them. For the woman who wanted to change her look, the possibilities were endless. A red beehive wig atop a head which bore a faint resemblance to Sandra drew Bills' attention.

"Don't even think about it," she warned as he raised his eyebrow. The arrival of her consultant, Jean Paul, saved him from further danger.

"Come sit with me, dear Sandra." He took her hands and guided her to a fashionable couch. He sat next to her, turned her toward him smoothly and motioned to Bill to sit on her other side.

"You, too, William."

"It's Bill." He sat down heavily next to Sandra.

"Surely it is, but we will have to work on that later. Today Sandra is my only priority."

While Sandra laughed, Bill chuckled despite himself. Jean Paul faced her and continued.

"Now Sandra, we have important things to do. You will be fighting that terrible 'C.' I'm sure you will win, dear," he said, still holding both of her hands. "But we must look good doing it. I understand you are in an election and need to look exactly as you do today even when you lose your hair."

Sandra nodded. Jean Paul moved her to a chair where he studied her hair in several different lights, stood up and ran his hand through it a few times. He then produced a series of wigs which she tried on until he was satisfied.

"When you return, the wig will be sized. You will need to stay with me for an hour or two while I do the final cut. No one will ever know you are wearing it."

Sandra nodded. "Thank you."

He turned to Bill and ran his fingers through the short, reddish-gray mop.

"William," he smiled. "If, heaven forbid, you ever need chemo, there will be nothing I can do."

"It's Bill," Bill deadpanned.

Jean Paul shook his head sadly and patted Bill's cheek. "Nothing at all."

They spent that night in New York. Since they had ridden the train, the next morning they sat in a quiet, nearly empty Amtrak car, eating bagels and drinking coffee. Sandra found the tastes that morning particularly vivid. Energized, she was ready to make plans. Bill, on the other hand, was absorbed with the beating the *Daily News* was again giving Elliot Spitzer. He had crossed paths with the former Governor at his political peak in Albany, and their meeting had not gone well. As Sandra watched him read, his satisfaction was obvious. He looked up and caught her eye.

"Enjoying yourself?" she asked.

"It's not my vengeance, but it'll do." He laughed, then paused. "I didn't mean to be a jerk, laughing while you've got this problem."

"Bill," she whispered, putting her hand on his arm to draw him close, then continuing in her polished courtroom voice. "Even if am on my death bed, you have my permission to laugh at that son of a bitch." She abruptly pulled away and returned to her bagel, leaving him alone and stunned for a minute.

He picked up his paper, laughing. "Elliot," he said loudly enough for her to hear, "I only need her."

A few days later, Sandra and Bill met with Dr. Matthews, who reviewed the history and treatment plan.

"Well," he started, "you are very likely cured by the surgery, but we cannot be sure. We know that chemotherapy in this situation improves the results. They have recommended the aggressive plan that they developed."

"Are they biased?" asked Bill, the slight tension in his voice allowing Dr. Matthews a faint glimpse of how he could be a formidable foe in the courtroom.

"Probably not in a legal sense," Dr. Matthews smiled. "They favor this treatment from an intellectual viewpoint. They really believe in it. As you get closer to New York—the center of the universe, the more you find aggressive medical care. In other parts of the country, you might find a more modest chemotherapy program offered."

"What do you think?" asked Bill.

"I agree with them. A young woman should get every statistical benefit possible. If you were older or had medical issues, we might think differently. We can certainly administer this treatment here. We are a small enough office to work the schedule so you will have privacy. We do that for many people in the community. It's hard to tell exactly how you will react, so I can't tell you how it will affect your campaign. I think you will be able to do much of it, but I would leave the first week as clear as possible until we see your pattern."

Sandra invited her campaign manager, Janice Simmons, and her close friend, Georgia Williams for lunch. Janice was a lawyer in the Republican party who had pushed hard for Sandra's nomination. Georgia, an English professor at Skidmore College currently on sabbatical, was a rare collegiate libertarian critical of Democrats and Republicans alike. The three had previously agreed not to discuss campaign business while eating, so the talk revolved around families and children. Over coffee, Sandra relayed the news of her breast cancer.

"The bottom line is that this is very curable, but I need four months of chemotherapy, which, of course, starts now and goes past election day. The question is how do I handle it? Do I let anyone know? Do I try to keep it secret?"

Janice started. "The campaign is in good shape. The rank and file Republicans are upset with Johnson for going on the Conservative ticket. He may get some of our votes, but I still think we win if we keep going. But we need to keep you in front of those small local groups that he is going to play to. If you let up, well, I don't think Johnson can win, but he might bleed us enough to let Smith sneak in."

Sandra stuck out her tongue. "I'm already pretty sick of eating chicken at every small-town meeting, and I haven't even started the chemo yet."

Janice laughed. "But it is the issue. We win if you can keep this going. The old boys need to see you in person and shake your hand if they are going to feel good about giving up on Johnson."

"What if they know I am getting chemotherapy?" asked Sandra.

"Well, usually medical issues hurt candidates," said Janice, "but we could probably make breast cancer different. We could cloak you in pink and turn it into a cause which might play well with some groups. It's still a hard sell, but it probably beats other illnesses. You might even get a few sympathy votes from Democratic women."

"Do you have a choice? Can you keep it secret?" asked Georgia.

"I think so," replied Sandra. "I will be getting my treatments at a small office where I can be treated in a private room."

"You'll lose your hair?"

"Yes, but I have ordered a human hair wig that looks identical."

"Good thing you're an upstate Republican," commented Georgia. "Those boys will never know what they are looking at. It might be harder to fool a room of downstate Democratic women. But how you will feel? Can you keep up with the campaign and stress?"

"I'll do what I have to. I won't be in the hospital unless something unusual happens."

"Then I think that is the right answer," replied Georgia. "As much as we like to think it doesn't matter, cancer still scares people. And your opponents will use that. Johnson will say it doesn't matter with a wink and a nod to the old boys who will jump ship and vote Conservative with no problem while they forget about their own rotting prostates. And worse, Smith and her liberal friends will have surrounded you with self-righteous sympathy which will be even worse for your campaign than Johnson's crap because it will make them look good while you have the cancer."

They all paused for a moment. Then Sandra spoke.

"That's a bit harshly put, but I agree. Besides, I've made my career as a lawyer, and I don't want to suddenly be identified as a breast cancer patient."

After a quiet moment, Georgia spoke again. "But, Sandy, the real issue isn't the campaign. What we really want is for you to be okay. You can forget this race if you want." Janice nodded.

"I don't want to. This cancer will hopefully just be a brief period of my life. I don't want it to control everything else."

"Good," said Georgia. "If there is anyone who can do that, it's you. And if you are going to do all this, you'll need an extra driver to get you to all those treatments and meetings. It's a good thing I'm free, although some poor parents are paying tuition to support me."

Sandra's first treatment was at seven-thirty in the morning. Bill brought her.

"How are you doing?" asked Dr. Matthews.

"Fine," she replied. "I just want this over."

"Sure. It will be good to know what you are facing. Did you have any questions after the teaching session?"

"No. Let's go."

Sandra was treated in a corner room. The large window looked out over the woods while in the distance movement on a busy road provided some life. Sandra felt a pinch as "her nurse" inserted the needle into the port. It's okay if she belongs to me, Sandra thought.

"You can put the numbing cream on next time if that hurt," Rebecca Lotito noted, referring to the lidocaine cream which many patients used.

"That little pinch is not worth the mess," Sandra answered.

First came the anti-nausea medications, clear liquids which produced no sensation when put into the intravenous line. Then came the Adriamycin, easily identifiable by its bright red color. This Rebecca injected over about fifteen minutes, watching both Sandra and the syringe carefully. Sandra found herself staring at the red liquid it as it entered the tubing then moved upward into her chest.

"Strange, isn't it?" Rebecca noted.

Sandra nodded. She disliked seeing the red liquid entering her body.

"How long will it stay inside me?" she asked.

"Most of it is gone pretty fast," replied Rebecca. "There will be very little in your blood by the end of today. You might see some red in your urine. The small amount in the cells is what kills the cancer. That will keep working for days."

Sandra nodded.

"Do you have kids?" asked Rebecca, changing the conversation. They compared notes until the syringe was empty. Sandra welcomed the distraction as Bill semi-read *The Wall Street Journal*.

Next up was the Cytoxan, a clear solution which produced no obvious sensation when infused.

"This one is not so bad," Sandra commented.

"True," replied Rebecca. "The lack of color helps. We will give you some extra fluid to make sure you flush out your kidneys and bladder. Remember to drink today."

The treatment finished by ten-thirty. Bill and Sandra left the office through the back entrance and returned home.

"You can go to work," she informed him. "I feel fine."

She vomited as his car left the driveway. It came on suddenly, then was gone. Over the next few days, Sandra had a mildly nauseous feeling despite her medications. The white cell boosting shot called Neulasta which she received the day after her treatment made her bones ache. She was tired but kept a steady half-time work and exercise schedule each day.

A week after her treatment she returned to the office for a visit with the Nurse Practitioner, Angela Pagano.

"Your blood counts are good, for our world. Your white blood count is low, but not dangerously. Your red blood count and platelets are just slightly low. So, from the blood viewpoint, you tolerated the chemo well. How about the rest of you?"

"I only vomited once, but have had mild nausea most of the week."

"That nausea is a problem," replied Angela. "Our medicines are very good with the vomiting, but the nausea is tricky. Sometimes cutting down the acid in your stomach helps. We can give you a stronger antacid pill, or you can take Tums. Many women also find that keeping some food in the stomach helps, you just need to watch out for extra calories. Some women try ginger products."

"I hate to take more medicine. I'll probably just live with it. Today seems better."

"Usually it wears off by the second week. How is your energy?" asked Angela.

"I was tired, but I'm lucky I can control my work week. I made sure this week was easier and cut back a little on my exercising."

"Good. Keep up the exercise but don't overdo it and don't measure yourself against how you were a few months ago. Just keeping up a regular schedule is great, even if the intensity is much less."

"I read somewhere that exercise and keeping your weight down helps keep the cancer away," Sandra noted.

"Yes, well it might help to a small degree, but who really knows for any one person. For sure we don't want women to feel that if they go through all this surgery, chemo, radiation, raise their children, work, do the dishes, keep the house, and manage to keep their marriage intact, they are failures if they gain a few pounds or don't make it to the gym every day. We also don't want them to feel like failures if they don't get to the nutritionist, Reiki practitioner, lymphedema specialist, cancer psychologist, and have time with the therapy dog."

Sandra laughed. "Put that way it does sound like a lot."

"It is a lot," Angela replied. "Our advice is to keep living the life you enjoyed before you had cancer. Get in, get the treatment, and get out of here. You also have the added burden of trying to keep this secret. That makes it harder to get support."

Sandra nodded. "I'll manage. I've got a great inner circle."

A week later Sandra's second treatment had just finished when Bill re-entered the treatment room after taking a phone call. He sat down in the chair across from her; his rare somber look was alarming. Her first thought was for the girls.

"I have some sad news," he said. "Kelly Smith died unexpectedly last night. They announced it this morning."

"My God, what happened?"

"They think an aneurysm in her brain burst. I heard from Dan Jones that last night she developed a severe headache then collapsed at home. They brought her to St. Peter's, but she was gone."

"Oh, God. Her poor children and husband . . ."

They sat silently together.

"It doesn't make much sense, does it?" she asked. "Here I am getting chemotherapy, worried about how I will get through the election, thinking I'm the sick one, and she dies."

He nodded.

The wake was four days later. Sandra felt time warp on that beautiful fall evening as they pulled into the modern funeral home in nearby suburban Clifton Park. Attendants directed them to a parking space while a police car with its lights flashing slowed passing traffic. As they walked across the pavement, they saw both friends and rivals in somber dress. They took their place in line, exchanging condolences with those nearby. Karen Jones, a prominent Albany lawyer who had been head of the Capital District Women's Bar Association and a well-known breast cancer survivor and advocate, approached Sandra and Bill.

"What a terrible shock. I'm sure it must be strange for you here tonight, Sandy. One minute you are trying to beat her and the next she is gone."

Sandra nodded. "It is hard to understand," she agreed.

"Kelly was very good to me when I had my cancer." Karen continued. "And later she always helped me with the Bar's Cancer Support Group. I remember I always thought I would be the one who was gone and now I've beaten the cancer, and she dies . . ."

Sandra paled. "You really can't make any sense of these things, Kelly."

"I feel bad for her family and the kids," continued Karen. "I remember when I had my treatments thinking I would never see my kids married or be a grandmother . . . that Jim would have to do it all alone, or worse, with another woman."

Bill moved to interrupt and wedged himself between them.

"How's Jim? Is that him over there?" He pointed at a man obviously searching for someone.

"It is him. Thanks, Bill. Bye Sandy, I'll see you inside."

The line moved slowly. When they entered the hall, the pleasant outside breeze vanished, replaced with a warm and oppressive air laden with the powerful fragrance of years of flowers. Pictures of Kelly Smith and her family on the display boards and screens chronicled a full and loving life. The extended family clung together, variously hugging or crying as they tried to comfort each other. Near the casket, the immediate family looked dazed as they greeted the many mourners. Bill and Sandra made their condolences and exited quickly, avoiding attention. Bill had his arm around Sandra, his expression keeping away those who might have otherwise approached. Outside they made a wide path around the local evening news reporter. As they reached the car, Georgia and her husband approached.

"Good work, Sandy," she said seriously. "Now get out of here."

After the quiet drive home, they sat together on the back porch as the sun set. Bill sipped a scotch and Sandra a green cancer-fighting smoothie from the Vitamix. She looked down at the green sludge, then at his deeply colored scotch. He handed her the rest of his drink, and she sipped it gratefully. A car came up the driveway, announced by the crackling of the stones Bill insisted they keep instead of blacktop.

"Who is that?" she asked. Bill smiled as the girls came in together.

"What are you two doing here?" she asked happily, hugging them both.

"We wanted to see you, and it seemed like a good time," said Julie. Sarah nodded.

The coolness of the fall night air had replaced the warmth of the evening, so they regrouped in the shelter of the living room with coffee and cookies. Sandra directed the conversation towards the girl's lives, and they caught up on collegiate life, welcoming the distraction of professors, exams, and a few scandals. When he judged the portion of the update suitable for him complete, Bill retired and left the women curled up together on the big sofa.

Julie turned the conversation towards her mother.

"Mom, we were sorry to hear about Mrs. Smith. We didn't know her, but it was very sad." Sarah nodded.

"It was very sad and shocking, too," agreed Sandra. "She seemed so healthy. I didn't know her well and obviously didn't agree with her on everything, but I admired her. I feel very sorry for her family."

Julie pushed on. "I'm sure it was hard for you, too, going through all your treatments and then having this happen. Particularly because no one really knows what has happened to you." Sarah nodded again, looking at once both serious and frightened.

Sandra paused for a moment and sipped her coffee reflectively.

"It's very thoughtful of you to say that. It has been hard to face my own treatments and fears. There have been moments when I felt panicked. But we all have these challenges in our lives, and I am so lucky to have your father, you, and some very special friends to help. You are right. To have this happen to Mrs. Smith somehow made it almost surreal, so I'm so happy to have both of you here."

"Will you tell people now?" asked Julie. "I don't mean to sound terrible, but Mrs. Smith's dying means you will definitely win the election, right?" She paused. "I know that sounds horrible."

"No, dear. Her death was awful, and no one wished it, but you are correct. It is possible there will be another person named to run in her place, but I am not even sure if they can be put on the ballot at this late date. I hope so, for the Smith family. It would be very hard to see her name on the election ballots and reported on the news. But it is very likely I will win now."

"So why keep it secret?"

Sandra smiled inwardly at her earnestness.

"Okay, honey, let's think about this. Why tell people now that I have cancer? Let's ask the key question." She paused.

"Whose needs are we meeting?" They chorused the oft repeated question used by Sandra's mother whenever an action was to be judged. They stopped to refill their coffee and take an extra cookie while they prepared their answers.

"I'll try," said Julie. "I think it would meet the needs of women with breast cancer if you went public. As you said before, this area is still a bit backward and seeing a woman doing well with this disease would be inspiring. It might keep other women who have the disease from giving up on their jobs and goals. I think it would meet your needs because people would understand how hard this has been for you. You deserve credit for this."

"What about the Smith family and their friends?" asked Sandra. "How would this affect them?"

"I'm not sure. Why would it?" replied Julie.

"It would hurt them," said Sarah abruptly. Sandra nodded.

Julie looked puzzled. "How?" she asked.

"It will take something away from them right now," answered Sarah slowly. "They have lost their mother and friend. You shouldn't take the moment away from them, too. I think it will almost be a 'me too' type of thing. Only not quite."

Sandra nodded. "That is what I also thought, Sarah." She turned to Julie. "I agree with what you are saying about being an example for women, but I am concerned that, even if I wanted that role, it might not be the right time."

"I didn't think of it that way. You are certainly a politician in some ways, but not others." Julie seemed satisfied.

But it was Sarah who would not let it end. "Even if it was okay from that viewpoint, I don't think I would want everyone to know. I'm not like you, Julie," she paused.

Julie responded quickly, smiling and tugging on her designer blouse, which contrasted with Sarah's faded Cornell tee shirt. "You think?" They all laughed.

"Seriously," Sarah continued. "I'm all for fighting for women, but I would have trouble if everyone knew my medical history. I could not do that. It's too private."

"Sure, I get that," answered Julie, who knew that Sarah, despite her reserve, was a tenacious advocate for women in science. She had been the only girl in her high school in computer science, ignoring comments from the boys in the class and equally ignorant remarks of both sexes afraid of hard science. Fatty, Sarah's name for the chauvinistic, protuberant, and slightly oily computer teacher, had once told her there would be more girls in class when the computers could talk. It was clear that her programs had to be twice as good as the boys to receive the same grade. Despite the testosterone laden environment,

Sarah had persevered. She was simply better and harder working than the boys. And, as Sarah pointed out, she spent no time on pornography. In college, Sarah had found a more welcoming atmosphere and even a few women professors with whom she bonded. In the summer, she worked teaching computer science to high school girls.

"It's even more than my medical history," added Sandra. "For me, keeping this quiet was the right thing even without the campaign. I don't want to be known as a woman who had breast cancer. I want to be known for who I am—a lawyer, hopefully a judge, your mother, and Dad's wife. I guess those are my needs."

"That's the answer then, Mom," said Julie as Sarah nodded.

The next morning as the girls slept, Sandra relayed the conversation to Bill.

"Sounds like they came down about as you would expect. Julie more outspoken and Sarah more private."

"What about you? What do you think?"

"I think you should be the judge, so to speak," he replied, laughing as the bagel she threw hit him square in the chest. He caught it and bit off a piece, looking satisfied.

9:20 John Evans: Pancreatic Cancer

John Evans still looked strong. Despite two months of intensive chemotherapy, his face was still hard, jaw square, posture straight, and the muscles in his forearms arms were still defined. He appeared every bit the athlete he was, making it hard to believe that within this sixty-two-year-old man grew a pancreatic cancer.

His week began each Monday at 6:00 a.m., training hard-core, middle-aged tennis fanatics who needed a pre-work endorphin release and the occasional high school student who wanted extra practice. He awoke 4:30 a.m., his eyes invariably opening just before his twenty-year-old square black travel alarm would click on and emit its high-pitched squeal. Years ago, his wife Caroline had tried to get him a new music alarm, but he refused. Later she tried to program his cell phone, but again he refused. There was a satisfaction in pressing the button on the top of the alarm and silencing it before it had a chance to cry. Breakfast was a single Thomas English muffin with strawberry preserve and coffee lightened with skim milk.

His early morning workouts were in a branch building of the YMCA, a low-level structure fashioned of corrugated aluminum located near the Wall Mart which fronted a vast parking lot, deserted at that hour. The lobby of the Y was old while the changing rooms contained rusted lockers and leaking water-stained fixtures. The bleak conditions were perfect for this no-nonsense program. Quiet stretching and warm ups led to the repetitive slamming of the balls building in intensity according to his carefully composed plan which pushed these athletes to their limits. Later in the morning, he would direct different groups. Middle-aged, non-working mothers from affluent Taylor Drive played at their plush homeowner's association clubhouse and compared notes about where they would have lunch. Seniors enjoyed tailored injury prevention exercises followed by a spirited game of pickle ball. In the afternoons, he coached the Saratoga High School Boys Tennis team.

In college, John had been an All-American Division I tennis star and entertained the professional circuit before realizing that he made the most of his talent and was not genetically programmed to reach that level. A brief stint in the corporate world led him to Saratoga High and almost thirty years of teaching American history and coaching. Caroline had been an English teacher in the school. They married after a brief courtship and raised two children. He was highly regarded by his students for his honesty as he reported both their talent and effort with precision. He always had a plan. At fifty-five, he retired from teaching and continued a highly successful second career as a coach and private trainer.

Nine months ago, he had noticed the first vague sense of heartburn, easily quelled with Mylanta. He changed his coffee from Starbucks to Dunkin' Donuts and, for a month or two, his symptoms were better. When they worsened, he made an appointment with Dr. Josh James, his primary physician who had been one of his first athletes at Saratoga High.

"Hello, coach. It's nice to see you." He would always be coach.

John relayed his symptoms. His examination was normal.

"Well, you certainly look great," concluded his former student. "But we should send you to the gastroenterologist for an endoscopy. This type of heartburn can be the sign of esophageal or gastric irritation or ulcers. It's important to know if that is the case. While we are waiting, I want you to try some Nexium." He paused before continuing. "I also want you to have a CT scan of the abdomen. I just want to be sure there is nothing else more serious going on."

The normal result of the CT scan was reassuring. His appointment with the gastroenterologist was in three weeks. The Nexium had worked, and he briefly considered canceling the appointment, but his constitutional drive to stick with a plan prevailed. His meeting with the Physician Assistant was uneventful, and an endoscopy was scheduled for two weeks later. By the time of the test, the discomfort had returned, and he was glad to be getting an answer.

The endoscopy took place in the modern building owned by the local gastroenterology group, a site dreaded by those over fifty who had not yet had their colonoscopies. A bright-eyed, young woman took John's information in a private cubicle. The modern waiting area included abundant information on colon health and treatment of heartburn. Behind this pleasant façade lay "the factory," an assembly line of stretchers containing patients in various states of sedation, all hoping not to be recognized by their neighbors. John was up to date on his colonoscopy, so he was spared the dreaded bowel cleansing prep and simply did not eat after midnight. His test went smoothly. Sensitive to the sedatives, he promptly fell asleep. When he awoke, the cheerful gastroenterologist reported the results.

"Good news. We found some minor irritations in the esophagus which should be easily treated with medication. I did some biopsies, and we will see you in the office next week to review the results."

Caroline was anxious about the good news. "Honey, I've never known you to have these symptoms before and you have been taking the medication. It just doesn't make sense that a few irritations could cause this . . ."

His appointment a week later was with the senior gastroenterologist in the group, Dr. George Arthur. When Caroline expressed her concerns, Dr. Arthur agreed.

"It is sometimes hard to sort out this type of complaint. You do have some gastric irritation, but gall bladder disease is also a possibility. Let's double your medications and get an ultrasound of the gallbladder. Call me in two weeks and let me know how you are feeling."

The ultrasound of the gallbladder was normal and doubling the medicine did not help. In fact, the symptoms worsened into a gnawing pain which spread into his back began and woke him at night. When she found him sitting in the chair in the living room, Caroline was panicked.

"This is not right. Dr. Arthur said to call him and let him know how you are doing. Promise me you will call him."

Another visit with Dr. Arthur led to more blood work and an MRI. The call came that night.

"John, I have some bad news. There is a mass on your pancreas, and we need you to see a surgeon. We have two choices in the area. One is at Albany Med and the other at St. Peter's. Or I can send you to Mass General in Boston."

"I have always liked Albany Med, but if you feel I need to go to Boston, I will."

Dr. Gordan Yung was caring but blunt.

"This looks like a cancer of the head of the pancreas. We need a special CT scan done here with a pancreas protocol to see if this is resectable. The main question will be whether it involves the superior mesenteric vein. If it does not, we will go ahead with surgery. I also want you to have an endoscopic biopsy with Dr. Gold. We will meet after those are done and decide."

"What if it can't be resected?" asked John.

"Then we will give you two to three months of chemotherapy to shrink it, then another CT."

PANCREATIC CANCER AND THE WHIPPLE.

The pancreas is a mysterious organ, often neglected in daily life. The best known of its functions is to secrete insulin into the bloodstream to control blood sugar levels. When this fails, the result is diabetes. Less well known is that the pancreas also secretes highly caustic juice containing powerful enzymes into the small intestine to help with the digestion of food. This enzyme-rich juice must be kept away from the tissue of the pancreas and nearby structures. Occasionally the secretion of this juice is blocked by gallstones, and it backs up into the pancreas. Sometimes the juice leaks into the pancreatic tissues from inflammation, usually caused by alcohol or a medication. The result is pancreatitis, a severely painful burning of the tissues by the enzymes which can incapacitate a person.

The pancreas is about six inches long and has three parts. Beginning in the right upper abdomen is the bulbous head which nestles into a curve of the small intestine, then the body which passes behind the stomach, and the thinner tail which reaches the spleen on the left side. Running down the middle of the pancreas is the main duct which collects the juice and carries it into the small intestine at the head of the pancreas. The pancreas lies at the crossroads of many of the body's critical supply lines. Partially digested food leaving the stomach passes by the pancreatic head on the start of a journey through the twenty-five feet of the small intestine. Bile from the liver which aids the digestion of the food empties into the small intestine alongside the pancreatic juice. The aorta passes the middle of the pancreas while branches of the main arteries supplying blood to the liver, stomach, intestines, and spleen run nearby. Critical veins, including the inferior vena cava and portal vein, add to the complexity. The whole area connects to the nervous system through a complex web of nerves from the celiac plexus. The many structures in this area make it difficult to examine using a CT scan or MRI. And anything that goes wrong affects multiple systems.

Most pancreas cancers start in the glands or ducts that secrete the enzymes and are called adenocarcinomas (adeno meaning glands). Rarely the cancers can start from other cells in the pancreas and are less aggressive. The cause of most cancers of the pancreas is not known. Smoking raises the risk. Some families have a genetic predisposition, including those with some *BRCA* mutations associated with breast and ovarian cancer.

Pancreatic cancers grow silently when they are small and confined to the pancreas. Symptoms develop when the cancers enlarge and spread. As they grow and invade the surrounding nerves, a burning pain going through to the back is common. Jaundice develops when the cancer blocks the biliary system and prevents the normal flow of bile from the liver to the intestine. Sometimes the small intestine itself can be blocked, leading to starvation and vomiting. As the cancers spread elsewhere through the blood, fatigue and weight loss are common.

Cancers of the pancreas are deadly. Two grim statistics tell the story: the number of new cases each year about equals the number of deaths, and the 5-year survival rate is 4 percent. Surgery can cure some patients with pancreatic cancer, but the operation is among the most difficult to perform because of the complex anatomy. The surgeon must remove the portion of the pancreas which contains the tumor without damaging the other structures or causing a leak of the toxic pancreatic juice or bile. Most commonly the cancers start in the head of the pancreas, meaning that area and a section of the nearby small intestine called the duodenum must be removed. If the cancers start in the tail of the pancreas, only that part of the pancreas must be removed, and the operation is somewhat less complex.

Early surgeons were taught that God had placed the pancreas in the back of the abdomen so that no one would operate on the organ. Even modern surgical residents learn the three rules of "eat when you can, sleep when you can, and don't mess with the pancreas."[118] One of the earliest successful surgeries for pancreatic cancer was performed in 1898 by William Halsted, the surgeon famous for pioneering the mastectomy for breast cancer. Halsted was Surgeon-in-Chief at the Johns Hopkins Hospital and had an interest in disorders of the gallbladder and bile system. He was among the first surgeons in the U.S. to remove gallstones, performing an amazing technical and filial act when he did this surgery on his mother. Halsted later used his skills in surgeries of the biliary system to remove a pancreatic cancer from a sixty-year-old woman in a series of procedures. Although she died a few months later, Halsted began the process of surgically "messing with" the pancreas. In 1909, a German surgeon named Walther Carl Eduard Kausch performed the first modern procedure, but for unclear reasons history never assigned him proper credit. That recognition came to Allen Oldfather Whipple, the Surgeon-in-Chief of Columbia Presbyterian Medical Center in New York, who advanced the surgery in the 1930s and 1940s.[119] Whipple reportedly performed his first operation as an improvisation when he was demonstrating the resection of a gastric (stomach) cancer to visiting surgeons and realized the patient actually had pancreatic cancer.[120] Whipple's final one-step procedure was a surgical tour-de-force which removed the head of the pancreas and nearby duodenum then re-attached the pancreatic and bile ducts back to the small intestine. The "Whipple" became the standard for surgical treatment of most pancreatic cancers. Since Whipple had a great interest in training future surgeons, it is appropriate that this distinguished surgeon is credited with teaching how to mess with the pancreas.[121] The Whipple for pancreatic cancer has been improved, and with modern supportive care, experienced surgeons can do the procedure safely. Since it is among the most difficult operations with the potential for serious complications, it is performed only on otherwise healthy people. The main problem is that most patients with pancreatic cancer cannot have the surgery because the tumor has spread to other parts of the body or invaded the many structures near the pancreas. Of one hundred people with pancreatic cancer, only about fifteen will be able to have the Whipple. Of those, three or four are cured—slim odds. Since the Whipple is the only chance for cure, patients with pancreatic cancers which cannot be removed often seek treatment with chemotherapy and radiation to get them to the surgery. It is a difficult journey, and very few reach the conclusion they so desperately desire.

John had the second upper endoscopy with a biopsy at Albany Medical Center. In contrast to the upbeat factory, this waiting area had a bleak institutional look and held sicker patients, some pale and faintly yellowed. As they entered the waiting room, John felt Caroline recoil slightly and took her hand. The reception window was covered with signs written with varying degrees of grammatical correctness, some hand-printed in large, black, block letters. The window slid open to reveal a young, bored woman.

"Hello, I am John Evans. I am here to see Dr. Gold for an endoscopy."

She looked up blankly. "Insurance card and ID, please."

She left with the cards and returned a few minutes later, handing them back with additional forms.

"Have a seat and fill these out. Someone will be with you shortly." The window shut.

They took one of the few remaining pairs of seats together. As John completed his paperwork, Caroline looked up. Directly across was a middle-aged man of immense proportions who overflowed his chair. He was apparently asleep, head lolled to one side with several areas of droll easily visible on his faded blue and holed Yankees shirt. Two massive, white legs with thickened patches of peeling, red skin and several bandaged, oozing ulcers ended in the largest and most disgusting, untied sneakers she had ever seen. To his left sat a slightly less massive and somewhat healthier but equally unkempt woman working a smartphone. The surly-looking, obese boy of middle-school age mimicking her actions on his own phone completed the family portrait. A few seats away, a well-dressed, young black woman held a gorgeous sleeping baby. The end of the row was occupied by a frail, older Asian man wearing a tired suit which only partially hid his distended belly, accompanied by his worried looking wife. Similar scenes were repeated in each of the several seating areas in the harshly lit large room.

Caroline looked down at her husbands' powerful forearms as he wrote, precisely filling each blank. I don't understand, she thought. What are we doing here?

John completed his paperwork and returned to the window. After a minute, it opened. He tried to hand over the forms but was rebuffed by the flat voice.

"They get those when they call you." The window closed again.

John returned to his seat. They held hands as the bleakness of the waiting room isolated them. After another thirty minutes, they went into the procedure area where John put on a gown to replace his shirt and waited by a stretcher for the arrival of Dr. Gold, a pleasant, reassuring man.

"I will try to get a biopsy for you and Dr. Yung. You are in good hands with him."

The endoscopy and biopsy were uneventful. Caroline collected John, eager to leave that place far behind. She drove them home through the city's rush hour traffic as he slept in the passenger seat, his breathing peaceful and strong.

He slept well that night, too, his body still sensitive to the sedatives. She lay next to him, alone with her thoughts. Can this be? Her own much-delayed sleep was a confused mixture of blurred images. In that brief but endless moment just before she awoke, she dreamed he had a terrible infection in his foot. They struggled to avoid amputation, but his limb slowly rotted before their eyes until the surgeon entered and told them it must come off. She felt the agony of his loss until she awoke suddenly in their bedroom. An ecstatic instant of pure relief that the dream had ended came crashing down when her now conscious mind remembered their infinitely worse reality.

They returned to Dr. Yung for the results of the biopsy and CT scan. Again, he was blunt.

"The biopsy confirmed this is pancreatic cancer. The CT shows it is not resectable because it extensively involves the superior mesenteric vein." He showed them the CT on the computer screen.

"Why does that matter?" asked John.

"You cannot remove the vein," replied Dr. Yung. "It drains blood from much of the small intestine. If you removed it, you would have to remove the small intestine. You need to start with chemotherapy. If that shrinks it, I can do the surgery. I will put a port in tomorrow, and we will make you an appointment with an oncologist closer to home."

The port meant another waiting room, this time a large and pleasant one with a central desk which reminded Caroline of an airport traffic control tower. More forms preceded another drive back home in rush hour traffic with a sedated husband.

She ate alone that evening, sitting at the table on the screened in porch which bordered their back yard while John slept. The normally pristine yard looked slightly ragged. Her salad tasted like cardboard, and she moved it around the plate before giving up and going indoors. Reading seemed impossible and, in desperation, she turned to the television. For some reason, her channel search stopped on an advertisement of a man driving a car. As she watched, the man faded away until the vehicle was empty. The voice announced pancreatic cancer had taken his life. Most die within six months, but PANCAN was fighting for them. Caroline sat stunned as Patrick Swayze followed in an advertisement for a rerun of *Footloose*. She stabbed the power button until the screen finally went blank.

The next stop was Dr. Matthews for chemotherapy. Once again, they waited, though this room was smaller and quieter than the last. As John again filled out forms, Caroline watched as a young, obviously ill woman entered the room from deep within the office and headed to the reception window. She shuffled on swollen feet in pink slippers with rabbit heads and wore matching pajama bottoms. Her discordant sweat shirt was emblazoned with obvious handmade bold lettering which read "CANCER SUCKS" and beneath it, in smaller letters, "SO DO THE YANKEES." Beside her was an older woman who Caroline guessed to be her mother. Surprisingly, they were laughing as they reached the window.

"I missed it. How did it go?" asked the smiling secretary.

"He took it well," replied the older woman.

"Yeah, but I thought he was going to pull those big ears off when he saw me with my shirt!" gushed the younger woman. "What a great guy!"

Caroline never heard the response as they were called into the room. Dr. Matthews sat with them and reviewed the events. The repetition of her husband's history brought Caroline a profound weariness, but John was determined to reach a conclusion.

"So, what is the plan?" he asked.

Dr. Matthews reviewed the treatment, a combination of chemotherapy drugs abbreviated FOLFIRINOX. John would come every two weeks to receive an intravenous treatment in the office and then wear an infusion pump for another two days of continuous chemotherapy. The side effects included fatigue, diarrhea, mouth sores, nerve damage, and low blood counts.

"It is a very hard treatment," concluded Dr. Matthews. "But you are in excellent health other than this problem, and it offers us the best chance to shrink the cancer. We will do two months of treatment, then repeat the scans to see if Dr. Yung can do the surgery."

"What if it doesn't work?" asked John.

"If it does not work and the cancer remains confined to the same area, we can try adding radiation."

"What are the chances it will work?" he asked. His voice was clear and strong. Caroline looked at him as he spoke. She loved his drive for clarity.

"About one in four."

He nodded and remained silent.

The first chemotherapy was brutal. John received six hours of intravenous chemotherapy under the watch of the nurses. He had declined a private room and enjoyed watching their quiet teamwork. Caroline was with him, nervous and hyper-alert. He received four different drugs: oxaliplatin, irinotecan, leucovorin, and fluorouracil (5-FU). He went home wearing a small portable pump which infused 5-FU into his body for the next forty-six hours. That part was easy.

Two days later, the diarrhea hit. First five, then seven, then twenty times a day. Each started with cramping, the call for a quick run to the bathroom but not real relief, just a temporary respite. Fearing dehydration, he drank water, juice, electrolyte mixtures, anything. Pills of Imodium and Lomotil and injections of Sandostatin all failed to slow it down. They took home intravenous fluids in endless bags. Caroline learned how to attach him to the IV and sat with him, checking his pulse and color. For seven days it went on. When finally, mercifully, his bowels stopped, he was depleted, and she exhausted.

"Can you do it again?" asked Dr. Matthews when he had recovered.

He nodded. "Three more times. That is the plan. On the good side, my stomach pain is gone."

The second treatment started the same. He sat in the reclining chair, Caroline by his side. She was relaxed, and John realized that she felt safe here amongst the nurses. They knew what to expect this time and started his medications and IV fluids before the explosion. The week was hard and some moments of utter exhaustion and cramping made him want to revoke his decision. Only four times, he told himself.

At one of the visits, he asked Dr. Matthews about his chemotherapy.

"Pancreatic cancer has traditionally been a tough cancer to treat. You know better than anyone how hard it is to diagnose. When it is found, it usually has spread elsewhere. So, we would like to have chemotherapy treatments which would kill it. But these cells are used to a tough environment. Thier normal job is to handle the pancreatic acid and enzymes. When they become cancerous, they can tolerate most of our poisons. This combination is basically trying to use several different drugs together."

"How do you pick them?"

"I don't. Physicians and scientists at major medical centers who are spending their whole careers studying one specific cancer design these programs. They try to figure out which compounds might work well together, then test them in clinical trials. They publish their results, which are criticized by other experts. The government has organized the major cancer centers into an online network called the National Comprehensive Cancer Network, or NCCN. The leading experts across the country evaluate all the studies, and the NCCN gives us guidelines for their use."

"If they make him so sick, they must be working," pleaded Caroline.

"We hope so," answered Dr. Matthews.

DRUG RESISTANCE: HOW DO CANCERS SURVIVE?

The drug combination FOLFIRINOX reads like a mini-history of chemotherapy. The fluorouracil (5-FU) is an old medication brilliantly designed by Charles Heidelberger in 1960 to mimic the amino acid uracil, which the cancer cells need to make DNA. When used by cancer cell instead of uracil, the 5-FU results in damaged DNA which destroys the cell. The leucovorin is not a chemotherapy, but a variation of the vitamin folate which makes the 5-FU work better. The irinotecan is a synthetic version of a drug found in the bark and wood of the Chinese plant *Camptotheca acuinata*. This drug kills cells by interfering with the function of one of the enzymes which control the structure of DNA.[122] Oxaliplatin was synthesized in the late 1980s by Dr. Yoshinori Kidani in Nagoya City University in Japan. It also works by damaging the DNA of the cancer cells. The Swiss pharmaceutical company Debiopharm acquired the license, then collaborated with Sanofi to gain FDA approval for use in a record forty-six days—an example of academic and industry collaboration.[123]

How do the cancer cells survive and even grow despite the coordinated attack of all these chemotherapies? "Drug resistance" has plagued patients, doctors, and the scientists working in cancer medicine for years. It is the reason why traditional chemotherapy has its limits; why we can cure a few cancers with chemotherapy, but not most.

Drug resistance is often thought of as something inherent in the cancer cell. While this is partly correct, many aspects of drug resistance have little to do with the cancer itself and belong in the field of pharmacology, the study of drugs and their actions. Chemotherapy drugs need to be properly absorbed, activated, delivered to the cancer, then metabolized and eliminated. Within each of these steps, there may be formidable hurdles which limit effectiveness. Absorption can be a problem; many of chemotherapy drugs are complex molecules which cannot be taken by mouth. If given orally, the optimal conditions for drug absorption must be identified (empty stomach, full stomach, the presence of other medications). Intravenous infusions can overcome this barrier but are not suitable for all medications and are obviously less convenient. Once the drug enters the bloodstream, its distribution throughout the body must be considered. Where in the normal tissues does it go? Does it enter the brain? Once inside the body, the drug may need to be activated or inactivated by enzymes then eliminated by the kidney or liver.

The absorption and metabolism of drugs may vary among people based on their genetic make-up—a field of pharmacology called pharmacogenetics. The drug 5-FU which is commonly used to treat colon, rectal, and other cancers, is a good example. 5-FU is not well-absorbed when taken by mouth and is given intravenously (although there is a modified oral version called capecitabine). Once inside the body, 5-FU is metabolized, or broken down, in a reaction which starts with an enzyme called DPD (dihydropyrimidine dehydrogenase). Many cells in the body, including those in the liver, gut lining, and white blood cells, participate in the process of inactivating the 5-FU. The more active DPD, the quicker the drug is removed from the body. A few people have little or no DPD activity. Giving these people 5-FU results in high levels of the drug and terrible side effects, including devastating diarrhea which can be fatal. The breast cancer drug tamoxifen is another example of pharmacogenetics. To be effective, tamoxifen must be activated by an enzyme in the body. Women who have genetically lower levels of the enzyme which activates tamoxifen might not get the full benefit of the medication. Testing for these types of genetic differences is challenging.

Absorption and metabolism of drugs can also be influenced by non-genetic factors. Larger patients usually need larger doses of chemotherapy. Patients with conditions ranging from diabetes to gastric bypass may not have normal absorption of oral medications. Patients with poor kidney or liver function might not be able to metabolize or eliminate medications. The dosing of some drugs is routinely adjusted for kidney function. For many drugs, there are unknown variables. The end result is that the drug levels delivered to the cancer in the patient are not the same as delivered in the lab. This form of drug resistance is actually a failure of dosing.

Once the proper amount of drug is in the bloodstream, the next requirement is that it reaches the cancer. Some cancer cells form tumors with rotten cores called "necrotic" by pathologists who see them under the microscope. Little blood or oxygen flow into these areas, meaning little chemotherapy will enter. At present, there are no particularly good answers for this problem. In some specific areas of the body like the liver, direct injection of drugs into the cancer is done. For cancers scattered throughout the body, this is not feasible.

Once most chemotherapies reach the cancer, they must enter and remain in the cancer cell. It is claimed that ten thousand to one hundred thousand molecules of a drug must enter the cancer cell for it to be effective. A few drugs simply slip into the cancer cells in a process called "passive diffusion." For most chemotherapy agents, the cell "ingests" the drug, particularly if the drug resembles a naturally occurring molecule. Resistant cancer cells may slow this entry. Some have developed very efficient methods to "pump out" chemotherapy using a multidrug resistance system (MDR, also called p-glycoprotein). This form of drug resistance is particularly devastating because the MDR pump works on many different chemotherapy drugs. Other cancer cells become resistant by increasing the breakdown of the drugs in the cell.

When they are inside cancer cells, many chemotherapy agents kill by triggering a process called "apoptosis" or "programmed cell death." The word derives from ancient Greek word apo, which means "away from," and ptosis, meaning "falling." The image of the cell "falling away" is a good one since the DNA of the apoptotic cell condenses and then disintegrates before the whole cell ends up as a small clump. The body uses apoptosis to remove unwanted tissue as it repairs or remodels itself. Apoptosis can also be used to eliminate cells which have DNA damage beyond repair, particularly from radiation or toxin exposure. Normal cells have evolved remarkable methods to assess damage to their DNA and undergo apoptosis if it cannot be repaired.

Cancer cells vary in their ability to undergo apoptosis. Since many chemotherapies work by damaging DNA, those cancer cells which can undergo apoptosis will be more sensitive. A good example is testicular cancer, which is extremely sensitive to chemotherapy. The chemotherapy damages the DNA of the testicular cancer cells, and they undergo apoptosis. Renal cell cancers are the opposite. They simply will not undergo apoptosis when exposed to chemotherapy; many have mutations in the genes which control the process. Other cancers are in-between. Since apoptosis is part of the complex control of cell division, it may help explain why rapidly dividing cells are more vulnerable to chemotherapy than slower dividing ones.

Pancreatic cancers are good at surviving chemotherapy. They are used to the toxic environment of the pancreas with its various enzymes and can limit entry and pump out chemotherapy drugs. Pancreatic cancers often have mutations in the *P16* gene which normally controls the cycling of the cell and the *TP53* gene which causes apoptosis. All these factors make pancreatic cancer resistant and add to its fearsome reputation.

They met two weeks ago to review the results of John's CT scan, hoping that the cancer would have shrunk enough to allow surgery.

Dr. Matthews was direct.

"Your CT scan looks worse. The cancer in the pancreas did not change, and it has now spread to the liver. We see about five small growths in the liver. They measure about an inch in size."

Caroline covered her face. John spoke clearly.

"That means surgery is out?"

"Yes. The cancer in the pancreas still cannot be removed because it involves the blood vessels. Even if it could be removed, there would be no point since it has spread into the liver."

"What are my choices now?" he asked.

"Basically, there are three choices. First, we can try more standard chemotherapy using different drugs. It is possible that these treatments might control the cancer for a while, but they cannot cure it.

This treatment would be milder than the one you had in terms of side effects, but it would still involve some. The second choice is that you could go to a major cancer center and see if they had a clinical trial testing new treatments. They are looking at immune treatments for these cancers, and you might be a candidate. The final choice is hospice care. We would work to make you as comfortable as possible."

"What would you do?" asked John.

They sat in silence for a few moments before Dr. Matthews responded.

"I like to think I would choose the option that would allow me to spend the best time I had remaining with my wife and family. I think that is with hospice. But I am not in your position, and it is always easier to say these things when they do not apply to you."

John nodded. "Thank you. We will think about it."

On the ride home, John turned left off Union Avenue, taking them away from home. She almost asked where they were going, but remained silent. After a moment, she understood. They drove into the country, out county highway fifty-three, on a route they knew very well. He stopped at their spot, the place overlooking the horse farm where they had ridden their bikes during an early date. Each spring they would ride here to watch the new foals as they nuzzled their mothers and stumbled on unsure legs. They had been here together the year Funny Cide was born and often tried to pick out the next big winner.

This time, he just stopped the car. The farm was quiet and the foals older, walking on sure legs.

"I don't want any more chemotherapy. I'm sorry."

"Why don't you try it, honey?" she asked.

"It's not a real plan. The chances of it working are almost zero. Even if it does work, it's no cure. I'll be trading the side effects for a little longer life. If it doesn't work, which is much more likely, I'll have traded my few good days for nothing."

They had returned today. She sat beside him, eyes red, as he spoke.

"I do not think taking more chemotherapy is a good plan. I understand the end of my life is here and I will have to face that fact. These treatments will not change that, but they will probably worsen the experience for all of us."

Dr. Matthews nodded. "I understand."

Caroline sobbed. John hugged her.

"I have been blessed with a wonderful life and family." He wiped her eyes with his handkerchief, then his own, and stood.

"I would like to stop in the back and thank the nurses," he added.

Then they were gone.

9:40 Frank James: Non-small cell lung cancer

"Bye, Lisa." Frank James ended his call as Dr. Matthews entered the room.

"Lisa sends her love," said Frank, smiling brightly. A tall man in his early fifties with movie star looks, the female office staff had nicknamed him George Clooney.

"You must be doing well if Lisa isn't here," replied Dr. Matthews.

Frank laughed. "I am. I feel great. I sent her to Canyon Resort for a little pampering after she hosted a family party for the new in-laws from France."

It had started five years ago with a phone call. The signal on Dr. Matthew's cell had not conveyed urgency, but the voice message did.

"John, it's Frank. I need your help with a medical problem. Call me when you get a chance."

Frank was Dr. Matthew's longtime friend, occasional golfing buddy, and professional confidant. They had grown up together, lost contact during their training years, and then reunited when their families and careers were both young. Frank was the highly respected regional director of a pharmaceutical company who kept an eye on Dr. Matthews' business, making sure his billing was correct and vendors fair.

"Frank, what's going on?"

"Let me put Lisa on the phone, too," he said. After she had joined, he continued. "I've been having some back pain for a few weeks. We thought it was just my golf at first, but Josh James, my primary, wanted an MRI. We just got the results. There is a spot in my thoracic spine, about T7, and they see a lesion in my lung as well. He has me set up for a PET scan tomorrow."

His story was shockingly straightforward. Frank had always been healthy, never a smoker, and only an occasional social drinker. The men in his family died of cardiac disease, not cancer. That an MRI could suggest lung cancer with spread to the spine was incomprehensible.

When they met the next afternoon, Frank moved slowly, trying to hide his pain. On the computer screen, the PET scan image of his body slowly rotated, bones and major organs faintly visible while the cancer showed as two bright spots, one on his spine and the other on his lung. The spine MRI gave a clear view of the two vertebral bodies damaged by cancer, explaining his pain.

"I know it seems impossible, but it does look like lung cancer with metastasis to the spine," Dr. Matthews told his friend. Lisa began crying softly.

"What's next?" asked Frank.

"First we need to get you out of pain. I'll adjust your medications, and we will get that area in your spine treated with radiation."

"Can we treat the lung too?"

"Yes, but not yet. We will want to get a biopsy of the lung before we give any treatment that would affect that area. The spine radiation will start tomorrow with Dr. Chris."

He paused. "The next question is whether the lung biopsy should be done here or in Boston. Obviously, we want you to go there at some point to discuss options and, if you are willing, I would like them to do the biopsy as well." Frank's territory covered Boston, and he was well known to several lung cancer specialists at Dana Farber.

"Why not here? Is the biopsy dangerous?" asked Lisa.

"No, Lisa. The procedure can be done at either place, but at Dana Farber they have dedicated pathologists and the ability to do genetic studies on these cancers. That could be very important in deciding treatment."

"What are the choices?" Lisa continued.

"The radiation will be given to the spine and should be very effective in treating the cancer there. Hopefully, it will help the pain. There is some damage to the bone, so we are not sure it will completely work, but I do think it will significantly help. After the biopsy, we will know more details about the cancer, and we can pick treatments for the whole body, probably starting with chemotherapy. We can also then give radiation to the lung area as well."

"What treatment would you use?" asked Frank.

"At this point, I would start with chemotherapy." He turned to Lisa. "Let me explain. Since Frank was never a smoker—"

"Well, that's not exactly true," interrupted Frank. "I did smoke an occasional cigarette in college, tried marijuana a few times but hated it, and have a cigar once or twice a summer in memory of my old man."

"If that counts, Frank, we would all have this. Anyway, the radiation will work well where it is aimed, but we also need to treat your whole body. Chemotherapy is the standard, but for some lung cancers in nonsmokers, there are new oral medications. There are genetic tests done on the cancer cells to see if they will respond to these drugs. At Dana Farber, they do these regularly. We may start with chemotherapy while we wait for the results of these tests, then use the oral medications later."

Lisa nodded. Frank spoke again. "Which chemo?"

"I suspect this will be an adenocarcinoma and we will use pemetrexed and carboplatin or cisplatin. They may also have some studies of newer agents."

"I know we have several in the pipeline."

"I would also add Avastin, but we will see."

They were quiet again, then Lisa spoke. "Can you cure him?"

"If this is what we think it is, Lisa, not now. No. We can treat it. With the chemotherapy and radiation, there is a good chance he will get into remission. Hopefully, we can use the oral medications to keep him in remission for a long time."

"How long?" she asked.

"We hope years, but we cannot know."

Frank took her hand. "Long enough for them to develop something else. We can fight this, honey." He looked at his friend. "We know what we are up against, but we also know we have tools to use. And more coming."

It was a quiet ride home. Lisa drove, fighting back the tears and bile while Frank gazed out the window. A shot of morphine had dulled the pain so he could make the twenty-minute ride. Lisa helped him from the car and into their living room where he found more relief in the recliner. She sat beside him on the sofa, her head resting on his arm. He felt her tears.

"I'm so sorry, honey," he said as she cried.

"It's not your fault. You have nothing to be sorry about. I just don't understand it. What did you ever do?"

"Who knows," he replied. "Listen to me. This sucks, but there's a lot we can do. The radiation will make me feel better, and I know the chemo will work. Plus, we have a lot of new drugs in the pipeline, you'll see." He picked up her chin. "Don't give up, Babe."

She mopped her eyes. "I won't. I'll go get your medicine from the CVS."

"That's my girl." He kissed her.

The CVS was busy, but the pharmacist called Lisa to the counter right away. She was a young woman with a worried look.

"Frank helped me a few years ago when I had just finished pharmacy school. I'm sorry to see him getting a prescription for morphine, particularly from Dr. Matthews. Here is my card. Please let me know if I can do anything. Anytime." She handed Lisa the bag and her card.

"Thank you," nodded Lisa, holding back her tears yet again. "We're not sure what he has yet."

Frank ate little that night. Lisa helped him to bed and gave him the morphine and lorazepam. After an hour, he fell asleep. She sat in the reading chair beside their bed and watched as he slept, his handsome face finally relaxed. She felt alone but afraid to involve anyone else. Not the children, she thought. They would need information and comfort. Not her mother, she would only worry. Not his mother, she was crazy. Not her sister, she had her own problems with a daughter who was suicidal. His colleagues? Their friends? What would she say? He had always been with her, but now, at this moment, she was alone.

What did we do? Why God? He's a good man; even the pharmacist loved him. Lisa stood and moved to the pictures standing in frames on their dresser. Their family, when son Anthony and daughter Francesca were small. The kids together. The kids with grandmothers and grandfather. Prom gowns and dates. Graduation. Frank honored at work. It was this last picture which stopped her. She and Frank were in a group of his colleagues standing in front of a company banner in the lobby of the Chicago Museum of Natural History, the excitement of the night captured in his smile.

She picked up the picture and looked at it, remembering the trip and the bold corporate confidence of the group.

You better have something for him, she told them, then returned the photo to its place.

The next morning, after a good night's sleep, Frank felt better.

"I like that morphine and Ativan," he announced as he opened his eyes. "I needed the sleep."

Lisa awoke instantly. "Good. Be careful," she responded. "I think you should take another morphine with breakfast before we drive to radiation. Have you moved your bowels? The morphine is constipating."

He looked at her. "My bowels? Gee, I remember when you wanted to have sex when we woke up."

"Shut up, you jerk. I'm worried about your pain and cancer and radiation, and that's all you can think of? Get yourself another nurse, then. Or another wife." She got out of bed, stormed into the bathroom, then went directly downstairs. After twenty minutes, she returned with coffee and a breakfast of toast and scrambled eggs.

"Get into the chair so you can eat," she ordered, helping him up. He moved painfully.

"I'm sorry," he said.

"Shut up and eat, then take the pill, and we'll get you ready."

He ate the eggs and toast.

"Thanks . . . it's good."

"I'm glad." He noted her voice had slightly softened.

"Any chance of a little kiss, then?" He smiled, a weak version of his famously handsome one.

"Bastard," she replied, but kissed him and helped him dress.

Dr. Chris, the radiation oncologist, was his usual buoyant self. After their meeting, Frank went for a CT scan and marking. The radiation staff was efficient, and Frank's treatment was planned, calculations were done, and his first dose given that day. After about an hour, Sally Kite, a serious young technician, wheeled him out of the treatment area.

"He had his first treatment and did well, Mrs. James. Tomorrow will be quicker, I promise," said Sally sympathetically.

"How are you?" Lisa asked Frank.

"Piece of cake," he replied. "They take all these pictures, put you in a lead room with the biggest doors you've ever seen and all these fancy machines, but nothing really comes out. It just buzzes and clicks. Right, Sally? Nothing to it . . ."

"Oh, no, Mr. James. We gave you the first treatment today," she replied earnestly.

"Don't pay attention to him," Lisa said. "He's teasing. He looks nice, but he really is a jerk."

That afternoon Frank was comfortable sitting in the chair.

"You look better," Lisa fussed. "Could the radiation have worked that fast?"

"No, I don't think so. This is the morphine. As long as I take it regularly and don't move, I'm not too bad."

They sat quietly for a minute.

"I have to let them know at work I'm going to be out for a while."

Lisa nodded. "And we will have to tell the kids and your mother."

"Let's start with work. I'll speak with Bill. I won't be able to hide this for long, but he will keep it quiet until we let the family know."

Frank was the manager for his pharmaceutical company's operations in the northeastern United States. He had been with the company for almost thirty years, starting as a sales rep and working upward. He was a natural; his tall, handsome look and easy manner instantly drew people toward him. In a competitive business where personality conflicts were common, Frank was universally respected.

Pharmaceuticals were in his genes. Frank's paternal uncle, also named Frank but always known as Frankie, had been a pharmacist and sole proprietor of "Johnson's Apothecary," a small business on Broadway in Schenectady. Frank loved the store. The front windows always held exhibits of local school sports teams and clubs while promoting the daily fountain specials and compounded remedies, clever marketing by Aunt Shelly, Frankie's wife. Customers entered through a pane glass and wood door which opened into an aisle running up the middle of the shop. On the immediate right was an old-style soda counter with eight stools, managed by Mrs. Kelly, a robust and seemingly ageless Irish wife of a police sergeant who worked at the station next door. Mrs. Kelly was known for her ice cream shakes, banana splits, and strict attention to manners. Opposite the fountain was the candy display, also Mrs. Kelly's territory. Her "pay before you touch" rule was strictly enforced, but many neighborhood children benefited from her largesse when they came into the store to pick up prescriptions for their family. The sweet scent of ice cream and candy made entry into Johnson's a childhood memory for many locals. After the fountain came the medical equipment section containing wheelchairs, crutches, and bandages, followed by the raised toilet seats which elicited adolescent jokes told out of earshot of Mrs. Kelly. Next were the neat shelves of skin creams, regular medications, band aids, and the like.

The pharmacy counter stood like an altar at the end of the center aisle. High on the wall behind the counter were old jars containing mysterious colored liquids and various herbs. Below came a row of impressive looking books and several scales in glass boxes. Beneath that were shelves of modern jars and boxes, all neatly ordered. Everything was meticulously cleaned, dusted, shined, and polished by the gate-keeper of the pharmacy, Mrs. Wilson. She was a thin Dutch woman whose angular appearance was in stark contrast to Mrs. Kelly. Mrs. Wilson knew everyone's medication history and the financial status of their accounts. While she kept these strictly confidential, she felt no such compulsion with her opinions on social matters. She was a great deterrent to the out of wedlock purchase of condoms and the reason Johnson's sold virtually none. Behind Mrs. Wilson, barely visible over a half-door, was the work area of the pharmacy where Frankie, always dressed in his white lab coat, prepared the prescriptions and com-pounded medications. On rare occasions when Mrs. Wilson felt the need for a second opinion, she would call Frankie out to the counter to dispense advice.

As a child, Frank dearly loved Mrs. Kelly's banana splits, yet the pharmacy counter was his favorite part of the store. It was not until high school that he understood the mysterious liquids were food col-oring and the herbs came from Aunt Shelly's garden. Though the harsh truth shattered his childhood fantasy that these were potions with special powers, it did not diminish his admiration for his uncle and his work. He saw the neighbors turn to Uncle Frankie for advice on the practical matters of their health and felt the respect and trust he earned their family.

Frank's father, Anthony, had died of a massive coronary when Frank and his older sister Cathy were in grade school, so he and his uncle had developed a special relationship. Frank had entered college planning a career in medicine but quickly realized he was not a devoted enough student. Frank knew this would upset his mother, who had never hid-den her fervent desire that he be a doctor, and he naturally turned to Uncle Frankie for advice. Frank first paid his respects to Mrs. Wilson, once again admiring the display wall, then helped Mrs. Kelly wipe down the counter while his uncle finished the last of his work. They retired to the Irish pub next door and drank his uncle's favorite warm Guinness while he shared his revelation and anxiety. The memory of his uncle's response had stayed fresh over the years.

"I'm not surprised, Frank," his uncle replied. "Medical school is a lot of bookwork. You're plenty smart enough, but I never saw you as leadass. You would rather be out with people, doing things."

Frank nodded. His uncle continued. "Pharmacy school is about the same, maybe even worse. At least in medical school those who can only study so much can be the cutters. We didn't even have that option."

"Are you sorry you did it? Pharmacy, I mean?"

"No, Frank. Look, in school I was a nerd. And I love what I do. Your aunt runs the show, deals with the people, and I take care of the pharmacy—it's the right place for me. We have a good business and a good life. We do all right. But that doesn't mean it's right for you."

He paused to sip more Guinness, then continued.

"My advice to you, Frank, is to get into pharmacy, but not as a pharmacist. Study your chemistry, but major in business. I'll put you in contact with some of these pharmaceutical guys, and you can work with them in the summers. When you finish, you'll be ready to take a job with one of the big pharmaceutical companies. If you get in the right place, you'll be set. These companies are going to take off, believe me. The advances in medicine are incredible. And you can be there to help deliver the new drugs. You're a natural for it. You'll have the science and business background and people like working with you."

Uncle Frankie paused, then continued dryly.

"The other choice is plastics, but stay away from Mrs. Robinson."

Frank laughed. "I would like that. Not Mrs. Robinson. The pharmaceuticals, I mean. Thanks, Uncle Frank. There's just one thing. I'm a little worried how Mom will take it."

"I'll talk to Sylvia."

Frankie had often talked with Sylvia. In high school, Frankie supported his nephew's desire to try out for football and basketball, something Sylvia could never understand.

"They'll pick on him, Frankie. Those big boys will hurt my baby."

"It's good for him, Sylvia. He's big and strong, too. And good look-ing. He needs to learn to stand up for himself without being a bully."

It was a fine line in Schenectady, where Italians were a minority and, outside the neighborhood, a fine target for the Dutch or the Irish. Overt violence was rare, but the divisions occasionally ran deep. As he went through high school, Frank found himself a leader in his neigh-borhood, and both admired and resented by others, a difficult position he explained to his uncle.

"Everyone likes me when I clear a lane for Jimmy Doyle and he scores. The neighborhood boys want me to stand up for them when some of his buddies call them guineas. The neighborhood girls are mad when I say hello to Jimmy's sister, but not as mad as Jimmy's friends. And coach expects me to keep everyone happy."

Frankie laughed.

"There's no easy answer, Frank. Did you ever wonder why we named the shop Johnson's?"

Frank paused. "Not really."

"Think about it, then come back and talk to me."

That was one of Uncle Frankie's lessons, slow down and think.

Frank answered a few days later. "I got it. It was good for business."

Frankie laughed. "Sure. We had a choice to make. If we made this an Italian drug store, we would never appeal to the rest of the city. So we gave it an English name, hired an Irish lady with a policeman hus-band to run the soda fountain, a Dutch woman who was tough as nails to run the pharmacy counter, put everyone's accomplishments in the window, celebrated every damn holiday, and made sure every priest or clergyman in town got a discount. We didn't win over everyone. Some of the diehards in our own neighborhood said we were disrespectful. Some of the Irish were annoyed. But we did one other thing."

"What's that?"

"We outworked everyone else."

Uncle Frankie's career advice had been good. Frank found the extraordinary chemistry of his industry, involving both drugs and people, fascinating. Uncle Frankie's lessons in balancing different viewpoints also served Frank well in his complicated world. And he worked hard.

THE BIRTH OF PHARMA AND DRUG DEVELOPMENT.

As the nineteenth century started in England, medical care provided by physicians and surgeons was largely useless and very limited. University trained physicians spoke Latin but had no modern diagnostic or therapeutic tools while surgeons practiced without anesthesia or antisepsis, and both practitioners were few in number. It was, therefore, the more numerous apothecaries who compounded medicines and delivered care in their communities.[124] Many well-known physicians and surgeons of the day, including Thomas Hodgkin, spent time working with apothecaries. Even though there were few useful treatments in this era, the public wanted to believe in medicines, consumer demand drove the growth of the business, and the reputable apothecary was considered a valuable member of society.

The growth of the modern pharmaceutical industry in England during the nineteenth century was preceded by the rise of "patent medicines," named after the "patents of royal favor" given to preparations provided to the British Royal family. The first patent medicines came to America from England, but almost immediately many similar concoctions were manufactured locally. The specifics of the preparations were usually secret, but often included some combination of alcohol, cocaine, and morphine. During the century, the sale of patent medicines reached a fevered pitch for use in a variety of ailments familiar to modern society: menstrual pain, gastrointestinal complaints, arthritis, breast development, and erectile dysfunction.

The modern pharmaceutical industry began in 1860–80 with the formation of companies like Burroughs Wellcome, Parke-Davis, Eli Lilly, Upjohn, and Abbott Pharmaceuticals.[125] Many of these companies developed large-scale facilities which included research labs combined with chemical factories and began affiliations with medical schools and universities. They used emerging technology like the Rotary Tablet Press to produce compressed pills of items such as malt extracts, vegetable, and iron preparations. Burroughs Welcome, for example, compressed extracts of sixteen different animal tissues into Tabloids, their version of pills.[126] Many of the pharmaceutical products these companies sold were patent medications, although they did usually try to ensure they were reproducible. Beecham's Pills were an example of a patent medicine which did have some laxative qualities, became popular and eventually helped support the development of the Beecham Group. Most importantly, this childhood of the pharmaceutical industry produced the first unequivocally useful medications such as aspirin, precursors of acetaminophen (Tylenol), and anti-serum for diphtheria.

World War II set the stage for the marked growth of the pharmaceutical industry and the development of modern medicines, particularly antibiotics. The U.S. government's War Production Board formed a coalition of eleven drug companies to produce penicillin for the troops. It is ironic that the same Board was supplying the GIs with the cigarettes which would unknowingly lead to an army of customers with tobacco-related cancer, lung, and heart diseases for these same companies. The post-War years brought additional promotion of the industry with more antibiotics and immunization against polio. The 1960s saw successful medications to treat cardiovascular disease, mental illness, and the birth control pill. The 1980s saw the addition of biotechnology to the industry and remarkable advances in the treatment of serious illnesses such as cancer, viral infections including HIV/AIDS, and cardiovascular disease. By the end of the twentieth century, treatment of many of the every-day conditions for which patent medicines had been offered could now be managed: erectile dysfunction, overactive bladder, gastrointestinal disturbance, and menstrual pain. The modern pharmaceutical industry had begun delivering on the promise of longer and better lives.[127]

Where does Pharma get these amazing drugs? One approach is to search "pond scum" or other natural products for candidate compounds, reminiscent of the use of herbal remedies seen in many societies throughout history. After World War II, the pharmaceutical industry began scouring the globe for medicines found in nature. The drug streptomycin was identified in soil from a New Jersey farm and became a powerful weapon against tuberculosis. Dr. Selman Waksman won a Nobel Prize for the discovery, although most of the work was done by his graduate student Dr. Albert Schatz, a reality Waksman kept buried for years.[128] Pfizer scientists reportedly screened one hundred thousand soil samples from around the world to develop their aptly named antibiotic Terramycin.[129] Some of these antibiotics had anticancer activity, leading the National Cancer Institute to sponsor similar searches in the 1970s for potential chemotherapies. The problem with this approach is that the molecules which killed the bacteria or cancer cell are hidden in the pond scum or soil mix. These molecules are complex structures which are very hard to identify, purify, and manufacture. The scientists who carried out these searches had a tremendous tenacity and the successful ones often some manner of good luck (or good students, like Waksman).

Another approach for obtaining new medicines is to modify key molecules already found in the body. Advances in biochemistry around the time of World War II allowed scientists to identify and modify many hormones, the type of synthesis that led to the birth control pill. In oncology, this technique was used brilliantly in 1957 when Charles Heidelberger and Robert Duschinsky synthesized the chemotherapy drug fluorouracil, called 5-FU.[130] They reasoned that since dividing cancer cells rapidly replicate their DNA and make large amounts of RNA, they would be using the raw materials such as the amino acid uracil at high rates. They modified uracil into 5-FU and found it would be incorporated into the DNA and RNA where it would kill the cell. This chemotherapy has been a mainstay for treatment of colon and a variety of other cancers.

Modern biotechnology allows the synthesis of entirely new medicines. Scientists can now identify the genetic abnormalities found in cancer and determine the abnormal proteins made by these cells. Understanding the structure and function of these abnormal proteins can lead to the design of molecules which block or reverse the abnormality. Unlike the creation of 5-FU, this technique requires teams of scientists but can yield amazing molecules for use as "targeted treatments" in cancer and other diseases.

Frank started as a traditional pharmaceutical representative, calling on physicians and hospitals while learning the culture of medical practice. As his talents became evident, he rose in the hierarchy and eventually even Sylvia appreciated his success, ultimately forgiving Uncle Frankie for steering him away from medical school. Her pleasure came with some burden for Frank, however, as she championed new products for his company. The most famous episode occurred ten years ago when she sought to convince him that asparagus extracts could prevent cancer. Sylvia had prepared asparagus in virtually every possible way and administered vast quantities to her family. One Sunday dinner at her home, it was featured in the soup, as a side dish, and found woven in the bread. Frank's then teenage son Anthony became the first to openly rebel. When Sylvia left the table he surreptitiously dumped the offending greens into a plastic bag taped to the underside of the table, an action gleefully reported by his younger sister Francesca. His mother reacted first.

"Anthony—" Lisa started ominously.

"Anthony, did you really do that?" interrupted Frank, saving his son from maternal wrath as Uncle Frankie and Aunt Shelly pretended not to pay attention.

"Dad, my pee smells terrible. I can't stand it!"

"Anthony!" Lisa spoke sharply. "You watch your mouth."

Frank held up his hand.

"Quiet! Grandma will be back soon. Listen, I'll talk to her about the asparagus and take care of it."

Frank's first true scientific project had been to act as the liaison between his company and several Boston hospitals for a trial of a substance called tumor necrosis factor, or TNF. The idea was exciting. Years ago, it was observed that some patients with cancers, particularly leukemia, who survived severe bacterial infections could see their cancers go into remission. A physician named Denton Cooley tried to grind up bacteria and give it to patients hoping to reproduce this effect with a mixture called "Cooley's toxin." Occasionally it worked, although the responses usually did not last long and the mix produced severe side effects. Yet it started a scientific search which eventually led to the identification, manufacture, and naming of the molecule called tumor necrosis factor. In the lab, TNF killed cancer cells and stimulated the immune system. Frank's company had obtained the rights to TNF and contracted with these hospitals to try it in humans. It was Frank's first introduction into the convoluted world of drug testing and regulation.

REGULATING MEDICINES.

The public wants medicines to be effective and pure but prefers that there are few restrictions placed on their development. Whether they are patent medicines, natural products from the soil, compounds made by brilliant revelation, or molecules designed by teams of scientists, the regulation of the manufacturing process has been a complex and changing balancing act. We have typically started with the belief that we can trust the industry and should hold it to high standards. In England in 1815, Parliament gave the Worshipful Society of Apothecaries a significant role in supervising the activities of the providers of medications. This early self-policing of the industry introduced "the distinctive

Anglo-American system of arm's-length state regulation."[131] Some control, but not too much, is a common theme in our struggle to find the right balance. At the center of that balance in modern life is the Food and Drug Administration (FDA)—the gatekeeper of drug regulation in the United States and an agency influential across the world.[132]

In the United States during the 1800s, the pharmaceutical marketplace was a confusing free for all, replete with products and patent medicines containing varying undefined ingredients sold with outlandish claims. Regulation of the industry seemed inevitable, and even the young pharmaceutical industry wanted to be able to distinguish itself from the purveyors of questionable mixtures. A first step came in 1906 when the Food and Drug Act required manufacturers to reveal ingredients on labels. But reporting ingredients is a far cry from making them safe, as many families discovered in the shameful tragedy involving "Elixir of Sulfanilamide" in the 1930s. This antibiotic was a remarkable advance in the treatment of many childhood infections, but it tasted bad. The logical way to expand its use was to sweeten the preparation. The S.E. Massengill company did this by dissolving the sulfa using the sweet solvent diethylene glycol. Although the company tested the taste and smell of the preparation, they did not do any safety testing, and the solvent killed one hundred people—including children.[133] This horrible event led to the 1938 Food, Drug and Cosmetic Act which gave FDA authority over the marketing of drugs and required that the agency review and approve the safety of new drugs.[134]

The expansion of the industry after World War II led to further regulations. In 1951, prescriptions were first required for many medications, and the FDA sought to improve clinical trials. At the time, most drugs were simply tested by physicians on their patients and the results reported (sort of) to the company. The importance of a scientific approach became evident in 1953 when a small German pharmaceutical firm marketed a remarkably effective sedative named Contergan. With few obvious side effects, it soon became the country's best-selling sedative and was used to aid sleep, calm stress, soothe children, and control the morning sickness of pregnancy. In 1960, when the pharmaceutical company William S. Merrell submitted a new drug application for the use of the sedative in the United States to the FDA, it was thankfully assigned to Frances Kelsey for review. Despite tremendous pressure, Kelsey repeatedly denied Merrell's application, insisting the company supply data showing the drug was pure, effective, and safe. Contergan, whose chemical name is thalidomide, was widely used in Europe, Australia, and Japan, and produced devastating birth defects when taken during pregnancy. These included deformed or stunted arms, legs, ears, and eyes. Across the world, ten thousand children with these deformities were born, but in the United States, there were only seventeen cases.[135] The heroic work of Kelsey and her colleagues saved thousands of Americans.[136] The event resulted in the 1962 Kefauver-Harris Amendments which strengthened the FDA and required affirmative approval of new drugs using proper trials.[137] Thalidomide itself went back on the shelf and was never again marketed as a sedative, but was a treatment for a variant of leprosy. In the late 1990s, the drug was used as a treatment of the bone marrow cancer multiple myeloma—a unique connection made by a determined Manhattan family, a brilliant Boston researcher, and a dedicated physician in Arkansas.[138] After careful clinical trials, the FDA allowed the use of thalidomide when prescribed for myeloma under strictly controlled conditions. Ironically, thalidomide became the first in a class of related drugs which radically changed the treatment of myeloma and several other cancers.

While Kelsey's insistence that thalidomide not be used in the U.S. until tested was a vindication of the scientific drug approval process, very rapidly new pressures again raised the longstanding question of how to maintain a proper regulatory balance. The dramatic changes in drug discovery and the biotech era brought the FDA entirely new classes of drugs requiring special expertise. The science of clinical trials and drug testing also became more complex. For example, a debate over the definition of what constitutes benefit began. In cancer treatments, prolonging survival is an obvious way to measure the effectiveness of a drug, but could take years to determine. Other measures, such as shrinkage or control rates, improved quality of life, or less toxicity, can also be valid but are more complicated to evaluate.[139] The sheer volume of these challenges increased with the rapid economic expansion of the industry during the Reagan boom years. The financial stakes of the approval process also increased as the rewards for getting a blockbuster new drug through the approval process became ever higher.

Public expectations for new medications also increased in the 1960s and 1970s. In oncology, the successful treatment of some cancers with chemotherapy put pressure on the FDA to allow more experimentation. Tensions between the scientists testing these medications at the National Cancer Institute and other leading cancer centers and the FDA occasionally spilled over into the public and led to changes in clinical trials.[140] Demands from a coalition of alternative practitioners, dissident scientists, and patients to allow the use of the Laetrile, a compound made from apricot pits, as an anticancer treatment forced the FDA into political and court battles.[141] As difficult as these issues may have seemed, it was the arrival of HIV/AIDS in the 1980s that changed the fundamental nature of the debate over drug regulation for patients with serious illnesses. The organization of AIDS activists and their willingness to use public demonstrations both challenged the FDA to be more flexible and served as a model for other groups, with breast cancer advocates leading the way in cancer medicine.

This debate continues today. New drugs are introduced rapidly and approved using a variety of mechanisms, including the so-called "fast track" designation. Clinical trials are designed using new endpoints. Post-marketing studies are done. Criticism of each of these programs comes regularly whenever unexpected side effects are encountered. Given that billions of dollars and lives are at stake, the balance between public safety and progress continues to be decided in the context of our scientific, political, and economic times.

For young Frank in the 1980s, the TNF trial was his introduction to the tremendous work involved in testing a new medicine. The basic lab science, perfecting the manufacturing, safety tests in humans, exhausting regulatory hurdles, and seemingly endless paperwork had taken years before the trial went forward. This was a phase I clinical trial, which meant that patients with a variety of cancers who had few other options would volunteer to get steadily increasing doses of TNF to determine the side effects and maximum tolerated amount. The strict purpose of a phase I trial was not to measure the effectiveness of the drug, but everyone was hopeful for good results in some patients. Frank arranged everything, including drug shipments, payments, training of the doctors and nurses, and endless meetings. It was an exciting time, and he loved the work.

Frank knew intellectually that most clinical trials of new drugs did not produce winners. He had been warned not to get excited but still found his adrenaline surge almost uncontrollably as the trial opened and the first patient was treated. The day before the opening he had lunch with Chris Stevens, a brilliant and acerbic southern lawyer who ensured that all the regulatory issues were handled properly. Since he insisted on briefing all the "ground troops" personally, Frank had met him on several occasions, and they both enjoyed the differences in their personalities. When Frank entered the downtown Boston Legal Seafood, he found Stevens visibly agitated.

"How are you, Chris?" Frank asked as the thin, smaller man rose from his seat and shook hands, his glass of neat bourbon nearly drained.

"Screwed, man. Screwed."

"Why?"

Chris signaled the waiter. "Another," he held up the glass. "Frank, anything for you?" Frank ordered a Diet Coke.

"Listen to this tale of woe, man, and leave the business while you still can . . .," Stevens finished the rest of his bourbon, then continued.

"I negotiated the rights to this drug which is supposed to thin the blood for people when they have had heart attacks or strokes or crap like that. Now, most people use rat poison."

"It's called Coumadin, Chris," Frank noted.

"Whatever, don't interrupt me when I'm on a roll. So, this rat poison is a pain in the ass because you have to watch what you eat and check blood tests all the time. It kills almost as many people as rats. Now this new miracle drug thins the blood, but you don't need to take any blood tests and can eat whatever you want. Sounds great, right . . .," he trailed off as the waiter arrived with the Diet Coke for Frank and a fresh bourbon for Stevens. He took another drink and shook his head.

"All we had to do was organize the human trials. We were all set to make the deal when we found out the FDA wanted more primate testing. Some government scientist wasn't exactly happy with some of the pre-clinical levels of something or other, who the hell knows what."

"Who does primate testing?" asked Frank, interested.

"Yeah, well that's the thing, not too many places. And the wait is long. But we found one lab in New Jersey that could do it. So, we figured go ahead with the deal, get the primate testing done quickly and move on." He stopped and shook his head.

"What happened?" asked Frank.

"What happened? We made the deal and the damn ape died, that's what happened. Now we're really screwed. The FDA is all over us. The human trials are on hold. I've got paperwork coming out my ass, and we're out big bucks."

"How did the ape die?" Frank asked.

Stevens looked at him incredulously. "You think I know how the ape died? I have no idea. Probably it was old. Probably it drank too much bourbon like me. Probably they had used it in too many tests. All we wanted was a damn ape blood level, and now we got this mess."

Frank's trial went smoothly, but TNF was a bust. Over the next year, the thirty patients treated with the medication reproducibly got quite sick with fevers and chills but only one had a temporary shrinkage of the tumor. He had lunch with Uncle Frankie and reported the results.

"Years of work, thousands of dollars, and we have nothing to show for it," he concluded.

Frankie smiled. "It's like betting the horses. Used to be you bet on single races and the daily double. By the end of the day, everyone was a winner, everyone a loser. 'Take a little, leave a little' we used to say. Now they have the 'pick six.' Most of the time, no one wins. But when someone does, they win big. Or maybe it's like the mega lottery they are starting in New Hampshire."

"Let's hope we don't get the numbers that don't exist," Frank replied, recalling the New York Lotto scandal of a few years prior.

His uncle laughed appreciatively. "I don't think most people understand the expense that goes into this. These drugs cost money, and if we want them, we're going to pay. I can tell you from my years and Mrs. Wilson's experience, people won't like it."

The public's love-hate relationship with the pharmaceutical industry was summarized again for Frank years later. He ran into Chris Stevens late one night at a company meeting. Frank had heard Stevens was defending the company against a charge of price-fixing after they had kept a generic competitor of one of their most lucrative drugs off the market. In marked contrast to Frank's distinguished middle-aged appearance, the thin lawyer had not aged well, but he retained his acerbic wit.

"Frank! Jesus, man, it must be about ten years. How the hell are you? I see you never took my advice and stayed in the business. Let me get you a drink." He indicated the hotel bar and swept him along.

After they had sat, Frank nursed a glass of wine while Stevens quickly downed the first of two bourbons set in front of him. He quizzed Frank on his career and seemed genuinely pleased to learn of his rise.

"You did a nice job with that dog of a study they gave you back in Boston."

"Dog?" Frank asked, puzzled.

Stevens laughed. "Didn't you know? No one ever really thought that drug was going anywhere. It was part of a package."

"Really?" Frank recoiled.

"Of course." He looked at Frank. "Listen, don't be shocked. It's not all science. We all know there are some studies that need to be done because we have gotten so far into the damn drug that we can't give up on the outside chance it leads to something. Sometimes we have to be nice to someone who believes in it despite all the evidence. Sometimes it's all part of some bigger deal." He paused to sip at his bourbon. "Anyway, you did a good job."

"How's your work? How's the case?" Frank asked, changing the subject.

"This time we're in the right. We simply used established legal proceedings to challenge another company."

"I'm glad you'll win," Frank replied distantly, still thinking of his TNF study.

"I didn't say that," Chris answered. "We've hired a boatload of fancy legal minds, all billing us endless hours, but that and being right doesn't mean a damn thing. What matters is the public. Which side of the coin are they on at this moment?"

"How's that?" asked Frank, again back in the moment.

"Frank, we are Pharma. They love us because we make the drugs that save them. They hate us because we are rich and arrogant and they need us to make the drugs that save them."

PHARMA AND PROFIT.

Profit drives Pharma. Balancing the inherent contradiction between the responsibility to cure and making money is a longstanding challenge for the industry. This tension has come to public attention as new drugs and profits for the industry have soared at a time when inequalities in the distribution of drugs and the limitations of financial resources in medicine have come under increased scrutiny.

This nature of the problem is not new. The antiserum treatment for diphtheria used in the 1890s is an early illustration of the contradictions in this industry. Thanks to vaccinations, diphtheria is now largely forgotten, but for most of history it was a feared killer of children. The germ *Corynebacterium diphtheria* causes the disease, which spreads in fluid droplets from coughing or spitting. The bacteria produce a toxin which causes a thick coating throughout the back of the throat which can literally strangle a child. The toxin also produces fever and can damage organs leading to death. An epidemic in Spain in 1613 caused the year to be named "El Ano de los Garotillos (The Year of Strangulations)." The French physician Pierre Bretoneau named diphtheria in 1826 after the Greek word for leather to describe the coating of the throat. He successfully treated a patient with a tracheostomy, cutting an opening in the trachea and inserting a tube to allow air to enter the lungs. The English blamed the French for the disease, calling it "Boulogne Sour Throat" after the city in northern France. Whatever the name, the terror spared no one, and in 1878 Queen Victoria's daughter Princess Alice and her granddaughter both died of the disease.[142]

Given the horrors of diphtheria, it was with great excitement during the 1890s that word spread of the work of Japanese scientist Shibasaburo Kitasato and German Emil von Behring. They injected guinea pigs with heat inactivated diphtheria toxin and found the pigs would produce an antibody which could be harvested from their serum and used to treat other animals. Von Behring won the first Nobel Prize in Medicine for this work.[143] Since pigs produce only a small amount of antibody, large-scale production uses horses. In England, the first pony to produce anti-diphtheria antibodies, named Tom, belonged to the British Institute for Preventative Medicine, a charitable organization established to advance medical science which would later become the Lister Institute.[144] Almost immediately, British pharmaceutical companies realized the importance of these treatments and proposed purchasing and profit-sharing arrangements with the Institute. When the offer was rejected, the companies found other horses and competed with the Institute. The companies were tremendously successful in direct marketing to physicians, providing them with information, testing services for their patients to identify the disease, and an assortment of nice gifts. The companies then branched out into similar ventures using a variety of other anti-serum.[145]

The diphtheria model was repeated multiple times by the pharmaceutical industry as it matured and prospered. Drugs discovered in university settings supported with public or government funds were then modified, produced, and marketed by companies. New medications were promoted to physicians using a mix of information, trade shows, professional organizations, thought leaders, and gifts. Ancillary testing or practice aids were employed to make the medication fit smoothly into the prescriber's practice. Everyone was happy. The scientists and universities were modestly rewarded, drugs marketed, patients treated and, of course, profits made. There were also some checks in the system. Universities and academic medical centers traditionally had some level of disdain for commercial enterprises. Individual scientists, physicians, and their organizations often resisted pharmaceutical pressures. In some situations, strong public health labs competed directly with pharmaceutical companies in the production of antiserum or vaccinations.[146] As the industry matured and grew through the mid-twentieth century, these balances remained intact, primarily because the profits were solid but not great. The industry was "pharma" with a little "p."

Everything changed with the growth of the biotech industry during the Reagan boom years. In 1980, Senators Birch Bayh (D-Ind) and Robert Dole (R-Kans) collaborated on a law which enabled universities and small businesses to patent discoveries and grant exclusive licenses to drug companies. The similar Stevenson-Wydler Act allowed the National Institute of Health to license drugs discovered in their labs to pharmaceutical companies. Prior to these laws, discoveries made in universities funded by the government or the NIH were in the public domain; now they were controlled by the developers. This change set the stage for unprecedented collaboration between academia and industry or, as some would argue, the unprecedented control of academia by industry.[147] Many of the checks on the industry which previously existed were swept away by a tide of scientific enthusiasm and money. Academic institutions or their faculty "spun off" biotech firms and collaborated with drug companies, securing their royalties and own place in the previously somewhat disdained commercial world.

Genentech was the first of the Pharma biotech firms.[148] In 1973, Drs. Stan Cohen of Stanford and Herbert Boyer of University of California at San Francisco together developed recombinant technology or "cloning," the ability to cut and paste DNA fragments and insert them into bacteria to produce large quantities of a protein. The technology both promised new treatments and raised complex issues. The risk of creating a new runaway "Andromeda Strain" infection technology was first debated in the scientific community, beginning with meetings like the Asilomar conference, and later the government and public. Was this technology safe? The potential commercial value of technology challenged the traditional relationship between academic researchers, their institutions, and the corporate world. Could these techniques be patented? How should they be licensed? Who would fund, produce, market, and profit from them?

Scientists and institutions responded in different ways. Dr. Cohen continued a brilliant but largely traditional academic career at Stanford, mixed with some outside work which included Cetus, the first biotech company famous for developing the PCR. Dr. Boyer took a radically different route. Almost immediately after publication of his science, Boyer was approached by Robert Swanson, an unemployed venture capitalist who had ironically tried unsuccessfully to interest Cetus in cloning. The two men formed Genentech: Genetic Engineering Technology. They obtained funding and entered the race to clone the genes which produced insulin and other hormones. Producing vast amounts of synthetic human insulin with a huge potential market and profit was the goal. In laboratories across the world, the most brilliant and driven scientists worked endless grueling hours to be the first.[149]

Genentech won. First, they cloned the gene for a molecule called somatostatin, reaping publicity and additional investment funds which allowed them to recruit even more minds.[150] Somatostatin is a small hormone which inhibits the production of other hormones in the body. While the cloning of somatostatin did not produce a highly profitable product, it proved the process was possible. Genentech scientists then cloned insulin. Since insulin is a large molecule, it was much more difficult to clone. Genentech used a technique which allowed them to avoid the "Andromeda Strain" safety issues and restrictions which plagued other labs. Human growth hormone followed insulin, sweeping the market when regular supplies were contaminated with a variant of mad cow disease and becoming a $2 billion drug.[151] The company then turned its attention to interferon, a drug thought to have almost miraculous anticancer properties and which promised a great victory in President Nixon's War on Cancer. As the excitement peaked, Genentech went public, and the rapid rise in stock price made multimillionaires of the cloners.[152]

Genentech's success in combining brilliant science with business vision in the 1970s and 1980s contributed to changes in the scientific and academic worlds and the pharmaceutical industry. Genentech's culture as a freewheeling biotech company appealed to a new generation of scientists who skipped traditional academic careers to be the "professor-entrepreneur." Boyer's academic colleagues criticized him for selling out to commercial interests, but the money made on successful products was enticing to those academic institutions who either joined or fought their way into the profit centers. Genentech was sued and forced to settle with academic institutions who felt they had supported this profitable research. Pharmaceutical companies had to look at biotechnology in a different way, leading to partnerships between small biotech firms, universities, and pharmaceutical companies. New areas of law and policy had to be developed.

The successful combination of academia and industry could produce great rewards, as with the Bristol-Myers drug paclitaxel (brand name Taxol).[153] Paclitaxel was first obtained from the bark of the Pacific yew tree harvested in 1962 near Mount St. Helens in Washington by a young botanist named Arthur Barclay from the U.S. Department of Agriculture for the drug discovery program sponsored by the National Cancer Institute (NCI). After about five years of work, the drug was isolated and named Taxol by scientists Monroe Wall and Mansuki Wani under NCI contract at Research Triangle Park, a new non-profit corporation in North Carolina. Like many natural molecules, paclitaxel was large and complex, and it took until 1971 to work out the structure. Although it was soon evident that it killed cancer cells in the lab with amazing power, it took eight more years and a brilliant researcher from Albert Einstein named Susan Horwitz to discover how paclitaxel worked—it prevented the microtubules which form the scaffolding of the cells from being dismantled. Despite the excitement in the laboratory, paclitaxel could not be used in people because it would not dissolve in water, requiring further work from NCI scientists. It was not until 1984, after twenty-two years of work, that the drug was tested on humans.[154]

The results of the clinical trials were dramatic by oncology standards. The NCI tested paclitaxel in women with advanced ovarian cancer and found it produced responses in 30 percent.[155] The major problem was getting a supply of the drug. Stripping the bark from the yew trees was not a good solution since it would take an entire tree to give about one dose for one patient. The first answer was a semisynthetic paclitaxel developed by French scientists which was obtained from the needles of a shrub member of the yew family. Recognizing this problem, the NCI funded the Florida State University Lab of Dr. Robert Holton which developed an improved version of the semisynthetic method of producing paclitaxel.

Until this point, the story of paclitaxel is an interesting history of drug development. Enter Bristol-Myers. Shortly after the NCI announced the results of its clinical trial, it awarded the rights to paclitaxel to Bristol-Myers. The company took over the NCI's existing contracts to produce the drug, reached a deal with FSU to further Dr. Holton's work, and trademarked the name Taxol. Bristol expanded production methods, and Holton's lab eventually developed a totally synthetic version of the drug. Within a few years, paclitaxel was the leading oncology drug worldwide, helping thousands of patients with breast and ovarian cancer live longer.

The profit was astounding. Bristol made billions of dollars and FSU hundreds of millions. The vast wealth generated battles: Congress investigated the granting of the rights to Bristol Myers; FSU and Bristol fought over their relationship; FSU and Holton each set up their own research company. At every turn, lawyers profited. Paclitaxel was so valuable that Bristol tried desperately to keep generic versions off the market, using patent delaying tactics which required them to settle $670 million in lawsuits.[156]

The NCI calls paclitaxel a success story.[157] Pioneers in the oncology world like Dr. Vincent DeVita maintain that without the combination of the NCI, academia, and Pharma, the drug would not have been marketed.[158] In this view, paclitaxel paved the way for Pharma's interest in oncology and drug development, beginning the rush of advances we see today. Others believe that the NCI spent millions of dollars of taxpayer's money to develop paclitaxel, then gave the profits to Bristol and FSU.[159] Whichever interpretation one favors, it is clear that Taxol put the capital "P" in oncology Pharma.

Today, the engine of academic science and industry is running full speed to bring amazing advances to patients. There are useful and ridiculous checks on the excesses of drug promotion and more transparency in clinical trials. Yet there is still very little control over the profits made on new drugs. Pharmaceutical companies in this country are free to charge any price they see fit. If the FDA approves the drugs,

Medicare will pay. Patent laws give them protection against competition. As in the past when the public wanted to believe in medicines, and the reputable apothecary was considered a valuable member of society, we also struggle with our feelings toward Pharma. We love them because they make the drugs that save us. We hate them because they are rich and arrogant and we need them to make the drugs that save us.

Frank was surprised at the emotion he felt making his first phone call to Bill Jones, his immediate supervisor.

"I'm sorry, Bill, that's where it stands," he concluded after telling his story.

"Frank. Don't worry about us. Take care of yourself, Lisa, and the children. And whatever you need, you know the resources of this company are behind you."

That emotion was only a prelude to telling the children. Anthony, in his early twenties, had recently graduated from college and was working his first job as a history teacher at Albany Academy while Francesca was a senior at nearby Union College, majoring in physics and hoping to go to Geneva to work on the CERN collider. Lisa had them come home, and Frank told them of his illness.

"What do you think, Dad?" asked Anthony. "Can you beat this thing? What can we do?"

Francesca cried and hugged Lisa.

"No, Tony. I can't beat it right now. What we can do is control it. The odds of that are good. We have to hope that other medications come along that are even better."

"But why you? You're not a smoker," asked Francesca.

"No one knows," answered Lisa.

"What you can do," Frank went on, "is to keep living your lives. You are great young people, and you shouldn't change anything about your lives."

Anthony and Francesca spent the night in their old rooms, which Lisa kept ready for them. After their parents had gone to bed, the siblings sat together on the couch, much as they did as children when Anthony read history and Francesca almost anything.

"Dad's going to die, isn't he?" asked Francesca, crying again.

"Don't say that," said Anthony replied, stroking her hair. "There are treatments to control it."

"And what when they don't work?" she demanded.

"Then they'll find more. You know how much he believes in them—"

"They better find more."

Next on the list was Uncle Frankie and Aunt Shelly. Lisa had set an afternoon visit when Frank would feel his best. Despite her eighty-five years, Shelly still had the grace not to press for the reason.

Radiation had gone smoothly that morning. Frank had taken extra morphine and a nap. It was a gray and rainy day as Lisa drove them through Schenectady to Prestwood Gardens, a retirement community on the opposite side of the city. As they passed downtown and crossed Broadway, Frank remembered his last visit to Johnson's Apothecary. It was about twenty years ago, and he was picking up Uncle Frankie so they could meet their wives for dinner to celebrate one of his promotions. When Frank arrived, Mrs. Kelly and Mrs. Wilson both greeted him with particular warmth. The store was in its usual immaculate state, but he noticed a few empty areas in the durable equipment section. After his uncle had finished closing and they were preparing to leave, he commented on the changes. Uncle Frankie looked at him closely.

"You don't miss much, do you?" Uncle Frankie paused and ran his hand over the soda counter. He motioned Frank to one of the stools and sat next to him. They faced outward, looking across at the candy and up the aisle to the pharmacy.

"I'm closing after the Holiday season, Frank. It's been a great run, but we can't do it anymore. Shelly and I are ready." He paused. "The time for mom-and-pop pharmacies is over. The margins are too small, risks too high, paperwork too much, and everyone wants twenty-four-hour service."

"Are you selling? A chain?"

Frankie shook his head. "No, we talked but it didn't work. They didn't really want a Broadway store without a parking lot and, truth be told, I was glad. I didn't want to miss out on a financial opportunity, but unless it was a tremendous offer, I didn't want a chain here. I would rather just be gone. We did work out a deal where they will take over our clients and in return give us a good price on anything we have left in the store."

Frank nodded. "How do you feel?"

"Mixed, as you might expect. This," he waved his hand across the expanse of the store, "was our baby. When your aunt and I couldn't have children, we needed something together. The store was an amazing place. We did things here that they never could do in those chains. Mrs. Kelly, she was social worker to half the poor kids in the area. And her husband, too. Ruth Wilson, well, she knew who was running out of meds and who wasn't taking what they should. She would be on the phone with their doctor's office. She made deliveries herself and even put Father Kelly to work delivering meds with communion." He chuckled. "That was quite a sight."

Frankie paused. In the quiet of the store, Frank noticed the clicking of the clock over the soda counter. Thirty years and I have never heard that sound, he thought.

"But we're also tired. Running these small businesses is a daily grind. We want some freedom to travel while we still can, so this is our time."

"I guess everything changes," said Frank, "but it will be different. You have always seemed like part of this street, almost forever."

"Yeah, then one day you're gone. Remember that, Frank. When you leave, whether it's your own small business or your company, everyone will say how much they will miss you, give you a pat on the back, then go about their lives. Maybe you'll get a plaque or some-thing, but soon you will be a distant memory. No, the measure of what you do and what you accomplish in your life is in each moment, how you treat each person or make each thing."

He stood up. "But enough of that, let's go meet the ladies for din-ner and a Guinness."

Frank smiled at the memory and unconsciously sighed. Lisa caught his movement.

"You okay?" she asked.

"Sorry, I didn't mean to worry you while you are driving," he replied. "I was thinking of the Shop."

"Nineteen years it's closed," she answered.

"Really?" he started to speak.

"And don't tell me how you can still smell the candy and soda fountain."

He laughed as Lisa pulled into the well-manicured development. At the door, Shelly and Frankie greeted them warmly. She was still thin, well-kept, and immaculately dressed, while he still had the studi-ous appearance of a pharmacist, accentuated by his reading glasses. Their apartment was meticulous. The living room held a display of the accomplishments of the grandchildren, bowls of candy, and a small precisely organized liqueur cabinet, reminding Frank of the pharmacy. They sat while Shelly served coffee and cookies.

"You look sore, Frank. What's the matter with your back?" asked Frankie after they were updated on the children. Frank and Lisa looked at each other.

"You don't miss much, Uncle. That's why we're here. We've had some bad news. I have a cancerous growth on my spine and am getting radiation. It looks like it started from the lung. I'll be going to Dana Farber soon for a biopsy and probably getting chemotherapy and more radiation after that . . .," he trailed off.

"Is it operable?" asked Frankie.

"No. We need to treat it with chemotherapy and radiation."

Frankie looked suddenly older, for once matching his years.

"Did they give you a prognosis Frank?" he asked softly.

Frank cleared his throat. Lisa held his hand.

"No one knows. We are very hopeful that this treatment will work on the spine and lung and we have some medications which we hope will keep anything else in check. We also have several new drugs coming out soon. There's a lot happening in the field right now."

"You're in a good place to know," Frankie nodded, some color returning to his face. "This industry is really something. I've gotta believe we'll have something like a cure soon."

Shelly spoke next.

"How can we help you?"

Lisa responded. "Sylvia doesn't know yet. We want to tell her, but we wanted you to know first because we know she will turn to you."

Frankie nodded. "She won't take any medical problem with you well, Frank."

"We're going to try to put on as good a picture as we can," he replied. "Still, she has never gotten over Dad."

Shelly spoke up. "We'll see her as soon as you tell her. She will be scared, but she'll do what she needs to. Frankie will tell her that." She looked at her husband. "Just like he always does."

They spent more time together, talking about nothing and trying to let the emotions of the news slowly settle. As they left, Uncle Frankie gave Frank a hug.

"Be careful when you tell Sylvia, Frank. Suzanne Somers has a new book out. You could be eating that damn asparagus again."

But Sylvia did not crumble. In fact, Lisa and Frank had been surprised by her reaction. They had gone to Sunday mass together, then brought her home for brunch. Afterward, they sat in their living room while Frank gave her the news.

"What does your doctor say, Frank?" asked Sylvia.

"He says they can control it with treatments."

She nodded. "Does Frankie know?"

"Yes, Mom. We told him and Shelly."

She nodded. "How did he take it? He loves you, you know."

"He said he was sorry but ready to help. He knows we have a lot of different medicines. He believes I can fight this."

She nodded again. Looking down for a moment, she spoke.

"When my Anthony died, I didn't want to let you out of my sight. Frankie made me let you play ball at school. 'He's a big boy. He knows how to handle himself,' he told me then. So, I let you play. When you wanted to go into business instead of being a doctor, Frankie told me it was the right thing to do. He said I had to believe in you. After what happened to Anthony, I was so scared of everything. But I did it. I believed in what you and Frankie said."

She looked up at Frank and Lisa.

"You tell me what to do, Frank. You and Frankie. You know I'll do anything for you."

"We know. Give me a hug, Mom. Then help us with the rest of the family."

After two weeks of radiation treatments, Frank felt ready to travel to the Dana Farber Cancer Institute and meet Dr. Michael Williams, with whom he had worked on several research projects. The appointment and biopsy were on Friday afternoon so that Frank could have his radiation in the morning before the familiar three-hour ride east on the Mass Pike.

"Good luck with the biopsy," commented Dr. Chris cheerfully as Frank and Linda were leaving the radiation oncology unit.

"Do you think I can drive?" asked Frank innocently. Dr. Chris almost instinctively answered yes, but quickly caught himself as Lisa turned and glared.

"Sure," he replied. "With a note from your wife."

Frank laughed. "Worth a try."

"Maybe not," responded Dr. Chris, still watching Lisa.

The ride was smooth, and they met Dr. Williams, a lanky man in his mid-fifties who reminded Frank of John Kerry.

"Hello, Frank. I'm sorry to see you in this situation."

Frank introduced Lisa.

"So, you're the saint who put with him all these years?" Dr. Williams drawled. "I've been wanting to meet you. I'm sorry this brought us together."

Lisa smiled. Dr. Williams confirmed the plan; then Frank had a mild sedative, a quick trip into a CT machine for a biopsy followed by two hours of observation and another chest x-ray. They stayed overnight and left early in the morning. Neither felt like enjoying Boston; they just wanted to be home.

The call from Dr. Williams came next week.

"The biopsy did show non-small cell lung cancer, a well-differentiated adenocarcinoma. I know you didn't want any of this, but at least this is a type we can treat. The genetic studies are still out. They'll be another few weeks."

"Can I start chemo?" Frank asked.

"Yes. And radiation to that spot in the lung as well. I'll speak to Matthews about it tomorrow."

LUNG CANCER: DRIVER MUTATIONS AND TARGETED TREATMENTS.

For many years lung cancers were divided by pathologists into two types: "small cell lung cancer," which often dramatically shrank with chemotherapy but later regrew, and "non-small lung cancer" which was usually resistant from the start. The best treatment for non-small lung cancer is surgery. Unfortunately for most patients, by the time it is discovered the cancer has spread to other parts of the body and surgery is useless. Once the cancer has spread, surgery or radiation is given to painful or important areas like the brain, weight bearing bones, or major airways, but "systemic therapy" for the whole body is required.

Systemic treatment for non-small cell lung cancer began in the 1960s with chemotherapy. After the chemotherapies which worked so well against lymphomas failed in most lung cancers, decades of additional effort produced a few drugs which were minimally useful. Since long exposure to toxins and carcinogens in cigarette smoke causes most lung cancers, they resist many chemotherapy treatments. These disappointing results suggested different treatment approaches were needed. In the late 1990s, the treatment of chronic myelogenous leukemia (CML) using the drug imatinib (Gleevec) became the model for one new approach, called "targeted treatment." The specific molecular abnormality in CML (the target) was identified, drugs were developed to treat the problem, and patients cured. Scientists working in lung cancer also hoped to identify their own targets which might lead to effective treatments.

The study of lung cancers in non-smokers revealed potential targets. It was well known that lung cancers in non-smokers were different from those in smokers. Non-smoking patients often developed a specific type called adenocarcinoma, meaning it started in the gland cells of the lung, and molecular studies produced fascinating results. The cancers of non-smokers could result from mutations in a few key genes, called "driver mutations" because they "drove" the cancerous process. The first key gene in this category was named *EGFR*, the epidermal growth factor receptor gene. The *EGFR* gene normally produces a protein which signals the cell to grow. The cancer cells of non-smokers could contain a driver mutation in *EGFR* which causes it to be constantly "turned on," leading to uncontrolled growth. This discovery led to the development of drugs to block the EGFR protein produced by the driver mutation. AstraZeneca's gefitinib (Iressa) was the first drug developed. It produced some dramatic responses in patients whose cancers had not responded to chemotherapy. Studies showed Iressa worked in cancers with a driver mutation in *EGFR*, but the benefit was short—a few months longer survival. Despite initial enthusiastic press reports, in 2005 the drug was removed from the market and later replaced with the more successful drug erlotinib (Tarceva), which added six to nine months of survival.

Targeted treatment for non-small cell lung cancer was a small step forward, not the tremendous leap seen in CML with imatinib (Gleevec). In CML, virtually all patients had the same mutation, allowing the treatment imatinib to work for everyone. In lung cancers, only a small percentage of patients have the *EGFR* mutation and can be treated with erlotinib (Tarceva) (more often Asian and women nonsmokers have this mutation). Even in those patients treated with erlotinib, the effectivenss is limited because the cancers develop additional mutations in either the *EGFR* gene itself or other genes. These secondary mutations can result in regrowth of the cancer and require scientists to search for a new target. Testing for these secondary mutations and targeting them for treatment is underway.

In addition to targeted treatments, other strategies were developed to control non-small cell lung cancers. As cancers grow, they develop their own blood supply in a process called angiogenesis (angio meaning blood vessel and genesis meaning birth). The normal body produces blood vessels to grow and heal, but the process is kept under tight control. Cancers pervert the process, resulting in weak and disordered blood vessels; one reason why they bleed easily. Medications which can halt angiogenesis can keep cancers in check when they are small, before they have developed their blood supply. Bevacizumab (brand name Avastin) is an antibody directed against one of the factors which promote blood vessels. Since these medicines do not usually shrink the cancers, evaluating their effectiveness is very complicated. Bevacizumab works modestly well in lung and colon cancer. While it was first thought to be helpful in breast cancer, later trials showed it was not useful. Predictably, bevacizumab is very expensive.

Frank would use all available tools. Radiation to the spine and lung, chemotherapy, and the drug bevacizumab. Once the cancer shrank, the chemotherapy would stop and the bevacizumab alone would continue. If his cancer had the target *EGFR* mutation, he would take erlotinib.

Since Frank's bones were damaged, his treatment also included a medicine called zoledronic acid to strengthen his bones.

When the radiation to his spine finished, Frank was walking almost normally. The next step was chemotherapy, given once every three weeks with cisplatin, pemetrexed, and bevacizumab. Frank and Lisa met nurse Amy Lange to preview the side effects.

"I know you know these medications from your work, Frank," Amy started, "but it is always different when you're the patient."

"Listen to her," Lisa enjoined. She turned to Amy. "He has been telling me how 'well tolerated' this treatment is."

Amy laughed. "We say 'well tolerated' is a good term when someone else is getting the chemo."

Accurately documenting side effects of treatments is not easy; they are numerous and vary greatly in severity. To standardize the reporting, each specific side effect is described in "grades." Grade 1 is a minor toxicity, grade 2 annoying but not dangerous, grade 3 more serious, grade 4 life threatening, and grade 5 fatal. Oncology nurses know this grading system has limits. Some side effects are difficult to quantify, like nausea or fatigue. Some side effects that seem minor are torturous, like mouth sores. The impact of some side effects varies with the person. Some people do not mind hair loss. Others, including those with very few strands at the start, are devastated.

Frank did not have any disabling toxicities, but for a week after each treatment he had nausea, pulsating pains in his back, tingling in his hands and feet, and fatigue. He was reviewing these with Amy when an old colleague making a marketing visit happened to see him and briefly interrupted.

"Frank! I heard you were out sick, but I'm sorry to see you here. Let me know if I can help with anything."

"Thanks, Bob," Frank replied.

Bob turned to Amy. "He always was a pain to work with, but he still looks good." He turned to Frank, "Seriously, you do look good, but if you ever need anything . . ."

"Are you tired of being told how good you look?" asked Amy after Bob departed.

Frank looked thoughtfully at her. "How did you know?"

"It's a burden," she replied. "Often our patients go out in the world and get told how good they look when they feel horrible. People just don't know how you feel. It might be easier if you wore a cast, then people assume you are hurting."

To his colleagues at work, Frank seemed upbeat, but he reported to Dr. Matthews that he felt dull.

"I just can't seem to quite get it together. I am interested in the projects, but get tired easily and find I just can't concentrate as well. I guess that's what they call chemo brain."

"It is probably a combination of everything. The chemo, pain, nausea meds, and the stress of all of this. Pace yourself. Once you get through these treatments, it will get better."

Frank and Lisa settled into a routine of the treatments every three weeks. Dr. Williams reported the genetic studies of Frank's cancer had shown the *EGFR* target mutation, giving him the option to take the pill erlotinib once chemotherapy was over.

Three months later, Dr. Matthews compared Frank's PET scan with his first.

"It looks much better, almost normal. You can still see some faint uptake in the spine where the radiation was given, but that is to be expected because the bone is still healing. The lung looks fine, only a small scar."

"What now?" asked Lisa.

"Now Frank takes the oral pill, called erlotinib or Tarceva. He will continue the bevacizumab every three weeks with zoledronic acid every other time. The next scan will be in three months."

Sunday family dinner was upbeat. Sylvia, Uncle Frankie, and Aunt Shelly were ready to declare victory. Anthony and Francesca were relieved but more realistic.

"I'm so glad for you it's over Frank," toasted Frankie. Sylvia and Shelly nodded.

"I still need to keep up with the treatments," reminded Frank, hoping to moderate their enthusiasm.

"It's amazing what they can do these days," agreed Sylvia. "To think the scan was all clear."

Frankie nodded. "The research those companies are doing is just amazing."

"What we eat causes most of these cancers," opined Sylvia. "If we ate better we would not have all these cancers. I was reading about some vegetables—"

Francesca saved the day.

"Be careful with asparagus, Grandma. Anthony has trouble in the bathroom afterward."

They all laughed except Sylvia, who turned to Anthony.

"What trouble do you have, Anthony?" Without waiting for a response, she delivered him a dissertation on roughage and bowel function. Anthony looked painfully attentive while Francesca gloated. Frank and Lisa escaped to serve dessert.

After coffee, Anthony drove the seniors home while Frank sat with his daughter.

"I think you should go to Europe for your big experiment next year," Frank said.

Francesca laughed. "It's not my experiment, Daddy. There are thousands of physicists there."

"Well, now you should go. I know you were nervous about leaving if I was sick."

She hugged him. "I will go Daddy, but probably not next year. I'm going to work with data from the project at SUNY in Albany. My advisor thinks it will take me about a year until I'm ready to go over."

"Honey, you do what is best for your future. Don't skip anything because of me."

She hugged him again. "I'll do the best thing, Daddy."

Frank settled into his new routine. Each day he took the erlotinib pill to block the target protein in his cancer cells. Once every three weeks, he received a bevacizumab infusion to prevent the cancer from growing new blood vessels. Overall, he felt good. Sure, he was still tired. The rashes came and went and sometimes his mouth was sore, but his brain worked well. Life moved on. Work projects came and went, people changed, some new ones did not know of his illness. Francesca went to Switzerland and returned breathless with the excitement of thousands of physicists uncovering the foundations of the universe. Anthony had found his niche teaching and became absorbed in his community, debating history and the merits of the Common Core. Frankie, Shelly, and Sylvia all kept aging.

Three years passed. Then, two years ago, Frank's recurrence came without warning when his scan showed a new area of activity in the lymph nodes in his chest. Another trip to Boston and another biopsy brought Frank and Linda back to Dr. Williams.

"The cancer looks the same under the microscope, but the DNA analysis shows a specific mutation which makes it resistant to the erlotinib. There are a few options. It looks like this is a small area. You could radiate it and keep on your current treatment with the erlotinib and bevacizumab. That might work for a while. You are also eligible for a study of a new drug. It's oral and has a side effect profile similar to erlotinib, which you seem to be tolerating well. The drug is designed to work when these new mutations develop."

"Whose trial is it?" asked Frank.

Dr. Williams named the company

"Well, I won't tell anyone at work. They're a competitor." Frank replied.

"Do you think this one will work? Is this a serious trial?" asked Lisa, think of TNF.

Dr. Williams looked up. "This is a real trial. I can't promise you it will work, but there is a sense that this could be very useful."

Frank had signed up for the study. Not wanting to make the rounds again, they told only Francesca and Anthony of the change. He was more tired and the sores in his mouth were worse than with erlotinib. Yet the pills worked and for the last two years Frank had continued the medication.

Life had continued as well. Francesca became engaged to a handsome French physicist, Jean-Paul, who brought his parents to meet her family and friends. The weekend had been wonderful.

"I have heard Europeans like asparagus," Sylvia had been overheard telling the politely attentive future in-laws. "Do you know it helps to prevent cancer?" Mercifully, their English was not quite up to the challenge and Sylvia's French was nonexistent, allowing Shelly to skillfully change the subject.

After the guests had left, Anthony and Francesca found themselves on the couch, leaning together.

"Congratulations, sis. He's a nice man. And I like his parents, too."

"Thanks. We've agreed to split our time between here and France. Dad seems to be doing well but I want to be around . . . you never know." She looked instantly worried and, for a brief instant, Anthony saw her as his eight-year-old sister.

"They keep coming up with new things . . .," he stroked her hair, just like always.

"They better."

The next morning the house was empty as Lisa patrolled, straightening various items. When she was satisfied, she went upstairs to pack an overnight bag for Canyon Resort. As she left the bedroom, she stopped and picked up the photo of Frank's group in Chicago taken all those years ago.

"When we need it, you better have something more for him," she told them as she put the picture back in its place.

Carol Feinman 3: Breast cancer (Boston, 1988)

They worked in Saint Martin. Not as much as if they had been at the Boston Marriott under Rose's watch, but enough. The early risers, Carol and Mary, took a morning walk on the beach. At nine, they joined Roger and the still dazed Sophia on the villa's veranda. Roger had arranged for both breakfast and lunch to be served there so they could work until midafternoon. In the evening, they would regroup on the beach to enjoy the late day sun. The work discussions were lively, and Carol found breast cancer only occasionally intruded into her thoughts.

They had Wednesday afternoon off. Sophia and Mary had gone shopping, leaving Carol and Roger on the shaded beach with a spectacular view of the sea. Although they had not spent much time together, Carol valued Roger's company. He was a complex man, gay and black in the largely white marketing world, fashionably dressed in staid Boston, and fastidious in normal times but able to drop his compulsions to help a friend or colleague. Roger carefully guarded his private life and relationship with Allen, a white computer scientist whom he adored. Although Carol had worked with him for three years and felt close to him, she would not describe their relationship as intimate.

Carol noticed he was reading *And the Band Played On*, Roger Shilts' history of the AIDS epidemic which had been published to great controversy the year before. Carol had not read the book but knew the reaction it provoked.

"Pretty serious stuff for this place, Roger," she commented.

He lowered the six-hundred-page paperback and looked pensive.

"Have you read it?" he asked.

She shook her head. "Just the reviews."

"It's an important book, but it also has personal meaning. Since Allen and I met in college before all this took place and were always together, we escaped AIDS. But we have known some who didn't."

Carol decided to take the opening. "How did you meet?"

He smiled at the memory. "We were both in college. Allen was at MIT, a nerdy looking white boy from the city and I was at BU, an overwhelmed black boy from the country. To make extra money, he worked at the computer lab. For some reason, I had taken a computer programming course. In those days, you had to type each command on a card, then bring all the hundreds of cards in a stack to the computer desk where they would run them through the mainframe. You had usually made some typos and had to identify and replace the mistyped cards. Anyway, I was having trouble with my program, and Allen was working there. At first, I thought he was the smartest person I had ever met, but also very annoying. It took me a while to get to know him."

"Did you see each other then?"

"Oh, no. In those days you had to be even more careful about letting on that you were gay. Plus, we were so different, but eventually it worked out." He paused, not yet ready to go further and turned back to the book. "Anyway, this book is about what happened in the first few years of the epidemic."

"Why read it now?" she asked.

"You mean why didn't I read it when it first came out?" His voice had a slight edge, and Carol was concerned she had said something wrong.

"No, I wasn't really thinking of the year. I more meant here, Saint Martin. This seems like a place where you go to forget . . . At least I'm here to forget bad things." She paused. "I'm sorry. I didn't mean to upset you with the question."

Roger turned on his side and faced her.

"No apology, dear. My mistake. You inadvertently touched a sensitive spot . . . One of my own issues and I reacted in the wrong way." He paused. "Many people in our world feel if you are gay then you should be actively supporting the AIDS issues, marching in Washington and all that. This book was a call to action from those people. They expected the rest of us to read it and join immediately. But not all of us can do that, and we get a little sensitive about being criticized for it. So, when you asked the question, I reacted before I thought. I owe you an apology for being testy, particularly when you have your own much larger issues."

He took a sip of his drink before continuing.

"For you, this is a place to avoid having to think of bad things. For me, it is a place to give myself the space to think about some things I need to consider."

Carol nodded. "Either way, it's a heck of a lot better than the Boston Marriott."

Roger laughed and closed his eyes, the open book resting on his chest.

As she looked out over the beach, Carol felt a sense of detachment. I walked past the bronze ducks in Boston, felt an itch, was diagnosed with cancer, and am waiting for radiation on a topless beach in Saint Martin with a gay man. Mine is a strange world.

HIV/AIDS: THE BEGINNING.

In the strange world where the biology of cancer and viruses intersect, gay men caught in the plague of AIDS in the 1980s ended up leading the way for women with breast cancer, teaching them to claim pink as their color and fight for their illness.

HIV (Human Immunodeficiency Virus) infection destroys the immune system. When the immune system fails and a person develops unusual infections or cancers, they have AIDS (Acquired Immunodeficiency Syndrome). For many people now infected with HIV, treatment controls the virus, and they can live for years without getting AIDS—Magic Johnson is one famous example. A baby infected with HIV in the womb was apparently cured with treatment and will hopefully live a normal life. Our ability to treat HIV is now often taken for granted. But for those who lived and died in early years of the HIV epidemic, the story was very different.[160]

The late 1960s and early 1970s brought fears of new diseases. In the movies, Michael Crichton's *Andromeda Strain* saw the earth nearly poisoned by an alien disease. In real life, scientists concerned with the potential for diseases created in molecular biology labs discussed limits on research. They were all looking in the wrong direction. In fact, HIV was taking hold in Africa and beginning its spread through the planet. Since this virus took considerable time to produce its effects, the spread was nearly silent. In his book, *And the Band Played On,* Roger Shilts describes the visit of the "tall ships," the beautiful sailing vessels that came to New York City from all over the world for the 1976 celebration of the two-hundredth year of American Independence. These boats carried sailors infected with HIV to a fantastic party in the center of the New World and may well have started the spread of the disease. Regardless of how it first arrived in the United States, HIV rapidly spread into that part of the gay male community which was celebrating its newfound identity and freedom with frenzied, often anonymous, sex in the bathhouses of New York and San Francisco. Soon thereafter, an HIV infected Air Canada airline steward with a voracious sexual appetite named "patient zero" began crisscrossing the country and was blamed for infecting many men, although his role is now debated.[161] These infected men, called "vectors" in the infectious disease world, further spread the virus. The virus entered blood banks across the country and thus into patients who needed blood products, especially hemophiliacs. It also entered into the bleak world of intravenous drug users and was shared along with needles. At the start of the epidemic, no one knew what was happening. The virus was unknown, never before identified.

When HIV first infects a person, they often have typical viral symptoms of fevers and fatigue. Occasionally a person gets very ill, but for the most part, the body handles the initial assault. The later effects of the virus are devastating. The HIV enters and steadily destroys immune cells called CD4 T-cells, which are responsible for activating the system. The loss of these cells disables the immune system, allowing infections and cancers to develop. In 1981, reports appeared of previously healthy homosexual men with two rare diseases: *Pneumocystis carinii* pneumonia and Kaposi's sarcoma. *Pneumocystis carinii* was a fungal infection previously seen only in patients with debilitating illnesses like widespread cancers (it was renamed *Pneumocystis jirovecii* pneumonia). Kaposi's sarcoma was a skin tumor described by a Hungarian dermatologist named Moritz Kaposi in the 1870s and usually found in elderly men. These illnesses pointed to a profound destruction of the immune system, and the patients soon died horrible deaths from infection or extreme wasting. The epidemic was here.

Roger had seen it happen. When Carol asked why he was reading Shilts' book, the question touched a raw nerve. Like many in the early 1970s, Roger had come to college knowing he was gay but afraid to declare himself. On campus, it took him almost two years to find acceptance and a community of gay men. As he explored his feelings, he had struggled with his deeply religious upbringing and the pain of separation from his family. But most of all, Roger thanked God he met Allen. From the start, theirs had been a monogamous relationship, neither could tolerate anything else. As the gay sexual liberation of that time began to accelerate, they stood together on the sidelines. Roger watched as some in his original group of college friends joined the party. John, the first openly gay black man he had met, had come to him two years ago. Roger would always remember John sitting in his living room, on the edge of the couch, cradling a Heineken bottle and nervously peeling off the label.

"I have the damn spots," he said. "You can't see them very well because I'm so dark, but they're on my belly. They've injected some chemo into them to dry them up, but it won't work for long. I'm scared, Roger."

"I don't know what to say, John," answered Roger. "Isn't there anything else they can do?"

"No. Nothing. Now I wait until something else terrible happens. Either I lose weight or get some infection."

He was inconsolable, but Roger tried. "John. You helped me all those years ago to figure out who I was. Now tell me how I can help you."

John looked up, at once both tired and defiant. "If something happens, don't let me die in the hospital. I've worked hard, established my own business, and made good money. When I go to pieces, I want to be at home. But I need someone to supervise the nurses and all that. I know it's a lot to ask from you, but I have no one else I can count on. Everyone else is either also sick or scared to death waiting to see when they will get pneumonia or spots. And my family doesn't give a damn."

Roger took John's power of attorney. His friend's decline came with shocking rapidity as six weeks later he had a seizure and was taken to Mount Auburn Hospital. A CT scan found several large masses in his brain which were collections of toxoplasma, disgusting clumps of parasites which could infect patients with AIDS. The treatments were not effective and John only partially recovered, remaining confused. The doctors were blunt, telling Roger that John should go to a special ward for terminally ill AIDS patients across town at Boston City Hospital. It was Allen who refused.

"You made him a promise, Roger, and we will keep it."

Allen and Roger brought John home to his apartment in Cambridge. The first two weeks were manageable. John was confused but could follow some simple commands, sip some fluids, and get to the bathroom with help. Roger and Allen established a bizarre rhythm to their lives, taking turns going to their own home or work and getting the occasional break together when John was quiet and the nurse present. As the swelling in his brain worsened, John deteriorated. For the last two weeks, he moaned in bed, confused and incontinent while they alternated cleaning and rubbing him. Life had no rhythm. Allen spent time sorting through John's personal effects, carefully packing those they would need into a few boxes which he brought to their home. For Roger, it was a blur of seizures and horrible images.

After John finally died and the funeral home staff in protective garb had taken his body away, they stood on the balcony together. Roger always remembered the clean fall air of that early Sunday morning.

"I can't believe it is over, Allen. He was here, and now he is gone."

"You did what you said you would."

"We did, Allen. Where would I be without you?"

"You could have done it without me. You know that."

They stood together as the bells of St. Paul Church rang mass. Roger felt the overwhelming need to escape that place of sickness and death. His clothes and even his skin seemed to reek of decay.

"Let's clean up the place and get out of here," he said.

"No," said Allen. "I made arrangements for someone to come and take everything away. I brought us clean clothes from home. All we do is shower, change into them, and go. We can leave everything here and walk away. All our stuff and John's paperwork is already at home."

They never went back. Breakfast, calls to a few friends to spread the word, several meetings with lawyers, and a funeral service finished the job.

For the last two years, Roger had kept moving, refusing to allow himself to think of what happened. When Roger learned of Carol's diagnosis, memories of John came back to him. Now he wanted to know what happened. He started with the book on the beach and the question of why so many had to die.

HIV/AIDS: LEARNING TO FIGHT A DISEASE.

From the first official reports of illnesses which would later be known as AIDS in 1981 until 2000, the epidemic killed 448,000 people in the United States alone.[162]

The answer to why so many died starts with the science of HIV, known as a "retrovirus." The basic structure of the HIV is a strand of RNA inside a protein capsule. It works like a poison pill. When an immune cell swallows the retrovirus pill, the viral RNA enters the cell. This viral RNA is converted into viral DNA which then inserts itself into the normal DNA of the cell and either kills the cell or directs it to act abnormally (presumably in the best interest of the virus). Since normally DNA is used to make RNA, the order in this viral infection is reversed, hence the name retro. The enzyme that makes this retro conversion from RNA into DNA possible is called "reverse transcriptase." The discovery of this enzyme and the concept that cellular information could go "backward" from RNA to DNA occurred in the early 1970s and was a major scientific achievement.[163]

Retroviruses have an important history in cancer medicine. When the viral RNA is converted into viral DNA which is then inserted into the normal cellular DNA, that insertion can damage normal genes and become a step in the development of cancer. In 1908, Drs. Vilhelm Ellermann and Oluf Bang found a form of leukemia in poultry was caused by a virus, much later determined to be a retrovirus. Over the years, several cancers in animals were found to be caused by retroviruses, but a search for human retroviruses proved challenging. It was not until 1981 that a human retrovirus was found to be the cause of a rare form of leukemia seen in Japan, called adult T-cell leukemia.

Isolating these viruses and understanding the interplay between RNA and DNA was just beginning as the AIDS epidemic started.[164]

When AIDS was first recognized, it was clear the immune systems of these people were being destroyed, but it was not immediately accepted that a virus was the cause. At the start, some workers believed drugs, so-called "poppers," were responsible. Once it became evident that a new virus was the cause of AIDS, the next step was to identify the culprit. Since studying viruses requires sophisticated technology, this posed tremendous challenges in the early 1980s. HIV was particularly difficult and dangerous to work with in the lab. Growing the T-cells which the virus infected was difficult. Techniques for sequencing DNA were tedious, and HIV mutates very rapidly. Working with RNA was even trickier. Ultimately advances in molecular biology like the PCR test would allow small amounts of HIV in a person to be measured, as is done to track chronic myelogenous leukemia (CML). But PCR was not developed by Cetus' scientist Kary Mullis until the mid-1980s. At the start of the AIDS epidemic, the key enzyme for PCR from the *Thermus aquaticus* bacteria in Yellowstone Park was still undiscovered on a shelf. The era of molecular biology was just beginning to unfold.

The scientific response to AIDS was disorganized. Unlike in Michael Crichton's *Andromeda Strain*, the government did not have an elite team in a Wildfire Complex ready to fight the infection. Although many individuals responded with alacrity, early efforts to identify the virus were underfunded, disjointed, and rife with seemingly petty bickering among the lead scientists and administrators. The international cooperation which had characterized the efforts to treat cancers seemed absent in the search for the AIDS virus. A rivalry between Drs. Robert Gallo of the National Cancer Institute and Luc Montagnier in France led to charges and counter-charges and ultimately required high-level negotiations to allow both men to be declared co-discoverers of the HIV virus.[165] Despite these obstacles, in 1985 the first commercial test for HIV became available, and in 1987 the FDA approved the use of the anti-viral azidothymidine (AZT).[166]

As formidable as the scientific problem seemed, the medical, political, and social issues surrounding AIDS were equally or more complex. Medical care of early patients with AIDS was difficult on the individual human level. The destruction of the immune system led to illnesses which most physicians had never seen, terrible infections like fungal pneumonia and brain parasites or complex cancers like aggressive lymphomas. Many of the treatment protocols had to be worked out and were themselves toxic. Front-line doctors, nurses, and aides watched as their patients died horrible deaths. In some cities like San Francisco, specialized hospital wards were developed to care for AIDS patients, but in most areas, these units and home services were in short supply. Parts of the medical establishment were in denial. Many blood bank physicians refused to recognize the wider threat of the illness. Even when it was known that the cause of AIDS was a virus which had entered the blood supply, these physicians were afraid to risk shortages of blood and unwillingly to spend money on some simple tests which could have indirectly pointed to possible contamination and possibly saved lives. Their inaction was inexcusable.[167]

The public health implications of AIDS were also complicated. Closing the bathhouses and promoting an awareness of the sexual transmission of AIDS could have helped limit the spread of the disease. While initially public health officials were hampered by a lack of understanding, they often later lacked the will to impose changes. Many in the promiscuous gay community, enjoying or profiting from sex, refused to alter their behavior. The bathhouses and sex clubs were closed in 1984, only after far too many men had been infected within them. The federal government under the Reagan administration was frozen by both the philosophy of downsizing government and an unwillingness to acknowledge the gay community. To some degree, a "blame the victim" mentality was probably present. State and city governments were often distracted by other issues or in disarray. Even in San Francisco, the center of gay rights, longstanding divisions in the gay political community delayed effective action.

And the public was largely oblivious. The death of famous heart-throb actor Rock Hudson in 1985 at age fifty-nine is often cited as the moment when the public noticed the devastation AIDS was causing. Certainly, the fascination with Hudson helped. Of course, there were other famous figures who also died of AIDs, including pianist Liberace in 1987 and African-American news anchor Max Robinson in 1988. The story of Ryan White, the boy with hemophilia who acquired AIDS from a transfusion brought publicity when he was denied entrance to school. The 1986 *Surgeon General's Report on AIDS* by C. Everett Koop was seen by many as a formal announcement of the epidemic.

In the end, however, AIDS was thrust into the public eye and political action demanded by the gay community itself. At the start of the epidemic, it appeared the gay community might "exit with a whimper" as so many died. There was no army of wealthy influential sponsors to promote the cause and overcome government disarray and public disinterest, as cancer had with advocate Mary Lasker and her Laskerites. Ultimately the energy and creativity of the gay world had to be rallied by individuals within that community. At the start in 1981, San Francisco nurse Bobbi Campbell went public with his Kaposi sarcoma, dying after three years of publicizing the disease. Brave men and women formed organizations like the Gay Men's Health Crisis to provide services and People Living with AIDS to promote political action. In early 1987, Larry Kramer, a playwright and journalist, called for a new and more aggressive political action which led to ACT UP (AIDS Coalition to Unleash Power), a transformative group. Later that year, Randy Shilt's book *And the Band Played On* detailed the early years in a call to action and AIDS activist Cleve Jones began the AIDS Memorial Quilt. Marches, protests, and sit-ins took place across the country as HIV/AIDS became the first illness actively fought in such a public fashion. The gay community profoundly changed the way the illness was seen by both the public and government.

There are many lessons from the early history of the HIV/AIDS. But one practical lesson is that if you want to fight a disease, you need money and public support. The gay community learned that lesson. And watching across the country were women with breast cancer.[168]

It was gray and cold when they landed at Logan International Airport on Saturday afternoon. As she rode in the cab along the Charles River, Carol thought the city seemed unaffected by her absence. Her apartment, too, was exactly as she had left it, modern, pristinely clean, but a little barren. There were very few messages on her answering machine. Her conversations with her mother and sister were subdued. They were glad she enjoyed her trip but embedded in their own lives. For a few hours, Carol felt a little lonely and disjointed while she tried to re-enter her own life, anxious about the treatment to come.

Radiation was easy. Carol learned the routine of undressing, laying on the treatment table, and watching as the machine moved over her. The hum and click told her it was over. As she had waited during her first treatment, she again briefly had her vision of the hospital stripped down to its girders and floors with all the patients on stretchers or in beds. This time in her vision, she was in the basement and could see the beam passing through her body. The image had ended when Asa cheerfully approached and helped her down.

"How was it?" she asked, smiling.

"I didn't feel anything," replied Carol.

"Not the treatment, St. Martin."

Carol laughed. "It was beautiful. The beach was spectacular, and we really had a great time. Even did some work, too."

"So, close your eyes and imagine you're on that beach when we give you those treatments."

Over the next six-and-a-half weeks, the radiation treatments took place Monday through Friday. After three weeks, Carol developed a mildly annoying irritation of the skin. During the last few weeks, her whole breast looked red. Fortunately, the final week of boost treatments focused only on the surgical site. Rose and Betty had watched her closely at the start, but by midway even they had relaxed. At work, Mary, a pale Irish redheaded who lived in fear of sunburn, proved herself an expert in various soothing creams. Although what Carol could apply was limited by Asa's instructions, she found Mary's attention to her "poor booby" welcome. At the conclusion, the always polished Dr. Morris reviewed her situation.

"Carol, you have done very well. The chances of the cancer returning in your breast are very small. We now turn you over to Dr. Spiegel. I am confident you will do very well with chemotherapy also."

"How are you?" asked Dr. Matthews. Thomas Jones, a lean forty-year-old man, meticulously dressed in jeans and cowboy boots, answered with a slow southern drawl.

"No problems."

"Do you agree?" Dr. Matthews asked his wife, Laura, an attractive, petite woman with dark hair, bright eyes, and obvious anxious energy.

"Yes, this time," she laughed. "Did you get his discs and reports from Texas? They said everything was good." Her southern accent was much less pronounced than that of her husband.

"I did. They do look good. And the blood work we did was good, too."

"Even the LDH?" she asked.

"Even the LDH." Six years ago, Laura had read that this lab test was important and requested it each visit. It was their established ritual that Dr. Matthews never specifically offered the LDH result until she asked.

Dr. Matthews finished his exam.

"I don't find anything, so we will see you in six months. Your next tests will be at MD Anderson in three months, right?"

"Yep," came the slow deep voice from the table.

"I have one more question," added Laura.

The melanoma had started seven years ago on the back of Tom's left calf. One of many moles scattered on his body, he later admitted it had changed about a year earlier. Tom had been busy; they had moved to the area from Virginia three years earlier so that he could work for the massive new Global Foundries computer plant. He was a skilled machinist with his own company which made custom ordered parts. Since most of his work was for Global Industries, when the company announced one of the world's largest construction jobs would begin just outside Saratoga Springs, Tom had proposed the move. It was exciting. Laura had found a job as an admission officer at nearby Skidmore College. They had two young children, Ben (five), Crystal (three), and Leo, their seven-year-old Golden retriever. Who had time to deal with a mole? So what if it bled a little from time to time?

It was Laura who spotted it early that summer. They were swimming at a neighbor's pool when she noticed the black spot on the back of Tom's left leg. At first, she thought it was a tick. After all, this was Lyme country. They had been warned that since the winters had been milder, deer migration patterns had shifted north into their area. With more deer came more ticks. Hardly a week went by that someone wasn't diagnosed with Lyme disease, some with pretty bad problems, too.

After the children were asleep, she pushed him onto the bed.

"Lay down on your stomach," she told him, "and don't move your legs."

"This sounds fun," he laughed, face down on the bed.

"Be quiet. I'm looking for the tick."

"When you've found that, let me show you something else," he continued.

Laura found no sign of a tick, but the irregular spot which was dark and bleeding did not look normal.

"How long has this been there? How long has it been bleeding?" she demanded.

"I don't know. A few months? So what?"

"Well, I don't like it. You're going to the doctor right away," she declared, the tone of her voice expressing both displeasure and anxiety while making it clear there would be no discussion.

"Don't worry, honey. It's a nothing, a scratch. It just hasn't healed."

The dermatologists in town were booked for months, so Laura made an appointment with Dr. Larry Cannon, a general surgeon whom she had once met at a Skidmore College function.

Dr. Cannon looked at Tom's spot.

"I don't know what it is, but I wouldn't want it on me, so we'll take it off. I'll be right back. Get on your stomach." He pointed to the exam table.

"That's what you said," Tom joked to Laura as he moved to the table.

"You won't be happy if I get his knife," came her reply.

A quick injection of lidocaine, an incision, and a few stitches meant Tom's spot was in a jar and off to pathology. Three days later, a call came from Dr. Cannon while Laura was out.

"Tom, the spot I took off was a melanoma. I need you to come in tomorrow at two, so we can make plans for more surgery. And I want you to see Dr. Matthews, the oncologist as well."

Tom was too surprised to ask any questions. When she returned, Laura had plenty.

"Melanoma? That's cancer. What surgery do you need? Why an oncologist?"

Tom shook his head. "I don't know, but we'll find out tomorrow."

Ben and Crystal chose that moment to run into the room together, followed by Leo.

"Mommy," cried Crystal, racing toward Laura for a hug. While she continued, Ben stopped short and turned toward his father.

"Can I see your boo-boo?"

"Sure, sport," answered Tom, turning his leg to show the bandage to Ben, as Leo joined in the inspection.

The next afternoon, Dr. Cannon was direct.

"The melanoma was a deep one, which means I need to take a wide area of skin and tissue to be sure it is all removed. I will remove an area two inches around the spot and an inch deep. I will also remove a few of the lymph nodes from your groin to see if it has spread. We will inject a dye near the melanoma to guide me to the right nodes."

"Will that get it all?" asked Laura.

"I sure hope so," replied Dr. Gannon. "But because it was deep, I want you to see Dr. Matthews, the oncologist, to discuss anything else he thinks we should do."

That night, at her kitchen table, Laura began to learn about melanoma.

MELANOMA.

Melanoma is the most fearsome of the skin cancers, the "one that travels" and can lead to death by spreading to vital organs. Sun exposure leads to melanoma, particularly when burns repeatedly damage the skin. As more people have recreational time to spend in the sun (or tanning booths) and show more skin, the rates of melanoma rise. In our modern world, melanoma is a leading cause of cancer death in young people.

Melanoma has long had the reputation of being unpredictable. The relationship of melanoma to sun exposure illustrates this mysterious complexity. The more common and less dangerous skin cancers, called basal cell or squamous cell cancers, almost always develop in the areas of the body exposed to the sun, such as the face, ears, arms, neck, or shoulders. While melanoma is often found in these areas, it can also develop on areas of the body where the sun never reaches. A second example of the complexity of melanoma is when it grows and shrinks (called regression) in "fits and starts." Many patients describe spots on their skin which seemed to stay stable, then grew and sometimes shrank. Occasionally melanoma can even be spread throughout the body with no obvious spot on the skin, meaning the primary spot had completely vanished or regressed.

Scientists have begun to understand these unusual features of melanoma. The cancer starts from the cells in the skin called melanocytes, which produce the pigment melanin to protect the DNA of the cell from damage due to sunlight. Sun exposure causes our melanocytes to produce little packages of melanin, called melanosomes. In a remarkable process, these melanosomes are then transferred to the other cells of the skin so they can also be protected (hair cells also receive the melanosomes). This is tanning. We all have about the same number of melanocytes in our skin; about every tenth cell in the skin is a melanocyte. Racial differences result from the different types and amounts of melanin our melanocytes produce.

Melanomas occur when the melanocytes become deranged. Molecular science has revealed some pathways by which the melanocytes become cancerous. Some melanomas start with a mutation in a critical growth gene, called a "driver mutation" (because it drives the process). About one-half of melanomas have a driver mutation in a gene called *B-RAF*. The proteins these driver mutations produce can be targets for treatment. Melanoma cells also accumulate other DNA damage and are among the most mutated of cancers. As melanomas develop such heavily mutated DNA, they may express many proteins on their cells. These abnormal proteins can attract the attention of immune cells which may destroy some melanomas and contain others, causing the regression and explaining the occasional patient who has widespread melanoma with no obvious primary spot. This ability of the immune system to attack some melanomas has led to several treatments.

Once the melanocyte becomes cancerous, it first grows "radially," meaning the cancer cells expand along the surface of the skin. This phase of growth can take several years, but at some point, the cancer cells will grow "vertically" into the deeper layers of the skin. In these deeper layers, the melanoma can gain access to the lymph channels (and then lymph nodes) or blood vessels (and then other areas of the body). Once the melanoma is removed, the risk of spread is predicted by determining the depth of invasion, a process defined by two famous pathologists, Drs. Clark and Breslow.

Dr. Wallace Clark, a pathologist at Harvard's Beth Israel Hospital, is credited with developing the first system for classifying the risk of the spread of melanoma in the 1960 and 1970s. Clark was a brilliant intellectual, determined physician-scientist, and teacher who was also an energetic advocate for melanoma research and treatment, spreading the gospel of sun avoidance and early detection. Clark worked during an era when debates about melanoma and the biology of cancer were beginning, and he brought a broad vision to this discussion. Clark used the faculty of the Harvard School of Visual Arts to help classify various types of melanoma by looking at pictures and describing whether they thought the melanomas were "stationary" or "angry" looking. Clark identified layers within the skin and showed that as the melanoma invades into deeper layers, the likelihood of spread increased.[169] Melanoma pathology reports typically list the "Clark's level" of invasion. The main difficulty with using Clark's system is that even experienced pathologists can have trouble making the distinctions between the levels, which are often ambiguous.

In 1970, Dr. Alexander Breslow, a pathologist at George Washington University, published a simpler method for assessing the risk of spread of melanoma using a scale attached to the microscope to measure the depth.[170] Called the Breslow microstage, this method is easy and very reproducible. Breslow's work also differed from Clark's in another interesting way. In contrast to Clark's broad, almost philosophic, approach, Breslow did detailed studies on a relatively small number of patient samples (ninety-eight) available to him at George Washington University.[171] He later expanded these studies to develop recommendations for surgery and show a very high cure rate for thin melanomas (those under .75 mm deep). Breslow's work allowed the development of proper treatment plans for many patients with melanoma. Sadly, his own life was cut short by cancer at age fifty-two.[172]

A biopsy report for a melanoma will include a description of the cancer, usually followed by both the Clark's level and the Breslow measurement. Other features often include a description of whether there is ulceration (a bad sign), regression (good sign), the number of mitosis (or dividing cells—more is worse), invasion of the blood vessel (a bad sign) and the presence or absence of lymph cells (more is better).

Dr. Matthew's office was crowded on the afternoon of their visit. People obviously undergoing treatment and their family members occupied most of the chairs. John Welt, the medical assistant, quickly called Tom and Laura.

"Is it always this busy here?" Tom asked when they were in the exam room.

John laughed. "I've been here almost ten years, and I can't figure it out. No matter how we work the schedule, one minute it's quiet, and the next minute a bus pulls up and we're full. We try our best to keep everything moving, though."

Dr. Matthews arrived about fifteen minutes later. He reviewed Tom's history and examined him.

"Well," he addressed Tom, "you certainly owe your wife one."

Tom nodded, and Laura smiled as Dr. Matthews pulled out a diagram of the skin.

"Let me show you some information about melanoma." After reviewing the diagram, he showed them Tom pathology report. "Your melanoma did go deep into the skin, about 4.2 millimeters. We should do a few things. I want you to have a PET/CT scan to make sure there is nothing we can see anywhere else in your body. I do not expect to find anything, but it will be good to know that and to have a baseline test. We often find little cysts or other things on these scans which are not cancerous and it is good to know about them for the future. After the scan, Dr. Cannon will remove the area around the melanoma to be sure there is nothing left behind, and he will check your lymph nodes."

"What about after the surgery?" asked Laura, her mind rushing forward.

"Have you read or heard about other treatments for melanoma?" asked Dr. Matthews.

Laura nodded rapidly. Tom shook his head.

"Okay. The worry about melanoma is that a few cells might have spread to other parts of the body. We cannot detect a few cells by scans, so we have no way of knowing if they are there or not. In other cancers, like breast cancer or colon cancer, we give chemotherapy treatments after surgery if the risk of spread is high. We call these adjuvant treatments, but most people think of them as precautionary or insurance treatments. You may know people, particularly women with breast cancer, who have taken these treatments."

Laura nodded rapidly, Tom almost imperceptibly.

Dr. Matthews continued. "In melanoma, chemotherapy is not very useful, but there is an immune stimulator called interferon which is used if the cancer has spread to the lymph nodes. If their lymph nodes are infected, many people take the treatment. If the lymph nodes are clear but their melanoma was deep enough, some people take the treatment. In that situation, it is not an easy decision. People go both ways."

"Why?" asked Laura.

INTERFERON.

The story of interferon has several chapters. Introduced in the 1960s as a cure for viral illnesses, it failed. Revived as an anticancer drug in the late 1970s, it failed again. Interferon ended as a fascinating substance of scientific importance with some modest clinical utility. Many of the characters in the interferon story are familiar: researchers, physicians, pharmaceutical companies, politicians, investors, and patients. Some characters in this story are unique: Flash Gordon (of comic strip fame), a child hidden from the Nazis who became a scientist and escaped communist Czechoslovakia, and a potent female team of a socialite cancer activist and virologist. The plot is set in the backdrop of nationalism,

Vietnam, and Watergate.[173] Perhaps most surprisingly, the tale begins at the end of the eighteenth century in the Darwin family, later to be famous for Charles and his theories of evolution.

Erasmus Darwin is known to history as Charles Darwin's grandfather, but he was a remarkable man in his own right. As an English physician from about 1760 until his death in 1802, Darwin was famous for his clinical skills. Even though he relied on the misguided treatments of his era such as bloodletting and various dubious potions, Darwin strongly endorsed scientific advances, including the cowpox vaccination to prevent smallpox. Darwin was also a leading poet, scientist, and inventor who was friends with leading intellectuals such as Benjamin Franklin. Among his publications was a massive twenty-year effort to catalog the biologic foundations of life and medical illness called *Zoonomia or Laws of Organic Life*. In this work, published in two volumes in 1794 and 1796, Erasmus Darwin advanced the first theories of evolution which his grandson Charles was to fully articulate sixty-five years later in *On the Origin of Species*. He also provided a detailed classification and description of every known disease. It was in this impressive tome that Darwin noted that the cowpox vaccination failed in patients actively infected with measles. "The contagion of the measles, if it be taken in sufficient time before inoculation so the eruption may commence before the variolous fever comes on, stops the progress of the smallpox in the inoculated wound and delays it until the measles fever has finished its career."[174] [175] Darwin's observation that infection by one virus could block a second viral infection was again observed in the 1930s and called the "interference phenomenon."[176]

How would the infection of a cell with one virus block a second viral infection? The most obvious answer is competition. The first virus blocks the entry of the second into the cell or takes over the machinery of the cell, and thus the blockade is a direct effect of the first virus. This answer was simple, appealing, and largely accepted by scientists until the mid-1950s. At that time several researchers, including Swiss Jean Lindenmann and Englishman Alick Isaacs working together in

London, proposed a different theory. They suggested there was a substance released as the result of the first viral infection which caused the inability of the second virus to infect. Lindemann named this mysterious substance "interferon."[177] The initial reaction from many academic circles was that interferon was nonsense, it did not exist.[178] Proving the existence of interferon was difficult, yet the scientific evidence, thin as it first was, would not vanish, and gradually the concept gained credibility. Today we know interferon is produced by cells in response to a viral infection as a communication signal for the immune system and has many effects, including blocking a second infection.

Despite their initial skepticism, many mainstream scientists soon realized potential uses for interferon and enthusiastically communicated them to a receptive public. Interferon would prevent or treat viral infections from hepatitis to the common cold. Flash Gordon used it in outer space as a cure for a deadly comic strip infection.[179] The race to develop this "viral penicillin" took on national tones. In Britain, memories of the discovery of penicillin by Ian Fleming in London and its subsequent loss to pharmaceutical companies in the United States encouraged a collaboration of government agencies and drug companies to develop this new weapon and avoid the same mistake.[180] After the alliance produced the first interferon preparations, company executives publicly lined up for inoculations to prevent infection with the common cold while their scientists sought activity against other viruses.[181]

Interferon failed miserably. It did not prevent the common cold and other viral infections, the bubble burst, and by 1964 the prestigious *British Medical Journal* declared interferon unlikely to be useful.[182] What happened? Why did this substance which worked so well in space for Flash Gordon fail those on earth? One part of the answer was that the drug was not yet ready for trials. Interferon was hard to identify, purify, and produce. It is not clear how much interferon the subjects in these experiments received. Additionally, the trials were not done to today's standards and the information collected was confusing at best. Most importantly, we now understand that there are many interferons in the immune system and none is a magic bullet.[183]

Although interferon failed to prevent the common cold and public interest waned, scientific work continued throughout the 1960s. Researchers learned interferons helped regulate the complex activity of the immune system. Work in other areas of medical science helped interferon research. For example, a system for producing interferon from human white blood cells infected with a virus was made possible by advances in blood banking science.[184] Until this time, most blood banks had collected and distributed whole blood for transfusion. The modern technology of splitting blood into red cells, white cells, plasma, and platelets was introduced, allowing white blood cells to be readily obtained. Other important steps for interferon research included standardized nomenclature and techniques to measure potency.[185]

The interferon research of the 1960s also produced some unforeseeable benefits. One of incalculable value was the arrival of Jan and Marica Vilcek to Manhattan. As a young boy, Jan Vilcek had been raised by his Jewish parents in Czechoslovakia during the Nazi occupation. The Vilceks escaped the horrors of the concentration camps by hiding with a local family. After the war and during communist rule, Dr. Vilcek became a physician-scientist interested in interferon, and his work led to an invitation to visit Vienna. Normally the communist authorities would not have allowed him to travel with his wife, but for some unexplained reason, permission was granted for them to go together. The Vilceks defected and moved to New York City.[186] While Jan Vilcek made substantial contributions to interferon work, he is most famous for his later discovery of infliximab (Remicade), a valuable treatment for Crohn's disease, rheumatoid arthritis, and other autoimmune disorders.[187] Interestingly, infliximab inhibits the action of tumor necrosis factor (TNF), another molecule used in cell signaling in the immune system. As the result of this discovery, the Vilceks became wealthy, donating to New York University School of Medicine and establishing a foundation honoring the work of immigrants in the arts and sciences.[188] The Vilceks also returned to the Czech Republic, where they shared their gratitude with the members of the family who sheltered him during the War—a family who, along with interferon, played an important role for those needing treatment for autoimmune disease.[189]

After it had failed to prevent viral infections, interferon was largely forgotten by the public. In the 1970s interferon was revived as a treatment for cancer—again with high expectations. Why? The scientific answer began with speculation that viruses had a major role in many human cancers. This theory came from the long-standing observation that the effects of viral infections on tissues often resembled cancers combined with the demonstration that some viruses could cause cancers in the lab. In 1957, the prominent Australian scientist Sir MacFarlane Burnet dealt with this controversy in a philosophic review of cancer in *The British Medical Journal*. Burnet noted that the notion that many cancers resulted from viral infection was appealing because it suggested approaches to prevention and treatment, but was overly simplistic. Interestingly, Burnet also noted this potential role of viruses also contributed to the fear that cancers are spread like infections, a deeply rooted public anxiety which has only recently faded.[190] It is estimated today that viral infections cause 11 percent of cancers.[191] Vaccinations to prevent cancer are routine, such the Human Papilloma Virus (HPV) vaccine. For the public in the 1960s and 1970s, the speculation about viral causes of cancer and hope that interferon might stimulate the immune system to fight cancer also gained it popular support.

A second scientific reason for interest in interferon was that it had some anticancer activity in the laboratory. Preliminary lab activity is common in cancer research and usually does not translate into a clinically meaningful effect. Reminiscent of the experience with interferon as an antiviral, this activity was misinterpreted by the press, public, and even many scientists. These results prompted the first use of interferon in clinical tests which were not well designed. The public reporting of these controversial results added to the enthusiasm for interferon among its advocates.

There are non-scientific explanations for the public enthusiasm for interferon. In *Interferon: The science and selling of a miracle drug,* Trione Pieters broadly argues the public resurrection of interferon fit into the counter-culture movement of the 1970s which arose in the aftermath of Vietnam and Watergate. Interferon had appeal as a natural, therefore less toxic, cancer treatment which used the immune system rather than establishment chemotherapy.[192] Whatever the role of these motives, during this time a relatively closed political-academic-social system controlled government funding for medical research. The work of HIV/AIDS activists which would break open the process was still in the future. Interferon needed inside champions and had the team of socialite Mary Lasker and virologist Mathilde Krim.

Mary Lasker was an influential supporter of medical research in the interferon era. Lasker was the wealthy widow of Albert Lasker, the father of modern advertising whose made his fortune in the promotion of Lucky Strikes cigarettes. She promoted the National Cancer Institute, the 1971 passage of the National Cancer Act, and was eventually awarded a Presidential Medal of Freedom and the Congressional Medal of Honor. Lasker led a legion of similarly minded woman, often referred to as "Laskerites," which included a virologist named Mathilde Krim, wife of Arthur Krim, the influential Chairman of United Artists and Orion Pictures and political advisor to several Presidents. Mathilde Krim used her scientific and social standing to promote interferon, including holding a workshop in her own home; ironically (and possibly incorrectly) reported to have been held on April 1, 1975—April Fools' Day.[193]

Lasker and Krim were successful. In 1979, Congress approved modest funding which led to further public interest in interferon as a cancer treatment. Once again, expectations were high as the media portrayed the drug as a cure for many different cancers and showed the anguish of desperate patients and their families. Although Flash

Gordon was missing this time, the cloning of the gene further raised expectations and allowed the production of large amounts of pure interferon in bacteria.[194] As the pinnacle of hype was reached, concerns over a black market for the drug prompted the American Society of Clinical Oncology to issue a caution over the expectations for interferon pending the results of more clinical studies.[195]

Of course, interferon did not cure cancer and became "the miracle drug looking for a disease."[196] Why did it fail? One scientific answer was much the same as when interferon failed to prevent viral infections: interferon is a piece of the immune system, not a magic bullet. A second answer in cancer treatments was also similar to the experience in viral infections: poorly done first clinical trials. The early test results in patients with cancer were loosely compared with historical controls.[197] Accurate testing required modern clinical trials in which the administration of the drugs was prescribed by a predetermined protocol, effects and side effects were accurately reported with standardized measures, and results compared with a proper control group. When interferon was studied in these modern trials, its effects were limited and often dismissed in light of the tremendous expectations. In fact, interferon did have benefits and received approval for use in a few cancers. Although rapidly replaced by other medications, interferon helped in a rare condition called Hairy Cell leukemia (the cells do look hairy), a common lymphoma called follicular lymphoma, and chronic myelogenous leukemia (CML). Interferons were also used in the treatment of non-cancerous conditions such as hepatitis and multiple sclerosis.[198] Interferon research contributed to work on other molecules involved in the immune system, including IL-2. And, of course, interferon helped bring us Jan Vilcek and Remicade.

What about interferon and melanoma? The immune system occasionally attacks melanoma. Dr. Clark had seen lymph cells mixed in some melanomas while other physicians had seen occasional remarkable shrinkages of widespread tumors. For these reasons, a clinical trial was done using interferon by the Eastern Cooperative Oncology

Group. Patients who had a melanoma removed that was deep or spread to the lymph nodes (and were therefore at high risk to have spread) would either get an intensive treatment with interferon or nothing. The decision would be made by "flip of the coin," and detailed analyses of side effects and results recorded in a modern clinical trial which involved multiple institutions, physicians, nurses, data collectors, and patient volunteers. The information was audited for accuracy, reported, and studied for years.[199] The results of this clinical trial of interferon in melanoma, and others like it, showed interferon clearly had some effects. On the plus side, the first reports showed patients who received the treatment had improvement in survival, the first medication to show this benefit in melanoma. On the negative side, the benefit was not large, and the side effects of the treatment were great—the idea that this would be a natural, non-toxic treatment was disproven. With repeated analysis over time, the survival improvements produced by interferon became smaller.[200] The balance of benefits and risks led many patients and physicians to debate the worth of the treatment.

Ultimately, interferon would be replaced in melanoma by more specific immune treatments. Yet the historical paradoxes remain. Interferon has important biologic activity which is hard to harness, was a highly-hyped cure which failed to deliver, yet brought other benefits. It is a treatment which was (and is) controversial when used in patients, even when tested in modern well-designed studies.

Dr. Matthews reviewed the interferon treatment protocol: intravenous injections Monday through Friday for one month, then injections under the skin three times each week for eleven months. The side effects included fevers, chills, fatigue, depression, low blood counts, and possible organ damage.

"So, this interferon is a hard treatment with many side effects. There is quite a bit of debate about who should use the treatment."

Tom looked dazed.

"That's a lot of information for one day," concluded Dr. Matthews. "Let's get the scan and the surgery over before you make any decisions."

Tom nodded. "That makes sense. Wait until we know more."

At check-out, Tom was surprised to recognize the secretary, Anna, as a member of their church.

"Hi, Tom. We have your PET scan all set. You don't have diabetes or sugar, do you?" she asked cheerfully, obviously a well-organized woman.

He shook his head.

"Good. You're thin and don't look the type, but you can never tell. They will test your sugar the morning of your test and cancel if it is high. Now listen, do not exercise for two days before the test. If you exercise, all the muscles will show bright, and they won't see a thing, okay?"

Tom nodded.

"Good. That would never be a problem for me, unless you count cleaning the house. Here is the instruction sheet. Dr. Matthews said you can call us to get the results the next day. Good luck."

After Tom had left, Anna walked into Dr. Matthews' office.

"His PET scan is next Tuesday," she reported. "They're a nice family. I know them. Will he be okay?"

Dr. Matthews paused. "With melanoma, you never know."

Anna shook her head, "I think of those children . . ."

The ride home took about twenty minutes as Tom drove the Ford Expedition in his usual careful style, Willie Nelson playing softly in the background. After a few minutes, Laura spoke.

"What do you think?" she asked.

He shrugged. "He seemed to know what he was talking about. I guess we just have to wait for the tests, then decide." Laura knew that was all she would get for now. This was how he worked, too. Methodically. It was his way.

Unlike her husband, Laura could not wait. That night at the kitchen table she returned to the internet. The National Cancer Institute website provided her with the basics, but it was a melanoma blog that captured her attention. Joe had been diagnosed a few years ago, at about Tom's age. His melanoma was also on the leg and had spread into the lymph nodes. Two years later he had a recurrence in his liver found by his doctors and removed. He was okay now. Something in the blood called the LDH had tipped them off. Two years, LDH, liver cancer? Laura could feel her anxiety rise and was grateful to see Leo walk in, looking for attention and insisting she turn off the computer.

The PET scan was in a trailer which was towed around the county, landing in Saratoga twice a week. The rig was parked near the radiology building. A temporary tunnel erected out of sheet metal connected the trailer door to the building. As he entered the trailer, Tom noticed the heavy electrical wires which ran along the floor, connecting the scanner to a power source in the building. The walk was gloomy and the wires, although certainly adequate from a safety viewpoint, were messy and offensive to him.

The technician was a pleasant, talkative man in his thirties.

"I'm Ken. Your tech for the day. What are we looking for?" he asked Tom.

"What?" asked Tom, puzzled.

"It says melanoma on the req, but where is it on your body?"

"Oh," replied Tom. "It was on my lower leg. Here on the left." He pointed.

"Okay. That explains why we are doing the whole body. Usually, we don't do the legs below the middle of the thigh, but your doctor wanted us to do everything." Ken enthusiastically described how the PET scan used radioactive sugar to detect cancer cells. Cancer? Tom thought. Is that what I have?

The test itself was painless, a brief injection followed by forty minutes on his back with arms over his head. With Ken's running commentary, the time passed quickly. When they finished, he walked Tom out.

"Good luck, man. I know many folks who have beaten cancer. They have many new treatments, so hang in there."

Tom nodded good-bye. Is he kidding? I didn't know I needed to hang in there, he thought.

The next morning Anna printed the PET scan report, crossed herself, read it, smiled, then brought it to Dr. Matthews between patients. Nurse Karen Lange made the call.

"Dr. Matthews asked me to let you know the PET scan was fine. Good luck with the surgery."

MELANOMA SURGERY.
The main treatment for melanoma is surgical removal. After the surgeon does a "wide excision" of the melanoma and the surrounding normal tissue, many patients are surprised at the depth and width of the hole left behind. This is usually not a cosmetic problem if the melanoma is on a limb or the trunk, but if it is on the face, scalp, or neck, it can be very challenging. The depth and width of the surgery is determined by the Breslow measurement (the depth) of the melanoma. Thin melanomas (under 1 mm deep) can have a smaller rim of tissue removed (1 cm away from the tumor in all directions) while deeper melanomas need larger amounts of tissue removed. The second step for the surgeon is to determine whether to remove the nearby lymph nodes so that they can be checked for cancer. Again, Breslow's work was crucial. If the melanoma has grown deeper than .75 mm, the "sentinel lymph node biopsy" is done. Radioactive and blue colored dye is injected into the area of the melanoma and travels to the lymph nodes which the surgeon can identify and remove. This surgery was pioneered in women with breast cancer to reduce the number of lymph nodes removed from under the arm. Once the surgery is complete, the final pathology report will give the information about the melanoma and the lymph nodes.

The outpatient surgery center was near the mall. As they sat in the bright waiting area with large windows, Tom watched the traffic move smoothly along the nearby highway. After Laura had left for the women's room, he sensed a large shadow off to his right. He looked up and saw George Hand, a well-meaning and friendly busybody from his YMCA basketball league whose voice had only two volumes, loud and deafening. At this moment, he was only loud.

"Hey Tom, what are you doing here? Me, I'm getting my knee scoped for the thousandth time. And where's Laura? Is she here, too?" The other patients in the waiting area, thankfully few, could not help hearing George's greeting and watched the exchange with interest.

Tom paused, not sure how to respond.

"Laura's using the ladies' room," was the reply he finally settled on. "She will be back in a minute. How's your knee doing?"

George sat down, and Tom endured a description of his high school basketball injury and the subsequent multiple surgeries. Fortunately, the saga exhausted the curiosity of the bystanders and gave Tom time to construct an answer when the conversation finally returned to his reason for surgery.

"Dr. Cannon's fixing a hernia in my groin."

George nudged him.

"Are you sure Laura didn't finally get you to agree to be fixed? You've got those two kids, and maybe she's had enough." He laughed uproariously. "I kill myself; you don't have to answer that. Anyway, that wouldn't be Gannon. I know because I asked him to do it for me when he took out my appendix a few years ago, but he said he couldn't. Had to go to the urologist for the snip, snip."

Laura returned and alertly confirmed Tom's version of events before they were called and left George alone with his knee.

"Thanks. I didn't want George to know what I was here for."

"I can't blame you . . . that guy is loud."

The surgery went well. Even though warned by Dr. Gannon, Tom and Laura were still surprised by the size of the wound on his leg, covered with skin taken from his buttock. The groin incision was more painful. At home, as Laura changed his dressings, Ben insisted on being present. Tom watched proudly as his normally exuberant son washed his hands and solemnly acted as her assistant. After the dressing change, Ben sat in the crook of Tom's arm as they watched television together, with Leo in attendance.

At their post-op visit a week later, Dr. Gannon was pleased.

"Your wound looks good," he commented as he removed the dressings. "And best of all, the pathologists did not find any cancer in the lymph nodes or anything left on the leg."

"What does that mean?" asked Laura.

"From my viewpoint, you are done. Dr. Matthews decides if you need any other treatments, but you don't need any additional surgery."

They returned to Dr. Matthews.

"As you know, the lymph nodes were clear. That is good news. You now have a choice to make about the interferon treatment—"

"I want it," announced Tom, uncharacteristically interrupting.

Dr. Matthews looked surprised, and Laura looked quickly at her husband.

"Are you sure?" he asked. "The data about whether it is helpful is not entirely clear. It is a long treatment and a hard one."

"I want it," Tom continued.

"Okay, but before you do, would you be willing to go a big center like Dana Farber in Boston or Memorial Sloan Kettering in New York City to meet with experts there?"

"What can they tell me that you didn't?" asked Tom.

"Well, I am a general oncologist in a small town in upstate New York. We take care of patients with many different types of cancer and blood problems. At these centers, they have hundreds of oncologists, all focusing on one specific cancer and doing research. So, you can meet a melanoma expert."

Tom looked unenthusiastic. "You know the story. You've told me, and I want it."

"Tom, let's go," advised Laura. "It can't hurt. We can show the kids Boston."

Tom nodded grudgingly. "That part sounds okay."

As Dr. Matthews stood up to leave, Laura held up her hand. "I have one more question. What was Tom's LDH?"

Dr. Matthews looked puzzled. "It was normal. Why?"

"I read a blog from a man who had melanoma and the LDH blood test showed it had spread."

"We check it regularly in people who have had melanoma, but it is not very accurate. For what it's worth, Tom's is normal."

Tom looked at her as they walked out.

"LDH . . . I'm impressed."

Anna greeted them at the check-out window.

"We'll get it all set for you at Dana Farber. I'll get the insurance approval. Thank God you don't have one of the HMOs. Your pathology slides will go right out, and you will bring a disc with your PET scan. How is that Leo of yours? What a beautiful dog. I bet the kids love him."

Tom smiled, glad to be distracted by talk of Leo.

"Here's mine," Anna continued, pointing to a picture above her computer. "I love the pugs."

John Welt walked by and joined in. "Mine's a maltese, Gracie." He pulled out his phone and proudly displayed the photo. "Five pounds of white fluff. My wife won't go anywhere without her. Carries her in a little purse. Hard to believe that once the kids left, that little thing could fill their space, but she does."

Tom and Laura combined the visit to Dana Farber with a trip for the children. Laura's sister Melody had agreed to come and watch them during the appointment. They stayed at the Courtyard in Cambridge where the idle talk in the lobby was of the Red Sox's mounting disabled list, and the addition of Kevin Youkilis with a season-ending thumb injury. The first day, they rode the T to the aquarium. Ben seemed equally excited by the trolley, fish, and hotel pool while Crystal was most pleased that she had a room with Laura and Aunt Molly, away from the boys. The following morning Tom and Laura drove to the Dana Farber complex. They pulled into the parking garage and were directed to the oversized lot where Tom wedged the Expedition into a space.

"This whole placed is cramped," he commented. "I guess that's what you get from an old Yankee city."

"Don't be a snob," Laura replied.

The main desk was busy as they checked in.

"Sorry we are a little disorganized," commented the pleasant young women behind the counter. "The construction around here is crazy." Laura read the brochure which explained the Dana Farber was in the process of building its new Yawkey Center, a fourteen story and two-hundred seventy-five-thousand-square-foot facility for adult outpatient care named after Tom and Jean Yawkey, the late former owners of the Boston Red Sox and long-time Dana Farber supporters. The Center would handle three-hundred-thousand visits and treatments each year.

"That's an amazing number," commented Laura. "What do you think Dr. Matthews' office does? Probably twenty treatments a day, so ten-thousand treatments a year? No wonder he wanted you to come here."

Tom looked at her, unimpressed.

"Global has two-million-square-feet and a two-hundred-twenty-acre site. You could fit three of these Yawkeys into the clean room alone. And more to come," he replied.

"Big man," she rolled her eyes and returned to reading about the Dana Farber.

Dr. Michael Angler was friendly and well-prepared, having reviewed Tom's chart. He examined Tom, and they discussed the options.

"You technically meet the criteria for interferon because your tumor was deep enough, but usually it is used only when the lymph nodes are involved. In the studies that have been done, the number of patients with deeper tumors like yours and clear nodes was very small. So, it is hard to make any definitive statements. Even when the nodes are involved, interferon does not benefit the vast majority of patients. Frankly, most of us are giving up on it and looking for better immune treatments. There are some studies ongoing, but you do not fit into any that we have at the moment. My advice to you is to get on with life and watch carefully."

"But there could be benefit from the treatment, right?" asked Tom.

"Sure, it's possible," answered Dr. Angler.

On the ride home, once the children were asleep, Melody asked about the visit. Laura answered.

"The doctor said pretty much what Dr. Matthews said. There might be some benefit from the treatment, but it is pretty small, and the treatment is hard."

"Some decision," Melody mused. "Do you know what you are going to do yet, Tom? Do you need to think about it more?"

Laura's knew his answer. Tom had made his decision even before they left home. As far as he was concerned, this had been a trip for Ben and Crystal to see the aquarium.

"I want it," he replied.

"Do you mind me asking why, Tom? It sounds like even the doctors are not sure," continued Melody.

Tom looked up in the rearview mirror at his sister-in-law.

"I don't mind your questions, Mel. You've earned answers. I don't think this treatment is that great, but all the doctors say it does work in some people. And I can't look at those two without being sure I did everything."

"Well, Bruce and I are on board for whatever you need. Bruce specifically said to tell you he has your yard work covered. He has a group of guys ready to pitch in."

That night, with the children asleep, Laura again challenged his decision.

"Tom, you don't have to do this for us. I know this treatment isn't that great. Even the doctors don't seem very excited about it. And Ben and Crystal are too young to know the difference. So, don't do it to prove something to us."

Tom looked at his wife thoughtfully.

"Listen, honey. I screwed up when I didn't get this taken care of before. Who ever knew about melanoma? I never even really knew what it was. And I don't like it. There's too much unpredictability with it. It's not like my work where you can mill down to the hundredth or thousandth of an inch. These guys really aren't sure what they are doing. So, I have only one rule now. I blew it when I ignored it before, and now I'm doing everything. Whatever there is. Whatever it takes."

Nothing had changed the next day when Dr. Matthews walked into the exam room.

"I want it," Tom said.

Dr. Matthews paused. "Okay. We can do it, certainly. But why? You know many patients don't choose it."

"I know what they said at Dana Farber," Tom replied. "But I also know that I have to do everything. I can't look at Ben and Crystal if I don't."

Dr. Matthews nodded. "That's the answer then."

The first month was daily intravenous injections of interferon, Monday through Friday. Laura always remembered they started on the Monday after the Travers Stakes, the biggest race of the Saratoga Racetrack season, although she could never remember who won that year. After Karen Lange gave the pre-medications, Tom usually fell asleep.

"How did you meet him?" Karen asked as Tom slept, his cowboy boots crossed.

"You won't believe it," she laughed. "We met in a bar."

"I didn't think people got married that way," agreed Karen.

"Usually they don't. I was in college and went out with a group of sorority sisters. On a dare, we went into this dive bar, called the Tin Can. Some local garage band was playing the old seventies' song, 'Love is the Drug.' You remember Roxy Music?"

"Can't you see? Love is the drug for me," sang Karen, laughing.

"That's it. So anyway, this guy," she gestured to her sleeping husband, "comes up and asks me to dance. He was obviously not a college boy and was by far the most gorgeous man I had ever seen. Turns out, he was on a dare himself. One his friends had bet him a Klondike bar I wouldn't dance with him. And the rest, as they say, is history."

"I'm sure there was more to it than that," replied Karen.

"You mean like bringing him to the sorority, convincing my daddy that his princess could marry a cowboy mechanic from Texas, helping him start his business, having kids, then moving up north?"

Tom woke up, dazed from the medications.

"What's up?" he asked.

"Nothing," replied Laura. "Just telling Karen how I found you."

The twenty-minute infusions of interferon were uneventful. Afterward, Tom was unable to concentrate for work and returned home where Ben and Crystal were happy to include him in their games, oblivious to his pallor. While eating dinner was a chore, it was only a prelude to the nights of repeated waves of chills, fevers, and sweats, all unrelieved by medications. At the start, Laura had tried to stay up with him, but he quickly insisted she needed her sleep to be able to work and care for the children. The job of keeping him company fell to Leo. In the dark and quiet house, they would sit together on the couch, enduring the cycles as they watched Turner Classic Movies, Leo nuzzling his master.

Midway through the third week, Laura reported the toll it was taking.

"It's a tough treatment, but he'll be more himself once this part is over," said Karen.

"I didn't want him to do this interferon, but he's doing it for Ben, our son. He's five.

"That's a good reason," replied Karen. "I've children of my own. I'd do the same."

"You know then," nodded Laura. "Tom grew up in a small town in Texas. His daddy died of a heart attack when he was ten. After he was gone, there just weren't any men in the family. We joke he had all women around him—his mom, two older sisters, and one aunt who was single. Only his dog, Bijou, was a boy. His mother remarried when Tom was about sixteen. His stepfather was a good man, but could never replace Tom's daddy, and it was too late anyway. Tom was leaving home as soon as he could, off to find his own work. But his daddy's death has always been a worry of Tom's. He wants to be around, particularly for Ben."

After the month of daily intravenous treatments, Tom began eleven months of interferon injections under the skin, one given three times a week. Laura gave these in the evening. As she would prepare the injections, Leo would move closer to Tom, watching carefully. The reactions to these were much milder, and most nights he slept. On the occasion when he was awakened by a fever or chill, Leo would instantly be there, sitting beside his master, ready to watch a movie.

The year for Tom was a blur of shots, fatigue, chills, work, and family. For Laura, it was a year of nursing, motherhood, and her work. Thankfully, she had Melody and Bruce, for whom it was a year of anxious helping. Only the children escaped. For Ben, the year was kindergarten and Miss Jennings; for Crystal, the Beagle School and Miss Carter.

Each month they checked in with Dr. Matthews. One visit midway through the treatment, Karen Lange walked in.

"Dr. Matthews is running a few minutes late, so I thought I'd say hello," she announced and sat down. "How are you two doing?"

"I'm just tired," Tom replied and turned to Karen. "Laura has the harder time with this treatment. She gives me these shots, watches me, and still does her work and everything for the kids. I don't know how she does it." He hugged his wife.

Karen nodded. "The list of side effects for these medicines can be as long as your arm, but they never mention what it does to your family."

Then it was over. For some reason, Laura always remembered Stay Thirsty won the Travers Stakes that year. She wondered what was next.

"It's out of our hands," Tom had replied when she asked the question out loud. "We have done all we can, and it's time to return to business."

Dr. Matthews gave his answer. "We will watch. Obviously, if you notice anything or I find anything when I examine you, we will check it out. Remember, you will still get the regular aches and pains and minor sicknesses of life, but if anything seems unusual or drags on we want to know about it. Every three months we will do labs."

"Even the LDH?" asked Laura.

"Definitely," he replied, smiling. "The question of when to do CT scans is more controversial. We do not like to expose you to unneeded radiation, so we do not just do them regularly for no reason. We do them if patients have symptoms, something on exam, or their labs are off. We can also do scans if a person is planning a major change in life, like moving, switching jobs or their spouse, or spending a year in Africa. Often they need to know everything is okay before they make the change. Finally, we can do a scan if the walls are closing in and you are getting too nervous to function."

"Well, Africa is out," Tom replied. "And so far, she seems determined to keep me. So, I'm good for now."

As they left, they stopped in back to say goodbye to Karen Lange.

"Now we watch and wait," reported Laura.

"No," corrected Karen. "Now you watch and live."

Living started with first grade for Ben and pre-school for Crystal. Laura watched as Tom walked Ben to the bus for his first day, the boy's serious look reminding her of how he checked Tom's bandage. As Crystal danced, Leo supervised, and Melody and Bruce looked on, the melanoma seemed over, lost in the excitement of books, backpacks, friends, and teachers.

At times, watching and living was hard. For Tom, it was the visions of the children without him that caused the panic. Fortunately, he had his work. Using his hands had always calmed Tom. After his daddy had died, he found cutting, sanding, and fitting wood together in the middle school shop soothing. In high school, his talents were recognized by one of his teachers who had encouraged him to study metallurgy. After graduation, Tom had left home for a job in a manufacturing company. In the evenings, he had studied drafting and eventually started his business. Returning to full-time work meant Tom could focus, leaving the fear of melanoma in the same place as he left the pain of losing his father.

For Laura, calm became increasingly harder to find. She found herself obsessing over Tom, examining his skin, scrutinizing his every move. Despite the hectic pace of her life, the children, and her work, the thoughts kept coming. Even Leo could not calm her.

Help came one Saturday at a chance meeting with Karen Lange at Roma Importing, where they both waited to order their families' favorites subs. The line was long, but the mood party-like as the smells of Italian food mixed with the laughter of the staff and clients.

"How is Tom?" Karen asked.

"Back at work. He can really focus on his job. I envy him for that."

"What about you?" Karen continued. "How are you managing?"

"You don't really want me to answer that while you are off work. You get enough of this all day."

"Actually, it's nice to see people out of the treatment area, so tell me."

"I'm busy with work and the kids, of course. But I'm also more and more scared and nervous about what might happen to Tom the further we get out from the treatment. It was almost better when he was getting the treatments. Is that natural?"

"We call it re-entry," replied Karen. "It's very common, almost everyone feels it. You need to get back to your regular life, but you worry. And often you miss the security of seeing us and getting the treatments, even though you hate them. It will pass, but it is a hard time. If you want to see one of our social workers, let me know."

Laura shook her head. "Just you telling me it's natural is enough for now. Can I ask you one more thing?" Karen nodded, and Laura continued. "Once in a while, I'm angry at Tom for not noticing this melanoma earlier and putting us through all this. I know it's not right to feel that way."

Karen nodded again. "That's common, too. Many family members or friends wonder how someone could miss a cancer. Usually, it's a man whose wife was afraid to go to the doctor while she knew a cancer grew in her breast. Those cases are very sad. But Tom is different."

"How's that?" said Laura.

"Well, from what I remember it was on the back of his leg and probably hard to see. The second thing is that you and he were very busy."

"That's true," agreed Laura. "We had the move, the kids, and work…particularly his business."

"We see many men like Tom who really get focused on work and ignore their health."

Laura nodded, and Karen went on.

"Truthfully, men like Tom or my Roger, are workers. And when they get into that work mode, that's all they do. Self-awareness isn't possible. Roger is a cop, always working overtime and taking extra jobs. He's a great guy, but wouldn't notice a spot on his leg or back in a million years. Tom probably didn't pay attention any more than Roger would. The same focus that's good for him now was probably bad for him then. That's just how they are, and we love them. Remember, you two did a great job together with the treatments. So, don't let the fear of melanoma beat you without the cancer even being present."

"Thanks. You're a dear. I don't know how you do what you do, but I'm glad."

Karen's words became Laura's mantra: don't let it beat you when it's not even there. Even so, she was still scared. Sometimes at night she would wake up and watch him breathe. And the next morning, she would wake the children and start the day, living and watching.

Then one year later, five years ago, it was there. Tom was lying down on the floor, building a Lego castle for an evil emperor with Ben, when by chance he slipped his hand into his jean pocket and felt the lump in his left groin. He must have looked puzzled because Ben asked him what was wrong. He recovered quickly and blamed an ill-fitting piece of the castle drawbridge. That night when he checked again and reported to Laura, there was no joking in his voice.

"Laura, I can feel a new lump near the scar in my groin."

"How long has it been there?"

"I just noticed it today, I swear."

She checked, and her eyes moistened. "Maybe it's nothing. Let's see what Dr. Matthews says."

"It's a lymph node," Dr. Matthews reported. "Sometimes you can have lymph nodes swell for noncancerous reasons, but we need to know. First will be a PET scan to see if there is any activity in this lymph node and check the rest of the body. Then Dr. Gannon will take it out."

As they drove home, it again fell to Laura to break the silence.

"I know you're going to say we have to wait for the scans, honey, but what are you thinking?"

"I think it's back in my groin. I don't know about anywhere else."

Laura cried as they passed familiar landmarks and noticed the school buses beginning their afternoon routes. Tom parked the Expedition in the driveway and turned to her.

"I will not leave you," he said, holding her hand. "I'll do whatever it takes."

Anna had arranged the PET scan. As Tom walked into the trailer and passed the now familiar wires, he recalled his first trip and shock at the word cancer. Ken was his usual enthusiastic self.

"We will check your whole body; so you can fight this thing, Buddy," he said.

Karen called with the results. Laura answered.

"Tom's scan was good. There was some activity in that node but nothing anywhere else. Dr. Matthews has spoken to Dr. Gannon, and he will remove it."

"Thank God," Laura replied. "We were worried. Karen, you do one other thing for me? Can you check Tom's LDH?"

A few keystrokes provided the answer. "It's normal."

The visit to Dr. Gannon was brief.

"I'll take it out, and we will get a quick look at it while you are still under anesthesia. If the pathologist says melanoma, then I'll take more nodes. If I do, you might have some leg swelling afterward."

"Is that dangerous?" asked Laura.

"No," replied Dr. Gannon, "but it can be uncomfortable, and you may need to wear a support stocking at times."

He left, and Tom dressed.

"What are you thinking?" asked Laura anxiously.

"Let's hope we don't meet George Hand in the waiting room again," he replied dryly. "He'll tell the whole room I'm getting my vasectomy reversed."

She punched him in the shoulder, then paused. "Amen to that."

Dr. Gannon removed one lymph node from Tom's groin which contained melanoma. The next fourteen were clear.

"There really is not anything more to do at this point," stated Dr. Matthews. "There is no program like the interferon for this situation—"

"And the interferon didn't work," concluded Laura.

"Not in the sense that it kept the melanoma away," agreed Dr. Matthews. "But I know your husband had very strong feelings about it, and you both did a great job to get through it. I don't know how you would be feeling if you were in this spot and had not done it."

They pondered this question.

"Worse than I do now," came Tom's reply.

"So, we watch and hope that was all there was," concluded Laura.

Dr. Matthews nodded.

That night Laura searched the internet for answers and found herself back on Jim's blog. To her horror, she learned his melanoma had returned. His LDH had once again risen, and this time there were many tumors. He was on an experimental treatment, hoping to live to see his daughter get married. Tom found her transfixed, staring at Jim's blog and crying. He looked over her shoulder, read for a moment, gently moved the computer away and closed the cover, shutting off Jim.

Laura looked up and saw the man who asked her to dance in that bar those many years ago.

He kissed her. "Listen, honey. I know we are in this fight together, but you do not need to seek out the answers. I will do that. Stay off the internet and away from Jim. You focus on our family . . . The children and yourself."

Laura sobbed. "But I want to help you."

"You will. But not by going on the internet. We can't share Jim's sorrow or anyone else we don't know. If we need to, I'll do the research, and we'll decide with Dr. Matthews. We will work the best if you keep our family together and have a clear mind."

For the most part, it worked.

It was another year later, four years ago, that Tom felt the bump on his chest. It was hard, about the size of a pea. He knew what it meant. Anna scheduled the PET scan and a visit with Dr. Matthews.

"The PET scan shows uptake in this mass on your chest and several spots on both lungs. These spots are small, under half an inch, but there are seven or eight of them. They almost certainly are melanoma, too."

Laura started to cry.

"What now?" asked Tom, his arm around her, visions of Ben and Crystal in his mind.

Dr. Matthews turned to Laura. "Do you need a minute, Laura? Are you ready to go on?"

She blew her nose, nodded, and looked at Tom. "Okay," she answered. "Go on."

"When melanoma returns, we try to remove it with surgery. We can't do that in your situation; there are too many spots in your lungs. So, we need to give you treatment for the whole body. The interferon did not work, but there is an even more powerful immune treatment which has produced some dramatic shrinkages in melanoma. It's called IL-2, and you need it."

❖   ❖   ❖

INTERLEUKIN-2: THE FIRST EFFECTIVE IMMUNOTHERAPY.

Interleukin-2 (IL-2) is "the first effective immunotherapy for human cancer." In 1984, Dr. Steven Rosenberg, a pioneer in the use of immune therapies at the National Cancer Institute and a developer of IL-2, treated a thirty-four-year-old woman suffering from widespread melanoma with IL-2. Her disease completely disappeared, and she was alive and well twenty-nine years later.[201] Although not as highly touted to the public as interferon, IL-2 has been critical to the development of immunotherapy for cancers, most particularly melanoma.

The immune system is a complex network of cells which seek out and destroy invaders (bacteria, parasites or viruses) or rogue cells (cancers). In simple terms, the cells of the immune system include myeloid cells which develop in the bone marrow (some called neutrophils, others called monocytes) and lymphoid cells which develop in the lymph system (called lymphocytes). The myeloid cells are the first responders to most attacks and handle invaders in a non-specific fashion by eating them—this is called innate immunity. The lymphoid cells join the battle later with specifically developed antibodies and killer cells directed against the attacker—this is called adaptive immunity. The 1970s and 1980s brought tremendous advances in the understanding of the immune system. One group of scientists led by Dr. Robert Gallo, later to become famous for his work on HIV, was searching for growth factors which would stimulate myeloid cells. In a nice example of the unpredictable nature of research, their work identified a lymphoid growth factor called TCGF (T-cell growth factor) which stimulated T-lymphocytes. Although Dr. Gallo was reportedly initially disappointed that the TCGF stimulated the wrong cells, it became a crucial reagent in many labs studying the immune system and searching for viruses. During this period, it became clear that communication between the cells of the immune system uses many different signaling molecules and TCGF was one example. As scientists identified and purified more of these molecules, they renamed them in a uniform system. TCGF became IL-2.[202]

The convoluted story of how IL-2 became the first effective cancer immunotherapy includes many familiar themes: academic research, corporate competition, and driven researchers making scientific discoveries. Academic investigators at Dartmouth who isolated and identified IL-2 laid the foundation.[203] Their work began an intense corporate competition to clone the gene and allow large scale production. Cetus, the first biotech company which had developed the valuable polymerase chain reaction (PCR) test, successfully mass-produced IL-2 using recombinant techniques (cloning). Once large amounts of pure IL-2 could be made, it could be tested in patients. Cetus bet its corporate future that Il-2 would be a blockbuster—a wager it ultimately lost.[204]

One of the key proponents of IL-2 was Dr. Rosenberg at the National Cancer Institute, who encouraged its development with both biotech firms like Cetus and the Food and Drug Administration.[205] Intensely driven to find effective treatments for cancer, Dr. Rosenberg began using IL-2. His first tests were disappointing. At low doses, Il-2 was safe but ineffective.[206] Dr. Rosenberg pushed on with higher doses, developing a program of IL-2 given by vein every eight hours for up to fifteen times and repeated two months later. As he and others gained experience with IL-2, they realized this treatment was different from chemotherapy. First, there were severe side effects of low blood pressure and kidney or liver failure which required patients to be carefully selected and treated in ICU-like settings. Once the treatment was over, the side effects resolved. Secondly, treatments were individualized, and each person was given as many doses as they could tolerate. Thirdly, patients with melanoma and kidney cancers were most likely to have a response; IL-2 would work in about 10–20 percent of these patients. Finally, and most importantly, IL-2 cured some of these patients—something almost never achieved with chemotherapy. The FDA approved treatment of metastatic melanoma with IL-2 in 1998.

Dr. Rosenberg and others tried improving the treatments by removing lymphocytes from the blood of patients, stimulating these cells in the lab with IL-2, and giving them back to the patient with the IL-2 infusions. These cells were called lymphokine activated killer cells or LAK cells. They were only modestly useful, but the concept was exciting. Dr. Rosenberg then found that by removing the specific lymph cells which were surrounding the tumors, stimulating them in the lab with IL-2, and giving them back to the patients, the results were better. These lymphocytes, called tumor infiltrating lymphocytes or TIL cells, are the lymph cells seen by pathologists like Dr. Clark years ago which appear to be trying to control the cancers. In further fascinating work, researchers also found that the ability of TIL cells to attack the cancers was improved when patients were first treated with chemotherapy to deplete their normal lymph cells. The chemotherapy seemed to remove any lymph cells which might have the job of restraining the TIL cells—a feature the normal immune system has to keep it in balance. In the terminology of war, TIL was an army of lymphocytes programmed to attack the cancer, stimulated with IL-2 in the lab, then turned loose on the battlefield with further IL-2 stimulation and without any restraints.

"These treatments are only done at a few centers across the country. You will need to stay there for a few weeks at a time. So, if you have family or friends at any one of them, that would be a good choice. You know Boston. We can send you back there."

Tom answered definitively.

"No. We are going to Texas. To MD Anderson."

Laura looked surprised. "Why Tom?" she asked.

"They do a lot of it there, and we can stay with my sister."

Dr. Matthews nodded. "We have a few patients who fly back and forth there. It is not an easy trip, but it is an excellent place. Anna will help you make the arrangements."

As they left, Laura turned to Tom.

"How did you know about MD Anderson?" she asked.

"I knew this was coming. I researched it."

The trip to MD Anderson took most of the day. They left the Albany International Airport, named because of an occasional flight to Canada, then flew to Charlotte and Dallas. It was dusk when they arrived at his sister's home, but the air was still hot. The next morning Tom drove their rented Ford Expedition to their appointment.

"It's huge," Laura sounded awestruck as they drove to the main buildings.

Tom smiled, "Yep. The biggest."

Laura looked at him, surprised. "The biggest?"

"Biggest cancer center in the country. Makes Dana Farber look tiny. You won't fit this into the clean room at Global."

"Is that why you wanted to come here?" she asked as he pulled comfortably into the parking spot.

Tom shifted into park but did not shut off the engine so they would stay cool. He turned to her.

"They were nice in Boston, and I'm sure they would try their best. But we're in a fight here. And in this fight, I want to be in Texas. And you can park a truck easily here."

The met Dr. Henry Chou, an intense Asian man who rapidly reviewed the plans. First would be scans, then surgery to remove the melanoma from Tom's chest, followed by preparatory chemotherapy, and finally the IL-2. After Dr. Chou had left the room, Tom looked at Laura.

"What do you think?" Tom asked Laura.

"I know I'm just a girl from North Carolina, but he doesn't look very Texan to me."

Tom laughed. "No, but he knew where to come."

That week, surgeons removed the growth on Tom's chest. The cancer went to the lab where it yielded his army of lymphocytes, the TIL cells. While his troops were readied, Tom received mild chemotherapy treatments to eliminate any of his lymph cells which might hold the attackers back. So far, so good. Then came the treatment with the IL-2 and his soldiers, the TIL cells. The battle was short and brutal.

Tom received his infusions in a brightly lit room in the immunotherapy wing. The view out the window was pretty; the treatment was not. Fevers, chills, and confusion. He was never so sick. After a week, he recovered. Partially.

Tom and Laura returned from Dallas to Charlotte then back to Albany. On the trip down, they had walked across the Charlotte airport for their connection, but coming back Tom had been forced to rest halfway in one of the airport's white rocking chairs. They sat until he regained his energy.

"How are you doing?" she asked after a few minutes.

"Good. These rocking chairs remind me of the ones on the porch of mama's house. All I would need is Bijou. I miss the kids and Leo."

Their arrival home was memorable. It was a beautiful summer evening when they pulled into the drive. As Laura and Melody watched, Tom ended up in the grass with Ben and Crystal on his stomach and Leo licking his face.

"Were they good?" Laura asked her sister.

"The best. How are you?"

Laura's eyes welled up for a moment.

"God, I hope it works."

Melody hugged her until Crystal and Ben pulled their mother down to Tom, who still lay on the ground laughing as Leo licked his face.

"You, too, Aunt Mel, in the pile," commanded Ben, imitating the southern drawl of his father.

Three weeks later, Tom packed once more. Since they had to leave early in the morning, they said goodbye to Ben and Crystal the night before. They were no longer babies, but they still looked young and vulnerable in their beds, surrounded by an army of stuffed animals. Next to his bed, Ben had carefully hung the black cowboy hat his daddy had brought him home from Texas. Leo was in his bed next to the door, guarding. Laura came in as Tom packed the last of his clothing.

"Got everything?" she asked.

"I guess," he replied reflexively, counting his underwear and socks. Except a miracle, he thought.

The first step at MD Anderson was a repeat CT scan of the chest to see if the initial treatment had worked. If the cancer had grown significantly, Tom would not get the second round of treatment. As he slid through the machine, Tom thought of Ken doing his scans back in Saratoga Springs, thousands of miles away. He's probably telling someone to hang in there right now. George Hand is probably next door getting another knee surgery, and I am in Texas, cracking up. And I haven't even had my second round of the IL-2 yet.

Two hours later, Dr. Chou reported the results.

"Very good. The spots are all smaller and no new ones. You get the second treatment."

It was the same. Brutal.

On the trip home at the Charlotte airport, they again stopped at the white rocking chairs. They were occupied, but a soldier waiting for his own flight noticed him struggling and offered up his seat.

"He's finishing cancer treatments," explained Laura. Tom sat down heavily, thanking him.

"Where are you heading?" Tom asked when his breathing had returned to normal. They learned the young man had finished a tour in Afghanistan and was heading home to Denver where he would meet his infant son for the first time.

"I can't wait. I've seen him on Skype, but it's not the same. He and my wife are with my parents. My mom's fighting cancer, too. Breast cancer. I know cancer really sucks." He turned to Laura. "Excuse my language, ma'am."

"Don't worry about that." Laura smiled. "What a great day for your family."

"Yes, ma'am. Well, my flight is being called. Good luck to you, sir."

After he had left, Tom turned to Laura.

"Imagine those soldiers in Afghanistan, thinking about their families and the babies they never met, fighting God knows who. At least I know who my enemy is and where I stand."

At their own home, they replayed the reunion scene in the front yard at Ben's insistence. This time it was fall, and Tom rolled in a pile of leaves with his son who had raked them for his father. Crystal joined in, throwing them in the air joyfully while Leo jumped like a puppy. It's over, Laura thought, IL-2 is finished. As she stood with Melody and Bruce, she imagined their soldier friend in Denver seeing his wife and meeting his son for the first time.

"Now we watch again," Tom said when they returned to Dr. Matthews.

"Right. The question for you is how to watch. You can have your scans here if you want. My suggestion is that if you can manage the travel, they be done at MD Anderson. I think in the long run you will be glad you had them read by their doctors. It is much more work, but it keeps you attached to them in a very direct way. They will continue to see you as one of their own. I hope you beat this, but if it ever comes back, you will want them thinking of you as their patient."

Tom nodded his agreement.

Laura spoke up. "What if it comes back?"

"We will do surgery if needed, reconsider IL-2 treatments, and look at the new immune treatments. We will basically start all over. But now is a time to watch—"

"And live, as Karen constantly reminds us," interrupted Laura.

"She's right, of course," Dr. Matthews concurred. "You two have done an amazing job."

So, they did it again, the watching and living. They would fly to Dallas for scans every six months and meet Dr. Chou, who Tom said looked more like a Texan each visit. In between they would see Dr. Matthews and Karen. Ben turned ten, his new black cowboy hat a few sizes larger. Crystal turned eight, an independent-minded young girl. Melody and Bruce continued as devoted aunt and uncle. To his utter shock, Tom learned George Hand had organized the YMCA basketball team to do his yard work during the treatments. Tom had tried to thank him in front of the guys, but George would have none of it.

"I'm fat, loud, and have no jump shot. And these guys can barely get up and down the court. But we can all do a little yard work. Forget it and get back to playing when you're ready." He paused, then continued. "Now listen, did I ever tell you about my knees?" It was a clear signal for the group to disperse.

Only Leo did not fare well. The office learned that Tom's devoted friend had died when he came for a blood draw with John Welt.

"You look good, Tom. How are you doing? Laura okay?" John asked.

"We're both okay, but Leo's gone."

"Leo? Aww. What happened?" John put down his tubes and sat.

"His kidneys failed him. The vet said there was nothing we could do. He looked so miserable we had no choice, so we put him down last week."

"That stinks. He was with you the whole time."

Tom nodded.

John went on. "They know when something is wrong with you. I remember when I had my back surgery, Gracie was so upset I was gone. When I got back, she stayed with me the whole time and was waiting each time I came back from PT. They know. When Gracie died last year, I felt so bad . . . How did the kids take it?"

"They were pretty upset. You said once Gracie filled a space in your life. When my daddy died, my dog Bijou filled a hole. When I got the treatments, Leo did the same."

"I know. I'm sorry Tom."

In the phlebotomy room, they sat together, the man who endured and the medical assistant who witnessed, and quietly mourned their dogs. At check out, Anna joined in.

"Hi, Tom. I'm sorry about Leo."

When Laura telephoned the next day for the results of Tom's blood tests, Karen took the call.

"Everything is good Laura, even the LDH. We were all sorry to learn about Leo."

"For as strong a man as Tom is, he was pretty upset. That dog went through the whole thing with him. They were good buddies."

For four more years it went on, this life of watching and living. For some reason, possibly because life felt so good again, the watching began to take more of a toll on Laura. Each visit to Texas brought back the terror of Tom needing more treatment. Ritual helped, so they took the same flights, rented an Expedition, and tried to park in the same spot. With each walk through the Charlotte airport, they stopped at the rocking chairs and thought of their soldier friend and his family, imagining how they were doing. At home, Laura found herself watching Tom, sometimes too closely. Don't make us go back there, she thought. The mantra "don't let it beat you when it's not there," no longer worked. It had been there, she knew. The visits to Dr. Matthews and the normal LDH helped a little, but eventually even they were not enough. Once again, Laura turned to Karen for help.

"All those things are normal. This stuff is hard when you have had cancer," Karen reassured her. "Everything can scare you. Most of the time it passes, and you can let it go, but sometimes it builds. We often see that in people when they are a few years out from their treatment. If that is the case, some people find it useful to regroup, face their worst fears, and ask what they would do if it did come back. There have been many new treatments and changes. If you are in that spot, ask Dr. Matthews."

Laura worried the discussion would upset Tom. Unlike her, he seemed in a good place, happy in the routine of his life. She asked him if she could speak with Dr. Matthews about it at their next visit.

"Sure. I think about it, too," he replied, to her surprise. "Ask him if you want. I don't mind. I know they have a lot of new treatments. I tried to keep up for a while, but now I really don't want to. So let's hear what he says."

MODERN IMMUNOTHERAPY FOR MELANOMA.
IL-2 and interferon can non-specifically stimulate the immune system, yet many melanomas seem to hide and escape the attack. The question for scientists was how.

Scientists had long known that the immune system needs to recognize both the body's normal cells ("self") as well as cells which do not belong ("non-self"). Making this distinction is critical. When the immune system fails to recognize non-self, infections or cancers can go unchecked. When the immune system fails to recognize self and attacks our own cells, the result can be auto-immune diseases like rheumatoid arthritis (attack on the joints), psoriatic arthritis (attack on the joints and skin), or lupus (attacks anywhere in the body). Beginning in the 1990s, scientists began to understand how the immune system made the distinction between self and non-self.

The cells which attack enemies like cancer cells are called T-cells. These T-cells are programmed to attack specific targets selected by another group of cells called antigen presenting cells (APCs). APCs present protein targets to the T-cells which will then attack the enemy bearing that protein. If the presentation goes properly, the T-cell will be programmed and attack the desired enemy. Like all important cellular events, the presentation process is carefully regulated and includes "checkpoints" which slow the process down. The checkpoint molecules act as control switches to suppress the activation of T-cells. If cancer cells switch on these checkpoint molecules, the immune system may fail to recognize the cancer, allowing it to grow or lay dormant for years. One important checkpoint is cytotoxic T-lymphocyte-associated protein 4 (CTLA-4), while other related controls are Programmed Death-1 (PD-1) and Programmed Death-Ligand 1 or 2 (PD-L1 and PD-L2).

Once the roles of these checkpoint controls were understood, scientists could make antibodies to block their action. Blocking checkpoints, called "check-point inhibition," has allowed the immune system to recognize and fight melanoma. In 1996, antibodies against the checkpoint CTLA-4 were tested in mice and allowed them to reject tumors.[207] Fifteen years later, in 2011, the FDA approved the anti-CTLA-4 antibody named ipilimumab, brand name Yervoy, for the treatment of widespread melanoma in humans.[208] As ipilimumab was developed, the other checkpoints were also targeted for antibody treatment, including PD-1, PD-L1, and PD-L2. In 2014, the anti-PD-1 antibody nivolumab, brand name Opdivo, was approved by the FDA for use in melanoma.[209]

The results of checkpoint inhibition using these antibodies have been impressive for some patients. Former President Jimmy Carter and others appear to be cured of widespread melanoma using ipilimumab and nivolumab. Although melanoma is among the most responsive cancers to this modern immune therapy, these treatments are being used for many other cancers as well.

Now four years after the IL-2, Laura posed the question.

"What if it comes back now? What will we do?"

Dr. Matthews discussed the choices of surgery, more IL-2, and the new immune treatments.

"Do you think it will come back?" Tom asked directly. "We won't hold you to it."

Dr. Matthews stayed silent for a moment.

"No," he said quietly. "I don't."

Tom looked at Laura. "Let's go with that, honey."

Sitting on the exam table was Charlie Phillips, a fifty-seven-year-old man who looked older than his years, dressed in camouflage hunting gear and an orange vest. Sitting in the chair was a similarly dressed woman about ten years younger whose blond hair was pulled back to reveal a face which at one time would have been strikingly pretty but was now weathered and lined.

"Doc, you remember Angel," said Charlie.

"Of course." Dr. Matthews shook both their hands. "How is the treatment going?"

"Fine," replied Charlie. "I feel good. We'll be back in two weeks for the next one, too. But after that, I'm not sure."

Charlie Phillips' first visit had been three years ago, in early December. He had finally gone to his primary doctor for his worsening cough. The chest x-ray had shown several spots in his lungs, CT scan uncovered more in his liver, and the biopsy proved it was lung cancer, squamous non-small cell type. His wife explained.

"He was coughing his lungs out, but he wouldn't go. I tried to make him, but he wouldn't. From the second Saturday after Columbus Day and for the next forty-four days, you can't get him to do anything else. He's finished work, they all have. So off they go, into the woods." June Phillips looked aggrieved. She had obviously come to hate hunting season. "The only way you would get them out is if they were dead." She looked at her husband. "I guess it almost came to that, didn't it, Charlie?"

"Shut up," he answered sourly.

She turned to Dr. Matthews. "They talk about football widows. I'm a hunting widow. Almost for real, too." She turned back to her husband. "You idiot."

Charlie Phillips shook his head, face reddening.

"Don't push it," he warned.

Dr. Matthews interceded by reviewing Charlie's medical history. Despite years of smoking, he had been healthy until the cancer. His cough was bad, but he otherwise felt well.

"We should begin with chemotherapy. If it works, your cough will get better. It cannot cure your cancer, but we hope to be able to shrink it and control it," Dr. Matthews began.

"Just like his father," announced June. "He smoked all his life, too, and ended up with lung cancer. The chemo didn't work for him."

"Will you shut up?" Charlie said. "That was years ago. They have all new treatments now. Right, doc?"

"We will start with chemotherapy and use that as long as we can. We are expecting some new treatments which use the immune system to be approved soon. Hopefully, we will have those to use after the chemotherapy. They have worked very well in some patients and seem to have fewer side effects generally," answered Dr. Matthews.

"Well, we start with the shotgun. Blast away, doc."

Anna Budney, the secretary, scheduled Charlie's first treatment.

"It's set for next week," she told Dr. Matthews. "But don't get between them two. I know them. They fight like cats and dogs. Have for years."

Charlie's chemotherapy was an intravenous treatment of paclitaxel and carboplatin given once every three weeks. He had very few side effects during the first five-hour treatment. A week later, he and June met Angela Pagano, the Nurse Practitioner. Charlie offered no complaints, but June did.

"He sits around all day and won't do anything. He's usually lazy this time of year anyway, but this is the worst. Watches movies and won't get off the damn couch. One more damn western and I think I'll shoot somebody."

"Shut up," replied Charlie. "I like them movies. And the ice ain't out yet."

Angela pieced together the story. Charlie worked road construction each spring and summer, then was unemployed in the late fall and winter, a schedule which suited him. Fall was for hunting and winter for ice fishing. He and June had been married for thirty-five years. Until recently, June had worked for the county court while their one daughter and her grandchildren had been nearby, so his absences had gone unnoticed. Last winter their daughter had moved to North Carolina and the county offered June a retirement package, so there had been more time together and more friction.

"I wanted to travel a bit, visit the kids, and see the country," June told Angela as Charlie slept during a treatment. "But this guy, he wouldn't give up ice fishing. Can you imagine, all day in a hut on the ice, smoking and drinking with some other smelly guys? One jerk even put a generator and TV in his hut, so they can watch football. That took away the only reason they came home, except starvation."

Charlie's cancer made the strain even worse.

"Now we'll never get out of here. He brought it on himself, smoking all these years even after what happened to his father. Once I got pregnant, I quit and wouldn't let him smoke in the house. Probably why he liked that ice fishing. He never was much of drinker, though, I'll give him that."

Finances didn't help.

"We were never rich, but we got by. He made good money in the summer, and I worked all year. But all these doctor visits and medicines are costing us big time. Gas, too. At this rate, we won't be going anywhere, even if he would."

Nor did the weather help, as that winter was one of the coldest in years with weeks of sub-zero temperatures.

"I keep speaking to my daughter down in North Carolina. It's cold for them, in the fifties. Can you imagine? I told him we could get his treatments done there and come back in the spring, but this guy would rather stay here. Idiot."

Angela reported to Dr. Matthews.

"I don't think there is much happiness in their marriage right now. They argue all the time. She wants to leave, blames him for not taking care of himself, and doesn't want to ruin her own life because of his problems and stubbornness. On the other hand, she feels guilty because he has cancer. I referred them to social work and helped them fill out the forms to get help with co-pays and travel expenses."

Anna added her assessment. "They fight all the time now, worse than ever. Last month, the neighbors had to call the cops. This won't last."

"And we think cancers are complex," noted Dr. Matthews.

The spring of 2015 brought the conclusion of chemotherapy and a new set of scans.

"Your scans look remarkably good," Dr. Matthews reported. "We cannot see any sign of the cancer. We know there are still cancer cells somewhere, but we can stop the chemo and check with another scan in three to four months."

"Good. Maybe we can go south now," answered June.

"Maybe you. I gotta work," replied Charlie.

"Maybe I will. It would serve you right." She looked at Dr. Matthews. "He's an idiot."

Three months later, Anna reported Charlie was a no-show for his visit.

"I left a message on his phone, but he won't answer. He's busy working. I used to see his wife in Price Chopper, but she hasn't been there for the last few months. I heard she left him and went to North Carolina to be with the daughter and kids. And I heard she had someone on the side, too. I bet she didn't want to leave him while he had the cancer. Once he got better, she was gone. People are funny that way."

Two months later, Charlie returned. He felt well and agreed to another set of scans, but only after hunting season finished.

"How is your wife?" asked Dr. Matthews.

"Gone," replied Charlie. "Ran off south to be with the daughter. Ain't coming back, neither. Took up with some insurance fellow she knew from the county. Bastard."

"I'm sorry," replied Dr. Matthews.

"Yeah, well, it's a jungle out there, doc."

❖   ❖   ❖

UNDERSTANDING THE IMMUNE SYSTEM.
It is a jungle out there. Every other life form wants what you have—your proteins, your energy, your DNA. And to get it, they will invade you, eat you, decompose you, or take you over. In the words of philosopher Thomas Hobbes, life is "nasty, brutish and short."

Survival requires defenses. To fight bacteria, viruses, and parasites, humans have an immune system. Scientists divide the system into the "innate" part, which recognizes and rapidly fights known threats, and the "adaptive" part which responds to new invaders. Plants primarily have innate immune systems which use defenses including antibiotic-like compounds and enzymes. Animals and humans have advanced adaptive immune systems which fight constantly changing enemies by making specific weapons like antibodies and attack cells for each new threat. An adaptive immune system is helpful for a long life in this ever-changing jungle.

Many species of animals have similar adaptive immune systems. The scientific term for this consistency is "conserved," and it implies the system evolved many years ago. Remarkably, biologists have been able to trace our adaptive immune system back to the first jawed fish. The jawless fish which first appeared 500 million years ago, such as hagfish or sea lampreys, used different mechanisms for their adaptive immune systems. When fish evolved jaws about 50 million years later, a change in the adaptive immune system occurred, referred to with some hyperbole as the "immunologic big bang." This dramatic change produced the basic components of the adaptive immune system found in humans today.[210] Prominent in the adaptive immune system are the lymphoid cells, including B-cells (from the bone marrow) which make antibodies and T-cells (from the thymus gland) which control the attack and engage invaders in direct combat. To be effective, these cells must identify and respond to new threats, then keep a memory of the invaders for future reference.

The adaptive immune system must be careful not to attack the body it is designed to protect. In the lingo, it needs to "recognize self." If the immune system mistakenly attacks the body, "auto-immune" conditions like rheumatoid arthritis or lupus can result. The scientific advances in molecular biology which began in the 1970s allowed scientists to understand how the system distinguishes invaders from self and how it controls signals to attack. One important early step which occurs in the thymus gland (under the breast bone) is the elimination of T-lymphocytes which might attack the self, a slaughter charmingly called "thymic education." Even after this drastic step, further controls are placed on those T-lymphocytes which patrol the body. In labs across the world, scientists have painstakingly detailed this beautifully complex system of strictly directing the immune defenders while limiting their activities.

Cancer cells are a type of invader which our adaptive immune system often recognizes and destroys. The importance of a healthy immune system is demonstrated by HIV infection, which leads to damage and an increased risk of cancer, particularly lymphomas and Kaposi's sarcomas. Possibly the most fascinating example of the importance of a healthy immune system is from a 2015 case study in the *New England Journal of Medicine*. A forty-one-year-old man in Columbia had been diagnosed with HIV infection seven years earlier and did not take his medication, leading to a severely damaged immune system. The man had become infected with a common human tapeworm, called

Hymenolepis nana, which lives in the small intestine. What is unique about this case is that the man's damaged immune system allowed the tapeworm cells to grow, develop mutations, and form a tapeworm cancer which then spread throughout his body. The poor man died from a non-human cancer caused by a failure of his immune system.[211]

Using the adaptive immune system to destroy cancers is an obvious goal. Scientists have long had relatively non-specific methods of stimulating the immune system, including injections of interferon, interleukins, and even stimulated lymphocytes themselves. These treatments would occasionally work but were either too toxic or ineffective for regular use in many patients. One major problem is that cancer cells are also self and our immune system is often unable to identify these home-grown terrorists. Recent advances have allowed manipulation of the system to encourage the immune system to better recognize cancers, a strategy called "checkpoint immunotherapy." This approach has offered the hope that the immune system might be manipulated to fight cancer while sparing the normal self.

"I told Mr. Phillips you would call him to have his scan in six weeks, after hunting season is over. Do you think he will keep the appointment?" Dr. Matthews asked Anna.

"Yeah. He will," she answered. "Did he tell you he took up with a new lady?"

"No," replied Dr. Matthews.

"She's different," Anna informed Dr. Matthews as Angela joined them. "She's from Alaska. A real hunter herself. Moved here with her daughter last year. And I hear the girl shoots even better than her mamma."

Angela laughed. "Is there anyone in this town you don't know, Anna?" She turned to Dr. Matthews. "If he needs more treatment, will we go back to the carbo and Taxol?"

"We could, but I think he might be a good person to try the new immune treatment," answered Dr. Matthews. "It should be approved soon."

Anna replied first. "Yeah, well, Charlie's into new things now."

The hunting season of 2015 was good, but Charlie's scans afterward showed growth of several spots in his lung.

"You should restart treatment," said Dr. Matthews.

"More chemo?" asked Charlie.

"No," answered Dr. Matthews. "I think you should try the new immune treatment which was recently approved. It is called nivolumab or Opdivo."

USING THE IMMUNE SYSTEM TO FIGHT CANCERS.

As scientists dissected the molecular workings of the immune system, specific methods for enhancing its anticancer effects became possible. One approach was to accelerate the immune system by mimicking activation signals on T-cells. A second approach was to release the breaks on the immune system by blocking control signals on T-cells, called "checkpoint inhibition." Both approaches used specifically designed monoclonal antibodies to perform the task and, if successful, would signal a fundamental change in cancer treatment.

To accelerate the immune system, scientists chose the target CD28, a signaling molecule on the outside of T-cells which helps stimulate them in a variety of situations. Activating T-cells with an anti-CD28 antibody seemed a reasonable way to enhance the immune system. On March 13, 2006, in a private research center at Northwick Park and St. Mark's Hospital in London, six healthy young volunteers were given an infusion of an antibody directed against CD28. All six almost immediately died of multi-system organ failure when their immune systems were unleashed in a terrible "cytokine storm"—cytokines being the term for the various signaling molecules in the immune system.[212]

Although all six survived after a period of ICU care which included dialysis and breathing machines for some, one of the volunteers lost his toes and some fingers, and all may have suffered other long-term damages. The anti-CD28 antibody was developed by TeGenero Immuno Therapeutics (now bankrupt) and tested by a clinical trials company called Parexel (still active). Investigations revealed no problems with the manufacturing of the drug. There was criticism of the treatment of all six patients in a group, but the main conclusion was that manipulating the immune system in this fashion had tremendous risk.[213]

The second approach, releasing the brakes on the immune system, is also named checkpoint inhibition. As part of the complex process of recognizing self and preventing immune attacks on the normal body, checkpoint molecules act as control switches to suppress the activation of T-cells. When these checkpoint molecules are switched on in the presence of an outsider, the immune attack on that enemy stops. Over time, the immune system may even fail to recognize the outsider. Cancer cells may activate these checkpoint controls to escape the immune attack, explaining the ability of some cancers to lay dormant for years.

In 1996, scientists led by Dr. James Allison at the University of California at Berkeley reported exciting work on one checkpoint of the immune system called cytotoxic T-lymphocyte-associated protein 4 (CTLA-4).[214] They found that when mice were given antibodies against CTLA-4 to inhibit the checkpoint, their immune systems could better reject tumors. The next step of creating human antibodies was done at Medarex, a biotech company founded by Dartmouth scientists in 1987. They used the remarkable combination of transgenic mice which had human antibody genes and hybridoma technology to produce the antibodies. One of their antibodies, called 10D1, was then injected into twelve cynomolgus monkeys. These monkeys are named because they are crab-eating and used in experiments because they are small and have many similarities to humans. When given to the monkeys, 10D1 stimulated the immune response to viral and tumor vaccines and produced very few adverse effects.[215] Now ready for human testing, 10D1 was named ipilimumab.[216]

Human testing of potential medicines requires expertise and money. When Dr. Alison and his group had initially reported their results with CTLA-4, there was little interest from pharmaceutical companies. Their reluctance was understandable. Ultimately, it took over a decade from the first clinical trials until the 2010 approval of ipilimumab (brand name Yervoy) as a treatment for widespread melanoma. Medarex's key work allowed them to be acquired in 2009 by Bristol Myers for $2.9 billion.[217] This proved to be a sound investment for Bristol Myers as within a few years of approval sales reached $1 billion per year.

Human testing of ipilimumab produced successes in melanoma and renal cell cancer, but also some lung cancers and prostate cancers. It was exciting but not surprising that melanoma and renal cancer would respond. Both had reputations as cancers whose behavior was hard to predict and which could undergo "spontaneous remissions" (shrinkage without explanation), hallmarks of cancers being attacked by the immune system. Both were occasionally dramatically sensitive to nonspecific immune treatments such as interferons and interleukins. The more surprising results in cancers like lung and prostate were powerful evidence of the widespread utility of this approach.

Human testing demonstrated that using checkpoint inhibitors was different from using chemotherapy. Side effects of checkpoint inhibitors were different. The release of the brake on the immune system allowed it to attack "self," producing autoimmune side effects (termed AIEs). These ranged from minor attacks on the skin (rash) or thyroid gland (requiring thyroid medication) to life-threatening attacks on the gastrointestinal system, lung, liver, or brain. Learning to recognize and treat AIEs was an important part of the early clinical research, particularly discovering the importance of the prompt use of steroids to quell the immune system. Satisfying the FDA that these AIEs were managable paved the way for approval of other immune treatments.

Results with checkpoint inhibitors were also different than with chemotherapy. While oncologists traditionally measured rates of shrinkage or complete disappearance to assess drug effectiveness, ipilimumab produced more variable patterns. Tumor shrinkage, stabilization, or even initial growth could all result in eventual control of the cancer. Recognizing this difference was obviously important for patients, but also made the approval process more challenging.

In addition to CTLA-4, scientists discovered other checkpoints which halt the immune attack. Cancer cells also evade immune attack by activating these checkpoints. Understanding these other systems was followed by the generation of antibodies to block these checkpoints, animal testing, and clinical trials in humans using the lessons learned with ipilimumab. These included the ominous sounding "Programmed Death-1" (PD-1) molecule and two others that attach to it, "Programmed Death Ligand-1" (PD-L1) and "Programmed Death Ligand-2" (PD-L2). On March 4, 2015, the antibody anti-PD-1 antibody nivolumab (Opdivo) was approved by the FDA for use in lung cancer.[218] The modern era of immune treatment for cancer had begun.

"What if I don't?" asked Charlie.

"If you don't do anything, you'll probably be fine for a few months, then get sick. I think you would probably last six to nine months, but it's hard to know for sure," answered Dr. Matthews.

"And this treatment is good?"

"It targets the immune system to try to make it recognize and fight the cancer. For some people, it has been very effective, but we can't know without trying."

"Well, I'll take it. You know, I got myself a new girl, name's Angel. She's from Alaska. Good hunter." Charlie smiled.

"This treatment can have side effects," continued Dr. Matthews. "Sometimes the immune system attacks the body. You can get different side effects depending upon what it attacks. Usually, they are mild, but once in a while—"

"Then let's hope the body's wearing orange," interrupted Charlie. "So it don't get shot."

Charlie received the nivolumab infusions every two weeks, and they produced virtually no side effects.

"This new glop beats that chemo crap, hands down," he reported after two months. "I feel great."

Anna added her observations.

"I seen him out last week with his new woman. She's younger, pretty in her day, and very quiet. But tough. She's why he feels so good, not this immune stuff."

Angela also met Angel, during one of Charlie's treatments.

"It's interesting," she reported. "She really cares for him. Her ex was a bad drinker, that's why they left Alaska. She told Charlie she wanted no alcohol around her or her daughter. He was never a drinker himself, so that was no problem. But you know what else?"

Dr. Matthews shook his head.

"He gave up smoking, too. After all these years. You were right," Angela commented, "when you said we think cancers are complicated."

After four months of ice fishing in a smoke-free shack, the early spring of 2016 brought the first set of scans on the treatment.

"Overall, not much change," reported Dr. Matthews. "A few spots are smaller. A few are a little larger. This is what we see with these immune treatments. We should keep going and check in the fall."

"After the season," Charlie reminded. Dr. Matthews nodded.

"This won't cure it, right? Just control it," he added. Dr. Matthews nodded again.

"Figures," Charlie continued. "I heard them companies have the cure but won't give it to you guys. This way is better. They get to keep making money. Maybe when Trump gets elected, we'll change that, too."

The fall of 2106 brought President-elect Trump, another hunting season, and more scans.

"Your scans show no changes. There are still a few spots in your lungs, but they haven't changed," Dr. Matthews reported.

Charlie nodded. "Sounds good, doc. I guess we keep going."

Dr. Matthews agreed. "How's life?" he asked.

"It was a good season. Angel's daughter, she's seventeen, what a pistol. That girl can shoot. I seen her use a Winchester 70, with low recoil load mind, and place all her shots in a eight-inch circle at two hundred yards. I took her out and she bagged a black bear. You never saw anything like it. She gets the bear and puts it on Instagram. Can you believe it? Before we got home, all her friends knew. Even the ones in Alaska."

This spring, Charlie's scans had again been stable. Life was good. Angel's daughter graduated from high school and joined the Army.

"She'll be teaching them boys how to shoot; you can bet that," Charlie noted proudly.

Charlie had continued treatment over the summer, giving up work to be with Angel. Fall came, the foliage was in full bloom, and it was once again his favorite time of year.

"What happens in two weeks, besides hunting season?" asked Dr. Matthews at today's visit.

"We're moving to Alaska. Angel has family there, and we can hunt and fish with them. For me, it'll be something new."

"Your labs are good," began Dr. Matthews.

Walter Grady, a large Irish man in his late sixties who stood six feet four and weighed three hundred pounds, nodded. His rich baritone voice carried a clear brogue.

"A guy goes into a theater. After he takes his seat, he realizes that sitting two seats away is a man with a dog. The movie comes on, and the dog laughs at all the funny parts. The guy is amazed. He turns to the man and says, 'This is remarkable. Your dog is laughing at the movie.' The man turns back to him and says 'Yeah, it is. He really didn't like the book that much.' "

The exam room filled with his deep laughter. Dr. Matthews smiled and shook his head. Grady, as he was known to all, had never failed to tell a story at each visit, regardless of the news.

After the room had quieted, Grady reported his health had been good. His recent colonoscopy was clear. His exam was normal.

"We'll see you again in six months with another set of labs," said Dr. Matthews.

Grady nodded. "Glad to do it."

As they walked to the check-out desk, Dr. Matthews asked, "How is your daughter doing with the store?"

Mr. Grady smiled. "She had a great summer. Hardly needed her old man at all. But it's still good I'm around. I thank thee and, of course, me wife."

Grady had turned sixty almost ten years ago. On that birthday, in front of a nicely lubricated crowd of well-wishers, his wife Molly announced she had made an appointment for him to have the colonoscopy his primary physician had been urging two days hence. As she presented him with the gallon jug he was to drink the following day; the assembly roared its approval and Grady knew he had no chance of escaping.

Grady had long evaded the colonoscopy, although he had known he should take it. After all, his own father had died in his late sixties of colon cancer. His father's cancer was far gone when diagnosed, and the surgeons had been forced to leave him with a colostomy. Grady had seen how "wearing the bag" had cost his father the ability to play the bagpipes and how the spread of the cancer had eventually cost him his life. Grady himself was known as a sharp businessman and knew the calculations, but he simply could not bring himself to do the procedure. Fortunately, Dr. Oakley also knew the history and had recruited Grady's wife to the cause.

The colon connects the small intestine to the rectum. The function of the colon is to remove water from the stool to make it firm. The colon is about five feet long and divided into four parts. The "ascending" colon starts in the lower right-hand corner of the abdomen at the end of the small intestine. The ascending colon goes upward to near the liver, where it turns and becomes the "transverse" colon, which extends across the abdomen to near the spleen. There it turns downward to become the "descending" colon. The final curving part which joins the rectum is called the "sigmoid" colon. Throughout the colon, cancers can develop in the lining, often starting with polyps. These cancers can be seen using a scope, but to view this lining the colon must be free of stool, hence the dreaded cleansing prep.

Grady drank his jug of the cleaning liquid, spent his night on the toilet, and escaped death. His colonoscopy uncovered a cancer growing silently within his ascending colon. A CT scan showed no sign of cancer elsewhere, and two weeks later Dr. Larry Cannon removed that part of his colon, joined the remaining pieces, and spared Grady "the bag." Shortly thereafter his wife brought him to Dr. Matthews. It was a memorable first visit.

Dr. Matthews introduced himself and took a seat. Before he could begin, Grady spoke.

"I've a story to tell."

Dr. Matthews set his chart down.

"A man reports to his doctor. 'My brother thinks he's a chicken.' The doctor tells the man to bring his brother in for treatment. The man replies he can't. 'Why not?' asks the doctor. The man looks at the doctor, somewhat puzzled. 'Doc, we need the eggs.' "

As Grady's deep laughter filled the room, Molly, a pleasant woman of obviously great tolerance, looked at Dr. Matthews helplessly.

"If you want me to take him elsewhere, I will," she added.

For all his humor, Grady listened attentively while Dr. Matthews spoke.

"Probably Dr. Gannon has cured you of the cancer, but there is a chance some of the cancer cells escaped from the colon and are hidden in your body. Your scans did not show anything, but they would not detect a small number of cells. The chance that this took place is increased because we found some of the cells in one of the nearby lymph nodes. Twenty were removed, and one was infected."

"And where might the buggers be?" asked Grady.

"The most likely spot is the liver. The blood leaving the colon travels to the liver first. While they can be anywhere, that is the most likely spot. If you are in good health and have cancer cells in the lymph nodes, we recommend chemotherapy."

"He'll take it," interjected Molly sharply.

Grady looked at his wife for a moment, then back to Dr. Matthews.

"That's settled then," he agreed.

"Good, let me tell you about it."

Dr. Matthews outlined the chemotherapy program called FOLFOX, given every two weeks. The first four hours would be intravenous treatment in the office, then for the next two days, Grady would wear a pump which would continuously infuse chemotherapy. The treatments would go on for six months.

When they had finished, Grady had one further question.

"Dr. Cannon took out the whole right side of my colon, right?"

"Correct."

"Why so much? The cancer was only a few inches long. Do they crawl up inside the colon?"

"It relates to the blood supply," replied Dr. Matthews. "Once you remove the cancer in that part of the colon, you also remove the blood supply to the entire right side, so it all has to come out. You can't leave it in without a blood supply. Thankfully, you don't need all of the colon.

"There is one other thing you need to consider. Since your father had colon cancer, I imagine you have thought of the possibility that there could be something inherited. Your cancer was tested in a preliminary way, and it is possible that there is an inherited genetic cause for your cancer. The next step is to do actual genetic testing on you. This does not change your treatment, but it could be useful information for your twins or your sisters. If we found a gene mutation in you, they could be tested to find out if they carry the mutation. Then they would know what to do."

"Like have a colonoscopy?" asked Molly.

"Yes," replied Dr. Matthews. "Some of these mutations may also carry a higher risk of uterine cancer, so women watch for that and may opt for a hysterectomy when they have finished having children. You and any of your family who want can learn more about it by meeting with our Nurse Practitioner, Tracy Callahan, for a counseling session. If you bring other family members, they can listen on your dime, and it won't appear in their medical records."

COLON CANCER GENES.

Colon cancer became an important model for scientists in the 1970s who were using the emerging new techniques of modern molecular biology to study cancer. While it had long been known that colon cancers could develop from small growths called polyps, scientists led by Dr. Burt Volgelstein at Johns Hopkins described a series of DNA events called the "adenoma (polyp) to carcinoma sequence." These scientists studied biopsies of normal colon, small polyps, larger polyps with pre-cancerous (dysplastic) features, cancers which had just started, and advanced cancers. They identified the DNA damage which accompanied each step and found a remarkably reproducible story. On their way to becoming cancers, normal colon cells developed mutations in critical genes in a general order. The progression Vogelstein and his colleagues identified started with a gene called *APC* (Adenomatous Polyposis Coli), followed by *K-RAS*, then *DCC* (Deleted in Colon Cancer), and finally *TP53*.

The adenoma to carcinoma sequence led scientists to define the specific effects which these mutations cause, called the "downstream events." For example, the *APC* gene controls a cell system called Wnt. The *APC* gene mutations increase the activity of the Wnt system and encourage colon cells to divide, a start to polyp formation. A second example of a "downstream event" occurs when the *K-RAS* mutation produces stimulation of the cell by permanently turning on growth signals called the EGFR pathway.[219] Understanding these events led to the promise of specific treatments, so-called personalized medicine.

The adenoma to carcinoma sequence also helps us to understand inherited colon cancers. A small number of patients are born with mutations in the *APC* gene, a condition called Familial Adenomatous Polyposis (FAP). These patients develop hundreds or thousands of polyps in their colons by the time they reach their twenties, and all will develop cancer. For scientists, the condition proved the importance of the *APC* gene. For patients, the detection of the condition can allow them to have preventative removal of the colon.

A more common inherited condition is Hereditary Non-Polyposis Colon Cancer (HNPCC) or "Lynch syndrome." The syndrome is named after Dr. Henry Lynch who described families with colon cancer without large numbers of polyps, and uterine cancer.[220] Lynch began his work in the 1960s and 1970s, a time when the concept of hereditary cancers was not well understood. Using molecular techniques, scientist found these families have a mutation in one of the several genes which repair DNA. When the repair mechanism does not work properly, defects in the critical genes in the adenoma to carcinoma sequence occur more rapidly. Detecting the Lynch syndrome may allow family members to make medical decisions. Most have regular colonoscopies, although some opt for preventative removal of the colon. Most women with Lynch syndrome undergo a hysterectomy after they are finished bearing children.

DNA tests for the rare Familial Adenomatous Polyposis (FAP) or more common Lynch syndrome (HNPCC) are readily available.

Grady traced his genes back to County Cork, Ireland, the land which his great-great-grandparents had left in their early twenties, miraculously just before the Great Hunger of 1845. The reason for their sudden departure was never entirely clear, but it was whispered that marriage and conception, not necessarily in that order, were involved. A job on the Improved Erie Canal attracted them to the Albany area and gave their eldest son, Grady's great-grandfather, the start he needed to open a bar in Watervliet, a connecting town for two branches of the canal. Grady's grandfather had also successfully owned the bar and fully expected it would remain in the family. His only son, Grady's father, had different plans. He had been a good enough baseball player to try out with Yankees, returning to the area only after several seasons as a journeyman in the minor leagues and a tour as a combat pilot in World War II. He had settled in Saratoga Springs, attracted by the racetrack and Grady's mother, herself a beautiful and tough Irish woman. Together they had opened a three-season grill and soda fountain which capitalized on the summer tourist season and the garrulousness of Grady's father.

That Grady's father had colon cancer was certain, but the medical history from earlier generations was murky. In that era, death was part of existence, and the specifics were not often known, or, if cancer was involved, were not shared. You got sick, the doctor came, the priest followed, you died and were buried. Why wasn't really an issue. It was your time, or it wasn't, but you went anyway.

So why did Grady's father develop colon cancer? During normal cell division, some errors in the reproduced DNA occur and must be repaired so that cancers do not develop. Although not known at the time, Grady's father had been born with a defect in one of the genes which repaired DNA damage in his colon. The baseball player turned fighter pilot who eluded inheriting a bar in Watervliet could not escape inheriting this same gene. In an era where wives did not present their husbands with screening colonoscopies, colon cancer caused his death. Along with the soda fountain and his wicked sense of humor, Grady had inherited the same mutation.

Tracy Callahan was the Nurse Practitioner. A local Irish woman who started at Saratoga Hospital as an aide, Tracy completed nursing school, worked for several years on the medical floors, specialized in oncology, then returned to school for her NP degree—all as she raised her own two lively boys, frequent summertime visitors to Grady's ice cream window. Tracy had also studied cancer genetics. She sat with the Gradys and their twin daughters, Meg and Missy, who were identical in appearance and opposite in personality. Meg lived in town, was a homemaker married to a fireman, and had two small children of her own. Missy was single and worked for an investment firm in Manhattan. Whatever their similarities and differences, the twins remained close.

"Most cancers are caused by a combination of many of our genes, how we live our lives, and whoever you believe is running this show," began Tracy. "However, some families are different. They can have a single gene mutation responsible for starting the cancer process. If we can find the gene mutation for that family, we can test the people in that family and tell who inherited the gene mutation. We can tell those who did get the mutation what to do about it. We can also tell those in the family who didn't inherit the mutation that they don't have that same risk. With me so far?"

The Gradys nodded. Tracy faced Grady himself.

"For colon cancer, these inherited gene mutations keep some cells from repairing damage done to the DNA. Our DNA is always getting broken, and we have all these ways to repair it. In the colon, there are several repair genes. If one doesn't work, you're more likely to get a cancer. Your cancer was tested to see if the cells repair the DNA or not. The technical name for that is MSI-testing, microsatellite instability testing. Your results show your cancer cells did not repair the DNA well, suggesting you might have a gene mutation. This test is not conclusive, but it means you and your family should think about genetic testing."

"Maybe me father had the same thing," Grady noted.

"Right. If we can find a gene mutation in you, that would nail it down. If you have a mutation, we call it the Lynch syndrome or HNPCC." She turned to the twins. "If we find something in your Dad, we could then see if you inherited the same thing. You should think about what that might mean for you.

"If we find a gene mutation in your father, there is a 50 percent chance you will have inherited the same mutation. We can test you to see if you inherited that mutation. We assume you two are identical twins, but we would still do testing on both of you. If the test came back positive and you had the same mutation as your father, you would be at risk for colon cancer. You would need regular colonoscopies right away. You would also be at risk for uterine cancer, so your gynecologist would want to do regular uterine ultrasounds. Most women who have the gene mutations have hysterectomies when they are done having children. On the other hand, if you did not inherit the gene mutation, you do not have these worries. You would have the risk of the average person since I don't think there is anything that might have come down from Mom's side."

Tracy paused before continuing.

"A few other things to know. If we do not find a mutation in your father, then we can't really tell you much. These tests are not perfect in detecting all the possible gene problems, and you will still have to be careful. Second, even if your father is tested and we find a mutation, you don't have to take the test now. You are not yet thirty and can think it over, even for years. Sometimes it's just not the right time. Finally, if you are thinking of applying for life or disability insurance, do that before you get the test. We have not heard of denials, but why take the chance?"

"Could it effect health insurance?" asked Grady.

"We doubt it. There are laws to protect you, and we haven't heard of any problems."

Grady's blood test was first. He had inherited a mutation in a gene called *MSH2*, meaning he had the Lynch syndrome. Tracy had called him with the results.

"No surprise, was it dear?" he responded.

"Not really," Tracy answered. "Still, it makes it more real."

"True. Well, I guess the twins will have to get tested now."

"Only if they want . . . they're young still."

"Molly and I will tell them, and they can decide." He paused. "We blame the damn English, don't we dear. We never should have let Henry be King of Ireland. He had some bad genes, that one, probably contaminated the pool."

The twins were tested together, and the whole family met with Tracy to receive the results.

She smiled as she told them there were no mutations in either daughter. When the hugging was over, Grady spoke.

"Now that that's finished, Tracy, give them the bad news," he intoned.

"Bad news?" asked Tracy, puzzled. The twins and Mrs. Grady looked up, alarmed. Grady turned to Tracy.

"Ah, tell the poor things they still have me backside and nose genes." He laughed uproariously.

It fell to Mrs. Grady to respond. "Grady, out of here right now before I give you a good kicking in your own jeans."

Grady's chemotherapy had started with a story.

"Did you ever hear the story of Mrs. O'Malley's boys? No? Well, they were eight and ten and headed for a life of trouble, so they were given jobs cleaning up in the church where Father Devin could keep an eye on them. Now the young rascals had just broken into the coin box for the poor when Father called them in for their first lesson. 'Where is God?' he asked the trembling youths. When they made no answer, he repeated in his most terrifying voice, 'Where is God?'" The boys emptied their pockets, crying. 'We took the coins, Father, but please don't pin that on us.' "

Baritone laughter again filled the room, and Mrs. Grady rolled her eyes.

"It's not too late, Dr. Matthews. I can still take him elsewhere."

Grady's chemotherapy was given every two weeks for six months. Each treatment was the same: three chemotherapy drugs (5-FU, leucovorin, and oxaliplatin) given by vein in the office over about four hours, then a pump (5-FU) which he wore for two days at home. The treatments were typically uneventful, and he enjoyed the company of the nurses. The office walls were decorated with prints and photos of Saratoga's rich history. Grady shared his extensive knowledge of the City with other patients, often comparing old *Harper's Magazine* articles or other memorabilia.

Grady was raised in Saratoga Springs, a small city of 30,000 located midway between New York City and Montreal at the foothills of the Adirondack mountains. Through the 1800s and early 1900s, it had been a world-famous resort known for summer horse racing, gambling, and its social and art scene. The post-World War II years of Grady's childhood had not been kind to the City. While the famous Saratoga Racetrack continued to draw the horse racing elite every August, the formerly vibrant Victorian downtown had decayed. The great hotels which lined the main street of Broadway went dark and were torn down. The Grand Union Hotel was one of the largest and most elegant in the world, capable of seating a thousand people for dinner. It was demolished in 1952; its exquisite chandeliers sold and the wood parquet floors ripped apart. As a small boy, Grady remembered watching from Dan's Soda Spa across the street as the cranes did their ugly work; the dust cloud that hung over Congress Park matching the depressed mood of the residents. When he finished high school in the late 1960s, the City was bleak. Downtown was empty store fronts, the statues in the park were neglected, and the large summer homes on Broadway and Union Avenue abandoned.

Even Grady could not articulate what brought him back to the Saratoga Springs of the 1960s and early 1970s. Most of his high school classmates fell into two groups: those born for small town life in upstate New York and those with the smarts or skills to leave. Only a few like himself chose to return after college. For some, it was horse racing that brought them home; for others, the flickering light of the local art scene. For a very few like Grady, the reason for returning was harder to define. He simply loved the place for what it had been and might again become. The beauty of Frederick Law Olmsted's Congress Park in downtown Saratoga reprised in miniature New York's Central Park or Boston's Emerald Necklace. The glory of Saratoga's brilliant past was still seen in the old buildings which yet survived, like the Hall of Springs, the Canfield Casino, the Batcheller Mansion, and the empty but still elegant summer homes. Even the mocking symbol of the Grand Union supermarket which stood on the site of the former Grand Union Hotel had the still standing and beautiful Bethesda Church as a backdrop.

Grady had gone to Sienna College in nearby Troy where he earned his CPA degree, then worked in Boston for few years. He remembered visiting home one spring, walking with his father down Broadway and stopping at Globe Hardware so the elder Grady could pick up a few items as he readied the shop for the season. Many of the storefronts were bare, although a few were freshly painted and their windows held works from the local art groups. His father caught Grady looking down the street.

"Don't be fooled, son. This old gal will rise again. We've had a few new families move in on North Broadway, rebuilding the summer homes. Skidmore College is planning a new campus in that area. And we've a committee going to rebuild the downtown. The Adirondack Trust bank is behind us, and even City Hall seems to be working together."

His father's words struck a chord in Grady. His fate was unknowingly sealed later that afternoon at the Grand Union supermarket when he ran into Mrs. Ryan, the mother of his high school buddy Seamus. During their childhood, Mrs. Ryan had provided many a meal for Grady and his friends.

"Walter Grady," she exclaimed in surprise. "Just look at you. You're taller than your father himself. And much more handsome, I might add."

"Hello, Mrs. Ryan," he replied. "It's very nice to see you. How's Seamus?"

"Well now, he's coming home this evening, and I know he'll be wanting to see you."

"I'd like to see him, too."

"Good, because by some miraculous coincidence his sister is also home with a few of her girlfriends from college, including one that Seamus seems quite taken with. So, he'll be looking to get a few boys together to go out with them. I'll expect you for dinner tomorrow, then.

Whatever was planned for that evening, in the end it was Grady and Seamus' sister Molly who married. They returned to Saratoga Springs, started an accounting firm, ran the restaurant, and raised their own identical twin daughters. And Grady's father had been right. As Grady and Molly's twins grew, so did Saratoga. The bleak downtown became a vibrant Victorian shopping district with unique boutiques and restaurants. Skidmore grew from a small women's college into a first-rate co-ed liberal arts school. The Saratoga Performing Arts

Center amphitheater was built and became the summer home to the Philadelphia Orchestra, New York City Ballet, and series of summer concerts ranging from Frank Sinatra to the Who. And above all, the famous Saratoga Racetrack continued to draw race horse fans like those who saw the famous Secretariat lose to Onion, furthering the Track's reputation as the Graveyard of Champions.

Molly described meeting Grady in one of their visits.

"The week before, I had a dream that I met a tall man who carried me away. So when we girls heard Seamus was getting us dates, I told them I would take the tallest one. That turned out to be Grady. I had known him as Seamus' friend, but never thought he was the man in the dream."

"She means she dreamt of the best-looking one, Doc," Grady corrected.

"That may be, man," responded his wife, "but you were picked for height. Seamus is five feet ten and the others were smaller. They were all thin as rails then, too, doc."

"And would you pick the tallest one again?" asked Dr. Matthews, teasing.

She looked Grady up and down appraisingly, paused, then smiled. "I guess."

"This reminds me of a story," started Grady. His wife groaned.

Undeterred, he began in his deep brogue. "A man was in and out of a coma for months while his devoted wife stayed by his bedside every day. When he came to, he called her. 'You know what? You have been with me all through the bad times. When I lost my job, you were there. When the business failed, you were with me. When I fell and got hurt, you were by my side. When we lost the house, you stood by me. And now when my health is failing, you are still by my side. You know what?' She grabbed his hand and asked, 'Tell me, my love?' The old boy raised himself and spoke, 'I think you bring me bad luck.'"

Grady roared with laughter.

His wife looked helplessly at Dr. Matthews.

"Can you double his dose of that chemo?" she begged. Dr. Matthews nodded.

No one day was terrible. The four hours with the nurses were pleasant; the medications made him sleepy but otherwise did not produce any severe reactions. The treatment area was usually quiet as patients talked or rested while the nurses did their work, the calm punctuated by an occasional burst of laughter. Once Grady witnessed the atmosphere shattered by a dreaded "chemo reaction." The patient next to him that day was a heavy middle-aged woman who had looked anxious and ill at the start of her treatment. Grady had felt sorry and planned to speak with her, but never got the chance. About five minutes into her treatment, her face became flushed as she motioned for the nurses. The next few minutes were a blur as nurses moved quickly and Dr. Matthews arrived. The immediate area was cleared of other patients, the red resuscitation chart rolled up, and the whole office came to a standstill as the drama played out. Grady learned later that these reactions usually resolve quickly, but for this poor woman it started a cycle which left her short of breath. A siren announced the arrival of the EMTs, and she was taken out on a stretcher.

In the eerie quiet after the EMTs left, the patients sat stunned. The office slowly returned to normal, but the atmosphere remained somber. A few minutes later another nervous looking middle-aged woman entered the treatment area with Rebecca. Grady spoke for the remaining patients.

"Maybe you ought to leave that seat empty." He pointed to the chair in which the reaction had taken place.

Rebecca nodded. "I think you're right."

The main problem with the chemotherapy was its duration. Although Grady escaped any serious side effects, particularly the dreaded nerve damage, the six months was a long time. At the end, he was tired.

"You did very well with the chemotherapy," reviewed Dr. Matthews. "It may take six or nine months until you are fully recovered, though.

You may still notice some fatigue and your bowels probably won't quite settle out until then. Your prognosis is good, but we still need to watch you. Dr. Cannon will do a colonoscopy in a few months. We will check your blood in four months and do a CT scan every year."

Grady's recovery took the full nine months. As the next three years passed, his grandchildren grew, the restaurant served a seemingly endless parade of customers with incessant demands, downtown Saratoga exploded despite the recession, the racing season added an extra week, jokes were told, and life lived. Grady's labs every six months and his yearly CT scan were normal while two colonoscopies were clear.

Then came Rebecca's call.

"Your CEA blood test is elevated, and Dr. Matthews wants you to come back in so we can repeat it. If it is still high, then you will have to have a PET scan to see if there is any sign of cancer. I'm sorry this is scary for you."

"It's not your fault. It's the damn cancer's fault . . . Anyway, let's hope it's a nothing."

❖ ❖ ❖

TUMOR MARKERS: SEARCHING FOR CANCER.

The CEA (Carcino Embryonic Antigen) was the first of several "cancer blood tests" or "tumor markers" which include PSA (prostate cancer), CA-125 (ovarian cancer), CA 19-9 (pancreatic cancer), and CA15-3 or CA 27-79 (breast cancer). The hope was that tumor markers might allow early detection, give information about the success of treatments, and offer targets for therapy. Each test has uses and limitations which depend upon the marker, the cancer, and the patient.

In the 1960s, Drs. Phil Gold and Samuel Freedman of McGill University discovered the CEA as they were searching for molecules which might allow detection of a cancer or its destruction by the immune system.[221] Since the surgical removal of a colon cancer also includes a large section of healthy colon, they isolated the CEA by comparing proteins in the cancer with those in normal tissue. They found the CEA in other digestive system cancers and fetal tissue obtained from spontaneous abortions, hence the name carcinoembryonic ("cancer" and "embryo") antigen.[222] Healthy tissue of the gastrointestinal tract, particularly the colon, produce small amounts of CEA. Most of this CEA is contained by supporting structures around the tissues, so it does not reach the blood and is secreted into the feces. Cancerous cells of the colon often make CEA in larger amounts than normal cells. Even more importantly, these cancerous cells have invaded the tissue and blood vessels, breaking down the normal barriers and allowing the CEA to enter the bloodstream.[223]

The CEA has been the most widely used tumor marker, although there is debate among physicians and insurers over when it should be measured. The CEA is checked to follow the progress of many patients with widespread colon or other digestive cancers. For these patients, the CEA blood test can be used as a "quick read" as they undergo treatment. Falling levels usually mean the treatments are working while rising levels signify the cancer may be worsening. The other common tumor markers are also used in this way.

The real hope for tumor markers was that they would detect early cancers and save lives. Unfortunately, when the CEA is elevated, it usually means the colon cancer has invaded and spread, otherwise the protein would not reach the blood stream. Additionally, mildly elevations can be seen in smokers or those with noncancerous situations, like bowel inflammations. Thus, the CEA is not a good test to detect early colon cancer and cannot replace the colonoscopy. Most other tumor markers have the same limitation, except the PSA which can detect some prostate cancers before they have spread.

The CEA has one use which is different from other tumor markers. It may save lives after surgery by detecting the recurrence of a colon cancer isolated in the liver. When most other tumor markers rise after surgery, the cancers they detect are widely spread and not curable. The benefits of this type of early detection are not great. For some patients with colon cancer, however, an elevated CEA detects the return of the cancer in only a single or few spots in the liver. This pattern of spread occurs because blood leaving the colon passes through the liver which can trap cancer cells. Since these metastatic cancers in the liver can be removed or destroyed and the normal liver will regrow, some patients may be cured or their lives markedly prolonged. This unique situation makes the use of the CEA test following colon cancer surgery valuable for some patients.

Grady's repeat CEA remained high, so he underwent the PET/CT scan. As he lay on the cold table for the forty-five minutes it took to complete the test, Grady thought of his father. His father had never complained about his illness, except that his colostomy made it very hard for him to play his bagpipes. Still, Grady thought, he must have feared dying. Somehow though, the thought of his father going through the same thing calmed Grady. He felt him nearby. Faintly, he even thought he could even hear bagpipes.

CANCER, SUGAR, AND THE WARBURG EFFECT.

The PET/CT scan is a useful tool to detect cancer. The test has two parts. The PET portion involves an injection of radioactive glucose which can be detected as it is used by tissues. The CT portion allows the radiologist to see the structures where the radioactive glucose is being used. The images from the PET and the CT scan can be fused by computer to provide a single picture of both the structures and activity. The scan relies on cellular use of glucose to make energy. Since cancers generally use more glucose, they appear brighter.

All cells use glucose to make energy. High school and college science students study the burning of glucose to make energy (in the form of ATP in the Krebs cycle for those who remember these lessons). This process is called respiration, a different meaning than the act of breathing. As they memorize multiple steps, students learn cells turn glucose into energy in two ways. The first is "anaerobic respiration," meaning without using oxygen, a simple but inefficient process which produces lactic acid and other breakdown products. We recognize anaerobic respiration (without oxygen) when we sprint and our muscles hurt from the build-up of lactic acid. The second way to convert glucose into energy is "aerobic respiration" (with oxygen), a more efficient process using oxygen. This is how we obtain energy for a long-distance walk without the pain of lactic acid build-up.

Cancer cells use anaerobic respiration (without oxygen) to burn glucose for energy. This is understandable when cancer cells are in environments with little oxygen, like the middle of a tumor. However, even when cancer cells have oxygen, they still use this less efficient anaerobic respiration (without oxygen) which produces less glucose and more lactic acid and other by-products. The use of anaerobic respiration (without oxygen) by cancer cells is called the "Warburg effect" as it was described in 1924 by Otto Warburg.[224] Since anaerobic respiration (without oxygen) is not efficient, cancer cells use up to two hundred times more glucose than normal cells. Therefore, they appear bright on the PET scan.

The PET/CT scan can be used both for diagnosis and to follow the effects of treatment. When cancers are killed by treatments, the glucose uptake decreases and they appear less bright, sometimes even before they shrink. The scan does have some limitations. Some non-cancerous tissues use a great deal of glucose, like rapidly contracting muscles (hence no exercising before the test) and infections with many active white blood cells. The brain uses a great deal of glucose and changes there must be measured carefully. The test is also expensive. The radioactive glucose rapidly decays and becomes useless, so manufacturing and distributing the material must be done efficiently, and test cancellations are costly. The complexity of the test also means the radiologist's reading takes considerable time. Despite these limitations, in 2000 the PET scan became *Time Magazine's* Invention of the Year and a key tool in oncology.

In addition to using the Warburg effect to see cancers on PET/CT scans, there have been many attempts to exploit the differences in glucose use to kill cancer cells. Various strategies to starve cancers of glucose have been tried, including a variety of diets and insulin therapy, all without success. The reason these strategies fail lies in the answer to the fundamental question of why cancer cells use anaerobic respiration. Warburg thought cancer cells might have a defect in their mitochondria, the energy producing organelle in the cell. Recently scientists have theorized that cancer cells use this less efficient method of burning glucose because it produces by-products which the cancer cells need to reproduce. In this hypothesis, energy production is not the key, and the cancer cell is greedy for glucose because it uses it to generate other metabolic products needed for multiplying. This theory has led to the discovery of ways cancer cells "turn on" the Warburg effect and will possibly result in blocking agents which work better than the unsuccessful attempts to manipulate the glucose levels.[225]

As Grady and Molly waited in the office the next day, Grady again found himself thinking of his father. Did he wait for results? Was he afraid like this? He never showed it, but what was he thinking?

"Where are you, man?" asked Molly, seeing him so deep in thought.

He looked at her. "I was thinking of me father, how he faced this."

"It's different now. There's so much more they can do," she replied.

"Ah, that's for sure . . ." He went quiet for a moment. "But the thoughts are the same."

She was saved from the need for a reply by the arrival of Dr. Matthews.

"The PET/CT scan shows only a single spot of cancer about one and a half inches in size in the liver. Nothing anywhere else. Usually, when we find the cancer, there are multiple spots. This means we can try to remove it with surgery. I want to send you to Albany Med to see Dr. Port. He is an excellent surgeon."

"Can that cure it?" asked Mrs. Grady.

"It's possible. He will want to do some additional tests to be sure there is nothing else he needs to look for in the liver area, but that is the goal."

"Then that is what we will do," Grady agreed. "The liver is where you said the little bastards would be . . . which reminds me of a story." His wife groaned. Dr. Matthews set down the chart to listen.

"A duck walks into a bar. 'Got any grapes?' he asks the bartender. 'No,' says the bartender. 'This is a bar; we don't have grapes here.' The duck leaves. The next day he comes back into the bar. 'Got any grapes?' he asks the bartender. 'No' says the bartender. 'This is a bar; we don't have grapes here.' The duck leaves. The next day he comes back. 'Got any grapes?' he asks the bartender. 'Look,' says the bartender. 'I told you, we don't have any grapes here. The next time you ask me that I'm going to nail your beak to the bar.' The duck leaves. The next day he comes back into the bar. 'Got any nails?' he asks the bartender. 'No,' says the bartender. 'Good . . . got any grapes?' asks the duck."

Again, his deep laughter filled the room. Even at the worst moments, it sustained him.

Surgery on the liver is not to be taken lightly. The good news is that after the removal of a portion of the liver, the remainder can regenerate. The bad news is that the surgery can be complicated. Dr. Port was a thin, middle-aged Asian man with a calm demeanor which the Gradys found soothing. He had ordered his own CT scan with a specific injection of contrast into the liver to study the tumor, and reviewed the results with the family. Grady and Molly were joined by the twins. Dr. Port spoke precisely.

"This is the only metastasis we can see. Fortunately, it is near the surface of the liver in what we call the right lobe. The liver has four lobes, and the right is the largest. I can remove that section of the liver, and you can live normally. It will take you several weeks to recover. You are a large man, and the incision will be a long one, so you will be restricted in your activities for several weeks."

Grady patted his ample girth. "Sorry you will have so much digging to do."

Dr. Port looked up. "We come in all shapes, sizes, and colors. But in the end, we all want the same things."

Two nights before the surgery it snowed, a true February nor'easter which left a blanket of white gleaming in the morning sun. Grady sat with Molly, eating breakfast and drinking coffee in their kitchen, which was brightly lit by the reflection from the outside snow. He fussed with his eggs.

"Eat, man," she said, standing behind him and rubbing his shoulders. "You'll need it."

"Thank you, dear, for everything." He held her hand on his shoulder.

"You'll be fine. I didn't give you that jug for nothing."

That evening the entire family, Missy, Meg, her husband, and the two babies sat together, remembering the old days. Missy recalled the day about ten years earlier when she had gone with Grady to pick up his new Lincoln. After the purchase, she had driven their old Dodge Caravan back home. When she parked it next to the new car in the garage, Grady had been directing her every turn of the wheel. In her anxiety, Missy had stepped on the gas and nearly killed her father. As he picked himself up from the garage floor where he had dived to avoid being crushed, it was the first time they had ever seen him at a loss for words. Over the years, epic battles between the strong-willed daughter and father over the responsibility for his near death had been refought on many occasions.

"You almost killed me that day, Missy dear."

"Stop now. It was a lesson to you not to boss her around," replied Meg, worried the battle could be rejoined even on this evening.

"Ah, and a lesson well learned." He patted Missy's knee. "I'll never tell you what to do again, at least not when I'm directly in front of ya."

Missy kissed him. "Daddy, I want you to go into that surgery tomorrow with a clear mind and an understanding that I never meant to kill you that day. And I'm sorry."

He hugged his daughter. "An apology certainly worth a small piece of me liver."

Meg looked at her mother, "Well, maybe there is something good out of this . . ."

Across town that evening, the bible study group opened with a prayer for Ann Grady and her husband. Like you did for Kathy Mulvaney, Lord, deliver us another miracle.

Grady was wheeled into the operating room and helped move himself over to the table. He remembered the bright lights and then nothing as the medications rendered him senseless. Dr. Hayes, the anesthesiologist, placed a tube into Grady's trachea and the machine took over his breathing while his heart rate and blood pressure were monitored. A catheter placed in his bladder drained his urine.

"You've a big one here," commented Dr. Hayes to Dr. Port, "but he's all asleep and all yours."

Grady's ample abdomen was painted with an antiseptic solution by Dr. Port and his two assistants, Drs. Leland and David, both experienced residents doing their training. Dr. Port drew his knife blade across the abdomen just below the ribs to cut the skin, then used his electrocautery to cut through the fat. This heated knife instantly caused the blood vessels in the fat to stop bleeding and produced small puffs of smoke which wafted upward. Beneath Grady's thick insulating layer of fat were his surprisingly strong abdominal muscles, also cut by Dr. Port's knife.

Dr. Port's next step was to enter the peritoneum, the thin membrane which covers the abdominal contents. For most of humankind's history, entering the peritoneum meant death from infection, but the team hardly gave it a thought. After Dr. Port cut the membrane, he reached in and felt the liver, checking to be sure there was no other sites of the cancer.

"I just feel the one lesion," he announced. "Check it, Leland."

Dr. Leland repeated the maneuver and agreed. "I don't feel anything else."

Dr. Port then took an ultrasound probe and placed it into Grady's abdomen, moving it over the liver. After a few minutes, he again reported.

"I can't find anything else. Just the one spot. Leland, prove me wrong."

Dr. Leland repeated the same motions with the ultrasound probe.

"I agree, Chief."

"Good, let's go on."

Having decided to continue, Dr. Port lengthened the incision under Grady's ribs and joined it to another incision right down the middle of his abdomen. After again cutting through the fat, the team placed retractors to pull all the tissue away. Grady had been right; it took a great deal of digging and work to expose his liver. Dr. David then removed the gallbladder as Drs. Port and Leland began to search for the arteries and veins which supplied blood to the liver.

Dr. Port paused. He had reached the point at which he would tie off and cut the duct which drained the bile from the right lobe of Grady's liver. Once this was done, there was no going back, and he would need to complete the surgery.

"We are at the Rubicon," he announced. Drs. Leland and David were quiet, but Dr. Hayes laughed.

"Something funny, Dr. Hayes?" Dr. Port asked, his voice fierce. Dr. Hayes, Dr. Port's longtime friend, knew the drill.

Unfazed and with a cheerful voice, Dr. Hayes replied. "I realize I am not the student of history that you are, Dr. Port. I am merely your faithful anesthesiologist. Still, I have some trouble visualizing Julius Cesar as a thin man of Chinese descent. Perhaps you could find a historical phrase more appropriate to your heritage."

Dr. Port looked at Drs. Leland and David.

"Either of you have any Latin?" he asked.

They both shook their heads.

"A pity," Dr. Port commented. "It used to be required of physicians like Dr. Hayes here. And even some of us surgeons. Correct Dr. Hayes?"

"Correct, Dr. Port. Our patient is ready. Vital signs are all good."

"Excellent," replied Dr. Port, his voice calm. "Alea iacta est."

Working together, Drs. Port and Leland removed the right lobe of Grady's liver by tying off the main blood vessels, then using their fingers to press away the left side of liver while they pulled the right side free, rapidly stapling all the bleeding areas. Finally, the lobe was free, and Dr. Port handed it off to the nurse. There was no time for a sense of satisfaction, however, as he quickly began packing the area to stop any bleeding they had missed with their staples. At his direction, Dr. Leland kept pressure on the remaining liver while Dr. David kept the view clear. Dr. Port looked up at Dr. Hayes.

"His systolic is 80, I have one unit in and the second is almost finished," Dr. Hayes noted, all business now, on high alert to be sure his patient survived this trauma.

Once Grady's blood pressure had returned to normal, and Dr. Hayes was satisfied, Drs. Port and Leland began the process of removing their packing and meticulously inspecting the area, using sutures and their coagulator to stop any bleeding points. While it was tedious work, Dr. Port was unflagging, a lesson not lost on Drs. Leland and David despite their many times working with him. He repeatedly washed the area with warm water, looking for more bleeding to correct. Finally, and only when he was completely satisfied, Dr. Port moved on. Two drains went through separate incisions in Grady's abdomen. A suction tube was placed through his nose into his stomach to keep it collapsed so it would not press on the area. Then Grady was sutured closed with several layers of stitches, and his breathing tube was removed. He left the operating room, minus his cancer.

Grady awoke briefly in the recovery room, but for the next week the big man was terribly ill. It was the trauma to his liver, the doctors reassured Molly, just give it time to recover. She recalled it as a long blur of pain, confusion, diarrhea, constipation, vomiting, and medications. For his part, Grady remembered none of it.

They met with Dr. Matthews six weeks after the surgery.

"It's been hard," said Molly. "He just started eating but still can't do much."

"Well, the good news is the pathology report showed that Dr. Port removed all the cancer. It was one spot that measured four centimeters or just under two inches."

"That's what Dr. Port said," nodded Grady.

"You will have a choice when you recover," continued Dr. Matthews. "You can be watched, or you can repeat a course of chemotherapy in case there are any cancer cells Dr. Port missed. The first time around we know from studies that the chemotherapy helps some people. I wish it had cured you, but it did not. This time around we do not know if the chemotherapy helps. There are not many studies of chemotherapy in people who have had this type of surgery."

Grady looked up. He shook his head. "I'm done."

Dr. Mathews nodded. Even Molly was silent, refusing to push Grady any further.

Late winter and spring were normally when Grady and Molly prepared for the summer season. The restaurant was cleaned, equipment repaired, and supplies ordered in anticipation of the first warm weather and longtime customers in search of Grady's famous hamburgers and ice cream, served with his booming voice and laugh. That year Grady was too weak, and Molly too preoccupied with his care. It was weighing on them both as they sat in the backyard, enjoying the first warm sunshine of April, when the twins walked in.

Molly stood up quickly.

"Girls, what a surprise! Missy, what are you doing here?"

The twins smiled at each other and Missy answered. "I'm back to help with the store. Meg and I will open it. She can't do it herself with the kids, but she can back me up."

Grady spoke up. "You don't need to do this, my darlings. I can hire someone to open it this summer."

It was Meg who answered.

"Forget it, Daddy. This store is in our genes, just like the backside and nose ones you gave us."

"Speak for yourself, sister, my nose is perfect," responded Missy. "And not another word, Daddy or I'll be looking for my Caravan."

For the second time on record, Grady was silent.

D r. Morris was wrong. Chemotherapy sucked. From the moment Carol entered that depressing waiting room filled with sick patients, a faint odor reached her, different than the smell of the ultra-sound jelly. It was a faint sense of something rotting being covered by disinfectant, and it made her gag. Betty and Rose seemed unaffected.

"Are you all right honey?" whispered Betty as Rose again went to the counter to turn in Carol's forms. "You look a little green."

Carol nodded. "I don't think I belong here."

She looked around. The chairs in the waiting room were arranged in groups of eight, forming three separate areas. Across from her in a wheelchair sat an elderly man with swollen legs. Next to him sat his wife, obviously a veteran of many visits here, knitting quietly. She looked up at Carol with kindly, tired eyes and faintly smiled. Next to her sat a young, muscular black man. Shifting restlessly while kneeling beside him was a handsome boy of four or five who had two model cars and would clearly rather have been anywhere else in the world. Rounding out their section of the waiting room was a strikingly pale woman who looked about seventy and was elegantly dressed, sitting alone, breathing shallowly as she tried to read. What are their stories? Carol briefly wondered, fighting to keep her own bile and anxiety down.

A nurse came over to the young black man.

"Your blood counts are good. Here is your prescription," she said, handing him a slip of paper. "I called it into the pharmacy, so it'll be ready this evening."

He rose quickly and nodded thanks. "Come on Jason, let's go." They left hand in hand, the large man and his miniature son.

Almost simultaneously, a young orderly in hospital dress arrived.

"Mr. Kurtz, sorry to see you again. They are ready for you in the hospital. Hi, Mrs. Kurtz. How's that blanket going?"

Mrs. Kurtz held up her knitting. Betty smiled. "It's beautiful," she said.

"Thank you," said Mrs. Kurtz. "I get a lot of time to work on it." She looked at Carol. "Good luck, dear."

As Mr. Kurtz was wheeled out, Janice appeared and once again ponderously brought them into the exam room, sat Carol on the exam table, and slowly went through the routine. Rose was apoplectic, but Carol found the atmosphere in the exam room a relief compared to the scenes in the waiting area, and her nausea subsided. After she had left, Rose erupted.

"Do you think she could possibly move any more slowly?" she asked acidly. "I thought the Commonwealth had slow workers in court, but she beats them all. No wonder they knit blankets here."

"Relax, dear," said Betty.

Yes, Rose, relax, thought Carol. I'm the one who will be getting the chemo.

Thankfully, Dr. Spiegel arrived shortly. He reintroduced Dr. Matthews, the oncology fellow.

"How did your radiation go?" he asked. "Did you have much skin irritation?"

"I really didn't feel much until the end. I did get a little burned, but it's all better now," replied Carol.

"She worked all the way through," added Betty.

"She is a strong woman," agreed Dr. Spiegel. "I can see where she got it from."

Dr. Spiegel reviewed the plans for treatment, answered Rose's questions, then excused her and Betty so he could check Carol's breast.

"It looks as if it is healing well," he commented. "I think once the skin finishes peeling and the color gets back to normal, you won't notice the scar very much."

"It's still numb under the arm."

"Yes, it will stay that way. Over the years, you may get some sensation back, but it will never be normal. Sometimes the arm can swell, called lymphedema. We used to see that quite often when surgeons removed more lymph nodes, but occasionally it can still be a problem. You should not have blood drawn from this arm, or blood pressures taken, unless absolutely necessary."

"I haven't felt any swelling," Carol replied.

"No, your arm looks good. Hopefully, the chemotherapy will also go well."

Carol nodded. As they left, she noticed that the elegantly dressed but pale woman was still reading.

Carol's chemotherapy would start the next Friday. On that day, she would be given her first intravenous treatment (methotrexate and 5-fluorouracil) and began two weeks of evening pills (cyclophosphamide). One week later, she would have the same intravenous treatments. Once the pills finished, she had two weeks off. The one month process was to be repeated six times. Carol had chosen Friday so that if she were sick, she would not miss work. She was scheduled for one o'clock and planned to work the morning before treatment, but Roger refused to allow her into the office.

"Not the first time, dear," he informed her emphatically. "You are starting a long journey, and you need to be relaxed that morning. Go for a walk, visit the Gardner, do something nice and quiet."

Betty would accompany Carol for her first treatment. Rose had an important court date, and Carol had assuaged her guilt.

"Mom can bring me. There should not be any problems. The real question is how I will feel over the weekend. So, if I know you are around, that will be very helpful."

"I will call you on Friday evening, then." Rose paused. "I'll be thinking of you at one."

"Thanks."

"Actually, if they still have that Janice working, I should probably think of you at two-thirty."

"I'm surprised you remember her name," laughed Carol.

"Yeah, well, I had about twenty minutes to study her name tag while she took your pulse or whatever."

Carol had mixed feelings about Rose's absence at her first treatment. Her cutting observations and obvious impatience could be embarrassing, but she was a powerful ally in the strange hospital environment. Her mother was supportive, but Carol knew that if anything went wrong, it would be Rose who moved quickly.

Thursday evening Betty had prepared dinner for the two of them, a comforting vegetable soup from Carol's childhood and a light chicken salad. After eating, they sat for coffee. Carol's thoughts drifted off to St. Martin while Betty watched, amused. After the spell had been broken, Carol turned toward her mother.

"Sorry, Mom, I was thinking of something else. I didn't mean to be so rude."

Betty laughed. "Not at all, dear, it looked like a nice place."

"St. Martin."

"I'm glad, then."

Carol paused. "Mother, do you remember Roger, my boss?"

"Of course, dear. Have you straightened him out yet?"

They burst into laughter.

"I guess you do remember him," Carol said, shaking her head in disbelief. Betty nodded, smiling.

"Well, anyway, no, I haven't 'straightened him out' at all. He is still gay. But I was thinking about him. In St. Martin, he was reading a book about AIDS and deciding how much he wanted to be involved in the politics of it all."

"Did he decide?" asked Betty.

"I don't think so, not yet."

"Why were you thinking of that now?"

"I'm not sure. Maybe because I'm wondering how much all this cancer stuff will be part of my life."

"Are you scared of the chemotherapy?"

Carol nodded. "The surgery and the radiation didn't seem so bad, but putting those chemicals inside my body sucks." She looked up suddenly. "Sorry, I mean stinks."

Betty smiled. "Honey, sucks is okay."

Carol woke later than usual on Friday morning. She felt well rested, and the brightness of the room again surprised her for a moment until she remembered the day. After coffee and thirty minutes with the *Boston Globe*, she decided to go for a walk. The fall air was crisp and the day clear. On impulse, she rode the Green Line a few stops, found herself near the park, and purposefully walked to the sculpture of the Mallard duck family. This being a school day, they were all alone.

"All right guys," she announced. "A lot has changed since I was here last. I have breast cancer. I finished surgery and radiation, and now have chemo. Do any of you have anything to say about this?" They all continued silently striving after their mother.

It's a strange world, she thought. You get an itch, have breast cancer surgery, go to a topless beach with a gay man, get radiation, and now talk to bronze ducks. At least they are not answering back. Yet.

The oncology waiting room was surprisingly quiet as Carol and Betty entered that afternoon. Although Janice still moved at a snail's pace, Carol was in the exam room and ready for Dr. Spiegel almost on time. He did not have much to say, but she felt his presence comforting. A few minutes later, a tall, blonde oncology nurse walked in and introduced herself.

"Hi, Carol. I'm Carol, too. Carol Jones. They call me 'CJ.' I'll be your oncology nurse."

CJ quickly reviewed the treatment plan with Carol and Betty, then brought them back into the treatment area. It was a large room, about seventy feet long and forty feet wide, with high ceilings and narrow frosted windows which ran to the top, offering light but no view. In the center was a low nursing station. On each of the long sides of the room were ten reclining chairs which faced the station, each with a small side chair. Although Carol later learned the room had been an early hospital ward, her first impression was that of a bizarre medieval church.

Carol sat in a reclining chair at the near end of the of the room, and CJ started an IV in her right arm and filled two tubes with blood.

"It will take about ten minutes to get your results," she said. "Then Dr. Spiegel can sign your orders. Once he does that, I can start the anti-nausea medications. It will take about half an hour to get the chemotherapy up, so that will give those meds time to work. So, relax for now. Nothing will happen for about twenty minutes."

Nothing except the show. Betty, sitting in the small chair on Carol's left, had started reading as CJ worked on the other side. Carol had a view of much of the room. About half the chairs were full. Directly across from her was a middle-aged man asleep in his chair, mouth open, with several IV bags hanging. He was alone at present, but the chair beside him had a bag on it. Next to him was an elderly woman getting a blood transfusion. The equally elderly appearing man asleep in the reclining chair next to her had no IV, and Carol surmised they were wife and husband. Further down that row, she saw a bald, wasted man of indeterminate age engaged in an intense conversation with a thin, severe looking younger woman who looked to be in her thirties, and whom Carol assumed was his daughter.

As she surveyed the room, Carol began to notice the faint smell of the lubricant jelly and had the first twinges of nausea. As her anxiety began to rise, a small, elderly woman pushing an IV pole sat down on CJ's stool, which still was next to Carol.

"Hi. I'm Marilyn," she announced. "I have leukemia and am in my fourth remission. That's a record around here. Of course, they keep giving me more treatment, but I don't mind because it keeps me alive. You're new here, aren't you?"

Carol nodded, and Betty looked up.

"CJ is your nurse, right? I saw her bring you in. She is nice, but a little hard, if you know what I mean. That's Fran over there," she pointed to a dark-haired nurse in her early thirties tending to the woman getting the blood transfusion. "She's my nurse, helping Mrs. Jones with her blood. Dr. Spiegel is my doctor. Is he your doctor, too?" Carol nodded again.

CJ returned to the room, holding a piece of paper and several syringes.

"Marilyn . . .," she began.

Marilyn got up quickly.

"I was just leaving," she said to CJ, then nodded to Carol. "Good bye, dear," she said and scurried back toward her chair at the other end of the room.

"I see you met Marilyn," commented CJ. "She is always around and talks to everyone. She is harmless and will go away if you tell her."

"Actually, she took my mind off it," said Carol.

"Good," laughed CJ. "These are your anti-nausea medications. First you get Decadron, a steroid. You might feel a little flushed or even a little sensation on your bottom; we call it 'bottom-burn.' If you do, let me know, and I can give it more slowly." She emptied the syringe into the IV over the next minute as Carol sat quietly and Betty watched. Carol had no reaction. Nor did she react to the rest of her medications. Both the methotrexate and the 5-FU infusions were boring. As she and Betty walked out, Carol felt slightly dizzy but otherwise felt well.

"That was easy," Carol commented to Betty after they returned to her apartment. They ate light sandwiches that Betty had made for dinner. After her mother had left, Carol phoned Rose.

"It went very well," she reported. "I did not get sick or anything. I just have to take the pills tonight before bed. I don't think this chemo is going to be a problem. Mom did well, too. And Janice sends her love."

About an hour before bed, Carol took the anti-nausea pill Compazine. Thirty minutes later, she opened the bottle of Cytoxan and removed two of the large white pills. To her surprise, she noticed an immediate harsh chemical smell followed by the overwhelming presence of the jelly lubricant. This is ridiculous, she thought, I am nowhere near the hospital. How can I be smelling that stuff? Her mouth turned dry, bile rose in her throat, and she began to perspire. Carol opened a window and allowed the cold, fresh air to clear her mind. Revived, she walked back into the kitchen. As she moved closer to the pills, however, the sense of nausea again rose within her. Bile is the right literary word, she thought. How am I going to swallow these things?

In the end, she brought the pills into the kitchen, opened the window and, as the outside air rushed over her, hurriedly swallowed them with cold water. They hit her stomach with a painful thump and seemed to slosh around in a mix of water and bile. They stayed with her that night in her dreams, casting a sickly pall over disjointed images of her life.

The next morning, Carol felt tired but okay. When Rose and her mother called, she was too embarrassed to tell them swallowing the pills had been so difficult. Saturday night was even worse. By Sunday, even the thought of opening the pill bottle produced sickness. Although she forced down the pills, Carol called CJ on Monday.

"I can't believe how well I did with the IV treatments, but these pills are terrible."

"This happens to some people," CJ explained, "and it can get worse if we don't treat it. I want you to start with some Ativan after dinner. That will relax and sedate you a bit and hopefully allow you to take the Cytoxan."

The little white Ativan pill was her friend, Carol decided. It relaxed her and let her swallow the Cytoxan pills, even if they still gave her bad dreams.

The next week Carol returned for more IV treatment. Again, the infusion went smoothly. Marilyn was not in that day, but sitting next to Carol was a man in his mid-thirties dressed in Red Sox sweats. He was asleep, but Carol could see under his matching Red Sox cap he was bald. Sitting next to him was a woman she took to be his wife.

They smiled at each other and struck up a conversation. Carol learned Nancy's husband was fighting a sarcoma, a cancer which had started in the muscle of his leg and spread into his lungs. Carol found it surprisingly helpful to talk with a young, non-medical woman also learning about chemotherapy.

"The pills are the hardest part for me," Carol concluded.

"I don't know much about pill chemo," she replied. "Each month Scott gets four days of IV chemotherapy. To control his vomiting, they basically put him in a coma. He checks in, says good-bye on Monday, and wakes up on Friday. I wrote down what they give him," she searched her pocketbook. "Here it is . . . a high-dose metoclopramide infusion with diphenhydramine and lorazepam."

CHEMOTHERAPY NAUSEA AND VOMITING BEFORE ZOFRAN.
Nausea and vomiting are among the most feared complications of chemotherapy. Vomiting is triggered by a portion of the brain located in the lower part of the brainstem (the region known as the medulla oblongata), called "the vomiting center" in a rare example of medical clarity. The vomiting center is under the control of a nearby portion of the brain called the "chemoreceptor trigger zone," which is activated by signals from the stomach or intestines when they are damaged. The vomiting center can also be triggered by other parts of the brain. An example is when a person sees something upsetting, as in the classic movie portrayal of the young detective vomiting at the brutal crime scene. There are many different signals used in the brain to transmit the vomiting message, but three are particularly important: dopamine, serotonin, and substance P.

Chemotherapy drugs can cause nausea or vomiting by irritating the receptors in the stomach which sends signals to the brain, acting like a bad meal. The sensitivity of the stomach is worsened by extra acid produced from the stress of the illness. Chemotherapy can also directly activate the chemoreceptor trigger zone or other parts of the brain to cause vomiting. As the drugs are given, "acute" nausea and vomiting can occur which usually lasts hours or a day. Serotonin is the main signal for this vomiting. Several days later, "delayed" nausea and vomiting may develop. Substance P is responsible for much of this type of nausea. Finally, "anticipatory" nausea and vomiting can appear in patients as they get ready for their treatments. In many ways, this is the most difficult to understand or control. Sometimes it will be triggered by the car ride to the treatment, the smell of the office, or even the sight of a particular person.

As chemotherapy treatments first began to cure lymphomas and leukemia in the 1970s and were widely introduced for other cancers in the 1980s, anti-nausea medications were relatively ineffective and had their own side effects. Dopamine could be partially blocked, and patients sedated, but the most important acute vomiting signals from serotonin could not be halted. The profound and pervasive fear of chemotherapy nausea and vomiting was justified, begging for the discovery of new medications. Something, anything, to block serotonin.

"Anyway, he comes out at the end of the week bleary-eyed, unshaven, and a little stale." Nancy held her nose.

"That sounds awful," Carol replied.

"Well, if he does well, he can get a bone marrow transplant. That's what we are aiming for." She looked at him lovingly. "Anyway, he cleans up nicely."

Carol forced her Cytoxan pills down, but it wasn't easy. Each night for two weeks she took the Ativan, prepared herself, then swallowed those vile Cytoxan pills. She could feel them sitting in her stomach as she waited for the Ativan to make her fall asleep. After her two weeks off, starting up again was even harder. Explaining it wasn't easy, either.

"Everyone takes pills," she told CJ. "I don't think I can describe this without people thinking I'm crazy. I don't want my family or friends to know."

CJ nodded. "It's hard to understand if you haven't been there . . ."

The large, Mediterranean-looking woman wearing a colorful, flowing dress held up her hand as Dr. Matthews entered the room, causing the many bracelets around her forearm to make a musical, ringing sound. She was seventy, but one minute looked fifty-five and the next much older.

"Before you say anything, I had a dream last night that you were here at work. All these patients were coming, and you were saying to them either you will die or you will live. And in my dream, I was waiting my turn, but it never came. So, what is it? Do I live or die?"

"Your scan and blood work are good."

"Amen," she cried. She climbed off the exam table and hugged the younger woman accompanying her, whom Dr. Matthews knew was her niece. As she rapidly widened her embrace to include Dr. Matthews, he was helpless to resist. After Dr. Mathews and the young woman were released, Thelma Lambros, in her beautiful voice, sang a brief verse from Tracy Chapman,

> Be and be not afraid
> Be and be not afraid
> Be and be not afraid
> To reach for heaven.

Thelma Lambros filled spaces. For many years she had been a well-known set designer capable of transforming any venue into a different world, real or imaginary, from the past, present, or future. As a child, she had been a singer with dreams of the stage and opera. Thelma was training her spectacular voice for classical music when an attack of lupus in her early twenties had damaged her lungs and taken away the wind and power she needed for performance. She channeled her creativity into the theater where her skills and forceful personality led to remarkable success on and off Broadway. After a wonderful career, Thelma had retired in Saratoga Springs where she enjoyed the ballet, orchestra, and arts community.

About eighteen months ago, Thelma had begun to feel poorly. It had been insidious, starting with a vague bloating and cramping whose arrival was hard to predict and unrelated to eating. Although Thelma had always been a self-described "spiritual eater" willing to try almost anything that seemed to satisfy her soul at the time, she first tried changing her diet. She ate fruits and vegetables regularly, eliminated her beloved late-night coffee and substituted herbal teas. Although for a time it seemed to help, eventually the symptoms returned. Constipation alternating with diarrhea became the norm. Thelma also felt a profound sense of fatigue. Usually a woman with boundless energy, her creative drive seemed dulled and the bright colors of her life somber.

Her friends had noticed Thelma seemed flat and, after their approaches were deflected, enlisted the help of her niece, Paola. In retrospect, Thelma was surprised at her resistance to accepting help. While she had always prided herself on being self-sufficient, she was also practical and recognized her limits with the goal of working around them. Somehow this illness had sapped her of this ability. She had slipped into apathy when Paola arrived.

Paola was the daughter of Thelma's half-sister. Raised in Manhattan, Paola had been exposed to her aunt's powerfully creative view of the world. Since Thelma had never married and had no children, she was included in many of her half-sister's family gatherings. Soon it was discovered that Paola and Thelma shared a special bond. "We have the same head, even in the little things," Thelma would say.

When Paola learned to flush the toilet, she covered her ears at the sound. After reading in bed at night, she needed to rebrush her teeth to fall asleep. Thelma shared these same innate idiosyncrasies, something that caused Paola's mother to comment that she was raising her own sister.

"I believe we were sisters in a past life," Thelma had told Paola when she was a teenager.

"Well, Aunt Thelma, you obviously kept the voice," responded Paola, whose singing was atrocious.

Despite her voice, Paola shared Thelma's love for the arts and had studied English literature. A writer of some note, she now taught at the University of Vermont in Burlington, about a three-hour drive from Saratoga. They often communicated by phone and text messages, but Paola had not seen her aunt in several months. She was surprised to find her drawn in the face but bloated in her belly and swollen in her legs. They sat together, sipping tea and eating the pastries Paola had brought, of which Thelma uncharacteristically took only little bites.

"Aunt Thelma . . .," began Paola, after they had caught up.

"Whenever you use that tone, dear, you want something. It's been the same since you were a child. What is it?"

"You look ill and tired. I want you to see a doctor."

Thelma looked thoughtfully at her niece.

"I am sick, dear. There is something inside me, eating away at my spirit. Worms, I think."

"Worms, Aunt Thelma?"

"Yes, dear, worms. I feel and see them inside me . . . when I close my eyes."

Thelma agreed to a visit with Dr. Stacey Gold, whose daughter Paola had mentored at the University.

Dr. Gold did an exam and an ultrasound in the office, then met with Thelma and Paola.

"Thelma, I believe you have some form of cancer, probably ovarian cancer. There is a mass in the right ovary putting pressure on your bowel and causing your constipation as well as producing fluid in your abdomen, what we call ascites. That is making you swell."

"I knew they were inside me," answered Thelma. "Damn worms."

❖ ❖ ❖

OVARIAN CANCER.

Understanding ovarian cancer starts with anatomy. The two ovaries are small, peanut sized organs located deep on each side of a woman's pelvis. Eggs released from the ovaries follow the fallopian tube to the uterus where they implant if fertilized. The uterus is joined by the cervix to the vagina.

Ovarian cancers are hard to detect at an early stage. This is not surprising given the ovaries are so small and deep within the pelvis. In contrast, the vagina can be seen on exam, the cervix checked for cancer with the PAP test, and the uterus seen using an ultrasound or scope. Thus, by the time they are detected, most ovarian cancers have spread beyond the ovary.

Ovarian cancers have a unique way of spreading, often going into the abdominal cavity rather than through the blood system. As they spread, they form clumps or plaques on the lining of the abdominal organs called the peritoneum. "Peritoneal carcinomatosis" is the name of this cancerous thickening of the lining. As the growth of cancer on the lining continues, masses form throughout the abdominal cavity. Symptoms result from a build-up of fluid in the abdominal cavity (called "ascites") or interference with the function of the bowel or bladder. Pain, bloating, constipation or diarrhea, fatigue, and distention of the abdomen can all occur in various measures. At the start of the illness, these symptoms resemble many other noncancerous conditions, making the diagnosis difficult.

The name ovarian cancer itself may often be wrong. Many ovarian cancers probably start in the fallopian tube rather than the ovary. Sometimes these cancers even develop in the abdominal cavity despite normal ovaries and tubes. In that situation, the cancers began in a small nest of ovary cells left behind in a woman's body as the ovaries moved to their final location when she was developing as an embryo. A similar situation can occur in men who develop testicular cancer elsewhere in their body with normal testicles.

The treatment for ovarian cancer starts with surgery; a complex operation called a radical hysterectomy with debulking. The goal is to remove as much of the cancer as possible. In the traditional operation, an incision is made from the pelvis up to above the umbilicus to allow inspection of the abdomen. Any fluid is removed and sent for analysis. If there is no fluid, washing of the cavity is done to find cancer cells. The diseased ovary and tube are removed along with the uterus and other ovary, called a "complete hysterectomy." In addition, the omentum, the large fold of the peritoneum which hangs down from the stomach like an apron, is removed since it is a common site for the cancerous spread. During an inspection of the rest of the abdomen, any visible cancer is removed, including involved parts of the bowel, bladder, or spleen as needed.

Surgeons who undertake this operation are usually gynecologic oncologists. These surgeons complete four years of medical school followed by three years of residency training in obstetrics and gynecology, then three to five years of training in gynecologic oncology, where they learn to perform these surgeries and administer chemotherapy treatments. Since these specialized surgeons are scarce, many women with ovarian or other female cancers will be sent to major medical centers for their surgery and return home to receive their chemotherapy.

Dr. Gold had ordered a CT scan and lab work then called Thelma with the results.

"The CT scan shows what the ultrasound found. You have a cancer of the ovary, and it has spread within the abdominal cavity. This is causing the symptoms you have been feeling. The CA-125 blood test is elevated, and that confirms this is ovarian cancer. The blood work also shows your kidney and liver function are excellent. That is a good sign. Getting to Dr. Ivanov for surgery is the right next step. Don't be put off by her manner; she is the best."

Dr. Valerie Ivanov was a petite woman with angular features in her late forties. She was attractive, but her blond hair was pulled back, producing a severe look accentuated by her gray pants and a black top under a lab coat. Thelma's first impression was that she moved precisely, like a dancer. If Dr. Ivanov was a ballerina, Thelma thought, she was a Russian, hard. After examining Thelma, Dr. Ivanov returned to the room where Paola had joined them.

"This cancer must come out; then you get chemotherapy."

"What will her recovery be like?" asked Paola.

"She will have pain and misery for one week, then she will get better," came the clipped reply.

"Dr. Gold said she might need a colostomy. When will you know?" Paola pushed on.

"At surgery time. She will have the colostomy if she needs it, then after chemotherapy, it will be reversed."

"Can it be cured?" asked Paola. "Is she doing this for a good reason?"

Dr. Ivanov answered sharply.

"You do this to live. Without it, you die. One in three cured; the rest live longer. Only you know if that is a good reason."

The room was quiet for a moment. Dr. Ivanov moved to get up.

"Please wait," asked Thelma "Where are you from?"

Dr. Ivanov's brows tightened. "Why? Is where I am from important to you?"

"Yes," replied Thelma simply.

Dr. Ivanov nodded. "I am Russian."

"Did you dance?" asked Thelma.

Dr. Ivanov sat down, surprised. "Yes, in Moscow, where I grew up before we came to this country. How did you know?"

"You move like a dancer," replied Thelma. For the next few minutes, they were lost in a discussion of the ballet. Paola saw the change in Dr. Ivanov's face matched the life in Thelma's eyes.

When they finished, Thelma asked one more question. "Why do you do this? Why such a difficult profession? Trying to save people like me?"

Dr. Ivanov became almost pensive for a moment.

"My grandfather. He fought in Leningrad against the Germans. Do you know this battle?"

Thelma and Paola nodded.

"He would never speak of it, but we all knew the slaughters which took place, the suffering. He lived, but he never understood why. Later in his life, he developed a cancer of his lung. We Russians all smoke, you know. But he took the treatments, again and again. He never gave in until he died. And he used to say to me, 'Dum spiro, spero.' It means 'where there is breath, there is hope.' "

Dr. Ivanov paused, the sternness, almost defiance, back in her face. "Now you go and get ready, then we fight."

Preparing Thelma for surgery required an EKG, echocardiogram, and breathing tests, followed by a visit with Dr. Martin, the pulmonologist whose office decor from the 1970s and country music seemed as far from Russia as the moon. As they sat in the waiting area, Thelma surveyed the scene.

"I feel forty years younger already," she commented to Paola. "And you should be an infant in this office. But at least they are playing Bonnie Raitt rather than Marie Osmond. I never could take her."

"Who?" asked Paola.

"Never mind," replied Thelma.

Dr. Martin spent considerable time with Thelma.

"Your heart seems fine, but your lung function is fairly limited. It is really remarkable that you have been able to do as much as you have with this damage."

"How did this happen?" asked Paola.

"It was the lupus when I was young," answered Thelma.

"That's true," agreed Dr. Martin. He spoke to Paola. "Lupus means the wolf. And that's what it is. It is an autoimmune disease that can strike at almost any organ and tear it apart. Sometimes, usually with treatment, it leaves as fast as it comes and never returns. Other times it can continue to ravage a person. One of my professors used to say about the disease 'you never lead the wolf; it stalks you.' He meant that you can't really prevent the attacks, you respond when it happens. I think we are getting closer to changing that with modern science, but it is still largely true. Anyway, your aunt was attacked by this wolf as a young woman. Thankfully it has never shown up again. But it did damage her lungs."

Dr. Martin turned back to Thelma.

"The surgery will be a challenge for you, but you can do it."

"I must," answered Thelma. "I need to be rid of these worms."

Thelma remembered entering the operating room on a stretcher, the space as bright as a stage during a performance. She didn't remember anything else. After she was anesthetized, the skin of her belly was cleaned, the drapes set up, and a catheter put into her bladder to drain her urine.

Dr. Ivanov first made a long incision down the middle of Thelma's abdomen. This initial incision took her down to the fascia, the layer covering the muscles beneath the skin. Working from the top of the incision down to the bottom, Dr. Ivanov deepened her incision to enter the abdominal cavity. Here she found the first problem: the cancer had grown in the omentum and stuck it to the front wall of the abdominal cavity near the naval. Before Dr. Ivanov could spread her incision to examine the entire cavity, she needed to free up this diseased omentum which hung down in the abdomen like a thick, sticky apron. It was the start of a long morning of dissection.

After Dr. Ivanov had freed the omentum blocking her incision, she spread open the skin, fat, and muscle to look inside the abdominal cavity. What she found was not good. Thelma had a large amount of cancer. Low down in the pelvis, Dr. Ivanov saw the cancer had started in the left ovary and spread to three areas along the large intestine, causing her constipation. There was cancer along the covering of the bladder. Higher up in the abdominal cavity, Dr. Ivanov found cancer along both side walls and the spaces near them called the gutters. There was cancer near the spleen. This would be a very long morning.

Dr. Ivanov began by removing the omentum, the thickened and diseased apron which hung down over the bowel. That was a few pounds of cancer gone. She moved the small intestine out of the way, packing it carefully onto Thelma's lower chest. Dr. Ivanov then cut her way into the area called the retroperitoneum, which means behind the peritoneum. This space contains the ovaries, tubes, and uterus. These were all removed, another pound of cancer gone. Dr. Ivanov then began work on the sidewalls of the pelvis, stripping the cancer-filled peritoneal lining off the walls. Another few ounces of cancer gone.

Dr. Ivanov then turned her attention to the colon (large intestine). She found cancer squeezing the left side of the colon and knew she would have cut the colon and remove that entire left side. This meant Thelma would have a temporary ileostomy; her small intestine would drain into a bag. After she recovered and finished her chemotherapy, Dr. Ivanov could later reattach the small intestine to the remaining colon, but now the flow of stool had to be diverted outside the body. If the stool reached the colon which was cut, it might not heal properly and delay chemotherapy. Before removing the left portion of the colon, Dr. Ivanov worked on other organs. She found the cancer had invaded the spleen, so that was removed. The appendix had some cancer on it, so it was also taken out. Dr. Yung, the liver surgeon, joined

Dr. Ivanov in removing several cancerous areas off the liver and taking out the gallbladder. A few more ounces of cancer gone.

Now that all the large clumps of visible cancer were stripped from Thelma's abdominal cavity, Dr. Ivanov returned to her work on the colon. She removed the left half of the colon with the cancer attached. The remaining right half of the colon she joined to the rectal area. She tested this to make sure it was well connected. Then Dr. Ivanov took the small intestine and brought it to the surface of the skin in the right lower portion of the abdomen so that the bag could be attached. Finally, she washed out the abdomen multiple times, put drains in place, and closed the incision.

Dr. Ivanov's work had taken four hours. It was reported as an optimal debulking, meaning all the obvious cancer along with Thelma's omentum, ovaries, fallopian tubes, uterus, appendix, spleen, gallbladder, and half her colon ended up "in the pan."

Thelma's recovery was hard. Her damaged lungs were the first problem. During the surgery, Thelma had been intubated, meaning a tube was placed down her throat into the main airway of her lungs to allow her breathing to be controlled by a ventilator. Dr. Martin had been worried that Thelma might need to stay on the ventilator after the surgery for a prolonged period. But surprisingly, after a night in the intensive care unit, she could breathe on her own again. To keep her lungs expanded, Thelma blew the ping-pong ball in the spirometer by her bedside up and down repeatedly. Her lungs may not have been able to carry her through Violetta in *La Traviata*, but she knew how to work them to avoid pneumonia.

Pain was another problem from the extensive surgery. A PCA (Patient Controlled Analgesia) pump meant Thelma could press a button to direct morphine into her system, but the morphine caused Thelma to hallucinate. The first night on the regular ward, she woke up confused and screaming, causing the nurses to rush into her room to comfort her.

The next morning, she explained to Paola.

"I was dreaming that the worms which Dr. Ivanov had cut out were coming after me, no matter which way I turned. They were slimy and evil, and they were hissing 'la donna e mobile.' I couldn't get away."

As terrifying as her dreams were, Thelma's worst problem was emptying her bowels into the ostomy bag. After Dr. Ivanov had cut Thelma's colon during the surgery, her whole intestinal system simply stopped working, producing terrible constipation, pain, and bloating. For the first few days, nothing passed, not even gas. Thelma desperately wanted food, but Dr. Ivanov would not let her eat until there was some movement. Being told by the nurses that it would help, she walked the halls of the surgical ward, sang, and prayed. After five days, her bowels finally came to life, and she passed her first stool into the bag.

"It is the first movement in the symphony of my recovery," she enthused to Carol, an experienced, no-nonsense LPN who worked nights.

Carol looked at her bag. "Honey, if this is some kind of symphony, then I'm your Beethoven. And I'm telling you what you got here is a few notes. You got some voice, but this end of your body still needs to get going."

When they finally did move, Thelma's bowels let go with a flood of diarrhea which made using her ostomy bags torture. Around the opening of her ostomy where her small intestine reached the surface, Thelma glued a ring to the skin. The bags would then be connected to this ring and disconnected when they were filled. But the ring was hard to attach to the skin, the diarrhea leaked around it, and the area became raw and irritated. After a few more days, Thelma was exhausted and miserable.

Carol came to her aid.

"Honey, you need help with this bag. It's time for Margaret."

"Margaret?" asked Thelma.

"She may not look like it, but that gal is your bag angel. Now that your bowels are working, you'll be needing her."

The bleached blond, five-six and two-hundred-pound angel was, in her own words, the nurse who dealt with shit.

"It belongs in the bag, and that's where it's going," she announced. "But first we better get your skin cleaned up."

Over the next few days, Margaret worked with Thelma to gain control of her ostomy.

"Why do you do this?" asked Thelma during one explosive mess.

Margaret looked up. "Do you mean why don't I work saving lives in the ICU or looking pretty in some clean office?"

Thelma nodded.

"I don't exactly know, except this matters. Shit matters, I guess. And most people won't do it, so I'll always have a job."

"She saves lives in her spare time," chimed in Carol, who walked in as her shift started. "Tell her about the flight to Atlanta."

Margaret laughed and continued working.

"Go on. You tell her," Carol continued.

Margaret shook her head, looking over Thelma's abdomen.

"All right. I'll tell you," continued Carol. "Ms. Bowel Nurse here was on her way flying to Atlanta with one of her friends when some fellow died in the seat in front of them. They did CPR and saved the guy. They were on the news, and someone filmed it and put them on YouTube, too."

Thelma looked up at Margaret. "That's really something."

Margaret nodded and rolled her eyes. "Yeah, well the guy was in the seat in front of us, and his wife was screaming and crying. We were trying to get over the wife and the seats to get him out. Finally, we did get him out and started CPR with him on the floor. They caught the whole thing on video, but all from behind me. So, for all fifteen minutes, the main thing you see is my fat ass moving up and down. Let me tell you, it fills the whole screen. Some jerk even set the thing to music. So much for being a sexy cardiac nurse saving lives."

Eventually, Thelma did master skin care and bag changes.

"It's much better, thank you," she reported to Margaret at their last visit. "Still, I will be glad to be finished with the bag when I get hooked up again. I imagine everyone is . . ."

"True," replied Margaret, "but not everyone has the same reasons. My last old man with an ostomy said what he missed the most was his twenty minutes a day on the toilet to read in peace."

When she was ready for discharge, Dr. Ivanov met with Thelma and Paola to discuss the next steps.

"I did an optimal debulking, which means I get everything out that was possible. But you now need chemotherapy."

TREATING OVARIAN CANCER.

Even the most aggressive surgery rarely cures ovarian cancer. The surgeon cannot find and remove all the cancer cells which have escaped into the abdominal cavity. In the early 1950s, chemotherapies which would shrink ovarian cancers were discovered. The next twenty years were an era of poorly controlled experimentation during which the enthusiasm fostered by cures of lymphoma and leukemia met reality in other cancers. Ovarian cancer was one of the resistant cancers. The poor results with surgery alone and the failure of early chemotherapy treatments led to the use of radiation after surgery. Radiation treatments given to the entire abdomen were very toxic and not highly effective.[227]

In the 1970s, chemotherapy for ovarian cancer changed with the development of the drug cisplatin. This compound was first discovered in the mid-1800s, but it wasn't until the 1960s that Dr. Barnet Rosenberg at Michigan State University realized its anticancer potential. Rosenberg had been studying the effects of magnetism on bacterial cells. To create an electromagnetic field, he used platinum electrodes in a broth filled with the bacteria *E. Coli*. The bacteria would not divide when the magnetic field was on, but they would enlarge—their cell division had halted. Rosenberg and his colleagues found that the magnetic field was not the cause of this effect; the platinum electrodes reacted with ammonium chloride in the broth to produce the drug cisplatin.[228]

Cisplatin is a very small molecule which links with DNA, causing the two DNA strands to be stuck together. These clumps (called adducts) of the DNA can lead rapidly dividing cancer cells to die when they try to reproduce their DNA. The cells sense the damage and commit suicide, called apoptosis. When cisplatin produced cures in testicular cancer, physicians hoped it might be the "penicillin of cancer." Although cisplatin did not fulfill this dream, it was approved by the FDA in 1978 and rapidly became a leading treatment for many cancers, including ovarian cancer, and used in combinations with other chemotherapies. Cisplatin has some significant side effects. It produces severe nausea and vomiting, which was particularly devastating before modern anti-nausea medications were developed in the early 1990s. It may damage the nerves, leading to numbness in the hands and feet or hearing loss.[229] Scientists produced a variation of cisplatin, called carboplatin, which had fewer of these side effects.

Paclitaxel (brand name Taxol) was a second important addition to the treatment of ovarian cancer. Paclitaxel kills cancer cells by preventing the microtubules which form the structural scaffolding of the cells from being dismantled, an important step in cell division. The drug was first harvested from the bark of the Pacific yew tree in 1962 near Mount St. Helens in a discovery program sponsored by the National Cancer Institute. Paclitaxel is large and will not dissolve in water, so it took until 1984 to work out the structure and develop methods to allow the drug to be infused and tested on humans. By oncology standards, the results were impressive: 30 percent of women with advanced ovarian cancer given paclitaxel had their tumors shrink.[230] The next major problem was getting a supply of the drug. Since a single dose would require stripping the bark of an entire yew tree, other solutions were needed. The first was a semisynthetic paclitaxel developed by French scientists which was obtained from the needles of a shrub member of the yew family. The second was a synthesis process developed at Florida State University. Paclitaxel was the first drug in the class called taxane.

The combination of a platinum and a taxane cured about 20 percent of women with ovarian cancer which was widespread throughout the abdominal cavity and allowed a higher percentage to live for several years. This partial success of intravenous chemotherapy and the understanding that ovarian cancers usually spread inside the abdominal cavity led to the idea that putting the drugs directly into the abdominal cavity might be even more effective. This type of treatment is called intraperitoneal chemotherapy (IP) and is usually combined with IV chemotherapy. The combination adds to the success rate, but also to the toxicity. Giving intraperitoneal chemotherapy is technically complicated since it requires placement of a catheter into the abdominal cavity. These catheters and the chemotherapy drugs are very irritating, leading to a high risk of painful abdominal problems.[231] So most gynecologic oncologists select only the healthiest patients for this combination treatment.

Dr. Ivanov was her usual blunt self.

"Thelma, you are a strong woman, but Dr. Martin and I do not think you could physically tolerate the IP chemotherapy. Your lungs are okay, but not great, and it will be too much. You should get the regular intravenous chemotherapy closer to home. You must meet one of the medical oncologists in Saratoga."

"I know Dr. Matthews," replied Thelma, to Paola's surprise.

"Fine, we make appointment."

On the waiting room wall in Dr. Matthews' office hung a sculpture which consisted of three metal boxes measuring three feet by five feet and eight inches deep. Each box had cutouts which gave views of different colors inside. As one came closer, writing was visible inside as well. Thelma stood and tried to read the words, which were part of the artist's story.

"I like these," she commented to Paola as they entered the exam room.

Dr. Matthews arrived shortly thereafter, and Thelma stopped him before he could begin.

"That sculpture in the waiting area is a remarkable piece."

Dr. Matthews nodded. "I enjoy it also. It was a gift."

"Do you do any art yourself?" she continued.

"No," Dr. Matthews answered. "I have no talent. But I do like that work."

"Well maybe you were an artist in a past life," Thelma offered.

"If so, starving. Anyway, I am glad to meet you."

Dr. Matthews reviewed her medical history and asked Thelma some additional questions about herself.

"Are you married?"

"Not presently."

"Oh, were you married in the past?" continued Dr. Matthews.

"Not when I should have been. I had a lover, but his family fought it," replied Thelma vaguely.

Dr. Matthews nodded, tabling that discussion for another time, and returned to the medical history. It later fell to Thelma's oncology nurse, Catherine Lotito, to sort out the details.

"She believes in reincarnation," Catherine reported later, after she had met Thelma.

"Reincarnation?" asked Dr. Matthews. "Okay, but what does that have to do with being married. Did she upset someone's family with this belief?"

"No. Actually, she wasn't referring to this life, although she wasn't married in this one. Thelma believes that her true love in a past life was Guiseppe Verde, the famous opera composer who lived around 1840. She's convinced that she was Giuseppina Strepponi, Verde's longtime lover. The story is that Verde's wife had died and he fell in love with this Strepponi, who was herself quite an opera singer. They could not get married since Strepponi didn't fit into Verde's circles, so they lived together. She was shunned. Finally, they did get married, but only when they were older."

"I see . . . I think."

"Well, there is more. Giuseppina apparently lost her voice due to overwork or possibly illness and couldn't sing in public, but used her voice to help Verdi compose."

"And Thelma lost her voice, too," mused Dr. Matthews.

"Sure, so she feels her life is really a repeated variation of the theme. There's a music term for that, but I forgot it. Didn't they explain this to you in medical school?" asked Catherine.

"No."

Catherine reviewed the treatment plan with Thelma and Paola. Thelma would have six treatments of chemotherapy, one every three weeks. The treatments lasted five hours: one hour of anti-nausea medications, one hour of carboplatin, and three hours of paclitaxel. During the first few days, the main worry was nausea and vomiting.

"Some people have no nausea, they leave and go right to Roma or Shirley's for lunch. Other people have a tougher time, and we need to adjust their medications."

"Can you predict who will have problems?" asked Paola.

"Not really," answered Catherine. "Except to say that alcoholics have very little nausea. They have damaged that part of their brain."

"I was never much of a drinker, just an occasional glass of wine," replied Thelma.

"Too late to start now," laughed Catherine. "You need years of it. But one more thing to know. Please don't eat your favorite foods around the time of your treatments or visits here. We do not want you to associate them with the chemotherapy. You might lose your taste for them, which is a shame. It's also why we don't have a coffee maker in the waiting room."

"I would never have thought of that," commented Paola.

"It was more common when we did not have such good anti-nausea medications, but it is still good advice. It's a shame when you lose a favorite food," continued Catherine as she reviewed the list of side effects. Allergic reactions, mouth sores, and nerve damage all needed placement in the proper context without causing fear.

"You did that very nicely, dear," noted Thelma when Catherine finished. "You have given that performance before."

"Many times," replied Catherine, acknowledging the compliment. "But each audience is different."

The first treatment went smoothly, Thelma had little nausea and did not vomit. She had some muscle aching but none of the nerve pain that made the treatment devastating for an occasional patient. During the second week she was tired, but by the third week felt her energy improve.

"I am back again for more," she announced as Dr. Matthews walked into the examination room before her second treatment. "I actually feel better. I think I have recovered from the surgery and this treatment is going well."

"I'm glad," replied Dr. Matthews. After they had reviewed Thelma's experience in more detail, he continued.

"Most people have the same experience each session, so we do not expect much difference the next time. It does begin to tire you out, however, and by the end you will be getting sick of us. However, there is an additional thing we should discuss today. I would like you to consider being tested for a mutation in the *BRCA-1* and *BRCA-2* genes."

BRCA MUTATIONS AS A TARGET: MEDICAL JIU JITSU.

All people have two *BRCA-1* and two *BRCA-2* genes. Some families have inherited mutations in these genes, and their women carriers are at high risk for breast and ovarian cancer. Since the mid-1990s, testing for *BRCA-1* and *BRCA-2* mutations has allowed women to know if they are carriers or not. Depending upon the results, this knowledge may cause them to undergo closer watching, preventative surgery, or relieve them of worry. This is the classic use of genetic testing for these mutations.

In recent years *BRCA* mutations have themselves become targets for treatment. This medical Jiu Jitsu starts with understanding that the function of normal *BRCA* genes is to produce proteins which help repair broken DNA. The BRCA proteins remove the damaged section of DNA and replace it with the correct sequence, a procedure called "homologous recombination." Breast and ovary cells rely on the *BRCA-1* and *BRCA-2* genes more than other cells for this type of repair. Women born with mutations in these genes do not have efficient repair of the damage done to the DNA in their breast and ovary cells. Mutations accumulate, and cancers of these organs result. Fortunately, there are other repair mechanisms besides BRCA-1 and BRCA-2, one of which is called PARP (poly (ADP-ribose) polymerase).

Cancer cells also need to repair their DNA. Although they are deranged, if they develop too much DNA damage, they will not be able to function and die. Thus, when an ovarian cancer develops in a woman with a *BRCA-1* or *BRCA-2* gene mutation, the cancer cell (which also has the mutation) cannot repair its DNA using the BRCA system. The cancer cell must repair its deranged DNA using the other pathways, like PARP. This reliance on PARP by the cancer cell leads to the key Jiu Jitsu move—cancer cells which have the *BRCA* mutation might be vulnerable to treatments which block the PARP system. This unique vulnerability of these cancer cells was reported in 2005 and led to the development of medications which inhibit PARP.[232] Olaparib is one example of these treatments.[233] How to use this class of medications is under study. Should they be given with or after chemotherapy to prevent or delay recurrence? Should they be used when the cancers return?

Dr. Matthews explained these issues to Thelma.

"So, the mutation turns the cell against itself?" she concluded.

"In a way—"

"It's just like *Rigoletto*, our opera. Do you know it?"

"I've seen it performed, but do not remember the details of the plot."

"Well, *Rigoletto* was also known as the '*La maledizione*,' or 'the curse.' In the story, Rigoletto, a sad, little man and unpleasant court jester if there ever was one, is cursed by a man he crosses. The curse causes Rigoletto to end up turning on himself and killing his own daughter, whom he loves."

"I see . . . I guess."

"Sure, you do. The curse, the root of the problem, causes the cells to kill themselves. Just like it did with Rigoletto."

"I see. Okay. Well, the other issue about this testing is that if we do find a mutation, it might have implications for your other family members. They could be tested to see if they carry the same mutation. I would like you to meet with our Nurse Practitioner, Tracy Callahan. She is an expert in explaining these issues—"

"Of course," Thelma interrupted. "Like I said, in *Rigoletto* la maledizione or the curse kills Rigoletto's daughter, so we must be prepared. But I'm quite sure this is not in my family."

Tracy Callahan, the Nurse Practitioner, was an Irish woman whose red hair contained a few white strands which she blamed on her young lads who were students in the local high school. She spoke with Thelma and Paola about the *BRCA* testing.

"Most cancers are caused by a combination of the effects of many genes, how we live our lives, and whoever you believe is directing this show. Or, if you are not of a faith, by chance. But some families are different. They can have a single gene mutation responsible for starting the cancerous process. If we find one of these gene mutations in a family, then we can tell those who did get it what to do. We can also tell those in the family who didn't inherit the mutation that they do not have the increased risk. It's the Angelina Jolie story, right?"

Thelma nodded.

"Dr. Matthews wants you to get tested because if you have a *BRCA* gene mutation there are more treatment options. But if the test was positive, it would also mean that your other family members would be at risk. So, we better figure out who they might be before we do the test. That way you can let them know the test is being done and find out if they want the result or not."

"Why wouldn't they want the result?" asked Paola. "I would want to know."

"Well," replied Tracy, "they might be buying life, disability, or long-term care insurance and not want to put this in the application. Or they might be at a point in life where they just do not want the information, like before their wedding or when they are pregnant . . . You never quite know. So, it is best to work it out ahead of time if you can."

By drawing out Thelma's family tree, Tracy concluded that only Paola and her mother would be at risk.

"That makes it easy," concluded Tracy.

"I guess our family tree looks more like a lopsided family bush," concluded Thelma.

"If there is a mutation and it travels with the voice, then I'll be spared," added Paola.

The third treatment visit produced the report of the testing.

"We received the results of your *BRCA* testing, and it was negative, so you do not have the gene mutation," Dr. Matthews reported.

"I knew that," replied Thelma, nodding.

"Did one of the nurses tell you? Or Tracy Callahan?" asked Dr. Matthews, puzzled. "We try to get these results out to patients quickly, but I thought it just came in late yesterday."

"No, my psychic told me. She said nothing like that was in my blood lines."

"Your psychic?"

"Yes, she has been my spiritual advisor for years. Her name is Mina. She's a Chinese woman in the City. You should really go to her. You would learn a lot about yourself and your past lives. Do you want me to make you an appointment?"

"Catherine told me something about your past . . . Did this woman reveal that to you?" asked Dr. Matthews, hoping to avoid answering the invitation.

"No. Actually, when I was young I went back to Bussetto in Italy with one of my friends," Thelma explained. "There is a small theater there named after Verdi. He never liked the idea of the place and was never in it, but anyway, we had tickets to hear *La Traviata*. It was over-sold, and we were seated on the side of the stage. It was then I knew for sure I was Giuseppina before I was Thelma."

"How is that?" asked Dr. Matthews, despite himself.

"When the lights were on, and our music began in our town, I just knew. When I went back to Mina, she confirmed it."

Ths fourth treatment visit brought converstions about God and reincarnation.

"Do you believe in God?" Thelma began as Dr. Mathews walked into the room.

"I was raised Catholic, so I was given a well-defined image of God," he replied.

"Do you believe in reincarnation?" asked Thelma, pushing. "Do you believe it is possible I was Giuseppina."

"I try not to take a theological position on the matter."

Thelma turned to Paola. "My oncologist is a chicken . . . in this life, anyway."

"That may be true," replied Dr. Matthews, "but I did want to report some good news for you. The CA-125 blood test which we took at the time of your third treatment was normal. It had been fifteen hundred before your surgery, thirty-eight after, and is now fourteen."

"That's wonderful," replied Paola and hugged Thelma, who was now crying.

After Thelma had recovered, she looked up.

"I'm sorry I called you a chicken. You're doing a great job."

Dr. Matthews took out his prescription pad and made a note which he handed to Thelma.

"Don't worry. Here, from your chicken oncologists, look up this fellow sometime."

On the paper was written the name Michele Peyrone, the Italian chemist who discovered cisplatin. As her chemotherapy infused, Thelma and Paola learned Peyrone's story from *Wikipedia*. He was born in Northern Italy to Vittorio and Teresa Peyrone on May 26, 1813. Peyrone's family was well-off, and he was well-educated, ultimately becoming a physician. Shortly after his graduation in 1835, however, a wave of cholera which passed through the area and the experience of treating patients drove him from medicine into chemistry. Peyrone studied in Paris and Germany before returning to Italy in 1849 for an appointment to the faculty of the University of Genoa and later Turino. It was in the 1840s in Germany that Peyrone began to study a compound known as Magnus' green salt, named after the scientist who discovered it. Peyrone synthesized a yellow variation of this chemical with the same composition but a different structure; called an isomer by modern chemists. Despite having the same chemical components as Magnus' green salt, Peyrone's isomer had different properties. Although he did not understand the differences at the time, Peyrone had discovered cisplatin, a molecule which would become one of the most effective traditional chemotherapy agents.

Near the end of her infusion, Thelma waved Dr. Matthews over.

"I probably knew him!" she enthusiastically reported. "He was in the same part of Italy at the same time as we were. He probably heard me sing, too!"

Paola laughed and turned to Dr. Matthews. "See what you did?"

"Leave my oncologist alone. He's not such a stiff after all," interrupted Thelma. "In fact, maybe he was Peyrone in his past life, ever think of that? I will ask Mina. Of course, it would be much better if he would come to see her."

Dr. Mathews waved good-bye before his lineage came under further discussion.

Thelma's last two treatments were hard, and the focus of her visits changed to practicalities. The cumulative effects of her chemotherapy had worn her down.

"It's miserable," Thelma announced as Dr. Matthews walked into the room for her final treatment. "I'm tired, my hands and feet tingle and, worst of all, I whine constantly. My stomach, my bowels, my hair . . . It's all I talk about. You've made me into this medical bore."

"You will be a medical bore for some time," Dr. Matthews answered. "Even though today is your last treatment, it will take three or four weeks for this one to be finished. Then your recovery can begin. That will take six to nine to twelve months. Plus, you will need to have your ostomy reversed and get over that surgery. Please do not expect too much of yourself. You have been through a great deal and recovery will take time."

"Hear that, Auntie?" chimed in Paola. "Be a bore for a while."

"Yes, dear."

A month later, already feeling less like a medical bore, Thelma returned to Dr. Ivanov.

"I am ready to have my bag removed,'" she announced. Dr. Ivanov ordered CT scan and lab studies. When these were clear, she returned to the operating room with Thelma, removed the ostomy and reconnected her bowel. On the ward, Thelma was pleased to see her old friend Carol.

"Hi, Carol. Do you remember me?"

"Course I remember you, Thelma. You got the nice voice and terrible bowels."

Thelma's recovery from this surgery was not easy, either. Once again, her bowels were torture. With help from Carol, she did get them moving enough for Dr. Ivanov to agree to her discharge. At home, though, the constipation returned with a vengeance. She relayed the story to Dr. Matthews.

"Finally, I was so bad we went to Urgent Care. Lovely people, but it was a theater of the absurd. One person to check you in, one to review all your medications, one to take your blood pressure, one to tell you your provider will be coming soon. Then in came some physician assistant who looked about twelve. She said she had never dealt with this before. I was so uncomfortable, but no one could do anything for me. They wanted me to go to the emergency room. Finally, they found an older doctor about your age, who also had white hair, to see me. He disimpacted me. A nice man, I felt sorry for him. But I've been better since."

Thelma paused.

"I never thought of my bowel as a separate entity, but it has its own personality and desires."

Once Thelma's bowels had recovered, she and Paola returned to Dr. Matthews to establish her follow-up routine.

"We will keep track of you with regular examinations. Dr. Ivanov will want to check you every four to six months. We will also do lab tests, including the CA-125 measurement. There is some debate about how often we should do CT scans or even if we should do them, but I like to check them at least each year for the first few years."

"What happens if it comes back?" asked Paola. "Will she need more surgery?"

"Not usually. Occasionally surgery is useful if there is just a single spot, but more often we would use more chemotherapy. The type would depend upon how much time had passed since your last treatment. If it has been more than one year, we would use the platinum again, combined with something else. If it is less than six months, we switch. In between, we wrestle with the decision."

"Well, it's not coming back. That's what Mina says," announced Thelma.

"I would like to agree with Mina on this," replied Dr. Matthews.

"Good. Can I make you an appointment with her?" asked Thelma.

"No, but I will see you in four months."

After the visit, Thelma and Paola returned home. They sat together, as they had on so many occasions over the past nine months, sipping tea.

"So, I'm finished with this," began Thelma.

"So it would seem, Auntie, but remember what Dr. Matthews said. You will need months to regain your strength."

"You have been very good to me, love. You brought me to the doctors when I would not listen to anyone else. You have been here for every surgery and treatment. I don't know what I ever did to deserve you, but I am grateful."

"We have the same head. How could I not?" asked Paola. "And don't forget, I will be back often."

Paola kept in touch, needing to hear Thelma's voice.

"What are you doing?" she asked on one call several months later.

"Drinking my tea and thinking."

"About what?"

"The worms, dear. Are they really gone? I don't feel them."

"I don't know, Aunt Thelma. I hope they are gone, but I guess we'll know after the next tests."

"It's a strange way to think of life, living test to test."

Today, when her brief recital ended, Thelma turned to Dr. Matthews.

"Tracy Chapman is a beautiful woman. I'm glad you are my oncologist," she said. "I have a good team. You know, when Dr. Ivanov said I needed an oncologist, I picked you . . ." Her trailing words almost demanded he pose the next question.

"How did you pick me?"

"My psychic picked you."

Dr. Matthews nodded, knowing he was being led somewhere. "And how did your psychic pick me for you?"

"You mean, did Mina see you in a vision or cards? Did she use her powers of divination?"

"Sure. I guess." He paused, waiting for the punch line.

"No, you dear, silly doctor, what do you think of me? I would never allow that . . . You take care of one of her cousins who lives up here."

And Thelma laughed, filling the entire room.

"It's great drama," announced Dr. Robert Fenton, a lean eighty-one-year-old with bright eyes and bushy eyebrows, who wore a striped suit and bow tie belonging to the 1970s.

Dr. Matthews laughed. "Do you have any side effects from the Xtandi?"

"None worth mentioning, but I am getting quite a bit of attention from the widows in the community being passed off as sympathy. I think they are worried that I won't be able to drive them at night or read their medical reports. You know, we all tend to do that, express sympathy while we are thinking of the impact another person's misfortune has on our own life. It's quite natural."

As Dr. Matthews stopped to consider this statement, Dr. Fenton continued.

"One of the great benefits of working with the mentally ill was that they do not usually hide their feelings in that way. They may be crazy, but I found they are usually honest."

Dr. Robert Fenton had been a psychiatrist in Saratoga during the 1970s, the period of deinstitutionalization when asylums were closed and the mentally ill released back into communities. He was an architect of the county mental health system built to care for these patients, a program acknowledged as a model for the rest of the state. Raised as the son of a Presbyterian minister and trained as a general practitioner, Dr. Fenton brought a no-nonsense approach to the practice of psychiatry, something still possible in his era.

Dr. Matthews had spent a month during medical school with Dr. Fenton. He remembered their first meeting. Dr. Fenton's hair was brown, but he still had his brilliant twinkle and bushy eyebrows.

"You will do all the admitting physical exams," Dr. Fenton explained, "except this one. Roger is a large, delusional, and occasionally violent man when he does not take his medications. I will do his exam. Your job is to slow him down if he comes after me so I can escape."

Matthews had nodded seriously, and Dr. Fenton continued. "Of course, that will leave you with a problem, so let's hope it does not come to that."

They survived the encounter, and Dr. Fenton had taken Mathews under his wing. The next morning, Dr. Fenton drove him to one of the small area clinics which served the mentally ill. This one was in a church basement in Mechanicville, a small railroad town about fifteen miles away. They first stopped at a factory just outside Saratoga Springs which employed many of their chronically mentally ill patients making small items.

"We need to check on Harry. He's been acting out a bit lately, and we want to head off any problems," explained Dr. Fenton.

Harry, a man in his late forties, was found at his workbench. Dr. Fenton shared a few minutes with him while Matthews waited in the background. After they had left, he reported the conversation.

"Harry just needs a little extra attention from time to time to keep him on his medications. Otherwise, he hides his pills. When that starts, the staff at his home must watch him swallow them, or he gets kicked out. He hates when they watch him, so things get out of control quickly. Then he loses his job here and ends up with us in the hospital for a while."

"Did you tell him to take his meds?"

"No, he knows that. I reminded him that we had a bet about the Milwaukee Brewers. For some reason, he loves that team and thinks this is their year to win the World Series. I reminded him that if he ended up in the hospital, he would miss their moment."

"Do you think he will take his meds?"

"I think he will. Like most people, from time to time he needs to be reminded why he does things he doesn't like. Of course, better pitching for the Brewers wouldn't hurt, either."

Dr. Fenton stopped at the men's room and paused before entering.

"Remember, son, in places like this you wash your hands before you use the toilet."

They proceeded with clean hands to Mechanicville and the basement of St. Michael's Roman Catholic Church where Dr. Fenton saw a series of patients, mostly women and a few unemployed men. Fenton asked each about their lives, families, and friends. He reviewed their medication lists, making changes and dispensing encouragement mixed with orders. It was a long session, and Matthews began to wonder whether they would eat lunch. Finally, at one-thirty, they drove across town where Carmella, the widowed mother of one Dr. Fenton's partners, waited. An elderly Italian woman who had immigrated from a poor village east of Napoli, she hugged Dr. Fenton and spoke happily in broken English.

"My doctor is here. Come, come." Dr. Fenton introduced Matthews.

"You be doctor, too." Carmella said. "Like my doctor, a good doctor. He come for lunch every week."

She brought them into her small white duplex. On the right was the living room where a shrine to the Blessed Mother was visible. They passed through the formal but simple dining room and into the bright kitchen with an attached porch where Carmella had set out three places for lunch. Salad was followed by pasta, meatballs and pork, fruit, and coffee. The meal was accompanied by Carmella's commentary, beginning with her grandson Joseph, a recent college graduate with a new beard.

"I told him you washa your face. He tell me, 'Grandma, Jesus had a beard.' " She looked at Matthews. "What you think I tell him?"

Matthews looked puzzled. "I don't know."

"I tell him 'I know Jesus. You're no Jesus. Now go washa your face.'"

"And did he?" asked Dr. Fenton, to which she replied with a wave of her hand.

She offered her opinion on St. Michael's Church, where she attended mass every morning.

"That Father, what he does to that altar is not right. When they fix the roof, they take down the old Jesus on the cross. When they finish, they put back just a cross. Why they do that? He says it's modern. I tell him 'you be gone and we still be here looking at that cross and wondering, why is Jesus gone?' God forgive me, that man may be priest but knows nothing."

She told Matthews about her own son's decision to go into psychiatry.

"My Sam tells me he wants to help these people. I say they crazy; you no help them. But he takes me to the house where they make a place for these people. He shows me the people. And I see what he does. I still no understand, but he and my doctor here," she hugged Dr. Fenton, "they help the people, so I happy."

The meal left Matthews ready for a nap, but at three-thirty they returned to the church basement where they stayed until seven. This group was different, mainly men with depression, anxiety, and some drinking problems. Dr. Fenton explained that most of them worked and needed to be seen later in the day. Matthews remembered sitting in the corner while Dr. Fenton met with a man in his late fifties who had suffered several bad depressive episodes and was heading into another. He could feel it coming and knew what it meant for both himself and his family.

"You will get through this, too, John," assured Dr. Fenton. "We have been down this road before, and we know there is hope at the end. We'll adjust your medications and see you each week."

On the ride home, Matthews asked him about the depression.

"Most of the time, what we see is complicated. It's some combination of people's genetic makeup, the way their lives and environment have influenced them, and the chemical patterns in their brain. But John's situation seems different. His seems like a chemical storm, and between times he is well adjusted and able to work. Maybe someday we will figure it out."

The rest of the month had been a blur. Psychiatry had the reputation of being an easy rotation, but Dr. Fenton had worked him hard. Matthews did admitting physicals on multiple patients each day and assigned reading in the evenings. Still, Dr. Fenton's lessons had been about more than medical science. In fact, one of Matthews' favorite story was told to him by another student.

"Dr. Fenton and I drove over to a house on the other side of town. The police met us there, and he told them to break down the back door. They did, and he went inside. After a few minutes, he came out and called the ambulance crew in. There was a catatonic old fellow they loaded up and brought over to the hospital. When I asked him how he knew he was in there, Dr. Fenton told me he drove by every day on his way to work and looked to see if the newspapers were taken in. When they piled up, he knew the guy was catatonic again. It happened once or twice a year. The police didn't even ask him for any paperwork . . . They just did what he said. I found out later from the nurses that Dr. Fenton kept the guy's subscription to the paper going."

During their time together, Dr. Fenton also compared Matthews' medical training with his own. He commented on how little he had to learn, offering as evidence a half-year course in parasitology. The lectures were Friday afternoons, and many in the class skipped them in favor of an early start to the weekend. Since the professor used the same final examination each year, Dr. Fenton and the other truants crammed only the needed information while reassuring themselves it was unlikely they would be called on to treat a parasitic infection without a textbook. The trade was not ultimately worthwhile, however, as during stressful times in later life Dr. Fenton reported he would awaken drenched in sweat from a recurring nightmare that the final exam material had been changed and he had failed. Clinical teaching was also different in his time. He described his first surgery lecture when their Napoleonic Chief of Surgery marched into the packed hall with a pint of expired blood which he sprayed over the students, particularly drenching eager surgeons-to-be in the front row. As the class sat stunned, the Chief administered his entire three-line lecture before striding out.

"This mess is from one pint of blood. The human body contains ten pints. When you see bleeding in the operating room, you will not panic."

Dr. Fenton's residency following graduation was true to its name as he lived in a small apartment attached to the hospital and worked the endless hours and nights of legend. When it finished, he felt he knew most of medicine and surgery. He had also made the greatest discovery of his life, Sharon. His face still brightened when he described their first meeting.

"She was taking care of a really ill woman with her partner, Carol. When I walked in and saw her face in the midst of all trouble, I knew she was the woman for me. Of course, I had gone into the room to check on Carol who I was dating at the time, so it took a little work to straighten it all out, but we all ended up friends. Make sure you get the right girl, son. It's more important than any possible residency program or job."

Dr. Fenton's career had started in general medicine in the rural Vermont mountains, and he relayed to Matthews the feel of practice in those days. Office visits were not scheduled, doctors simply posted their hours. He made house calls, which he considered a romanticized effort of limited use.

"There wasn't much we could do on a house call that a good nurse couldn't do as well or better. I did learn a few things. You never leave your medical bag open, particularly on the floor, or some dog will relieve himself in it. And always make sure you have seen the kitchen before you accept anything to eat. House calls are useful when your patient is dying because you can comfort them and their family. In those days, we never told patients they were dying; it was considered cruel to take away hope. Even now, though, I think the families really do need help."

After a few years of general practice, Dr. Fenton had found himself drawn to psychiatry while Sharon had become interested in secondary education. They left Vermont, and Dr. Fenton did psychiatry training while she completed her master's degree. Later, Dr. Fenton organized the county mental health system, saw patients, and mentored medical students while Sharon worked for the State Education Department, making her mark in countless policy decisions.

Matthews' psychiatry rotation had been one of his favorites. Over the years, he kept in touch with Dr. Fenton. He knew that Dr. Fenton had retired when he was in his mid-sixties. Sharon, who had multiple sclerosis for many years, was slowly losing her mobility. Had she been healthy, Dr. Fenton might have continued working. Still, Matthew's teacher admitted the practice of psychiatry had changed, and in the modern medical world he felt a kinship with the dinosaurs who survived after the asteroid impact. But retirement was not to be feared, he announced. Both he and Sharon immensely enjoyed their grandchildren and looked forward to traveling while she was still mobile.

Shortly after his retirement, Dr. Fenton had a routine physical and labs. His PSA was mildly elevated at 4.5. A repeat was similar at 4.8. His initial inclination had been not to take much action, but his primary physician, Dr. Paul Oakley, had recoiled.

"Listen, Bob, you might have a prostate cancer that we could treat. You're in good health."

THE PROSTATE SPECIFIC ANTIGEN (PSA).

The science of the Prostate Specific Antigen (PSA) is well understood. PSA is a protein secreted by cells lining the glands of the prostate. It makes the semen more fluid, allowing the sperm to "swim freely," and helps dissolve mucus in the cervix to allow them to "find" their egg. While most of the PSA is inactivated in the prostate, some enters the blood stream. When cancers grow in the prostate, they tend to secrete more PSA and break down the barriers which keep it in the prostate, thereby raising the level.[234] Credit for the 1979 discovery of the PSA is given to Dr. T. Ming Chu and his group at Roswell Park. They showed the PSA is very specific for normal prostate tissue and prostate cancer and is not found in other body tissues. They published their report at a time when many researchers were searching for "tumor markers," and their discovery remains one of the most significant.[235]

The clinical use of the PSA is less well understood. The PSA is useful to track the results of treatment in men with widely spread prostate cancer. As the treatment works, the PSA will decline. If the treatment is not working, the PSA often will rise. The real hope for the PSA test, however, was that it would be useful to detect prostate cancer before it spread so it could be cured. This is called "PSA screening," and it is a controversial area in medicine.

The concept of PSA screening is simple: testing healthy men will detect prostate cancers and allow treatment before the cancers become lethal. The reality is more complex. Prostate cancer is very common, and most men will develop it if they live long enough (90 percent at age ninety is a commonly quoted phrase). For many men, the disease is so slow growing that they will die of other causes. For these men, finding the disease earlier might cause them to undergo treatments with side effects they did not need. For other men, the disease is more rapidly growing and finding it earlier might make a difference. Distinguishing these two groups is difficult. Further complicating the situation is that both surgery and radiation treatments have significant side effects and neither work all the time.

The debate over PSA screening has played out in the press. The United States Preventative Service Task Force has voted "no" to the test. Many other groups have voted "yes." The public is often confused by the back and forth.

Next was a visit to the urologist who felt an abnormal area on the right side of the prostate and wanted to do a biopsy. Bob had again been somewhat reluctant, but the urologist insisted.

"You're young with many years ahead of you, so we should check this out."

Bob found the concept of the biopsy upsetting, but later readily admitted the procedure had been surprisingly easy.

"It is quite remarkable that they can stick a probe up your rectum and pass multiple needles into that little gland without causing more problems."

The results had returned the next week: prostatic adenocarcinoma with a Gleason score 7 (3+4) involving three of twelve biopsies—all on the right side.

THE GLEASON SCORE.

Most men with prostate cancer learn their "Gleason score." The score is named after Donald Gleason, who was born in 1920 in Iowa and raised in Litchfield, Minnesota, where his father ran a hardware store, and mother was a teacher. After Gleason obtained his medical degree and served in the Army at the Minnesota VA, he moved with his wife to Paris where he tried to become an artist, drawing in charcoal. Ultimately some combination of poverty, lack of artistic success, and a job offer from the VA lured him back to Minnesota. It was there as a young pathologist that Gleason's artistic and medical careers combined when he was asked to develop a standardized grading system for prostate cancer.

The Gleason score is the "grade" of the prostate cancer, determined by the pathologist who compares the cancer cells to normal cells. Low-grade cancers look more like normal cells while high-grade cancers look more bizarre. The grade of the cancer may predict the behavior of the cancer, but is different from the "stage" of the cancer, which refers to how large the cancer has grown and how far it has spread. For example, a man could have a high-grade prostate cancer which is therefore aggressive but found at a very early stage ("fast growing but small"). On the other end of the spectrum, a man could have a low-grade cancer which has had the time to spread widely ("slow growing but metastatic"). The combination of grade and stage determines treatment.

Gleason approached his task by trying to forget anything he knew about the behavior of prostate cancer (his words), then looked for patterns in the cancers that would predict behavior. His approach was influenced by a seemingly unlikely source, the work of scientists using the Minnesota Multiphasic Personality Inventory (MMPI). The MMPI is a psychological test used to distinguish personality traits and mental illnesses using a set of standardized questions. The MMPI was not based upon any specific theory of mental illness, and sought to develop questions which could distinguish between various groups of people. In a similar fashion, Gleason discerned patterns of prostate cancer in the specimens he evaluated, then determined whether these patterns allowed the separation of the behavior of the cancers into groups.

Gleason published his original drawings in 1966, showing the progressing grades of prostate cancer from cells which appeared nearly normal to those which appeared bizarre, work likened to the art of Midwestern artist Mark Tobey.[236] [237] His simple scoring system appealed to pathologists who were familiar with searching for patterns in tissues. In Gleason's system, the pattern seen in most of the cancer is graded on a scale of 1 to 5, then a second grading from 1 to 5 is done for the remaining cancer, and the scores are added. A typical score will be in the format 3+3=6 or 4+5=9. A Gleason score of 6 typically represents a slow-growing cancer, while a Gleason score of 8 or higher is a more rapidly growing tumor. A Gleason score of 7 is in-between, and 4+3=7 will be more aggressive than a 3+4=7.

The Gleason scoring system has been modified over the years, but the basic principles remain the same, a testament to his artistic and medical vision. Over the years, however, scores have risen somewhat in a form of "grade inflation."[238] In part, this may be due to differences in selection of men for biopsy. Yet even when the same pathologists examine the same slides from earlier years, they tend to score them higher.[239] It has been speculated this upgrading results from subtle changes in the work lives of modern pathologists. In Gleason's era, pathologists did most of their work in isolation from clinicians, often reviewing cancer specimens with their colleagues but only occasionally with treating doctors. As cancer treatments became more complex and multidisciplinary, the team approach to cancer care developed. The American College of Surgeons began requiring credentialed cancer programs to hold regular conferences where pathologists, radiologists, surgeons, medical oncologists, and radiation oncologists discuss patients. These meetings resulted in better communication among the physicians caring for cancer patients, but also exposed pathologists to the results of their Gleason scoring. As pathologists saw that lower scores meant less aggressive treatment, it is possible they subconsciously upgraded the scores.

Dr. Brian Cummings, a urologist in his late thirties, had trained at Memorial Sloan Kettering Cancer Center and moved to the region five years ago after the hospital purchased the latest robotic equipment.

"Your cancer is not fast growing, but unless you know something about your health that we do not, it will kill you if you do not treat it. Surgery is best. Radiation will probably hold it off for a decade, but won't get rid of it. I can do the surgery using the robot, and you will be out of the hospital in a few days, catheter out a few days later."

"How about sexual function?" asked Sharon. Her multiple sclerosis now confined her to a wheelchair, but her mind remained sharp. Dr. Cummings looked up.

"I'm not the model he bought, but an occasional drive is still nice." She smiled at her husband.

Dr. Cummings nodded.

"In your case, I can do a nerve sparing procedure, and that usually avoids impotence. Your cancer is on the right side of the gland, so I should be able to spare the left nerve bundle."

"How often is that successful?" asked Sharon.

"Most of the time. Many men who have the surgery are already impotent from other reasons. When you read the numbers, you need to take that into account."

"What would you do if this was you?" Sharon asked.

"No question, have the surgery. It is the only way to get this cancer out of you and has the highest chances of cure."

The next stop was the radiation oncologist. Dr. William Fine was a reassuring and cautious man almost Bob's age.

"There are no great studies comparing radiation and surgery. And really, how many men are going to agree to have that decision made by a flip of the coin? Plus, the technology is changing so fast that any study which took ten years to do would be outdated. Here is the story. If the cancer is in the prostate, either radiation or surgery will probably do the job. Which is best? Surgery might have a slight edge in cure rate, but it is small. Which one has fewer side effects? With our modern techniques, there is no question. Compared with surgery, radiation is much easier. Urinary incontinence is unusual unless the prostate is very large, which yours is not. Even then, it usually resolves quickly. With radiation, sexual functioning usually initially stays the same, although over time it can decrease. If it does, Viagra and the like are usually effective."

"So why would anyone pick surgery?" asked Bob.

"Some people are afraid of radiation, some people just like the idea of cutting it out, and some younger men want to be sure they have the procedure with the highest cure rate."

"What would you do?" Sharon asked.

"At my age, almost your husband's age, radiation. If I was younger, surgery."

"And if the cancer is already outside the prostate?" asked Bob.

"If the cancer has spread, then it will come back regardless of whether you choose surgery or radiation. In that case, it's more reason to have selected radiation and avoided the trauma of surgery."

PROSTATE CANCER: CHOICES OF TREATMENT, OR NOT.

The debate over how to treat prostate cancer confined to the gland is agonizing for patients and divisive for physicians. There are several facts which all agree are true. The prostate gland is in an inconvenient place in the body and is difficult to remove surgically. The removal of the gland, even by the best surgeons, can result in loss of control of urine (usually temporary) and the ability to have an erection (often permanent). Radiation treatments can be given to the prostate to destroy cancer, either in the form of pellets placed in the gland or beams aimed at the gland. Radiation avoids the risk of surgery and will not cause the loss of urinary control, although it can produce erectile dysfunction which occurs gradually years later. Since many prostate cancers are slow growing and in older men, watching may be an option.

Which choice is better? The ideal scientific answer to this question would be a clinical trial in which men with prostate cancer have either surgery or radiation or no treatment by "randomization," the proverbial flip of the coin. This clinical trial has never been done. People are not often willing to allow such a drastic medical decision to be made by a flip of the coin or computer generated random number. Physicians usually have strong opinions, often influenced by their training as well as their intellectual, personal, and economic investment in a specific technology. Hospitals, healthcare systems, and insurers may all have different viewpoints on the choices. Doing such a trial would also require a long period of follow-up to determine the results. During that time, the technologies will have changed, and the answer may no longer be relevant ("that was old radiation" or "that was old surgery"). This is the dilemma.

We do have some comparisons. Surgery has been compared with no surgery in men with prostate cancer in a few randomized clinical trials. One of the first trials was done in Scandinavia beginning in 1989. This trial did show that the surgery helped some men, particularly when they had longer life expectancies and more aggressive cancers.[240] Since this trial was done before PSA testing was widespread, it is argued that the results do not apply to the smaller cancers detected by PSA testing. A similar trial done in the United States beginning in 1994, a time when PSA screening was common, did not show much benefit to surgery.[241] Both studies are hard to interpret for the same reasons. Since most men refused to participate, the small numbers of men in the studies may be different from those who did not enter. Many of the men in the studies died of non-cancer related causes. Even as the studies were ongoing, the technologies were changing with robotic surgeries and improved radiation treatments with fewer side effects. On balance, most experts feel that trials like these have shown benefit to surgery for young men with more aggressive cancer, recognizing the definitions of young and aggressive are not precise.

What about radiation? Is it as good as surgery? We do not have any direct comparisons between surgery and radiation, so the best we can do is an indirect comparison. One example again comes from the Scandinavians who studied radiation therapy in men with cancers which appeared confined to the prostate. They gave half the men radiation treatment with some anti-hormonal therapy and the other half the anti-hormone treatment alone. In this study, the radiation produced a similar benefit seen with the surgery studies.[242] On balance, most experts feel that radiation and surgery are probably equal for most men, with surgery possibly being a little better in young men with more aggressive cancers, again avoiding a precise definition of young.

What about no surgery or radiation? "Watchful waiting" is one approach in which the man will never have surgery or radiation to try to cure the disease. He will only use treatments to control the cancer if it gets worse. A man might opt for this if he and his physicians feel that the risks of surgery or radiation are too great, the cancer is slow growing, and the man's life expectancy is not long enough to make the attempt at cure worthwhile. This is a reasonable idea for elderly men with many medical problems, but more difficult for men who think of themselves as healthy with a long life ahead.

A second strategy of avoiding surgery or radiation is to continue to watch the cancer and use surgery or radiation to attempt cure only if it seems to progress and if the man otherwise stays healthy. This approach is called "active surveillance" and involves repeat PSA tests and biopsies. The potential advantage is that if a man has a slow growing cancer, he might avoid any treatment. The potential disadvantage is that he might miss the chance for cure and will have many tests. The strategy is best suited for men who are not sure if they are elderly or not and not sure if their cancer is a threat or not. This strategy has not been compared with surgery or radiation.

Where does this leave a man with prostate cancer? Young men usually opt for surgery and elderly men for no treatment with everyone else in the middle finding the answer that best suits them.

Sharon and Bob sat together for dinner that night. He had made a roast and mashed potatoes, one of her favorites. The thinly sliced meat was easy for her to eat, although he had cut it in this fashion even before her illness, a tribute to his puritanical upbringing as a minister's son.

They ate in the kitchen of their old farmhouse, the home in which they had raised their two children. The roughhewn table at which they sat faced a picture window looking onto large field ending in dense woods. Outside it had begun to snow and the gray and white view contrasted with the warmth inside.

"It's good, Robert," she remarked. They ate in silence for a few minutes.

"What are you going to do?" she asked.

"I'm not convinced either treatment will make any difference, but the radiation seems less barbaric. If you can feel the lump, I have to think the cancer is probably already outside the prostate."

"What if it is not?"

"That's the rub. That's why the radiation." They finished their dinner as the wind increased, blowing the snow sideways. He cleared the plates and made the coffee.

"I think we should move," he said.

"Why?" she asked, surprised, but not shocked.

"This is a warning to us. Once your prostate starts to rot, who knows what's next. But we have a chance to get ourselves set up in a new life before something happens to either of us. This," he pointed out the window, "has been a wonderful home. But we can't keep it if both of us are having problems. It's too hard."

Sharon nodded. "I'm sorry. I was supposed to take care of you when your prostate went."

"I was hoping it wouldn't quite go so soon. But even if the radiation works, something else could be close behind. It's time."

"I know you're right . . ." Her trailing words were accompanied by tears in her eyes.

"Remember Ella," he reminded softly. "This is better."

Ella had been their neighbor down the road for many years. She and her husband had been about ten years older, and their children acted as elder siblings to the Fenton's. Once grown, Ella's children had moved away, and their once vibrant home had become quiet. After her husband had died, Ella continued to live there despite the protestations of her children. Bob and Ella had worked out a system by which she alternated the porch light she left on each night so that he would know she was okay. One night when the light had not changed, Bob found her dead on her living room floor. Although Bob and Sharon understood that Ella herself would not have been unhappy with this outcome, her solitary passing left her children with a mixture of sorrow and guilt.

Sharon nodded. "The children will be happier knowing that we are safe, but I will miss this."

Bob's radiation went well. The morning trip to the hospital pleasantly reminded him of his years of rounding. The treatment itself produced a mild sense of fatigue. He had quizzed Dr. Fine on the equipment.

"Where is the source of the radiation? You don't get it from Cobalt anymore, do you?"

Dr. Fine laughed. "No, in the early days, we used an actual radiation source like Cobalt to produce the energy. A few of those were even around until about a decade ago. Today we use a microwave, a bit more powerful than the one in your kitchen obviously, to generate power to accelerate electrons. The electrons smash into metal, and that collision produces the photon energy beam. The equipment shapes the beam and aims it at the target. Of course, there is radiation scattered around, so we need all this lead," he gestured toward the doors and walls, "but there is no pile of radioactive stuff like you would find in a nuclear reactor. We can turn it off at the end of the day and walk away."

"It's amazing that you can send all that energy into my prostate and I hardly even feel a thing."

On his last day, Bob said goodbye to the staff and received his graduation diploma. Outside the snow was gone and although spring had not yet arrived, the air felt warm and expectant. True to his word, he had begun preparations to move. He and Sharon had met with the director of the local assisted-living complex and selected an apartment.

They started sorting through the memories, valuables, and detritus of their lives. Some items were easy to discard. Bob finally disposed of his last remaining medical school texts, while Sharon contributed years of various committee meeting minutes. Other objects were valuable, such as photographs of the children, letters from close friends, and small keepsakes of their trips. For Bob, one sealed box of letters from patients and their families remained. It was never opened, but he knew he could never dispose of it. A vast number of their possessions had some significance but no defined purpose.

"What do we do with this?" asked Sharon, a smile on her face as she sat in her wheelchair and lifted a small old aluminum lawn chair with a faded and frayed cloth seat and backing.

Bob unfolded the chair and sat, his buttocks touching the ground as the cloth sagged.

"Spent a lot of time in this baby," he mused. They called it "Grandma's chair." The summer after his father's death, Bob's mother would call every evening, needing to hear his voice. He took the calls in the lawn chair, usually with a beer in hand, so he could watch the kids playing in the yard. The children knew Grandma was on the phone and made the association. As time passed and Grandma moved nearby, the frequency of calls declined, but the name remained. It had accompanied them on many beach trips and his now grown children still recognized the battered chair.

"We can't keep it," he determined.

"The children will be upset," she warned.

"Just a minute," he answered, leaving for a moment. He returned wearing his old sun hat and equipment vest, both veterans of many trips, and carried his camera, which he handed to Sharon. "One final photo which we can give it to the kids and be rid of all of this."

The camera encouraged Bob to first document, then ruthlessly dispose of many of their possessions. His mission was to simplify. A month later, after multiple trips to the waste disposal on Washburn

Avenue, they surveyed their work. The house and the remaining furniture were bare.

"It looks so clean," she remarked. "Almost a shame to leave."

"It does have a certain Spartan look," he agreed.

They had one more party for their children and a few close friends. It was vintage Bob, a roast sliced very thin, plenty of vegetables, and his famous berry pie, always a little tart.

Two of the grandchildren, Johnny and Katherine, both about eight, were engaged in a fight over the last remaining ball in the house when Bob intervened. His daughter Karen watched from a distance.

"You both cannot play with this ball. You have proven you are not capable of sharing. Is that correct?" he demanded. The children nodded, their fear of Grandpa's resolution to the problem offset by their rivalry and curiosity over his solution.

"I have a coin. I will flip it, and you will both agree to be bound by the results. Heads will be for Johnny and tails for Catherine. Understood?"

The children nodded. Tails was the result and Bob handed Katherine the ball. She promptly ran off with it, but not before sticking her tongue out at the now teary-eyed Johnny. Bob looked at Johnny.

"No point in crying, son. Some days we win, and some days we lose. Today you lost. Now go make the best of it, but stay away from Katherine."

After Johnny had sulked off, Karen came over.

"Not very Solomon-like, Daddy," she commented. "And I don't think it teaches them to play together."

"There are facts of life, dear. We all can't play together, sometimes we win, and often we lose." He paused and looked around. "But, as my father would say, despite those realities we still can live the life God has planned and love."

To their friends, the move seemed to happen quickly. One day they were in the old farmhouse, the next they had moved into the Springs, an assisted living facility with a variety of housing options to facilitate their motto of "Aging in Place." Bob and Sharon agreed to age, but not always in place. He had purchased a Saab into which she fit comfortably, and they embarked on a variety of trips. It was a good life, although Sharon continued her slow, almost imperceptible decline. Bob's health was fine. He saw Dr. Oakley each year for his examination and PSA.

Seven years after his radiation, Bob's PSA rose. He visited with Dr. Chris, the young radiation oncologist who had replaced Dr. Fine. Bob enjoyed his youthful enthusiasm.

"Your PSA is up somewhat. It had been 0.6 but now is 1.2," Dr. Chris reported.

"What does that mean?"

"It can be due to some inflammation in the prostate, or it can mean there is active cancer somewhere. We should repeat it in a few months. If it is up, then we would look elsewhere with a bone scan and CT scan. If it rose enough or we found cancer, we would have you see your urologist or a medical oncologist for hormonal treatment."

"I don't have a urologist. I never needed one after the biopsy," Bob replied.

"Then we can send you to Dr. Matthews, the medical oncologist. But let's just see where it is in three months."

Bob nodded. "Sharon is not doing well, and I would rather not have to burden her or the children. It doesn't seem like an immediate threat to me, correct?"

Dr. Chris agreed. "True. I don't think you need to deal with this now."

Three months became six months, and the lab slip still sat in Bob's draw. Dr. Chris' office called to remind him. Nine months later, he went.

The PSA was 2.6. Dr. Chris offered him a bone scan and CT scan.

"Not now. Sharon is not well. She is remarkably determined, but I don't think she has long to live."

"And you don't want to worry her," completed Dr. Chris.

"Yes, but it is more than that. She has always been a dutiful woman. She was a good student. She raised her children carefully. Even at work. Why, when we sold the house we had to destroy books of meticulous notes she had from all her committees. She always felt it was her responsibility to look after me, too. Knowing I had something going on while she is unable to help would be a special kind of torture for her. Better we wait."

Sharon's death was as comfortable as they could make it. A series of urinary tract infections brought immobilizations which caused her to lose muscle strength. Each time she had struggled to regain function, until one night she told Bob she could take no more.

"I'm tired, Robert. This body just won't do it anymore. My brain is tired, too, and I feel I'm losing myself and you."

"You are not losing me, dear. I'm here," he replied.

"But I'm not me anymore. So, we are not us. And I do not wish to change us in this way. We have adapted all we can . . . There is no place left for us to go."

He sat holding her hand. The familiar slight bend in her nose caught his eye. He recalled how in childhood Sharon had suffered an injury to the nose and needed a surgical repair. A few days later a young man had come to Sharon's house to speak with her. He, too, had a bandaged face.

"I want to thank you for what you did for me," the man said.

"I didn't do anything." Sharon had replied. "Who are you?"

"When your surgeon fixed your nose, he took out some of your bone and used it to rebuild mine. It was broken in a boxing match. I paid $800 of your $1000 bill." Then he left.

Sharon had asked her surgeon, who confirmed the events but refused to give any other information about the pugilist. The surgeon had done an excellent job, and Sharon was left with only a slight asymmetry which Bob adored. The story was famous in the family, and now it seemed to Bob both ancient and recent. Where had time gone?

They moved Sharon's bed into the living room so she could enjoy the view of the outside. The children alternated as a steady stream of their closest friends visited. Assisted care became hospice. When the urinary infection returned yet again, they made her comfortable.

After her death, Bob returned to Dr. Chris. His PSA was now 4.6.

"I know you are numb and grieving, but I think you should have a bone scan and a CT scan to look for any signs of metastasis. It is time for you to meet with a medical oncologist to discuss treatment."

"I'll think it over."

But he did not. He simply ignored it. In truth, he was overwhelmed by fatigue. Sharon's funeral had been a beautiful tribute to her life. The paperwork of death was done. Their apartment was efficiently returned to its former layout by the staff of the facility. Their friends had drifted back to their own lives and the children to their own homes. Bob had expected sadness, but not this fatigue. It was weariness so profound it seemed to have entered his soul. He had seen it before in his patients with depression, but he did not think he was depressed. He wanted to do things, but he was so tired.

One night, Bob had awakened from his sleep. That was not unusual; since Sharon's death he had slept fitfully. He pulled on his robe and walked from the bedroom into the dark living room where he sat on the couch.

"Robert." Her voice came from the chair in which she often sat before her decline. He saw the chair in his peripheral vision but was afraid to turn toward it.

"Yes, dear," he answered, almost before he was aware of it. The analytic part of his brain immediately announced he was hallucinating, that she could not be there. But other parts of his brain quickly quieted that rational thought, enjoying the feeling she was with him.

"Stop ignoring it. It's not like you. And dress properly, dear."

He nodded, despite himself, and then she was gone. I told you it was a hallucination, announced the rational part of his brain, which then quieted as the fatigue and sadness returned him to bed. He awoke that morning and, despite himself, looked carefully at the chair.

Surprisingly, he felt a little more energy. To honor Sharon's wishes, he made the appointment for the tests and a visit with Dr. Matthews, his former student. Over the years, professor and student had occasionally met and always enjoyed their conversations about life and medicine. Dr. Matthews was pleased to see Bob wearing his trademark bow tie.

"It's a pleasure to see you again, Bob, although not for this. I'm sorry about Sharon."

"I've been surprised at how hard this has been for me. It has taken me a while to get here. You and your family are well?"

After Bob had been updated, Dr. Matthews turned toward the business at hand.

"It looks like the PSA has been slowly rising over about the last three years. It is 8.3 now. Your CT scan is fine, but the bone scan shows areas of metastasis in the ribs, skull, and spine. They are small but real. If you do not do anything about them, they will start to give you some symptoms, probably in the next year or so. Typically, we would suggest you begin hormonal treatment to try and control the cancer. It will probably work for a while, often a few years, and possibly much longer."

HORMONE TREATMENT OF PROSTATE CANCER.

Testosterone stimulates prostate cancer, exactly how is an unfolding scientific mystery of importance to men with the disease. In simplified form, this is a "lock and key" system, similar in some respects to the stimulation of breast cancer by estrogen. Testosterone is a key which enters the prostate cell and fits into a lock, called the testosterone receptor. When the key is in the lock, the mechanism causes stimulation of the cell. In normal prostate cells, this stimulation causes development and function. In cancerous cells, it contributes to dangerous growth. Scientists examining this system have focused on several key areas: the production of the testosterone (the key), the fitting of the testosterone into the testosterone receptor (the key in the lock), and the action of the lock to stimulate the cell (the mechanism).

Since testosterone stimulates prostate cancer, the elimination of that hormone means most of the cancer cells die. The elimination of testosterone is done in two ways: "surgical castration" (the removal of the testes), or "chemical castration" (using medications to prevent the production of testosterone by the testis). Both methods work equally well and are called "hormone therapy" or "androgen deprivation." The loss of testosterone from either method causes the side effects: hot flashes, loss of sex drive, and eventually loss of muscle and bone strength. Chemical castration needs to be continued for years and is much more expensive than surgical castration, but much more commonly used in affluent societies. With either method, at some point, the cancers will regrow.

It is tempting to start hormone treatment as soon as the recurrence of the cancer is detected by a rise in the PSA. Those who prefer to begin treatment immediately argue that these treatments can prolong the time the disease is controlled (called progression free survival) and even produce a longer life. Some physicians advocate using both hormonal treatment and chemotherapy together as soon as possible to produce the longest control of the cancer. Other physicians have argued against using these treatments before they are clearly needed because of their side effects. Since the data is not conclusive, many patients and doctors struggle with the decision. Those who prefer not to start treatment point to the fact that there is very little data to suggest that early treatment prolongs life.

Once the spread of the prostate cancer becomes evident on scans, however, treatment is usually required relatively soon to prevent symptoms.

"Do you have many patients who refuse hormonal treatment?" Bob asked his former student.

"Sure, at the start. Many men who have had surgery or radiation and then have a rising PSA refuse hormone treatment. They don't want the side effects. That is really what you did. But once the PSA starts to rise rapidly or they get a positive scan showing there is active visible cancer, they take the treatment. Once in a long while someone refuses even at that point, and we manage as best we can."

"Sounds like I am at the point for treatment," Bob mused.

"Are you concerned about the side effects? Loss of sexual function, hot flashes, and the muscle and bone loss?"

"Truthfully, my interest in sex has faded away. The widows in our community are paying me considerable attention, but as long as I can drive at night, most of them would probably prefer a castrate man. I have overheard several of them complain what an ordeal Viagra was for them. So, no . . . I can't say that is the issue. Hot flashes don't sound life threatening. I don't expect I'll be around long enough to worry about the rest. I'm seventy-five after all. I'm not sure why I have delayed. I guess it is just inertia."

"How are the grandchildren? Don't you have two in high school?" Dr. Matthews asked.

Bob looked puzzled for a moment. "Yes, Katherine and Johnny."

Dr. Matthews smiled. "You know, I have been impressed how much influence grandparents can have on children that age. And I remember what one of my professors taught me in medical school."

Bob still looked puzzled, and Dr. Matthews continued.

"He taught me that sometimes you have to remind people why they need to do the things they need to do."

Bob nodded. "Well, that's true."

Grandpa did not have difficulty with the injection, called Lupron. An occasional hot flash and some mild fatigue were all he noticed as his PSA declined steadily to 0.7. Bob used his time well and his enjoyed his grandchildren's high school sports, plays, concerts, tests, proms, college selections, and graduation. Periodically he checked in with Dr. Matthews for his injections and PSA measurements. On one visit, Bob shared his satisfaction.

"Since you reminded me of what was important, I want to tell you a story. My granddaughter Katherine, Karen's daughter, is a junior this year at Hamilton College. She is spending a term in Oxford studying economics. With her week off she invited me to London. She had arranged tours for us. I had a wonderful time. I never imagined that would happen."

"I'm sure she appreciated your wisdom," Dr. Matthews replied.

Bob laughed. "That's exactly what she said. We were at Stonehenge at the time, and I warned her not to mistake age for wisdom, but I was pleased."

Six years passed. Grandchildren became young adults and reached milestones. Friends aged and were lost. Bob lived to celebrate his eightieth birthday. It was a remarkably long period of good results until Bob's PSA once again rose. As usual, he was reflective.

"I never planned on making it this far. Sharon used to speak of our lives as ships on a voyage across a vast ocean. As you sail, various other ships will join you or break off for their own destinations. Sometimes on your journey, you will have many companions, sometimes just a few ships. I always found that image comforting. This month I had a flotilla." He paused. "But many of my friends are gone, and I still miss Sharon. More recently, I have imagined myself in a line of soldiers advancing across a field, looking forward. You concentrate on what is ahead, but every so often you look at each side, and you realize your line is getting thinner. It's fairly thin now."

MORE OPTIONS FOR PROSTATE CANCER.

In men with widespread prostate cancer, eliminating testosterone usually causes most cancer cells to die, the survivors to become dormant, and the

PSA to decline. At some point, however, some of the cells will start to regrow. On average, "hormone treatment" works for several years. For some men this treatment controls the cancers for decades, while in others it works for only a brief time, a perplexingly wide range. Once they regrow, these cancers are commonly referred to as "hormone refractory," and were formerly treated with chemotherapy. Although chemotherapy can still be used, scientists have recently identified several ways these resistant prostate cancer cells work around the hormone treatment to activate the testosterone pathway. New treatments have been developed to further deprive the cancer of testosterone stimulation, thus continuing the hormonal treatment of the cancer. Immune therapies are also available, providing another option to the traditional chemotherapy drugs.

Most testosterone is from the testis. Leuprolide (Lupron) shots or castration (surgical removal of the testes) markedly reduce the level, but a small amount of testosterone results from the conversion of other hormones into testosterone. This stimulates the cancerous cells, particularly resistant cells which are more sensitive to testosterone. One way to control these resistant prostate cancers is to stop this extra testosterone production. Older medications like ketoconazole were not very effective and had many side effects. A new generation of drugs, led by abiraterone (brand name Zytiga), accomplish this more effectively with fewer side effects. A second approach is to block the action of testosterone (key) on the receptor (lock). While an older medicine called bicalutamide (Casodex) occasionally worked, a newer medicine enzalutamide (Xtandi) has proven more effective.

An entirely different approach to treating widespread prostate cancer is to use the immune system. Scientists have long recognized that prostate cancers cells had unique proteins on their surface, often somewhat related to the PSA. The goal has been to teach the immune system to recognize and attack the prostate cancer cells bearing these proteins. In 2010, the Food and Drug Administration (FDA) approved a new immunotherapy, sipuleucel-T (brand name Provenge), for the treatment of patients with widespread prostate cancer.

Sipuleucel-T treatment requires collecting specific white blood cells from the patient (called mononuclear cells) using a dialysis-like machine and taking them to the lab. These cells are trained to recognize one of the proteins on the prostate cancer cells, called prostatic acid phosphatase. These cells will present the protein to the immune system as a target, in the lingo they will be "antigen presenting cells (APCs)." Three intravenous infusions of the cells are given once every two weeks. If this works, the immune system of the patient will fight the cancer. In some respects, sipuleucel-T is an anticancer vaccine. The key study of this approach did show that men who received it lived modestly longer, a few months on average, but some had more sustained control of the cancer.[243] Sipuleucel-T is expensive, at about $100,000 per person, and complex, but it proved the concept that the immune system can be unleashed against prostate cancer.[244]

Bob started with the addition of the older medication bicalutamide to block the action of testosterone on the prostate cancer cell. After a few months, Dr. Matthews reported the results.

"The scans show some worsening. The bones still look good, but you have some nodules in the lungs. I doubt you would notice any symptoms from them at this point, but they do signal that we need to change the treatment. Chemotherapy is an option, but we would rather avoid that if possible because of the side effects. The immune treatment, sipuleucel-T, generally takes quite a while to work and I am concerned that we might not be able to wait that long in your situation. I think we should use the new agent Xtandi."

Bob's eyes twinkled, and he became the old teacher once again. "I still go to Psychiatry Grand Rounds occasionally and hear about the new antidepressants which block all these various pathways. Your analysis sounds like the rationale I hear them using for picking one:

review some amazing science, then guess. I used to think psychiatry lacked a truly scientific approach, but I now realize oncology is not as far ahead as I thought."

Dr. Matthews laughed.

"True. The next step is to add some more science to these decisions, what they are calling 'personalized medicine.' Even without that, we sometimes we get lucky. I still remember a lesson from my rotation with you. We had an older man who had a severe depression and was almost vegetative. You had told me that the MAO inhibitors worked well in these types of patients, so I wrote that in my note. You signed it 'agree with above' which pleased me to no end. And it worked. I heard later he did very well."

The teacher smiled, pleased.

"I have no complaints. My life has been full. To the degree any science can prolong it, I am grateful. But, as my father used to say, 'in the end we live the life God has planned for us.'"

11:40 William Denton: Multiple Myeloma

William Denton looked tough, a lean sixty-seven-year-old in camouflage pants and a black tank top with arms of cord-like tattooed muscle and a lined face drawn tight. But it was his eyes that made him fierce; they were dead, devoid of emotion. Over the years, Dr. Matthews had come to know the temperate sides of Denton's character, but he still paused before he entered the room, knowing he would find this hard man sitting completely still on the examination table.

"Good morning, Mr. Denton."

"Morning, doc."

"Your bloods are good. How are you feeling?" Dr. Matthews paused. "We have been concerned these treatments might be wearing you down."

"Better this week. Some old sergeant kicked my ass." He shrugged almost imperceptibly, and Dr. Matthews, although puzzled, knew the conversation was over.

Thirteen years ago, William "Will" Denton, age fifty-four, had presented with multiple myeloma. His chronic back pain had worsened, and his spine surgeon had ordered yet another MRI, hoping not to find anything which would require an additional operation. The MRI had shown the longstanding damage his hard life had done to his vertebral bodies and discs but also several surprising new areas where the bones had been destroyed by a cancer. Blood tests uncovered anemia and poor kidney function. A bone marrow biopsy which showed large numbers of abnormal "plasma cells" made the diagnosis of multiple myeloma.

Multiple myeloma, usually just called myeloma, is a cancer of the bone marrow's plasma cells which normally make antibodies to fight infection. As the cancerous plasma cells grow, they can destroy sections of bone, producing "lytic lesions" which show on x-rays as clear spaces and can cause terrible pain. The cancerous plasma cells can also occupy the bone marrow and prevent normal blood cells from forming, leading to anemia (low red blood count), thrombocytopenia (low platelets), or leukopenia (low white blood count). The plasma cells often also make a uselessly abnormal antibody which can damage the kidney and is detectable in blood and urine tests. The triad of bone pain, anemia, and kidney disease has been learned by generations of medical students as a clue to myeloma. If not treated, the disease is usually fatal in a few years, although there is a great variation and some patients may have a "smoldering myeloma" which progresses only minimally over many years.

Will Denton learned this quickly. Although he looked strong, his myeloma needed immediate treatment because of the damage to his kidneys done by the antibody. Dr. Mathews had explained the situation to Will and his sister Karen, an attractive and outgoing woman a few years younger than her brother. Even years later, Dr. Matthews remembered how silently and motionless his patient sat. After Dr. Matthews had finished, he had looked down in the chart to retrieve some paper and make a few notes. When he looked up, Denton was gone, and only his sister remained.

"Is he okay? I didn't hear him leave."

She laughed nervously. "You won't. I'm sorry. Please don't get upset. That's how he is."

Will's sister briefly told his story.

"Will has had a hard life. We grew up on a farm in Schuylerville, just the two of us and our parents. Will was older, a good kid. We had never left the area; we couldn't with the farm. After high school, he got drafted into the War. He left a simple farm boy, off to serve his country. When he came back from Vietnam, he was very bad. He doesn't talk about it, but he was terribly hurt. He had constant back pain and what they now call post-traumatic stress. Of course, we didn't know, nobody did . . ." She paused. "Those first few years were bad. He is much better now, but I know he still gets the dreams. He never married, but he is close to me and my husband. And he adores my daughter."

Dr. Matthews nodded. "Do you think he will take treatment?"

"Yes. I know he trusts you because you've taken care of some of his friends. He will do whatever you ask, just in his own time."

Dr. Matthews nodded again.

"Why did he get this?" she went on. "Will didn't deserve this."

CANCER AT WORK.

Establishing the cause of most cancers is difficult. Proving the now obvious link between cigarettes and lung cancer was challenging in the 1950s and 1960s. Proving tobacco causes less common cancers like those of the head and neck, bladder, esophagus, and pancreas came even later. In general, proving something causes cancer (called a carcinogen) requires multiple scientific steps. Scientists need to measure exposure to a possible carcinogen and correlate it with disease statistics. They must show in the lab that the substance can cause cancer in animals, then provide evidence this happens in humans. Further complicating matters is the different sensitivities of people depending upon their genetic makeup or other factors in the environment. In addition, not everyone exposed to a carcinogen develops cancer. We all know dedicated smokers who never get lung cancer. On the other extreme, some people who were not exposed might get cancer, the obvious example being nonsmokers with lung cancer. Sometimes we do not recognize an exposure; the risk of second-hand smoke was not recognized for years. Sometimes we prefer not to acknowledge an exposure; many marijuana smokers do not want to consider it a carcinogen.

Some cancers have occupational causes. The first famous example of an occupational cancer was London surgeon Percival Pott's description in 1775 of scrotal cancers which developed in chimney sweeps. These young boys were sent into chimneys to clean them and came out covered in soot, which contained many dangerous chemicals. The carcinogens covered their scrotums, and they rarely bathed, leading to high rates of scrotal cancers which they called "soot-wart." Percival noted it was a painful end to a short, hard life in which the boys were treated with great brutality.[245]

Mesothelioma, a cancer of the lining of the lung or abdominal cavity caused by asbestos, is a well-known example of a modern occupational exposure causing cancer. Asbestos is an excellent insulator and was used in many different products in almost every structure built until the 1970s. Asbestos fibers look like small needles; the longer and thinner ones are the most dangerous. When inhaled, the fibers enter the airways and eventually slice their way through the lung tissue to become lodged in the outside lining of the lung, called the pleura. Once in the pleural lining of the lung, they can cause a series of damaging events which years later can lead to the cancer mesothelioma, named because these lining cells are classified as mesothelial tissues after their origin in the embryo. In smokers, the fibers can also markedly raise the risk of lung cancer.[246] The link between asbestos and lung cancers was first made in 1935 in textile workers while mesothelioma was documented in 1960 in miners in South Africa. In 1964, a landmark conference on the effects of asbestos was held in New York City which led to surveys of pathologists in Canada and eventually the U.S. designed to detect the disease and correlate it with exposure to asbestos.[247] The proof that exposure to asbestos could lead to mesothelioma came in series of studies which took tremendous effort and generated considerable controversy. The scientific difficulties included the different types of asbestos, varying levels of exposure and sensitivity, differences in other factors like smoking, the long delay from exposure until illness, and the mobile and variable lives of humans. Political and legal issues made this analysis even more complex.

Proving an occupational exposure to a substance causes cancer is difficult. In our recent history, we have the example of debate over the cancers seen in those who rushed to Ground Zero after the 9/11 attacks and were exposed to many toxic substances.

Will's fellow soldiers knew the cause of his myeloma. One Vietnam veteran, a large and heavily bearded man who recognized Dr. Matthews as Will's doctor, offered the answer as they pumped gas together at Stewart's.

"The VC had all these tunnels under the ground. They could pop up out of those tunnels and suddenly be all around you. The systems were amazing. You can't believe how they lived in them, just like ant cities . . . The women even had babies down there. The only way to secure an area was to send someone down into those damn tunnels. Can you imagine? Being lowered in feet first with a pistol, a flashlight, and a knife . . . into the darkest spider infested hell you can ever imagine? Covered in filth and slime and sweat? Will was a tunnel rat. One of the best. Small, silent, and quick . . . The guy had balls enough for all of us. And you know what he got for it?"

Dr. Matthews shook his head, the gas tank of his Acura long full.

"Shit. That's what. While he was crawling around in them tunnels, this town held a war protest parade down Broadway with people carrying candles. When he got home, the VA gave him crap. There was no Wounded Warrior stuff then. And now cancer. From all those damn chemicals. Where do you think that Agent Orange ended up? The rain washed it into those stinking tunnels. Will was swimming in that Agent Orange shit. And you wonder why he got cancer?"

Finally, his large truck was sated, and Will's friend returned the hose to the pump, not yet finished with his story.

"You know, doc, you should check the oil on an old Acura like that. Here, let me do it for you." Dr. Matthews opened the hood, and the large man pulled the dipstick, wiped it, and returned it into the engine while he continued speaking.

"The other thing about Will was he stayed. After his term was up, he took another. He wanted to finish the job. He only went home when they made him."

He withdrew the dipstick again, looked at it with satisfaction, and closed the hood.

"It's fine. Remember, doc. When you see Will now, think of him as a young man. He was a real hero. But for him, my name might be on the Wall, too."

Many veterans and their families have found understanding Vietnam as difficult as penetrating its jungle. The story of Agent Orange is no exception.

VIETNAM, AGENT ORANGE, AND CANCER.
The Vietnam War was a defining event in the 1960s and 1970s, yet today it occupies only a portion of a chapter in the typical high school history book. The U.S. involvement in Vietnam began in the 1950s as advisors were sent to help the French prevent the spread of communism from North Vietnam into South Vietnam. By 1962, the French were gone, and the United States had eleven thousand advisors in place. In August 1964, President Johnson persuaded Congress to pass the Gulf of Tonkin Resolution, granting him broad powers to expand the use of U.S. combat troops. Johnson believed the "domino theory" which held that the fall of Vietnam to the communists would lead to the fall of other countries in the region. Johnson's brilliant political and military inner circle knew they could win against their primitive opponent using modern tactics. They began with a vast bombing campaign called Operation Rolling Thunder. The troops followed, and by

1964 the numbers rose rapidly, peaking in 1969 at five hundred forty thousand. This "never formally declared" war turned into a disastrous quagmire as the North Vietnamese proved a formidable foe, the South Vietnamese were unable to stand by themselves, and the conflict tore apart our own country. Americans opposing the Vietnam war clashed with their government, a sharp contrast to the national pride which characterized most prior wars. U.S. combat involvement ended in 1973, and the North overran South Vietnam in 1975.

Caught in the middle of the combat in Vietnam and the protests at home were the soldiers. Ultimately about three million U.S. soldiers served in the combat arena, over fifty-six thousand died, and three hundred thousand were traditional physical casualties. U.S. soldiers were young, their average age of nineteen compared with twenty-eight in World War II. Most of these soldiers were drafted rather than being volunteers. Furthermore, they were sent in as individuals rather than units, which often made their experiences unique rather than shared. After a year of service, they were also discharged home as individuals, often with little support and into a country in turmoil which did not properly acknowledge their service.[248]

One high-tech strategy employed in Vietnam was the extensive spraying of herbicides, called Operation Ranch Hand. The military purpose was to strip away the dense jungle in which the enemy could hide and to destroy their food supply. From 1962 to 1971, the United States government sprayed about nineteen million gallons of herbicides on Vietnam and covered about 10 percent of the country. Most of the herbicide was Agent Orange, a specific mixture of various crop herbicides. Other colors designated different mixtures, such as Agent White, Blue, Purple, Pink, and Green. The sprayings were carried out by soldiers from a variety of platforms including slow-flying airplanes, helicopters, river boats, and back-mounted units. As a military strategy, the herbicide program was not particularly effective. The repeated killing of plants did serve use around the perimeters of military bases and along convoy routes. In other areas, the enemy adapted, and the jungle rapidly regrew. As a crop elimination strategy, the spraying mainly deprived the local peasants of food. From a public relations viewpoint, it was a disaster.

Since Operation Ranch Hand involved many soldiers, it was poorly controlled and not well documented. The exact amounts of Agent Orange sprayed and the exposure that individual soldiers or airmen sustained are impossible to determine. The spraying ended when it was discovered that Agent Orange could cause birth defects in lab animals and, even worse, was contaminated with high levels of dioxin, a chemical making the news at home as a terrible poison. In 1971 the U.S. Military ended the program, and in 1975 President Ford issued an executive order renouncing the use of herbicides in war except to control vegetation around bases.[249]

When concerns over the effects of these poisons arose, the U.S. responded in early 1970 by sending the Herbicide Assessment Committee to Vietnam to investigate. This team raised questions about the effectiveness of the program, reporting most of the destroyed food crops belonged to the locals rather than the enemy and raising concerns about potentially serious health problems.[250] Later that year, a larger committee sponsored by the National Academy of Science studied spraying and issued their report in 1974, after the program had ended. While the committee focused on crop and environmental damage, they did examine effects on the local population. They noted several acute irritations from the herbicides but were not able to study potential serious adverse health effects. They did note the emotional importance of the spraying, particularly in the more educated urban centers of Vietnam. The "point had been reached where a poet or writer seeking to express complex emotions about the impact of the Americans in Vietnam, or perhaps of the war in general, would often select herbicides as a symbol."[251] The introduction and the extra comments added by committee members in the report reflect the divisions within the U.S. over the war.

These studies had little effect on the American soldier or airman who sprayed or breathed the chemicals. Only after the War ended did Agent Orange become a public issue. The controversy began in earnest in 1977 at the improbable location of the Chicago Veteran's Affairs office of Maude deVictor, a VA employee who researched benefit claims for Vietnam veterans with illnesses including cancer. After deVictor had become convinced that service related chemical exposure was to blame for some cancers, her information became public and was included in the documentary *Agent Orange: The Deadly Fog*. At the same time, a young Vietnam veteran named Paul Reutershan, dying of a cancer he was convinced began with exposure to Agent Orange, was galvanizing veterans and uttered his famous line "I died in Vietnam and didn't know it."[252]

Claims that Agent Orange was responsible for cancer and other serious health effects in Vietnam veterans reached a receptive public. The 1960s and 1970s had seen the growth of the environmental movement, often linked with other protest and social justice groups with anti-government and anti-corporate outlooks. Dioxin and related chemicals had gained notoriety. The infamous city of Times Beach, Missouri was abandoned after the roads were sprayed to control dust with waste oil containing high levels of dioxin.[253] Whether this evacuation was needed is debated, but dioxin and danger became firmly linked in the public mind. Although the early years of the Reagan administration produced some political backlash against environmentalists, the public had become convinced of the relationship between pollution and disease. Legal proceedings begun by Reutershan which culminated in a 1985 settlement between various chemical companies and veterans' groups also served to reinforce the impression that Agent Orange had caused serious disease.

In 1991, Congress passed the Agent Orange Act, directing the Secretary of the VA to ask the National Academy of Science to study the scientific knowledge about Agent Orange and the herbicide program in Vietnam. The result was an eight-hundred-page analysis by the Institute of Medicine which concluded that exposure to herbicides was associated with some cancers (soft tissue sarcoma, non-Hodgkin's lymphoma, and Hodgkin's disease) but not others (colon, rectal, stomach, pancreatic, skin, brain, and bladder). Some were inconclusive (hepatobiliary, nasopharyngeal, bone cancer, female reproductive, renal, testicular, and leukemia). The committee also concluded "there is limited or suggestive evidence of an association between exposure to herbicides and . . . multiple myeloma."[254] Regular updates allow the VA to compensate exposed veterans who develop cancer, yet the scientific debate continues. Critics have called the report an effort in political expediency rather than good science.[255] In the end, the jungle has regrown, and the truth can never be known.

Will never blamed Agent Orange for his myeloma, but Karen relayed his feelings about it with a story.

"After he had been home for a few years and was doing a little better, Will bought himself a truck. He and Daddy used to plow snow in the winter and Will did landscaping in the summer. He was good, too. Had an eye for plants, and it kept him outdoors and active, generally away from people. Sometimes he would put down their lawn treatments for them. As business got better, a man from the Conservation Department came by and told him he needed a license to apply the chemicals. He told the man he left his license in the jungle in Vietnam, and he could go read it there, with a few more words I won't say. Anyway, that fellow was really scared and never came back. The sheriff showed up, and so I filled out the forms and pretended I was doing that part. That made the sheriff very happy. But truthfully, I was glad when he gave the chemicals up a few years later and stuck to the cutting and planting."

After his diagnosis, Will began chemotherapy with injections of liposomal doxorubicin (meaning the doxorubicin was in fat globules, brand name Doxil) and bortezomib (Velcade). He took dexamethasone (Decadron) pills by mouth. Later, monthly infusions of zoledronic acid

(Zometa) strengthened his bones, and other medications prevented infection and blood clots.

The treatments worked. Over the first month, Will's back pain returned to his normal constant reminder of the tunnels in Vietnam. He could ride his Harley again, the deep roar announcing his arrival and departure from the office. Laboratory measurements of his kidney function became normal while the myeloma protein in his blood and urine vanished. Four months later, another bone marrow biopsy showed the cancerous plasma cells were gone. The enemy was on the run.

Next was high-dose chemotherapy and a stem cell transplant.

HIGH-DOSE CHEMOTHERAPY FOR MYELOMA.
The first effective treatment for myeloma with the chemotherapy melphalan combined with the steroid prednisone reduced the disease in about half of the patients; an achievement called a "partial remission." Rarely, the myeloma would appear to be gone; called a "complete remission." Since the definition of partial and complete remissions depends on the ability to measure the myeloma, as laboratory techniques improve, achieving a complete remission becomes harder. While a complete remission means the disease is not detectable using the best available techniques, it does not mean cure.

With these early treatments, the partial remissions usually did not last very long, usually months. Higher doses of melphalan produced longer partial remissions and a few more complete remissions, but patients suffered destruction of their bone marrow, leading to low blood counts with serious infections and bleeding. This led to the use of high-dose chemotherapy followed by a "bone marrow transplant." In this procedure, bone marrow stem cells are extracted from the patient and frozen. The patient is then given high-doses of chemotherapy to destroy the myeloma; a treatement which also destroys the normal bone marrow.

After the chemotherapy is finished, the frozen bone marrow is thawed and infused back into the patient so that the bone marrow regrows. Technically, this is not a "transplant" since the cells come from the patient rather than another person. The first extraction procedures involved inserting many needles into the bones of the pelvis while the patient was under anesthesia. Later the stem cells were collected from the blood by using a dialysis-like machine, a much easier procedure. Following the high-dose chemotherapy and the infusion of the stem cells, it usually takes two weeks for the bone marrow cells to regrow the marrow. Patients need supportive care including transfusions and antibiotics and suffer side effects like nausea and vomiting, rashes, diarrhea, and severe fatigue. Full recovery often takes months. In 1996, a European clinical trial was reported in the *New England Journal of Medicine* in which patients received regular chemotherapy followed by either high-dose treatment with bone marrow transplant or further regular dose chemotherapy. The results were clear: the high-dose chemotherapy produced a longer remission for most patients, but cures were extremely rare (if they occurred at all). The treatment was hard but safe. For younger healthy patients, high-dose chemotherapy with bone marrow or stem cell transplantation became the preferred treatment.[256]

For a few years following this study, it was clear that high-dose chemotherapy and bone marrow transplantation was the best treatment for younger, healthier patients with myeloma. As new treatments that were far superior to older drugs like melphalan emerged, debate arose over the role of high-dose treatment and stem cell transplant. Possibly these new agents could be added to the high-dose chemotherapy and stem cell transplant to produce a cure. Or, since high-dose chemotherapy and stem cell transplantation did not cure patients, possibly these newer agents could produce the same results without that ordeal. These are two very different strategies.

Some oncologists declared total war on myeloma. A well-known example is the Myeloma Institute at the University of Arkansas founded by Dr. Bart Barlogie, whose stated aim is of "attacking myeloma on every front at the outset of treatment and utilizing novel combinations of all therapeutic agents and methods of treatment that have been shown to be effective against the disease."[257] In this type of program, patients undergo the most aggressive treatments, often including two rounds of high-dose chemotherapy and stem cell transplants, followed by more treatments to suppress any other remaining myeloma cells. On the other side of the spectrum are oncologists who omit or delay high-dose chemotherapy in patients with slower growing myeloma which responds to newer medications. On balance, most oncologists feel that high-dose chemotherapy and stem cell support is still the preferred option for younger patients who can tolerate the treatment but are somewhat less aggressive than their colleagues in Arkansas.[258] Everyone hopes that modern molecular tools will help individual patients make the best choice.

Cancer is often fought using the vocabulary of battle. President Nixon announced the "War on Cancer" as soldiers fought in Vietnam in 1971. In the fight against cancer, the weapons from that era were the sharp edge of the scalpel, radiation from the nuclear age, and chemotherapy that began with derivatives of mustard gas used in World War I. Symbolically, the first cancer research institute of Nixon's war was built by converting the U.S. Army's Fort Detrick biological warfare facility.

Strategies for war evolve. World War II was a conventional war in which the U.S. mobilized its industrial might to produce a vast armed force fighting an enemy we could recognize. In Vietnam, the United States began with strategies based on conventional warfare: massive bombing raids, tanks, large military bases, projects like operation Ranch Hand. Yet Vietnam was a different war in which the enemy was less well armed, but often hidden or unidentifiable. On the front lines, it soon fell to the individual units and soldiers to adapt to a different reality where the enemy could look like the friend, live in tunnels, and attack from anywhere with weapons which ranged from advanced tools to simple but brutal traps.

Will understood the need for different strategies. When Dr. Matthews explained high-dose chemotherapy and stem cell transplantation was not a cure, he nodded.

"Sure. The big blast won't get them all. It will take them time to come out again, but they'll be back."

"You will have to be in an isolation room for at least a few days, possibly even a few weeks if you have a complication. Do you think you can tolerate that?" Dr. Matthews asked.

"I'll do whatever I have to. The war screwed me up, but I've made my peace with that. It's old history now. But what pisses me off is that even though the government screwed it up, we still could have won. They sent us in not knowing what the hell we were doing and we had to figure it out. Do you know they sent military scientists to try and tell us how to clear out those tunnels? They tried to blow poison gas in, crap like that. Every time we had to listen to those idiots I wanted to kill them. The only way to get those tunnels was to drop a five hundred right on them or go inside. There was no other way. And we were doing it. Just when we about had it done, they gave up. They sent us to that place, and when we finally figured it out, they gave us up."

In the silence, Dr. Matthews sensed Will was not quite finished.

"I understand. Tell me what you need me to do and I'll do it. I know this big blast of chemo won't get all the bastards and then later we'll use more to try to keep them down. I accept that. Going into some hospital room is no problem. No way that's going to make the dreams worse. They are what they are now."

Karen agreed, reassuring Dr. Matthews.

"Will has been the same for years. He struggles with the dreams, and he has his limits, but he's okay. We know he'll never have a normal life, but the life he has is good, considering where he was . . ."

She paused for a minute, took a deep breath, then went on.

"Will had been home about a year. He was really bad then, screaming at night, looking for his gun. My father couldn't understand. Daddy had been in World War II and came home to the farm. Sure, he had some adjustments, but nothing like Will. At the start, Daddy was calm. But as time went by and Will didn't get better, he began to get frustrated. I was scared it was going to boil over. Then one day, Daddy collapsed in the kitchen. Will did CPR on him until we got him to the hospital and saved his life. Daddy recovered and lived another twelve years. You know what?"

"What?" asked Dr. Matthews.

"In all those years, they never spoke about it. But when he got home from the hospital, Daddy was different to Will. He had patience like you wouldn't believe. Daddy's doctors wanted him to walk. He and Will would walk the farm and hike the Adirondacks for hours. Mom and I used to joke the two of them could cover more miles with fewer words than any other pair, but I think Daddy saved Will, too."

The bone marrow transplant team requested a formal psychiatry consult, and Dr. Lawrence Issel offered his perspective.

"When you think about it, it is remarkable that Mr. Denton is as well as he is now. He certainly was exposed to great trauma in Vietnam. He had no preparation and no formal support afterward. We did not understand PTSD at all. Vets like him got no treatment. Thankfully, he had his family. He still suffers from flashbacks, but he has found his own coping skills, even if they are not always verbal. He has come to equilibrium, and you have to admire him. I don't think this hospitalization will be an issue for him, but his life should be a warning for all of us who send young men into battle. Without his family, friends, and his own determination, this fellow could have turned out very different."

Will had a "double transplant." A trip to Memorial Sloan Kettering Cancer Center in New York for two weeks in the hospital was followed in three months by a second. He never said much about it, other than it had to be done. As soon as he could, Will started walking again. His muscle strength recovered quickly, but he was left with nerve damage and numbness in his feet, called neuropathy. Thankfully, it slowly improved to the point that the deep roar of the Harley again shook the parking lot.

"What now?" asked Karen as she and Will sat with Dr. Matthews.

"Your doctors in New York are studying the use of thalidomide in this situation. They think it may be useful to keep the myeloma in remission, but probably will not definitely know for a few more years. So, we can keep the treatment going or you can take a break."

"No point in stopping now," replied Will. "We've got them on the run. Let's keep the pressure on."

Will tolerated his thalidomide well. The numbness in his feet was a little worse, but he managed. Little else about him changed, as Dr. Matthews learned from a colleague with children in high school. One of the social studies teachers, described as a bored and flabby middle-aged ex-jock, had made the mistake of announcing to Claire's class that all the soldiers in Vietnam were high on pot. Shortly after, a student reported the teacher's car was blocked by a large motorcycle while a small man in camouflage was seen talking to him. The student was too far away to hear any words, but the teacher's normally ruddy face was pale, and he sat in his car for quite a while after the motorcycle roared off. The next history lesson had a different tone.

Will's remission lasted for almost four years. Every three months, he met Dr. Matthews for labs. On one visit, he also met medical student Cindy Jenkins, a tall, blond woman from California with an open and direct manner. Dr. Matthew saw her notice the tattoo on Will's arm.

"Mr. Denton served in Vietnam during the War," Dr. Matthews explained.

"I was there, too, in college. Of course, that was very different." Cindy remarked.

Will looked up, but remained quiet. Cindy continued, undeterred by his silence.

"My parents did not want me to go. My father said they all prayed they would never have to go there. He said he was so thankful the War ended before he was old enough to get drafted. But I wanted to see it, so I went for a semester in my junior year."

Will looked at her. "And?"

"It was a beautiful country. Do you want to see some of the pictures?" Not waiting for a reply, she pulled out her phone and sat down beside him. Dr. Matthews finished his paperwork and left them together.

"They were all very nice to us. They like Americans." She progressed through photos of college students in beautiful outdoor scenes, eating and socializing.

"Do they talk about the War?" Will asked.

"Not the young people we were with. Every once in a while, you will see a bomb crater. Actually, you see more of them once you get to know what they are; the plants have all regrown over them. But generally, the young people never even think about it. We went to a museum about the War. We even brought some of the Vietnamese students with us, they really didn't know much about it."

Will looked surprised.

"Did you meet anyone older? Who fought in the War?" he asked.

"A few older people. They were the ones who would talk about it. They also really liked Americans."

She showed him another group of pictures.

"Here is the War museum we went to. It had a display of how they fought. It showed the suffering of the people." She paused. "Were you in the fighting?"

He nodded, looking at the photos intently.

"The museum showed a lot about that, the tunnels they dug, the traps, and the way they survived in the War. The bombing and the poisons. It looked terrible. Even the Vietnamese students we were with were surprised."

They sat together for almost thirty minutes until she finished her tour.

"It's a beautiful place now," she said. "And the people seem happy, even if they don't have much compared with us. When I first got back, I would go shopping and think we have too much . . . So much it makes us not as happy as we should be. Anyway, that's my Vietnam trip."

"Thank you," he said.

"You're welcome. It must be strange for you to see Vietnam so different, so peaceful."

He nodded.

"Would you ever go back?" she asked.

Will frowned as he considered the question carefully before replying.

"No. Some things are better left alone."

Cindy met Will again a few weeks later, searching him out as he received an infusion to strengthen his bones.

"Mr. Denton, I was looking for you," she said as she pulled up a chair, not waiting for his response. "I have some different pictures for you this time." Rebecca watched the interaction, interested.

"Remember you told me about that hike in the Adirondacks? You said a California girl should see your mountains. Well, we did it. Look at this picture from the top of the Goodnow Mountain fire tower. You can see all the mountains from there. It was awesome! Of course, it had just rained and we were covered with mud. And the mosquitoes. I never saw so many!" Her enthusiasm was so contagious that Will seemed pleased.

"You know what I thought when I was at the top?" she asked.

Will shook his head.

"I saw all those miles of woods, and I wondered where you were. I knew you'd be walking out there."

Will Denton laughed and smiled, a bright, broad smile that Rebecca had never seen before.

As the staff sat together at the end of the day, Rebecca mentioned Will's smile. "Who would ever have thought that a man that hard could be made to smile by a medical student so different from him?"

"There is only one explanation," answered Dr. Edwards, breaking into off key song. "I wish they could all be California girls . . ." He ducked as Rebecca launched an empty folder in his direction.

The end of Will's remission had come six years ago, when he was sixty. He felt well, but his lab studies showed a return of the protein in his blood. Dr. Matthews again met with him and Karen.

"We have a few choices. Possibly we can use the same approach we used six years ago, aggressive chemotherapy and then another stem cell transplant. You know better than anyone the pluses and minuses of the stem cell transplant. I think your body could probably tolerate it, except that you have had some nerve damage. That might get worse. The other choice would be to use chemotherapy without the stem cell transplant."

"I can do it again," came the answer.

Chemotherapy led to another remission, but Will could not undergo another stem cell transplant. The treatments which had so successfully controlled his cancer for years had damaged his stem cells, and not enough could be harvested for the procedure. His doctors at Memorial Sloan Kettering Cancer Center offered him another choice: allogeneic stem cell transplantation. In this procedure, Will would receive high-dose chemotherapy, but the stem cells given after the chemotherapy would be from his sister. This would be risky, and there was a one-third chance Will would die from the procedure. If he survived, he would face "graft-versus-host disease" as his sister's stem cells would attack his body, threatening his skin, digestive system, and organ function.

Will declined this option. Dr. Matthews asked why.

"Part of the battle is knowing what weapons not to use," came the response from the man who took a pistol, a knife, and a flashlight into the tunnels.

MODERN TREATMENTS FOR MYELOMA: NOT YOUR PARENTS' CHEMOTHERAPY.

In the fight against myeloma, improvisation, individual determination, scientific brilliance, and remarkable organizations have produced new classes of weapons: immunomodulators (thalidomide) and proteasome inhibitors (bortezomib) and antibodies (daratumumab). These agents typify the new era in cancer medicine and represent a return on the investment in molecular science made in the 1970s and 1980s.

Immunomodulators are one class of new drugs. In addition to their effects on myeloma cells, these drugs block the formation of blood vessels (angiogenesis), enhance immune function, and change the supporting cells of the bone marrow. Thalidomide was the first of these drugs. It came to be used in myeloma in a remarkable way.

In 1995, Manhattan lawyer Beth Wolmer was trying to save her husband. Dr. Ira Wolmer, a cardiologist, had been diagnosed with myeloma at age thirty-five and had worsening disease despite bone marrow transplantation. Left without further treatments, Mrs. Wolmer improvised. She contacted Dr. Judah Folkman, a well-known researcher at Harvard Medical School studying the growth of blood vessels in cancers. Mrs. Wolmer learned of his interest in thalidomide, a drug with a terrible history of causing birth defects in thousands of children in Europe. Originally widely marketed as a sedative and aid for morning sickness during pregnancy in Germany, only the diligence of FDA employee Frances Kelsey had kept it from being approved for use in this country. After the disaster, thalidomide remained a treatment for leprosy until Mrs. Wolmer connected Dr. Folkman with Dr. Bart Barlogie at the University of Arkansas, who agreed to try it in patients with myeloma.[259] Although the drug did not help Dr. Wolmer, it was very useful for other patients, as Dr. Barlogie reported in a 1999 *New England Journal of Medicine* article dedicated to the Wolmers.[260] The success of thalidomide led to the development of more potent drugs in this class, including lenalidomide (Revlimid) and encouraged the study of the mechanisms of its action.

A second class of weapons added to the arsenal against myeloma are "proteasome inhibitors," like bortezomib (Velcade). These drugs block the action of proteasomes, structures throughout the cell which degrade proteins, acting as a cellular garbage disposal system. When the proteasomes of multiple myeloma cells are inhibited, proteins build up, and the cells die. Bortezomib resulted from a disorganized collaboration of familiar groups. The work began in a Harvard Medical School lab and a spin-off biotechnology company, progressed through name changes, venture capital funding, collaborations with pharmaceutical companies, studies at the National Cancer Institute, Dana Farber in Boston, MD Anderson Cancer Center in Texas, Memorial Sloan Kettering in New York, and University of North Carolina. Critical support also came from advocacy groups, including the prostate group CaP cure, the Multiple Myeloma Research Foundation, and International Myeloma Foundation. This circuitous path led to bortezomib's 2008 approval by the FDA.[261] Although the development of bortezomib was very different from that of thalidomide, it also introduced a new class of treatments.

Antibodies became a third class of weapons for myeloma with the approval of daratumumab (Darzalex) in 2015. Antibodies are familiar from science or health class, where students learn they fight infections. Antibodies are produced by immune cells called B-lymphocytes and have two ends. One end will attach to a specific target; in the case of infection on the outside of an invader. The opposite end will then attract other immune cells to destroy the enemy. The immune system makes specific antibodies for each infection. This specificity is called "adaptive immunity" and is important to fight new invaders and keep the antibody from attacking normal cells. Vaccinations ensure the immune system is ready to produce the desired antibodies when an infection strikes.

The use of antibodies as cancer treatment became possible in the 1970s when scientists Cesar Milstein and Georges J.F. Kohler developed the ability to make antibodies directed against a target they would select using a remarkable technology called "hybridoma." Mice were injected with the target, and the B-cells of the mice would respond by making various antibodies against the target. These B-cells were harvested. The next amazing part of the process was to use an electrical current to fuse the mice B-cells with myeloma cancer cells grown in the lab. The fused B-cells/myeloma cells would grow forever and produce antibodies against the target. This brilliant mix of Mickey Mouse and Frankenstein won Milstein and Kohler a 1984 Nobel Prize.

Although antibodies captured public attention as "magic bullets" against cancer, progress was not immediate. The science was difficult, and there were competing interests. The 1980s and early 1990s were the era of peak enthusiasm for new drugs like paclitaxel (Taxol), often used in complex combinations, and high-dose chemotherapy with which bone marrow or stem cell transplant. Targeted approaches to cancer were also generating excitement. In contrast, antibodies were seen by many as large, clunky molecules which would probably have little clinical effect.[262] The development of the antibodies trastuzumab (Herceptin) for breast cancer and rituximab (Rituxan) by Genentech in the late 1990s markedly changed these views. The 1999 founding of GenMab, a company in Copenhagen dedicated to the design of antibodies, eventually produced the antibody daratumumab for myeloma.

Daratumumab attaches to a molecule called CD-38, which is found on myeloma and normal plasma cells and sends signals into the cell. Since CD-38 is on few other cells, it was a logical target for antibody treatment of myeloma. Scientists at GenMab produced anti-CD-38 antibodies using the hybridoma technology of Milstein and Kohler updated with "transgenic" mice, rodents with altered DNA that made human antibodies. These human antibodies against CD-38 killed myeloma cells (a summary of thousands of hours of brilliant laboratory science).[263] Daratumumab was selected from the various antibodies by Genmab scientists in 2005, clinical studies reported in national oncology meetings in 2012, and approval granted by the FDA in 2015 (a summary of thousands of hours of brilliant clinical research). GenMab contracted with the pharmaceutical company Janssen to market the drug, which has extended the lives of many with patients and is being studied in combination with other treatments.

For most patients, this brilliant science does not yet offer cures, but rather allows the journey and struggle to continue.

For the last six years, Will had continued treatment with various combinations of lenalidomide, bortezomib, the older drug cyclophosphamide, and the old standby dexamethasone. The enemy would be put down, the treatments reduced to limit collateral damage until the rising protein levels signaled the need for more. More recently Will needed other weapons: pomalidomide, another variation of thalidomide, and carfilzomib, a variation of bortezomib.

Life went on. Claire graduated from Saratoga High School on a beautiful June day at the Saratoga Performing Arts Center. Will was there to see her, also witnessing the awarding of a degree to an old member of the class of 1940 who had left to join the Army in World War II. Clare went to Cornell to study biology and regularly returned to see her uncle. Between visits, she even wrote him letters, the only form of communication he would accept, suspecting she was the only student on campus regularly using postage stamps. Will continued hiking and camping in the Adirondack mountains, although the distance he could cover decreased. Karen reported he was occasionally accompanied by a woman, but Will wouldn't say much about that. In town, memories of Vietnam were renewed when the New York State Military Museum exhibited video interviews of veterans by Skidmore college students. Will visited but offered no comments.

Throughout the years, Will had few bad days, but the cumulative effects of the treatments took their toll. Although he would still be mistaken for a fit man, the neuropathy was with him constantly as a burning pain in his feet. Walking had become harder, and he sometimes carried a stick. The nerve damage had also thrown off his balance, and the roar of his now garaged motorcycle was no longer heard.

"Why not put on a third wheel?" asked medical assistant John Welt, also a rider.

"You can't tame a beast," was all Will would say about that.

Will was being worn down. The fatigue and nerve damage were problems, but the appearance of his feet particularly bothered him. Several nails were missing, the skin was discolored, and they looked somehow diseased. There was nothing he could do about it; the chemicals were responsible. No matter how coated the skin and trimmed the nails, they still looked bad. Will had always been proud of his feet. Even in the war, he had always kept them clean and dry, coating them with Vaseline and sealing any cuts with crazy glue. That had been one of the lessons he had learned from his first sergeant. And it had worked. Whatever else had happened, he had left Vietnam with all his toenails and no fungus. My brain was fucked, he used to say, but I had fine feet.

Rebecca first sensed Will's fatigue. She was administering his treatment on the second anniversary of the Boston Marathon bombing when an attractive, young television announcer declared that the bombing had put things into perspective. Rebecca looked up.

"What do you think, Mr. Denton? Do you think this bombing put life in perspective?" she asked.

She expected his usual short, hard answer. Instead, she was surprised by his expression as he looked at her.

"I don't know," he replied, almost gently. "I don't think I'm good at perspective."

"No. I don't think you need it." It was the first time in more than ten years that Rebecca felt she was even faintly supporting him.

Later she reported to Dr. Matthews. "I think even he is getting worn down."

"He has been doing this a long time. It must be wearing him down. His markers are stable, but if he stops they will rise again quickly. But I'll ask him about it and see if he wants to continue on."

Sargent Walter Hubert, USMC (ret) supplied the answer. If there ever was an old marine, it was this still solid eighty year old, with hair cropped so short the gray was invisible. By chance, Will sat next to Hubert as he rested quietly during a treatment. As Rebecca took Will's blood pressure, Hubert noticed his tattoo.

"Where did you see action?" Hubert asked.

"What makes you think I saw action?" Will answered.

"You look like a man who saw action."

Will grunted. After Rebecca had left, he spoke.

"Nam."

Hubert nodded and rolled up his sleeve. Around the middle of his forearm was a tattoo, a simple braid.

"See this?" he said.

Will nodded.

"My nephew went there to fly a helicopter. When he left, I put on a rope bracelet to keep until he came back. One day, three helicopters took off and went into some clouds. Only two came out the other side, not his. They never found him. When the rope began to fray, I had it turned into this. He was a good boy . . . A good man."

Will nodded. "A lot of good ones didn't come back. Some of the best."

They sat silently together. Rebecca disconnected Hubert from his intravenous.

"How long you been in this fight?" Hubert asked Will after she left, gesturing around the room.

"Twelve years. You?"

"Only a few months. They say this stuff will clean me up for a while. But I'm eighty, so who gives a shit. My fight is almost over no matter what happens here."

Hubert got up and looked at Will.

"Good luck to you, soldier. You know you ain't finished yet."

Will nodded. He wasn't. Not yet.

Carol Feinman 5: Breast cancer (Boston, 1989)

Suddenly chemotherapy was finished. The last injection was followed by a final week of pills. Roger had organized a small party on the evening Carol swallowed the last of the evil things, and everyone seemed relieved she was finished. At her appointment a week later, Dr. Spiegel ordered a three-month follow-up visit preceded by a set of scans. As she left, Carol met CJ, who was carrying a tray with an intravenous bag and a syringe filled with red liquid.

"Thanks for everything, CJ."

CJ nodded. "My pleasure. Chemo is better to give than receive."

Carol laughed. "True. Well, I'm glad it is over . . . And that you were the one who gave it to me."

"Listen, I have to drop this off, but if you have a few minutes to wait, I would like to talk to you."

Carol agreed and sat in the waiting area. The check-in counter and furniture were the same as the first day she had arrived and Janice still slowly lumbered, but Carol noticed there were different people in the room. She thought of Mrs. Kurtz and her knitting and wondered if Mr. Kurtz was still alive. She had not seen the black man with the young boy recently and had heard Marilyn was in the hospital again with her leukemia.

CJ came out. "I have half an hour. Would you like to get coffee in the cafeteria?"

After they were sitting, CJ began.

"You did a great job getting through the chemo, Carol, but I wanted to give you some advice. Even though you think it's over, it's not really. You'll feel the effects of this stuff for months. You'll be tired easily. You can ache all over. Are you having periods?"

Carol shook her head. "Not for a few months now."

"Hot flashes?"

Carol nodded.

"The periods will probably come back. Until they do, you may have the hot flashes. Remember, this wasn't birth control, and you could get pregnant."

"I wish that was a worry."

CJ smiled. "It will be again at some point. And it'll take months for your hair to regrow."

Carol nodded. "I'm glad you're telling me this."

"There's more," CJ went on. "Everyone else wants this to be over. The people who were being nice to you will probably stop. Your family and friends who love you will expect you to be yourself again. Everyone is back to normal . . . Except you. You've got to figure out what just happened. We call it 're-entry.' Some of our patients get depressed for a while, so keep in touch."

CJ was right. Things had changed, starting with her family who almost seemed to be ignoring her. They had been so supportive during her treatments that Carol thought they were upset with her. Perhaps they still resented her decision to avoid mastectomy. Carol planned to clear the air when they met for coffee at Betty's home, but Rose started with a tirade about Cynthia and Alisa.

"Cynthia is taking tests to be placed into accelerated math and science. She loves to read so she'll probably do well, but who knows. The way these other mothers talk makes me think I am the only one with average children. Everyone has the most gifted child in something or other. And Alisa, I'm lucky to get her to put her clothes on each morning and go to school, much less compose an opera or something."

"They're very bright children," challenged Betty. "You shouldn't speak of them like that."

"Mother, they are seven and five. I challenge anyone to tell me what someone will be doing with their life based upon some test at that age. But the way these mothers talk about little Johnny and Jane is ridiculous. You would think half of them have written books or taken calculus already. Meanwhile, Alisa can't find her toothbrush. I have bought four of them this month alone."

"Maybe she's using them," Betty responded.

"Sure. Either she is painting a masterpiece in the basement, or she wanders around and forgets where she puts them. I'm betting on the second."

Carol laughed. As the conversation turned to complexities of Betty's dental issues, Carol slowly realized that Betty and Rose were not ignoring her. They had simply moved on and returned to their own lives. Rose was busy, and Betty was acting every bit her age. For them, her treatment was over.

The office had also resumed its usual routines, her illness forgotten there as well. For Carol work was now different. Projects which would have previously seemed fun were now irritatingly trivial. For the first time, she had trouble focusing. Carol knew she was struggling, just like CJ had said. She wasn't quite sure where to turn.

A notice for a cancer support group in the elevator at Beth Israel had caught her eye during her treatment, and she had saved the information. At the time, she was too busy managing her chemotherapy to attend, but now the idea held appeal. The group met on Wednesday evenings at the nearby Harvard Community Health Plan. On her way home from work, Carol left the Trolley two stops early and walked over to the HCHP building. It was a summer evening, and people enjoying the weather filled the street. The group was held on the second floor in a conference room belonging to the primary care group. She passed a few doctors and nurses in their offices finishing up paperwork, turned the corner and stopped suddenly. Through the open door, she could see a thin, older woman in a wheelchair sitting beside a man she immediately took to be her husband. Next was an equally ill-looking, elderly man with yellowed skin. She paused outside the doorway.

"Can I help you?" asked a pleasant, young woman with black hair and brown eyes, wearing a tag which identified her as an HCHP oncology nurse.

"I'm not sure . . .," Carol trailed off.

"Were you thinking of attending the cancer support group?" asked the nurse.

Carol nodded.

"I'm Donna Reedy, the nurse assigned to the support group." She steered Carol into a nearby office where she quickly learned her history.

"I thought this might be a good place to meet some other people who are going through the same thing," Carol concluded.

"Sure. Listen . . . This is not the place for you. I know it was advertised as a support group. But those people in there will suck the life out of you. They are all old, dying of cancer, some bitter and angry at their doctors. It's the last place you want to be, trust me."

"I had no idea," Carol responded, recoiling.

"No reason you should. Next month we will be starting a new group just for young women recently diagnosed with breast cancer. Most of them will be in chemo or just starting, but one or two will have finished. Give me your number, and I'll call you. You might have something in common with them, but please, stay out of this room."

It was still warm when Carol escaped and walked the two miles home. Passing Beth Israel, she could see lights on inside the oncology unit. I hope I never need to go there again for chemo, she thought. In a shop window, she caught sight of her reflection, still strange to her because of her wig. I want my hair back. My own hair. And I want to wear a hat with it. Not just any hat. I'm going to London to buy a hat at Harrods. When my hair comes back, that's what I'm doing. Going to London to buy a hat at Harrods.

In the end, it was Roger who came the closest to understanding. It had been a quiet day at work, and he had come over to her desk.

"Buy you lunch?" he asked.

"Sure," she replied. "What's the occasion?"

"No occasion. Absolutely no reason other than I would enjoy it."

They found a spot at the Italian restaurant around the corner. After they had ordered, Carol asked Roger about a recent trip to his small Arkansas hometown, light-years away from life in Boston.

"Bittersweet. Mother is still alive, but she has dementia. She smiles and looks happy, but doesn't remember me."

"Is she in a nursing home?"

"No, my sister takes care of her in her home. Her husband is military and away a lot, thankfully for my visit. He and I have never come to terms. But my sister is very good with Mom, and I must give him credit for letting her stay in his home, even if he is a bastard to me."

"How about the town?"

"Still small and dusty. A few stores, some the same, but the people I would want to see are gone. The adults who helped me are dead and the kids I grew up with and liked left, except my sister. The ones who stayed behind I'd rather not see."

"Why do you go back?" she asked.

He paused. "To remind me of myself. Where I came from and where I have come. That's all."

She nodded. "How about you?" he asked.

"I'm struggling, Roger," she started. "I know my treatment is finished, and I'm doing well. Believe me, I'm grateful. But things don't seem quite the same. I don't know how to explain it, but somehow it seems like everyone else is back to normal, but I'm not."

"Is it your family? Work?"

"Everything." Carol paused. "Everything is the same on the outside, my family, friends, work. But I'm not quite me."

Roger smiled softly. "I don't really understand what you went through, but I think I understand what you are feeling. Do you remember on the beach when you asked why I was reading about AIDS?"

Carol nodded.

"Allen and I had a friend who died of AIDS. His family had disowned him, and so we took care of him at his home. It was one of those terrible deaths. When it was finally over, and we had gone to our home, I couldn't sleep. One night I went outside for a walk and found myself sitting on a bench. It was perfectly quiet except I could hear the noise of the traffic signal changing, again and again. And I sat there thinking that this terrible thing had happened, this wonderful man was dead, and my world was changed forever. And I was so mad at that stupid traffic light; it just kept going on its cycle like nothing mattered. I wanted to tear it off the pole."

"What did you do?"

"Nothing. I went home and went to bed. Deep down, I knew it wasn't the light's fault. It was me. I needed to come to terms with it."

"And did you?"

Roger looked thoughtful.

"No. I never did come to terms with any of it. Never made sense of his death. Never really came to terms with that dusty little place I grew up in, either. But time passes, and you feel better, Carol. Just let time pass and be yourself. That's all I can say."

A few weeks later, Carol had her first follow-up visit with Dr. Spiegel, preceded by a CT scan and a bone scan. Although she had taken both tests shortly after her diagnosis, Carol had no memory of them. It's probably a good thing, she thought, recalling that first breast ultrasound and the nauseating smell of the jelly.

The CT scan was uneventful. She was given a large bottle of a chalky drink and told by the smiling receptionist to enjoy it. Although the injection of dye which followed gave her a flushed feeling, the ride through the donut was quick. Not bad, she thought.

The bone scan the next day was different, almost weird. That morning she entered a small room to be injected with a liquid taken from a worn-looking lead container bearing a radioactive symbol. The technician, a kindly man in his early sixties who looked as aged as the bottle, caught her eyeing the insignia.

"Scary, huh?" he offered in a faint brogue, his bushy eyebrows rising.

"Sort of…," Carol replied. "Yeah, it is scary."

"This radiation is nothing. Don't worry about it, dear. When you hear the siren and see a big flash, now that's radiation."

Carol laughed.

"Remember what they taught you in school during those atomic bomb drills?" he asked as he pushed the plunger.

"Get under your desk and . . .," replied Carol, smiling.

"Put your head between your legs, and kiss your arse goodbye," he continued, roaring with laughter and so genuinely pleased with himself that Carol could not help but join in.

Although we tend to think of bones as static structural supports like the steel beams of a skyscraper, they are living organs which are constantly being remodeled. Cells called osteoclasts are continually removing old bone while others called osteoblasts lay down new bone. As we age and the breakdown exceeds the buildup, the infrastructure decay is called osteoporosis. When cancer cells grow in the bone, they often hijack the osteoclasts to create holes in the bone. This leads the osteoblasts to try to repair the damage, often in a disorganized fashion. The material injected into Carol contained a radioactive phosphate used in the repair, called technetium-99 methylene diphosphonate (99mTc-MDP). It will show sites of cancer (or active repair in the case of a fracture). To allow time for it to enter the bones, the radioactive phosphate needed to be in Carol's body for three hours before the picture was taken.

Three hours. Carol wondered what to do with three hours. Before this, three hours would have been nothing. A movie. A date. A bike ride. Now it was three hours to see if the cancer was in her bones. She decided to walk. Taking a right out the hospital onto Brookline Avenue she soon found herself near Fenway Park. It was almost eleven, and she noticed the green sign reporting that tours of the Park left every hour, including the new press box and clubhouse. Why not? Even though I don't like baseball, I should take the tour. After all, I live in Boston, she thought as she paid her $4.50. With her were two families with five excited school-age boys, three college age couples, one Asian couple, obviously tourists, and one grandfather with his teenage grandson. The guide, appropriately named Red, was a man in his late sixties who obviously lived and breathed Red Sox history. He introduced himself and asked the boys who their favorite players were.

They ran down the list of stars: Wade Boggs, Dwight Evans, Jim Rice, Bob Stanley, and Roger Clemens.

Without warning, Red turned to Carol.

"How about you, Miss? Do you have a favorite baseball player?"

Damn, she thought. Here I am waiting for some radiation to get into my bones to see if I have cancer and I have to come up with the name of a baseball player. I don't even like baseball. Why did I do this?

"Kevin Costner," she blurted out.

Red laughed.

"Oh, he's cute," responded one of the college girls enthusiastically. "I loved him in *Field of Dreams*."

"Me, too," replied one of the other girls.

The Asian couple nodded excitedly together.

"We have seen this movie. Very nice."

The ice broken, the group moved through the tour, and Carol found herself distracted by Red's history of the Red Sox Nation. By the end, Carol understood the Curse of the Bambino, why Red Sox hate Yankees, Tom Yawkey, Ted Williams, the Impossible Dream, the Boston Massacre and, of course, Bill Buckner, whom she already knew. The tour ended with a view from the new box seats where she took photos for the couples and families. Then Carol made her way back to Beth Israel where she stood in front of a nuclear camera and had her own picture taken.

Betty had insisted on coming with her for the visit with Dr. Spiegel. Rose had offered to attend, but Carol had encouraged her to remain at work, and she had needed little prodding. She's back in her own life, thought Carol. In the days leading up to the visit, Carol kept her anxiety about the tests to a minimum. But returning to the oncology unit was depressing, particularly when she noticed the faint smell she associated with her treatments. As she entered the waiting room, she did not recognize any of the patients or their families. The worn reception desk looked even more ragged and, most distressingly, was staffed by new receptionists who did not recognize her.

"What happened to Katie?" Carol asked the first woman, an attractive, young blond with perfect, bright teeth dressed in an almost seductive, cutting-edge suit. Her name tag read Dawn.

"She got married," said Dawn. "And moved to Worcester. God, I hope he was worth it. Can you imagine living in that dump of a city? The main store is Spags. Ever been to it?"

Carol shook her head, unable to respond to the question otherwise.

"Yeah, well, let me tell you, that store sucks. Junk everywhere, but they love it in that town. Excuse me, I mean, I know they told me not to say that type of thing, but it's true. It sucks. The motto is 'Spags has no bags.' Who wants to shop at a store with no bags? You got to bring your own box. Are you kiddin me? I want nice attendants when I shop. You know, the ones that spray perfume on you."

"Dawn, check her in," interrupted her partner, a plainer and serious young woman named Sarah.

"Oh, sure, excuse me. I don't usually work here. I'm on loan from plastic surgery. Now, who are you?"

"Carol Feinman. I'm here to see Dr. Spiegel."

"Let's see, here you are, and here's your chart. I'll let Janice know you are here. Nice talking to you."

Carol nodded and sat with Betty. Remarkably, Janice appeared almost immediately and slowly walked them into the room. Carol sat on the exam table and stuck out her arm. Janice took her blood pressure, pulse, and temperature, made some notes on the chart, then looked at Carol.

"One hundred twelve over sixty-eight, pulse seventy, no fever. Dr. Spiegel will be in." She turned and lumbered toward the door, paused, and looked back at Carol.

"You look good, girl."

Carol smiled. "Thanks, I'm happy to see you."

"Yeah, sure," Janice waved as she walked out.

Carol sat on the exam table, feeling a slight chill in her gown. They waited quietly for a few minutes, then heard a soft knock on the door. Instead of Dr. Spiegel, in walked Dr. John Matthews, the oncology fellow.

"Ms. Feinman?" he asked. Carol nodded.

"I'm John Matthews, one of the oncology fellows here. We met a while back. Dr. Spiegel is running behind today because of all the changes at the front desk. He wanted me to tell you all your tests were fine."

Carol and Betty hugged each other.

"Have you been feeling well?" Dr. Matthews asked.

Carol nodded. "Better, now that I know the tests are good."

"Good. Well, Dr. Spiegel will be in about twenty minutes. Is there anything you need?"

Carol and Betty shook their heads, and he left.

After he had left, Betty turned to Carol.

"He's cute. What about him? He'll be a doctor someday."

"Mother," Carol replied in an exasperated tone. "He is already a doctor. A fellow here. We met him before."

"All the more reason. Now that you're done with this cancer treatment, I think you should think about this. You have spent a lot of time in this hospital, and there are probably many nice men here you could meet. Maybe we could ask that girl at the desk about him. I bet she knows."

Carol groaned.

The ensuing silence was broken by the thump on the door announcing the arrival of Dr. Spiegel. He greeted Carol and Betty warmly. After he had examined Carol, they all returned to the room.

"As you know, your tests were all good. We did not find any signs of cancer. We'll check your bloods again in three months and repeat the scans again in six months."

"Didn't I hear on the news a few years ago that someone was working on a blood test for cancer?" asked Carol.

SEARCHING FOR CANCER IN THE BLOOD.

The "cancer blood test" has been a holy grail in oncology. The ideal cancer blood test would allow early detection and surgery. After removal of the cancer, the test then would tell if the surgery was successful. If cancer cells had spread, chemotherapy could be given and the test repeated until all the cancer was gone. The cancer blood test would allow patients and their doctors to know the status of their disease. Treatments would be based the test rather than group statistics. Watching for recurrence might be either unnecessary or, at the least, very simple. For years in labs across the world, scientists have sought this test for a variety of cancers.

The first cancer blood test or "tumor marker" was the carcinoembryonic antigen (CEA), discovered in the 1960s.[264] The colon and other tissues of the gastrointestinal tract produce small amounts of CEA, but most never reaches the blood since it is blocked by the supporting structures and ends in the feces. Colon cancer cells often make CEA in larger amounts than normal cells and break down the normal barriers, allowing the CEA to enter the blood.[265] Despite early hopes, time has proven that the CEA is not an ideal cancer blood test. It does not detect early colon cancer because it is often normal until the cancer is widespread, while elevations occur in smokers or those with non-cancerous bowel inflammations. Nor is the CEA useful for deciding whether to use chemotherapy after colon cancer surgery. Since a normal CEA test after surgery does not mean patients are "cancer free," chemotherapy is still prescribed based on the stage and features of the cancer, using group statistics. The CEA has some modest benefit when used to watch patients after colon cancer surgery. A rise in CEA can occasionally detect a recurrence in the liver which can be removed, but it more commonly signifies widespread, incurable disease. The clearest use of the test is to follow the results of treatment in patients with widely spread (metastatic) disease since a decline in CEA usually means shrinkage.

The Prostate Specific Antigen (PSA) is another well-known cancer blood test, discovered in 1979.[266] PSA is a protein secreted by normal prostate cells. Prostate cancers tend to secrete more PSA and break down the barriers which keep it from the blood, thereby raising the level. Unlike the CEA, the PSA can detect early prostate cancer which is curable by surgery, although using PSA as a screening test for prostate cancer is controversial. Unfortunately, as with the CEA, a normal PSA after surgery does not mean a man is cancer free after surgery or radiation. The PSA can also be used to try to watch for recurrence, although its use in this setting is also limited. Like the CEA with widespread colon cancer, the PSA is useful to track the results of treatment in men with widespread (metastatic) prostate cancers.

Similar tests exist for other cancers. The most commonly used tumor marker for breast cancer, the CA27-29 or related CA15-3, is less useful than either the CEA or PSA. The test does not detect cancers early and cannot replace a mammogram. After breast surgery, a normal test does not mean there are no cancer cells, so decisions about chemotherapy use cannot be made using the results. During the follow-up period, the CA27-29 is often used to detect recurrences. Unfortunately, it produces false-positives and usually detects recurrences only when they are widespread. Given these problems, most professionals societies have discouraged the use of the CA27-29, although many individual oncologists continue to order the tests. As with the CEA and PSA, the CA27-29 can be used to follow patients with widespread disease during treatment. Blood tests for cancers of the pancreas and ovary face similar limitations.

Cancer blood tests like the CEA, PSA, and CA27-29 rely on detection of the proteins using antibodies, a process called an immunoassay. The era of molecular science raised the possibility of more specific techniques to detect actual cancer cells or their traces in the blood. The search has produced some apocryphal stories of scientists who undertook the quest. One is the tale of a brilliant researcher who reported his cancer blood test in a prestigious medical journal, gathered investors, and staked his reputation and personal fortune in a new company. As others tried to duplicate his work, however, they discovered non-cancerous conditions could give positive results. These findings were devastating—a test which might falsely diagnose a person with cancer would be useless. The great man's ego refused to allow him to accept the scientific flaws in his work. As he attempted to refute his critics, whispers of fraud began, and his publication was retracted. As the intense pressure of the business and academic worlds mounted, he unraveled and, in desperation, ran his test on himself. To his horror, it was positive. Now convinced there was a cancer lurking in his own body, he underwent a series of tests to search for the disease. As the results came back negative, he insisted on progressively more invasive tests to find the cancer. More procedures generated small abnormalities which would normally be discounted, but which he could not ignore—finding his non-existent cancer would be the validation of his work. His search drove him to madness.

These cancer blood tests demonstrate the complexity of this holy grail. Even as improved lab techniques accurately detect a small number of cancer cells, it is important to know if those cells have the potential for harm, will or will not be controlled by the immune system, and most importantly, can be treated.

Dr. Spiegel knew the blood test Carol had heard about was called "NMR spectroscopy." In this test, the specific patterns of proteins and fats in the blood indicated cancer. The procedure was complicated, questions arose about its accuracy, and it was abandoned.

"You did. It didn't end up working. So, the best we can do is say that your scans and labs are normal and keep watching. But it's good news. I will see you again in three months after your next blood work."

Rose called that evening. She was pleased with the reports and quickly moved the conversation to Carol's future.

"Are you getting out with your friends from work?" she asked.

"Translation . . . Are you dating anyone?" replied Carol.

"I know it probably seems early after your treatments, but I think you should get out and meet people," Rose continued.

"Did you have anyone in mind? Some eligible lawyer friends?"

"Not really."

Probably hard to sell a sister with breast cancer, Carol started to say, but cut herself off. It was unfair to Rose and she did not want to expose herself. "Listen, Rose," she continued. "I have some nice friends. I just need more time."

Despite the clear scans, it was still hard to fit in. Donna Reedy had started her new support group specifically designed for younger women with breast cancer. Carol had gone to the first meeting but found it dominated by two married women with young children. As she listened to their fears of not being able to raise their children, Carol felt a mix of sorrow, depression, and anger. I may never even know that feeling, she thought, and left during the break. Outside she met another woman escaping the group. Nancy Pyle, self-described five feet and twelve inches tall and north of two hundred pounds, was undoubtedly the strongest woman Carol had ever met. She had recently undergone a lumpectomy and radiation for breast cancer but had not needed chemotherapy. Nancy was a martial artist who had occasionally worked the women's professional wrestling tour.

"Women wrestling in front of a bunch of guys who long to be Aristotle, even though they probably don't know who he is," she explained.

"Aristotle?" asked Carol, puzzled.

"Yeah, the philosopher. You probably didn't know he ended up being ridden around naked in a field by a woman with a whip. Someone even wrote a play about it."

Carol laughed, amazed. "I didn't know that."

Nancy had remained determined to continue her athletics despite the advice she had received from her surgeon.

"He told me not to lift anything over twenty pounds and said if I exercised I might get swelling in the arm, lymphedema. He took out twenty of my lymph nodes. When he said they were clear I told him I wanted them put back in."

Carol laughed again. "What did he say?"

"He told me that wasn't possible and would I please not kill him. He said I might need him later. He's a little wisp of a thing."

Nancy invited Carol to her gym for a workout.

"Exercise is better than that group. Keeps my mind off this stuff."

"I'm not much of an exerciser," Carol warned her.

"Don't worry. You can do as much or as little as you want. Just don't wear anything pretty."

Nancy's gym was in West Roxbury. When she entered, Carol knew this was not a health club—there was no nonsense here. Large determined-looking men and a surprising number of women grunted to lift heavy metal. The place was clean but worn and smelled of work and sweat. A few of the weight lifters nodded at Nancy as she walked Carol to a clear area of the gym where she spread a mat and started a stretching routine. After they had warmed up, Nancy took Carol through a series of martial arts forms. Carol marveled at the speed and grace of the big woman.

"Each position is a kata. Just concentrate on first holding the position and imitating what I do as smoothly as you can," Nancy ordered. After twenty minutes, Carol was both tired and rested while Nancy increased the speed and complexity of her movements. Twenty minutes later, she produced a set of jump ropes. Carol had enjoyed jumping rope as a child and joined in.

"Pretty good," Nancy commented.

"I'm out of practice, but it feels good."

Nancy's workout continued with a series of light weight work, most of which was beyond Carol's capabilities. Still, she enjoyed the feeling of using her body.

Carol continued to exercise with Nancy and occasionally at a trendy club in her neighborhood where the clients and dress were different. A few weeks later, she noticed a pain in her lower right chest, over her ribs. It was sharp and worsened with twisting or when she took a deep breath. When she stopped at Rose's for a visit, her sister noticed her wince as she bent down to greet Cynthia.

"What's the matter with you?" she asked. "Why are you hurting?"

"I pulled a muscle in my chest," Carol replied, enthusiastically describing her new exercise routine.

"How long have you had it?" Rose asked.

"A week or so."

"You better call your doctor right away. Pain like that might be something more serious. How do you know it's not the cancer?"

"Cancer? I never thought of that . . . I pulled it, Rose."

"Don't be stupid Carol. It's different now. Anytime you have a pain that doesn't go away, you need to get checked."

The pain was worse that night as she lay in bed. Damn Rose, Carol thought. It was getting better until she brought up cancer. It can't be. I just had all those tests, and they were fine. They would have shown something. But Dr. Spiegel said there were no perfect tests. I don't want more chemotherapy. Will I ever have children? When does this end? It was a long night, tossing and turning, making tea, pressing on her ribs, and trying to take deep breaths to test the pain before she finally fell asleep.

The next morning, Carol called the oncology unit and was relieved when Sarah answered, sparing her a conversation with Dawn. Dr. Spiegel was away, but she made an appointment to see Dr. Matthews that afternoon. Sarah was alone at the desk when she checked in.

"Are you the only one here?" asked Carol.

Sarah rolled her eyes. "Dawn is back in plastic surgery. They finally figured out maybe she wasn't the right person for this job."

"Is Janice here?" Carol asked again, seeing another nurse escort an anxious-looking couple into an exam room.

"She'll never leave. She's just off for the week." Sarah looked around, then whispered. "Dr. Spiegel loves her and would never let them fire her."

"Really?" said Carol, surprised.

"Sure, she moves so slowly that everyone blames her for the schedule running behind, but actually it gives him more time."

Carol laughed.

"Don't tell," Sarah added. "Anyway, since Dr. Spiegel is away, you'll see Dr. Matthews. He runs right on time."

Dr. Matthews entered the room and introduced himself again.

"Hi Carol, I'm John Matthews, the oncology fellow. We've met before."

"I remember."

He took her history, listened to her breathing and pressed on Carol's ribs, easily finding the area of tenderness.

"I think you pulled a muscle. It will probably take a few weeks to get better since with every breath you stretch it. But let's do an x-ray to be sure we're not missing anything. At the least, that will make your family happy. Then you can take some ibuprofen."

Carol laughed, "You remember my family."

"Sure. Your mom and sister. Take it easy for a few days, but don't give up exercising. Some of the nurses here are studying the stresses women have when they go through these treatments and are finding exercise helps. Just lay off the arms for a week or two, then go back gently."

Carol again met CJ as she left.

"How are you?" CJ asked. "And why are you here?"

"I'm here today because I pulled a muscle in my chest. Dr. Spiegel is away, so I saw Dr. Matthews. He's sending me for an x-ray but doesn't think it is anything. Overall, I'm okay. It's like you said. I'm struggling with figuring all this out, but I've been doing better lately."

"I'm glad you're doing okay," replied CJ. "You've seen Dr. Matthews before, right?"

"Yeah, a few times. He's nice. Is he single?" she asked.

CJ laughed. "Yeah, and not even gay. He's one of the prize cows around here."

Rose called that evening, and Carol gave report.

"I like that Dr. Matthews," she added.

"Who?" Rose asked.

"He is the oncology fellow we met with Dr. Spiegel that first visit. The tall, brown-haired one with a beard."

"I don't remember him." replied Rose.

"Well, he remembered you. Anyway, he's nice . . . I'm going to follow your instructions and ask him out."

"Good luck," Rose went on. "There is a rule that doctors can't get involved with patients."

"But he's not really my doctor. Dr. Spiegel is my main doctor. He's sort of an assistant."

"Listen, Carol," said Rose in her best legal voice. "Don't get your hopes up. These guys are very serious about this sort of thing. He's probably not going to want to risk anything."

Dr. Matthews called the next day while Carol was at work.

"Carol, it's John Matthews. Your x-rays were fine. The ribs all looked good. I think you can keep taking the ibuprofen for a few days. Let me know if it doesn't get better."

"Thank you."

"You're welcome."

"Can I ask you a personal question?" Carol paused.

"Sure," he replied.

"Would you consider seeing me again . . . but not as a patient . . . Socially?"

"I would like that . . .," Dr. Matthews stammered. "I mean, you're wonderful. I would have to think this through, though. It would mean

I could never be your doctor and I would need to, well, there are a number of issues . . ."

"My sister, the lawyer, said you couldn't. I didn't mean to put you in an awkward position."

Dr. Matthews regained some of his composure. "I would very much like to see you, Carol, but I need to think this over. You are a special person, and I don't want to do the wrong thing. I'll call you back tomorrow."

The call did come the next day, apologetic but clear.

"If we had met under any other circumstances without being doctor and patient, I would definitely want to see you. But I can't, Carol. I'm sorry."

"I understand. I knew it was a long shot but wanted to try. Can you still be my doctor when I need you?"

"Of course," he sounded relieved.

"I'm glad for that . . . Well, you might see me tomorrow . . . as a patient. I have some insurance paperwork to bring by the office."

CJ smiled when Carol told her the next day.

"I'm not surprised. It was worth a try, but he strikes me as a pretty serious guy. He wouldn't break the rules."

"Too bad," Carol mused.

"I don't know," replied CJ. "Do you really want to bring an oncologist to a party? That'll kill off any conversation."

1:00 Jeff Stiller: Head and neck cancer

J eff Stiller was forty-five but looked eighty. He was a thin man, with unkempt, jet-black hair. His pupils were constricted, yet he could focus. His old clothes were clean and the often-present sharp odor of urine absent. He was sitting in the chair, rocking slightly.

"How are you, Jeff?" asked Dr. Matthews, sitting down across from him.

"Not bad," he answered.

"Do you feel up for your treatment today?" asked Dr. Matthews.

"That's why I'm here, ain't it."

"Did you pick up your pain medication yet?" asked Dr. Matthews. In answer, Jeff held up the white bag and jiggled it.

The story was bleak no matter how it was told. In medical jargon, Jeff Stiller was a forty-five-year-old man with recurrent tonsil cancer metastatic to the lungs and liver being treated with paclitaxel and cetuximab who had severe narcotic addiction. In plain English, his life was a mess and would soon be over.

Six months ago, Jeff had been brought to the hospital from the homeless shelter in the horrible grip of narcotic withdrawal. The psychiatrist, Dr. Lawrence Issel, had been called in consultation and met with Jeff's younger sisters, Beth and Amy, to assemble the story.

"I think it started in grade school. Probably about sixth grade," began Amy. She looked at Beth, who nodded without making eye contact. "I remember he started to get into fights with the kids, especially the ones he thought acted smarter or higher class. He could be a bit of bully sometimes, but other times he was great. I remember once on the bus some of the other boys were picking on a small kid, throwing his hat back and forth. Jeff grabbed one of them by the throat and choked him until they gave the little kid back his hat. They never did that again. Then sometimes he would pick out some smartass kid who didn't really do anything to him and give him a tough time, for no reason that I could see."

"How did Jeff do in school?" asked Dr. Issel.

"By the time I really remember, he wasn't doing well," continued Amy. "That was probably junior high for him. Dad was drinking more and fighting with Mom. It would have been pretty hard for him to do any homework, even if he wanted to. Jeff wasn't stupid. He was always good at figuring things out, just not reading or studying."

"Was there violence in your home? Did your father ever beat your mother or Jeff?"

"No, they yelled a lot, but he never hit her. But he would go away for a few days at a time."

"I saw him hit Jeff once," said Beth. "He found Jeff with some pot and went crazy . . . Cuffed him on the side of the head. Told him never to use that stuff, that it would lead to more drugs."

"How did Jeff react?" asked Dr. Issel.

"He swore at Daddy, called him a hypocrite for drinking and a jerk, that kind of thing. But he didn't hit him back. I remember I was scared, because in high school Jeff was a strong guy, probably could have knock Daddy flat." Beth fell momentarily silent. "He was a good athlete, too, particularly baseball. Could hit the ball a mile and liked to play catcher . . ." Her voice trailed off as she became lost in memory.

"High school was really tough on Jeff," Amy continued. "Just before Daddy was killed, Jeff just wanted out of the house. Beth tried to help him, but it was hard for her, too. I was lucky in some ways because I was the youngest."

"Your father died around that time in a car crash, correct?" Dr. Issel asked, looking at his notes.

"When Jeff was a senior," agreed Amy. "It was ironic. He was such a drinker, and he was killed by a drunk driver . . . The one time he was stone cold sober."

"What happened to your family then?" asked Dr. Issel.

Amy answered. "Mom got very depressed for about a year, but she recovered. Jeff finished high school, but just barely. He hung around for a while, working odd jobs, then moved south. He had actually mellowed out and was good to be around. I missed him when he left. I was the lucky one because I was the youngest. Beth looked out for me until Mom was better. I hate to say it, but with Daddy gone, the house was quieter, and I could relax and study."

"Was Jeff using drugs when he left?" asked Dr. Issel.

Amy looked at Beth for an answer.

"Yeah, we both were," Beth replied slowly. "Jeff liked his pot, and I slipped in few of mother's pills. We also had a neighbor who had a supply of pain pills. We never let Amy get any, though. We kept her away from all that shit. I ended up in rehab, and you know about Jeff, but Amy made it."

Amy nodded. "It's true. They took care of me . . . And now I have a good husband and family."

RECEPTORS FOR PLEASURE AND PAIN.

We know pleasure and pain go together, as when John Mellencamp sings "Hurts So Good." Scientists know receptors in the brain determine both pleasure and pain.

Receptors are the locks of the cell. When the right key fits into the lock, a mechanism turns, and an action takes place. In medical terms, the right key is an "agonist." If a false key is in the lock, the mechanism jams, and nothing happens. The false key is an "antagonist." In the brain, there are locks, called mu-opioid receptors, for which the keys are narcotics. These mu-opioid receptors are in both the pleasure and the pain centers of our brain. When the narcotics fit into the receptors, pain goes away, and pleasure happens. The faster the narcotic arrive, the more intense the action. Injections are more potent than pills; smoking more potent than swallowing.[267]

Frequent use of narcotics produces problems. One problem is that with repeated use the receptors change and require more narcotics to produce the same result. In medical terms, this is "tolerance." The pain relief or pleasure of one pill now requires two pills. Two become three; three become an injection, then a bigger injection for the same response. If the narcotics suddenly stop, withdrawal symptoms of chills, vomiting, insomnia, and aching begin. In medical terms, this is "physical dependence," and it is prevented by slowly reducing the quantity of the narcotic.

A second problem is even more dangerous. With the repeated use of narcotics, other parts of the brain learn to associate these drugs with pleasure. These other parts of the brain may undergo physical changes which cause them to desire that narcotics be present. This is "narcotic addiction."[268] These physical changes in the brain may be facilitated using "gateway drugs"– compounds which lead to the use of more addictive drugs. For example, marijuana use often precedes abuse of other drugs and nicotine may prime the brain for cocaine addiction. [269] [270] Once these changes take place, reversal is very difficult.

Adolescent brains are the most vulnerable to addiction because they are the most malleable; the scientific term is "neuroplasticity." The reality is that 90 percent of Americans who become addicted to drugs started smoking, drinking, or using other drugs before age 18.[271]

Jeff spent his twenties in North Carolina, moving there for construction jobs building the new South. If you put in a good day and didn't complain, there was plenty of work. Malls and houses were springing up, the weather was great, and the money came and went easily. By his late twenties, Jeff had even moved in with Mary, a spunky emergency room nurse who insisted he toe the line. Marijuana and hard liquor were out; beer was okay if he kept it under control. He could not give up the cigarettes, even though she made him smoke outside the apartment. Jeff played catcher on the local softball team and had even started to help with Little League, where he bonded with the surly boys who tended to fight in the dugout. For three years, he was happy.

The fall had come out of nowhere on a beautiful day with a crystal blue sky. They were working on the roof of the house when for some reason Jeff could never remember, he slipped. He awoke in the emergency room taped to the backboard. Mary had been on duty when they brought him in, a memory that stayed with her forever. It was a miracle he had survived, the doctors said. She knew it was true because she saw the x-rays of his shattered frame. Mary's agony was worsened by the knowledge she was pregnant, a revelation she shared with Jeff as he lay immobilized some days later.

Jeff had suffered fractures of his spine, both legs, and ribs. His first hospitalization included a blood clot, pneumonia, antibiotics, a drug reaction leading to peeling of his skin, and pain. Terrible pain. The staff did the best they could to keep him comfortable; no one doubted that he needed the narcotics.

MORPHEUS: GOD OF NARCOTICS.

At the beginning of the nineteenth century, seventeen-year-old Freidrich Wilhelm Adam Serturner was an apprentice in a modest pharmacy in Panderhorn, Germany. In addition to his many duties, Serturner was attempting to chemically extract the alkaline part of opium. In 1803 Serturner completed his apprenticeship and moved to nearby Einbeck, where he succeeded in isolating a crystal with ten times the effect of opium. He named his creation after Morpheus, the Greek God of Dreams.[272] Although it took over a decade before his accomplishment was widely recognized, Serturner had brought to the world its premier narcotic: morphine.[273]

Prior to Serturner's work, medicinal control of pain had relied heavily upon opium, a weaker narcotic whose name in Greek means "juice of the poppy." Although the origin of opium is debated, it became particularly popular in Islamic cultures where alcohol use was discouraged. Cultivating, manufacturing, and distributing opium facilitated the expansion of the British and American empires and led to the Opium Wars with China.[274] While opium was a long-standing medicinal agent for pain, diarrhea, and anxiety, the various preparations varied widely in effect. For example, Laudanum, a popular recipe of Serturner's time, consisted of raw opium of various purity dissolved in 50 percent alcohol. Serturner's extraction of morphine was thus significant for both its powerful pain relief properties and ability to be synthesized in a consistent formulation.

In 1818, Serturner's discovery was widely publicized when French physician Francois Magendie wrote of its use to treat pain. Morphine became increasingly available when commercial production began with the pioneers of the pharmaceutical industry like Heinrich Emanuel Merck in Darmstadt, who was building Merck Pharmaceuticals.[275] Although morphine was first given orally, the development of the hypodermic needle in the 1850s by Charles Gabriel Pravaz and Alexander Wood allowed rapid administration for severe pain, particularly trauma. A series of European wars probably known only to scholars of that period expanded the use of the drug: Crimean War (1854-56), Prussian-Danish War (1864), Prussian-Australian War (1866) and the Franco-Prussian War (1871-2).[276] In the United States, the Civil War did the same.

Serturner's selection of Morpheus as the namesake for his discovery was prophetic. Morpheus appears in the Roman Ovid's book of mythological poems, *Metamorphoses*. In one romantic tragedy, Ceyx, the King of Thessaly, was drowned on a voyage. At home, his wife Alcyone sensed something was wrong and pleaded to the Goddess

Juno for aid. Juno, in turn, sent her messenger Iris to Somnus, the God of Sleep, ordering him to tell Alcyone the sad news and offer her comfort. Somnus chose his son Morpheus for the job. The winged Morpheus flew to Alcyone, appeared to her in the form of her dead husband Ceyx and told her of his death. Unfortunately, Morpheus' soothing effect was short-lived as Alcyone soon committed suicide by throwing herself into the sea. At the conclusion of this sad story, the benevolent Gods did allow Alycone and Ceyx to metamorphose (hence the title) into halcyon birds and fly away together.[277]

Just as the comfort which Morpheus gave to Alcyone was brief, and the long-term result was tragic, so it is with Serturner's creation. Morphine is an effective way to relieve acute pain, yet it comes with a grave potential for long-term addiction. While addiction to opium had been recognized for years, the increased danger with morphine was not immediately evident. Serturner himself may have become addicted to morphine as he apparently underwent some personality changes during his later life, although the historical record is very incomplete. Certainly, he would have been at significant risk given his young age, the tendency in that era to self-test new medical discoveries, and the ignorance of the problem.[278] These risks of morphine addiction were also mythologically foreshadowed when Ovid described Morpheus' home as a cave in a land of perpetual darkness, shrouded in fog. At the bottom of the cave flows the River Lethe, also known as the River of Forgetfulness, which separates the living world from the underworld and whose waters produce "a draught of long oblivion."[279] In the story of Ceyx and Alcyone, the messenger Iris nearly succumbed to the stupor of the place and fled to escape.[280] Others have reported that Morpheus slept in a bed of poppy, in a dangerous land guarded by a gate and terrible monsters.[281] Whatever the image, with morphine's power comes danger.

Although the ensuing years stripped Jeff of his memories, his bleak life after the fall was recalled by Amy and Beth. Dr. Issel summarized.

"It's a sadly familiar story. Jeff left the acute care hospital, spent a period in rehab, then went home with his girlfriend. He was left disabled from his fall, permanently unemployable, and in constant pain. Given his history, it is not surprising he became addicted to narcotics. That started a long spiral downward. He became socially isolated, outcast from the health care system, and accused of being a drug seeker. He became increasingly angry. His girlfriend stuck with him for a long time, but the pressures of her own life and their young son were eventually too much. Finally, when he had trouble with the law, she sent him home to live with his mother. It made sense since the Medicaid services in New York State are much better than in North Carolina. But it did leave Mary with guilt, her son without a father, and Jeff without a family of his own. It is the sad story of addiction."

THE SPREAD OF NARCOTIC ADDICTION.

Addiction to morphine and other narcotics in the United States expanded rapidly in the last half of the nineteenth century—the period following the Civil War. The degree to which battlefield narcotic use contributed to the rise in addiction after the War is debated.[282] Surgeons liberally administered narcotics to relieve pain from brutal injuries, amputations, and infections; many used the newly invented syringe and needle for injection. What is less well known is that morphine and opium were also used to control diarrhea, a common and devastating problem given the poor sanitation of the time. The constipating effects of narcotics, today advertised on television as a delicate problem with a new treatment, were used to advantage in this situation. With well over a million wounded or dead from battle and disease, there was no shortage of suffering, and the net result was that many soldiers received narcotics. While some certainly became addicted, the frequently used descriptions of narcotic addiction as the "army disease" or "soldier's disease" are incomplete. From the individual veteran's viewpoint, alcohol addiction and the curse of post-traumatic stress were probably greater problems.[283] [284] From a national perspective, historian David Courtwright notes there were many additional contributors to the rise in narcotic addiction.[285] Most addicts were women, many prescribed chronic morphine for conditions which would not be considered appropriate for narcotics today, such as menstrual and back pain. Many non-prescription patent medications containing narcotics were advertised as cures for everyday ailments and found in any well-equipped medical chest.[286] Addiction was available to everyone.

Morphine was only the first of several new and powerfully addictive drugs introduced in this era. In 1860, a doctoral student named Albert Nieman completed the thesis assigned to him by German chemist Friedrich Wohler when he extracted cocaine from coca leaves. Cocaine was a blockbuster; used as a local anesthetic agent in eye surgery for cataract extraction in place of ether, which could raise blood pressure and cause nausea. It was widely mixed in drinks, extracted with alcohol, and included in secret recipes like Coca-Cola. Park-Davis in Detroit was a large producer of cocaine and extensively detailed physicians on this wonder drug.[287] In the 1870s, Bayer scientist Heinrich Dresser synthesized a compound with a "heroic" ability to relieve pain: heroin.[288] Beginning in 1898, heroin was marketed as a cough suppressant. Even as these drugs were widely used and many people addicted, physicians simply did not understand the problems. It was not until the end of the nineteenth century that the physiology of withdrawal symptoms was well described.[289] When morphine addiction was recognized, heroin and cocaine were proposed as treatments, until doctors realized their even greater addictive potential. Morphine then became the treatment for cocaine and heroin addiction. In this confused and poorly regulated period of American medicine, well-meaning doctors readily administered narcotics to their patients and often themselves.

The problem of physician self-administration of narcotics deserves particular attention. William Halsted, one of America's preeminent surgeons, was an addict.[290] Halsted graduated from Yale and then Columbia College of Physicians in 1876. Following an internship at

Bellevue Hospital in New York, he studied the latest European surgical techniques in Vienna. This era was the "age of surgery" following the discovery of anesthesia in 1846 by Boston dentist William Morton and the introduction of germ theory in 1862 by Lister in London, which saw previously impossible surgeries. Halsted returned from Europe to Bellevue where he rapidly gained a reputation as a brilliant surgeon. It was in New York that Halsted also began experimenting with the use of cocaine as an anesthetic agent. He rapidly became addicted and disgraced when, in a drug induced state, he abandoned a patient in need of emergency surgery. After treatment in an asylum, Halsted was moved to Baltimore in 1886 by William Welch, the physician hired to create the new Johns Hopkins Hospital. Halsted became the Chief of Surgery. Despite his continued struggles with addiction to cocaine and morphine, Halsted made tremendous contributions, pioneering the use of strict operating room cleanliness and developing meticulous suturing techniques. He introduced the radical mastectomy, an extensive surgical removal of the breast and surrounding tissues to treat cancer.[291] Halsted also established a demanding surgical training program, leading to Johns Hopkins being the model cited in the famous Flexner Report on medical education. There is interesting speculation about the degree to which Halsted's battle with addiction furthered his compulsiveness and demanding personality, thus shaping the course of surgery at John Hopkins and hence America.[292] Possibly these forces also contributed to his development of the extensive radical mastectomy. At the very least, Halsted's demons caused him the horrible personal anguish universally found in an addict's story.

"Mom took good care of Jeff," said Amy. "He went to treatment, sometimes. She kept track of his medications and made sure he got to his appointments. It was a full-time job but gave her something to do. He lived with her in our old house, and she liked the company. It wasn't always easy. He was a handful, particularly when he got angry. He was short tempered and could turn on you pretty quickly."

"That's for sure. I had my own problems," said Beth. "I was in and out of rehab . . . Mainly alcohol, but some pills, too. I tried to talk to him about it, but he said we were different. His problems were from the fall; mine were my own. He always blamed that fall."

TWENTIETH-CENTURY ADDICTS: CRIMINALS OR PATIENTS?

A hundred years after Serturner's synthesis of morphine, the early 1900s saw narcotic addiction in the United States become a major issue with themes and policy decisions which have influenced successive generations to the present.

One theme which emerged during this era was that the enthusiastic application of addictive drugs for medical purposes leads to widespread addiction. At the turn of the century, the prescription of morphine by physicians to patients in higher social classes had created numerous addicts. Among the working poor, heroin pills were crushed and inhaled, producing rapid highs followed by profound lows. This cycle was repeated in the 1960s with LSD, the 1990s with OxyContin, and now with medical marijuana, each era seemingly forgetting the lessons of the last. In the early 1900s, the overlap between drug, alcohol, and tobacco addiction also became increasingly evident. Later these addictions would be linked in other ways: morphine and LSD were used to treat alcohol addiction, and narcotic addiction treatments were modeled after alcohol programs.[293]

A second theme exposed in the early 1900s was that the treatment of narcotic addiction is difficult, expensive, and unpopular. The medical science of supplying addicts with decreasing doses of narcotics and using long-term maintenance treatments was not well understood. Outpatient treatment of addiction was illegal, and addicts were confined to hospital wards or asylums, linking addiction with severe mental illness.[294] Today we understand more about the physiology of addiction, yet treatment remains a difficult problem requiring long-term therapy. The options for many (or most) addicts remain limited or nonexistent, particularly outpatient facilities. The early linking of addiction to the chronically disenfranchised mentally ill has meant both are underserved by government and the private sector; there are as few fund-raising "Runs for the Drug Addicted" as "Runs for the Mentally Ill."

Perhaps most importantly, the early 1900s saw the first wide-spread debate over whether narcotic addiction is a medical or criminal problem. The debate included the introduction of the sensational-ized "cycle of addiction," which emphasized criminal behavior and the dangers to society, particularly of lower social class or minority group addicts. The result was that addiction in America became a criminal problem requiring a legal response. This policy decision was different from other nations and had profound consequences.

Two laws passed in 1914 illustrate the nation's first attempt to repress narcotic addiction using the legal system. On the state level, the New York Legislature passed the Boylan Law (or Towns-Boylan Act) which regulated the prescription of habit forming drugs by phy-sicians by requiring the use of specific forms and record keeping.[295] The law was named after Senator Boylan, who himself credited it to Charles B. Towns, a drug crusader who had developed a system to treat addiction and promised a cure in a few days.[296] The law was widely interpreted by physicians, pharmacists, and law enforcement as forbidding the prescription of narcotics to addicts. On a national level, Congress passed the Harrison Narcotic Control Act of 1914, a tax and revenue act. Although the intent of Congress was probably not to limit the prescription of narcotics by physicians, this interpre-tation emerged in a series of Supreme Court cases which effectively criminalized the supplying of narcotics to addicts.[297] Neither law had a provision for allowing the treatment of addicts with tapering doses of narcotics or maintenance treatments.[298] The enforcement of these laws by the Treasury Department's newly minted Federal Bureau of Narcotics further limited the individual physician's ability and willingness to prescribe narcotics to addicts. In fact, the Director of the Bureau, Harry Anslinger, proclaimed physicians were both addicts and a source of addiction.[299] Addicts could only legally be given narcotics within a hospital ward, a position endorsed by the American Medical Association.[300] Since there were few inpatient treatment facilities, most of which had marginal effectiveness, treatment options were scarce. From this starting point, the United States entered a half century of expanding restrictions culminating in the 1956 Narcotics Control Act, which imposed a minimum five-year sentence for the first offense of selling narcotics.[301]

The criminalization of narcotic addiction in America had multiple effects. On the positive side, these laws reduced the medical use of narcotics and thus the number of new addicts created by doctors, although by the time these laws were being enforced physician awareness was already accomplishing the same goal.[302] The introduction of restrictive narcotic laws decreased the use of some specific drugs like cocaine and heroin. On the negative side, these laws certainly resulted in the chronic undertreatment of cancer pain and the suffering described in the 1980s by the World Health Organization and other medical authorities. In addition, addicts were denied treatment by these laws, promoting both the illegal narcotic industry and corresponding law enforcement response. The American experiment with Prohibition which produced widespread illegal alcohol was repeated with drug legislation as efforts to control narcotics encouraged criminal suppliers. In 1922, *The Druggists Circular*, a pharmacist trade publication, described the Boylan Law as a misguided effort which forced panicked New York drug addicts to turn to illicit suppliers and resulted in a reign of terror.[303] In later years, jails were filled with both addicts and low-level suppliers while worldwide criminal organizations grew. These restrictive laws were also used to repress minorities. In the 1920s this included labeling Chinese Americans as opium users and black Americans as cocaine

addicts with correspondingly terrifying images.[304] America's criminalization of narcotic use over this time contrasted with the British experience, where a much more powerful medical establishment promoted
a model which allowed prescription of narcotics to treat addiction.

Changes in America's narcotics laws and attitudes occurred in the
1960s, an era forever associated with drugs. LSD, one of the sixties'
most recognizable drugs, was given the same medical introduction into
society as morphine, cocaine, and heroin. LSD had been discovered
in 1938 by Sandoz scientists W.A. Stoll and Albert Hoffman, the latter credited with the first "trips" which included his dramatic four-
mile bicycle ride through kaleidoscopic colors.[305] LSD was used by
psychiatrists to treat disorders ranging from alcoholism to depression
to schizophrenia and promoted in the 1960s by Harvard professors
Timothy Leary and Richard Alpert for its mind opening properties.
The antiestablishment turmoil of the period aided the spread of LSD
and then heroin into the young, white middle class. The Vietnam War
contributed to addiction, causalities, and suffering in all social classes.
America's response to drug use and addiction in the 1960s became as
confusing and multifaceted as the time itself. On the one hand, treatment and the medical aspects of drug addiction were acknowledged
in the 1966 Narcotics Addiction and Rehabilitation Act, the Supreme
Court's recognition of addiction as an illness, and the acceptance of
the methadone maintenance. In part, this shift may have been due to
heroin use in the white middle class which challenged the image of it as
an inner-city ghetto problem. On the other hand, as the decade ended
the 1970 Controlled Substances Act created the system of narcotic
drug control which remains in effect today. Drugs were listed in five
schedules from most dangerous (Schedule I: heroin, LSD) to least dangerous (Schedule V: cough syrups) and differing penalties were outlined for addicts and suppliers within the groups. Marijuana was first
included in Schedule I with heroin and LSD. [306] The Act set the stage
for President Nixon's 1971 "War on Drugs" which increased penalties;
described as a strike at his hippie and black enemies.

During the last quarter of the twentieth century, the balance between treatment and repression vacillated as the Carter years promoted some tolerance, the Reagan years more restriction, and the Clinton years a moderate approach. By the end of the twentieth century, the severe criminalization of addiction which began the century had ended, although the debate over the proper response to narcotics continued. Yet the end of the twentieth century also brought a new and greater threat. For rising out of Morpheus' cave in the land of perpetual darkness was a cousin who would give new meaning to the phrase "a draught of long oblivion." The same forces that produced heroin addiction at the start of the century unleashed the era of oxy addiction at its end, an epidemic propelled by parts of the new muscular pharmaceutical industry.

Amy continued Jeff's story. "Mom died about ten years ago. Well, you know that, since Dr. Matthews took care of her. Lung cancer. At first, Jeff did okay in the house alone, but then he went downhill. He got in trouble with the bills and took in some renters. They were trouble, too. Eventually, it all led to the police and Jeff ended up in jail for selling drugs . . . Oxy was his favorite."

TWENTY-FIRST-CENTURY ADDICTION: THE KILLER FROM PURDUE.

The introduction of OxyContin in 1995 added a devastating new dimension to narcotic addiction in the United States. Oxycodone had been developed in Germany in 1918 as part of the search for a less addictive narcotic. It was a variation of opium called "semisynthetic," meaning the molecule was part natural and part manufactured. In the 1980s, as interest in treating chronic pain grew, a long-acting (or time-released) version of oxycodone was developed, brand name OxyContin. The theory was OxyContin would slowly release narcotic into the system, and thus the patient would receive long-acting pain relief with steady low doses which would not encourage addiction. A few inadequate clinical reports were used to support the idea.[307] Once again, the medical system adopted a treatment without complete testing, ignoring the lessons of the past. Just like heroin pills at the start of the century, OxyContin could be crushed to produce a rapid high. In some ways, it was the same old story: a new narcotic is introduced with great enthusiasm resulting in new addicts, more pain and suffering, followed by a medical and legal response. But this chapter was different. When one of America's pharmaceutical giants threw its full force behind the marketing of OxyContin, the addictive potential multiplied. Morpheus was on steroids.

Purdue Pharmaceuticals' promotion of OxyContin caused immeasurable suffering. As reported in 2003 by the United States General Accounting Office (GAO), never before had such a coordinated advertising blitz taken place for a drug with so much potential for abuse. In its unprecedented promotion, Purdue expanded and incentivized its sales force, hired physicians, sponsored twenty thousand presentations to health care professionals, financially supported pain management groups and even JACHO, the agency hired to inspect health care facilities like hospitals. Purdue specifically targeted general practitioners and encouraged them to use OxyContin as a maintenance treatment for patients with moderate to severe non-cancer pain. The results were impressive. In 1996, physicians wrote 316,000 prescriptions for OxyContin costing $44 million. By 2002 it was 7,200,000 prescriptions costing $1.5 billion.[308] As Purdue unleashed the OxyContin epidemic, the graph of sales, hospital admissions, and deaths due to opioids rose in parallel.[309] Initially hard hit were the rural regions of the Appalachian states where poverty made the profits on the sale of the diverted drug ("Hillbilly Heroin") especially enticing.[310] The epidemic of addiction fueled by OxyContin soon spread to all age groups in both rural and urban areas. Adolescent and young adults were the most common nonmedical users, overdose deaths were most common in the forty-five- to fifty-year-olds, and the greatest increase in opioid mortality was in the fifty-five- to sixty-four-year-olds, the targets of the original Purdue campaign.[311]

The initial response to Purdue's actions was pitiful. The FDA cited the company for minor advertising violations. In a well-publicized plea agreement in 2003, Purdue pleaded guilty to a felony charge of misbranding OxyContin and paid $600 million in federal criminal and civil penalties, a small portion of the $2.8 billion in revenue OxyContin brought in over that period.[312] Some additional state lawsuits have been settled for smaller amounts while others are ongoing. None of these actions addressed the epidemic. From the time of Purdue's payout until 2011, the use of prescription opioids doubled while the number of high-intensity users continued to rise—those most likely to progress to heroin use. By 2013, over sixteen thousand deaths were due to prescription opioids. Treatment programs remain underfunded and underutilized. The Centers for Disease Control and Prevention (CDC) has declared the epidemic an emergency. States have begun to require the use of narcotic registries and electronic prescribing. The small ray of hope is that the "new starts" of addicts are slightly decreased, hopefully signaling changes in prescribing patterns and public expectations.[313]

The themes seen with America's experience with morphine, cocaine, heroin, and OxyContin have been repeated multiple times: addictive drugs are enthusiastically introduced for medicinal use, addiction develops, treatments are limited, the problems of social disruption and criminal activity lead to legislative and legal responses which generate more issues. The American definition of drug addiction has included illness, prejudice, moral weakness, and criminal behavior in variable proportions. Today is no different. In addition to our pharmaceutically driven opioid epidemic, marijuana is being introduced for dubious medical reasons and will inevitably produce more addicts, social disruption, and probably more criminal activity. Our current politicians define drug addiction using imagery of cartels threatening our borders mixed with tearful renditions of agony in their own circles. Addiction remains difficult to treat while programs are limited and underfunded. And many Americans continue to live in Morpheus' land of perpetual darkness, shrouded in fog.

Amy sat quietly for a moment, crying softly.

"About five years ago, maybe a year before Jeff got cancer, we couldn't take it anymore. The house was in my name, and so we were responsible for what was going on there. We had to sell it. My husband took the money and set it up so every month Jeff got some and there was no way anyone could touch it. It was enough for him to rent a small apartment."

"How did that work?" asked Dr. Issel.

"At first, not good," replied Amy. "When he started getting the mouth pain, before we knew what it was, it was a terrible time. He would go to the emergency room, and they would think he was drug seeking. The sad thing was, even when they looked in his mouth, they couldn't see the cancer. It was hidden at the very back of his tongue. So, Jeff was taking more drugs to ease the pain. He was in and out of trouble with the landlord. He was just about to kick him out when Jeff got diagnosed. The poor guy, his wife had died from cancer, and he felt sorry for Jeff."

HEAD AND NECK CANCER.

Most cancers of the mouth, tongue, tonsils, sinuses, throat, or voice box start from the "squamous" cells which line these regions. Squamous cell cancer of the tongue would be an example. Squamous comes from the Latin squama which means scale because under the microscope these cells look like the scales covering a fish. These squamous cell cancers are very different from other cancers in the head and neck area that derive from entirely different cells, such as cancers of the brain or the thyroid.

Once the squamous cells become cancerous, they usually form a heaped-up ulcer and invade into the tissues below. As they do this, they often spread to the nearby lymph nodes. Thus, a person might present with a growing ulcer on their tongue and a hard and swollen lymph node in their neck. Often the person or their doctor first notice the swollen lymph node, and later the primary source is found when a complete examination of the mouth, sinuses, and back of the throat is done using a flexible scope.

Squamous cell cancers of the head and neck are often caused by tobacco, either smoked or chewed. The toxins in the tobacco damage the cells and start the vicious chain of events which lead to cancer. Alcohol use seems to propel the process. Over the past twenty years, scientists found the human papilloma virus (HPV) is an important cause of these cancers, particularly in nonsmokers. While HPV infection is common and does not cause most people any serious effects, some subtypes of the virus can infect the cells of the mouth in ways which may start the cancerous cascade. Other factors, such as the genetic makeup of the person and other viral infections, play roles in this process. HPV infection is best known as the cause of cervical cancer, and vaccination programs to prevent that cancer will also prevent some head and neck cancers.

The treatment of a squamous cancer of the head and neck region is complex. If the cancer is small, surgery is done if the cosmetic result will be reasonable. Radiation is also used in this situation. The cure rate with either treatment is equal and quite high. If the cancer is large, not amenable to a reasonable surgery, or spread into multiple lymph nodes, then radiation and chemotherapy together are preferred. Obviously, many patients will fall in between these extremes, making the judgments of the surgeon and radiation oncologist critical. Advances in surgical techniques, radiation, and chemotherapy constantly change the balance between these options.

When the choice of treatment is radiation and chemotherapy, the patient faces a predictable ordeal. The radiation treatments are usually given daily over a period of six to eight weeks. The treated area is the site of the primary cancer and the nearby lymph nodes. The first few weeks are usually smooth, but by the third or fourth week, the lining of the mouth and throat are burned and inflamed. Swallowing often becomes painful; solids are usually impossible and even liquids difficult. Many patients have a feeding tube inserted into the stomach to maintain their nutrition. Chemotherapy treatments add to the misery. The drug cisplatin is often used; producing nausea and fatigue and requiring careful monitoring. An alternative to cisplatin is the antibody cetuximab; it produces a rash, often worse on the face or neck. With either choice, by the end of the two months most patients are miserable and depleted, having mouth pain and losing weight. It takes many months to recover. Hopefully, the results are worth the struggle.

"And after the cancer was diagnosed? How did Jeff do?" asked Dr. Issel.

Jeff's treatment was seven weeks of radiation daily, Monday through Friday. The base of his tongue, mouth, and both sides of his neck received radiation. On the first day and three weeks later he received a dose of the chemotherapy cisplatin. The staff had been worried about Jeff's ability to get through this very difficult treatment. The radiation produced terrible burning of his mouth while the chemotherapy made him tired and nauseous. After three weeks, he could not eat. Fortunately, Jeff had agreed to the placement of a feeding tube which went directly into his stomach, into which he put can after can of tasteless nutritional broth.

"He did really well, considering what he went through," answered Amy. "In some ways, Jeff was better with the treatment, like it gave him something to do."

Beth nodded. "He even was careful with his meds . . . Didn't abuse them or anything. He tried really hard. His mouth was really burned from the radiation, and he couldn't eat. It looked terrible, but for some reason he could stand that pain."

"He particularly liked the oncology nurses," added Amy. "They were good to him. I think one of them reminded him a bit of Mary."

"Did Jeff ever try to contact Mary?" asked Dr. Issel.

After a brief silence, Amy responded.

"Once, early after he moved back with Mom. She basically told him never to call again."

"That bitch," added Beth. "She only wanted him when he was fun."

"Well, it's hard to blame her sometimes," counseled Amy. "When he got here, he was more than a handful, particularly when he was doing drugs. And she was trying to raise the baby. I did call her when Jeff got the cancer."

"How did she respond?" asked Dr. Issel.

"At first, she seemed mad that I called, but then she calmed down and asked if she could call me back. She did a few days later. She told me she was sorry for Jeff. That she had once loved him and remembered the fun they had. But those days were gone, a memory of an old life. The accident and his drugs had almost cost her everything: her nursing license, home, and even the baby. She had made a new life. She was still working as a nurse, had a husband, and her son was in high school."

Amy paused.

"She told me that her son was raised by her husband as his own. She said he was a good boy, with Jeff's fun side but none of the anger. The boy knew his father had left, but they never spoke of him. She told me she could not let anything about Jeff back into their life, that it was better to let it stay buried. She asked me not to call again."

"Did you ever speak to Jeff about the call?" asked Dr. Issel.

Amy wiped her eyes. "No, I never . . . Once Jeff told me he wished he could see the boy so he could show him what it was like to fuck up your life. That would make him stay out of trouble, he said. Even then, I couldn't tell him."

"How did Jeff do after the treatment finished?" continued Dr. Issel.

Amy picked up the story. "At first he was okay. But the further away the treatment got, the more he seemed to fall back into his old ways. The same things. More drugs, crack, the wrong friends, trouble with the law, back in jail. Finally, when his building was sold, the new landlord threw him out."

"Personally, I think the old landlord sold because he couldn't deal with Jeff, but he didn't want to throw him out either," added Beth.

"He couldn't stay with either of us," finished Amy. "We hated to see it, but he ended up in the shelter. He would vanish for days. Thank God it was a mild winter that year and he didn't freeze to death . . . Sometimes I think maybe it would have been better than this. I hear that's a peaceful way to go." Amy started crying again, and Beth took over.

"Last year sucked. He would show up at the shelter after being away for a few weeks, stay a while, then go God knows where. To Albany, I think. Or maybe Troy. When he got back there this time he was coughing so bad, they took him to the emergency room. They were worried he might infect everyone with TB, they said. He looked like sh—well awful. I guess you know the rest. The cancer is back, and the doctors say he doesn't have long . . ."

It was true. When Jeff came from the shelter to the hospital emergency room, he was vomiting and coughing. The staff feared he might have active tuberculosis, and put him in isolation until a CT scan showed that it was cancer, spread to his lungs and liver. Withdrawal came next, and Jeff was kept sedated while the demons inside him raged, demanding more drugs, infuriated when they were not delivered.

It was during this admission that Beth and Amy had told Dr. Issel of Jeff's story.

"Here we have enough pain to go around for everyone," he noted to Dr. Matthews sadly. A few days later, it was Dr. Matthew's turn to sit with the sisters.

"Jeff's cancer has spread to his liver and lungs," began Dr. Matthews. "We cannot cure the cancer, the most we can do is to attempt to shrink and control it. We call this palliative treatment, meaning we are trying to prolong his life and make him more comfortable, but not give him bad side effects. The treatment is a weekly dose of chemotherapy called paclitaxel and an antibody treatment called cetuximab. The treatment can be done in the office each week. It takes about two hours, and the main side effects are fatigue and a skin rash. First, he would need to recover from his pneumonia, get his medications stabilized, and find a place to stay. And, of course, he would need to agree."

Amy spoke, "Neither of us can take him. I'm sorry, but I can't bring him into the house with my children. Beth can't do it either."

"That's all we need, him with me as I'm trying to stay out of my own trouble," agreed Beth.

"Our social work team tells me the shelter will take him back as long as he is not acutely ill," replied Dr. Matthews.

"How long?" asked Amy. "How long does he have? To live, I mean."

"It's hard to know, but usually six to twelve months. Sometimes the treatments work well and the time is longer," replied Dr. Mathews.

"Is it worth it, then?" asked Amy. "All this treatment?"

"That is a very personal question. Some patients opt to go directly to hospice care, but most people want to try the treatment. Since occasionally the chemo and the cetuximab can be very effective, they want to see if it will work for them."

CETUXIMAB.

Once a squamous cell cancer of the head and neck has recurred after the first treatment, the prognosis is poor. If the cancer is found again in the same area, more surgery or radiation can occasionally be an option. If the cancer is spread, chemotherapy, antibodies, or immune therapy become the treatment, with the goal of prolonging life and easing symptoms. Cetuximab (brand name Erbitux) is one of the antibodies.

Antibodies are proteins produced by immune cells called B-lymphocytes to fight infections. Antibodies have two ends. One end will attach to a specific protein (hopefully on the enemy) while the opposite end will then attract other immune cells to attack and destroy the enemy. The immune system produces specific antibodies for each infection. This specificity is important to keep the antibody from targeting normal cells for destruction. Vaccinations ensure the immune system is ready to produce the desired antibodies when an infection strikes. Beginning in the 1970s, antibodies were made by scientists against a target they would select using a remarkable technology called "hybridoma." In this procedure, mice are injected with the target, and their B-cells make antibodies against the target. The mice B-cells are then electrically fused with myeloma cancer cells in the lab. The fused B-cells/myeloma cells grow forever and produce antibodies against the target which can be purified and used in the lab or clinic.

In the 1980s, scientists John Mendelsohn and Gordon Sato at the University of California San Diego's Cancer Center proposed making antibodies against a specific target on cancer cells called the EGFR (Epidermal Growth Factor Receptor). The EGF Receptors are a group of related "locks" on the outside of cells which can stimulate growth when the proper "key" attaches—the keys are called "receptor ligands." Mendelsohn and Sato proposed that antibodies against the EGFR might slow cancer growth, perhaps by interfering with the key entering the lock. In scientific terms, they were hoping to block the receptor ligand. To summarize a decade of hard lab work, they made a monoclonal antibody called C225, later known as cetuximab or its brand name Erbitux.[314]

In 1993, the University of California licensed cetuximab to a company called ImClone which began a clinical trial in patients with widespread colon cancer with the goal to obtain FDA approval. Unfortunately, ImClone's key study of cetuximab was flawed; many patients were not appropriately evaluated, and the doses and administration of cetuximab and the companion drug irinotecan were not well controlled. ImClone's glowing reports to investors were also flawed. Ultimately, the FDA refused to approve cetuximab based upon this study, and ImClone's founder and CEO Sam Waksal went to jail.

Later clinical trials proved cetuximab was effective. When the antibody attaches to the EGFR, some cancer cells die while others may become more sensitive to chemotherapy. The treatment does have some side effects. Particularly annoying is an acne-like skin rash. As it turns out, skin cells have high levels of the EGFR. Fortunately, the rash usually fades when the treatment is temporarily stopped and usually the cetuximab can later be resumed. Cetuximab is particularly useful for the treatment of colon cancer or head and neck cancers.

Over the next week, Jeff recovered enough to understand. His answer was direct.

"Cut it out. Split me open and just cut the fucker out."

"I wish we could," replied Dr. Matthews, "but the cancer is in many small pieces, and we could never get them all without removing your liver and lungs. So, the chemotherapy is the only choice."

"Well, I ain't givin up. I'll take the fucking stuff. Let's go."

Organizing Jeff's treatment was not easy. One problem was Jeff's scarred veins, the result of years of drug abuse. The answer was a port, preceded by a lecture from one of the inpatient unit's oncology nurses, Kim Johnson.

"Listen, Jeff," she said, standing by the edge of his bed. "You need this port to get the chemotherapy, but everyone is nervous that you will use it to inject drugs. "

"I won't."

"I remember how you did with the first treatment, so I believe you. But if you do, you die. The shelter will throw you out. You will end up in jail. And you will suffer in the prison sick ward where the cancer will finish you off. With this, you got a chance. You understand that?"

Jeff nodded. "Where'd you get your bedside manner?" he asked.

"My mother is a nurse at Comstock. I know what it's like inside. So, you better not end up there. Got it?"

Jeff nodded again, "Yes, ma'am."

A second problem was narcotics. Again, Kim delivered the ultimatum.

"You again?" Jeff said when she walked into the room. "Look at this . . ." He pulled down his gown to show the new port. "I didn't screw it up yet."

"Very nice," Kim replied. "But now I am here to talk about narcotics. The shelter cannot supervise narcotics, so we need to arrange for you to get your pain meds. Here is the plan. You will pick them up at the hospital pharmacy each week before your treatment. That way we avoid the problems with your local pharmacy. With your record, they won't supply you anyway. If you lose them, you are out of luck. Done. If you use any more than the allowed amount, you are out of luck. Done. Got it?"

Jeff nodded.

"You know what happens if you mess up with the narcotics?"

Jeff nodded. "I die like a dog in Comstock."

"Right," she grinned. "Seriously, I know you can do it. You did it before."

The third problem was cost. Cetuximab is only available as the brand name product Erbitux, at a price of $3600 per dose. The paclitaxel was generic, so the purchase price was $350. Since Jeff was an inpatient and insured by Medicare and Medicaid, the hospital was paid a fixed amount each day which would not cover the cost of the cetuximab. Once Jeff was discharged and treated in the outpatient oncology unit, his insurance would pay the price of the drugs with a modest markup. Dr. Matthews was called by the administrator responsible for finance.

"Is this something this patient will need regularly as an inpatient? We could take quite a beating on it if it continues. It would be better for us if he could get it as an outpatient."

"Hopefully, it will be a one-time inpatient treatment, then he will go to the shelter," answered Dr. Matthews.

"In that case, I can approve it this time."

The pharmaceutical company made money; the distributor took a small percentage, and the hospital broke even when Jeff was treated as an outpatient. Jeff paid nothing. The taxpayers, who had funded the basic science, paid the bill to Medicare and Medicaid.

Amy had come into the hospital to sit with Jeff during his first treatment.

"It's the Martha Stewart drug," Kim told Amy as she started the cetuximab.

"Martha Stewart?" asked Amy. "What's she got to do with it?"

"Well, when they were first testing the drug, it failed. Martha Stewart heard it from a friend, the company's owner. She knew the stock price would go way down, so she sold her stock."

"She got arrested, right?" asked Amy.

"Yeah, they call it insider trading, when you know something before the public does and buy or sell stocks. It's illegal."

"Pretty stupid to go to jail for that."

"Yeah, well it was really stupid of her," continued Kim. "First of all, the amount she saved was small coin for her, only a hundred thousand or so. But the real killer was the drug was good. They had just screwed up the testing, so the FDA held it up. But once they did the clinical trial the right way, the drug was approved, and the stock went up. Martha never needed to sell. She really went to jail for nothing."

Jeff had heard their conversation.

"Well, we got that in common, me and Martha."

The treatment had few side effects. After three months, the scans showed Jeff's cancer shrank slightly. The routine seemed to help him focus, and he moved out of the shelter into an apartment. Recent scans had shown more shrinkage.

Dr. Issel updated Dr. Matthews on Jeff's addiction. "I think he is doing as well as we could hope. His oxycodone usage on his maintenance methadone is modest, and he seems to be reliable. Equally important, he seems engaged in the lives of his sisters to the degree that is possible."

"His cancer is under control right now, too," replied Dr. Matthews.

"So today is good," continued Dr. Issel. "Sometimes that's all we can ask."

Today, as Dr. Matthews finished his exam, there was a knock on the door. Amy had arrived to sit with Jeff during his treatment.

"I'm so sorry," she explained. "My son had his physical exam, and we ran late." She set down a bag which contained clean laundry for Jeff.

"Your brother is doing well and ready for his treatment," Dr. Matthews replied.

Amy smiled. "Good. You know, they gave my son the HPV vaccine. The doctor said it might help to prevent cancers like the one Jeff has in some people."

Dr. Matthews nodded. "The vaccination prevents cervical cancer in women and may also prevent some head and neck cancers, the ones caused by HPV infection. Jeff's was not that type."

Jeff looked up. "Yeah, I needed a fucking vaccine for life. There ain't one of those."

With that, they headed back for his treatment.

"**G**ood afternoon, Mrs. Flint."

"Hello, Dr. Matthews," responded Denise Flint, a matronly seventy-eight-year-old woman. Sitting next to her was Claire, her twelve-year-old granddaughter known to Dr. Matthews as a serious student in middle school.

"Hello, Claire. How are you today?" he asked. Her book was opened to a page showing the Grand Canyon.

"Fine, thank you," she replied in a clear voice, making direct eye contact.

"Claire is studying geology," announced Mrs. Flint. "She has a presentation to give next week."

"We call it earth science now, Grandma" corrected Claire.

Denise Flint had been sixty-six when she noticed blood in her urine. That was twelve years ago, about a month before Claire's birth. She was their miracle baby, conceived by Denise's daughter and her husband two years after they had abandoned a long period of prayers, medications, and *in vitro* fertilization attempts. Denise had not wanted to upset them, so she told only her husband, Bud, about the bleeding. He had taken her to their family doctor, then the urologist, and finally the CT scan.

Dr. Shepard, the urologist, had given them the news.

"The CT scan shows a mass in the right kidney. It looks like cancer, and we should remove it. It is near the center of the kidney, so we need to remove the whole kidney. Fortunately, you have two, and since you have been in good health, your left kidney should function just fine."

Denise scheduled the surgery for two weeks after Claire's delivery.

"They both came out at the same time, but we kept Claire," was Bud's joke.

Dr. Shepard had performed the surgery laparoscopically, using tools which allowed him to remove the cancerous kidney without ever having to place his hands into Denise's body. She was brought to the operating room, given general anesthesia, and placed on the table in a slightly bent position with her right side up. After cleaning the skin, Dr. Shepard made three small incisions, called key-holes or ports, into which he could insert his equipment. He made one incision under her lower ribs, one in the middle of her abdomen, and a third lower down below the first. After making the first incision, Dr. Shepard filled the part of Denise's abdominal cavity which contains the kidney with carbon dioxide, which gave him room to work. Dr. Shepard then placed a camera, scalpel, and suction device into separate ports. He then started his dissection, clearing all the tissue around the kidney, clipping the arteries and veins to prevent bleeding, then separating the kidney from the adrenal gland. Once the kidney was free, Dr. Shepard maneuvered it into a bag which he sealed and removed from the body through one of the incisions, which he had first widened. After he was sure there was no bleeding, the gas was let out, the wounds were closed, and Denise sent to the recovery room.

Dr. Shepard was pleased with the results.

"The cancer did not break through the capsule of the kidney and came out easily," he reported to Bud after the operation and repeated to them both the next day. "I think I got it all, but I want you to see Dr. Matthews when the final report is available to be sure there is nothing else we need to do. We will watch you with a CT scan in six months, then each year."

The pathologist reported the cancer measured three centimeters, about an inch and a half, appeared to be slow growing, and was contained within the kidney. Dr. Matthews had little to add.

"For some cancers, we give treatments after surgery to kill any cells which might have escaped. You probably know women with breast cancer who have taken chemotherapy or hormonal treatments after their surgery. They often refer to it as insurance. We call it adjuvant treatment. Men and women with colon cancer often do the same type of thing, a period of chemotherapy after surgery. In these situations, you must be sure that the risk the cancer has spread is high and that the chemo will lower it. The risk your kidney cancer has spread is low, and there is not anything we need to do now. We will check a CT scan each year for five years."

"That sounds good to me," answered Denise.

"She's an optimist," Bud reported to Dr. Matthews. "She never complains. It's good to be married to an optimist."

The five years went quickly for Denise and Bud, the time marked by the milestones of their grandchildren. For Claire, it was her first solid food, steps, and riding the school bus. For her cousin Katie, it was middle school and the start of high school, figure skating, and soccer. For the eldest cousin Sophia, it was high school graduation, swim team, and college.

Five years after her surgery, Denise's yearly CT scan was clear. She was seventy-one years old and felt well. Bud and Claire had accompanied her to the visit.

"Claire has today off from school, so we're taking her out to lunch, then going to the library," explained Denise.

"Your CT scan is fine. At this point, you don't need any more scans," said Dr. Matthews. "The chances of the cancer returning is small enough that they are not recommended."

"I'm glad," Denise answered, becoming reflective. "You know, I never thought I would have this life. Growing up our family was poor, and my parents could never go anywhere. This winter, Bud and I went to Florida for a month to his brother's place. You might not believe it, but my granddaughter Sophia came to visit. She actually spent her break from college with us. It was so lovely. She said we went to all her swim meets and school concerts, and now it was her turn to pay us back."

"It's true," agreed Bud. "And the other old folks in the place were so jealous. They all wanted her to program their remotes and cell phones. I had to beat the geezers off. Fortunately, there were plenty of canes nearby, so I had weapons."

"Stop it, Bud. Sophia was very nice to all of them," continued Denise.

"It was like that movie 'Night of the Living Dead.' All of them coming at you, 'fix my remote, fix my remote.' " Bud held out his arms and rocked side to side, imitating a zombie.

"Grandpa, behave," said five-year-old Claire sternly, putting her hands on her hips and rolling her eyes at Dr. Matthews. "He's naughty sometimes," she added by way of explanation.

"She melts me," reported Bud, hugging Claire. "You know what they say about grandchildren?"

Dr. Matthews shook his head.

"They are the reward for not killing your own children when they were teenagers," Bud concluded, laughing at his joke.

One year, nine swim meets, four band concerts, endless time in the ice rink, and three school plays later, Denise noticed a mild discomfort after she ate, particularly when she made the fried dough which Bud so loved. Dr. Gannon found gallstones and planned to remove them, but her pre-op chest x-ray showed a spot. This led to a CT scan which found many spots on her lungs, "nodules" was the radiologist's term. They were small, ranging in size from a quarter of an inch to half an inch, and scattered in both lungs.

Dr. Gannon called Dr. Matthews.

"Her gallstones are only minimally symptomatic and don't need to come out right now. They can wait for you to figure out what's going on. I'll just put her on a low-fat diet."

Dr. Matthews met Denise and Bud.

"It is confusing, but we think the spots are likely to be the kidney cancer spread to the lung, even though it has been seven years since your surgery. But we need a biopsy to know for sure."

Denise spoke first. "If it is the kidney cancer, what can we do about it?"

"We have many new treatments," began Dr. Matthews.

"Surgery?" interrupted Bud.

"Not surgery," replied Dr. Matthews. "We have other treatments—"

"But you can treat it," interrupted Bud again.

"Yes, we can—"

"Good. I needed to hear that," he nodded.

The biopsy was done in radiology using the CT scan. A week later the pathologist called Dr. Matthews.

"It's the kidney cancer. I looked at her slides from seven years ago. I wanted to be sure, so we sent it out to Mass General, and they agree. Just goes to show how unpredictable those renal cells are . . ."

Dr. Matthews relayed the news to Denise and Bud, who were both shocked despite his warning.

"I don't understand. How did they get there if Dr. Shepard took out the kidney cancer all those years ago?" asked Bud.

"The seeds were already sown before Dr. Shepard removed the kidney. They were lying in the soil of the lung until something caused them to grow and they reached a size we could detect."

METASTASIS: THE SEED AND THE SOIL.

In the late 1890s, William Paget, an assistant surgeon in London, was puzzled. How was it that when widespread cancer developed, some organs "suffered" (his words) more than others? It was recognized at the time that cancer cells could spread through the lymph or blood systems. Some thought the cancers could then recruit nearby cells to become cancerous. Paget performed a formidable analysis of seven hundred thirty-five patients who died of breast cancer and found it most often spread into the liver. He concluded it was as if "when a plant goes to seed, its seeds are carried in all directions. But they can only live and grow if they fall on congenial soil."[315] Paget thus articulated his famous "seed and soil" theory of metastasis.

The modern scientific restatement of Paget's theory belongs to Ian R. Hart and Isiah J. Fidler of the National Cancer Institute. In 1980, they reported experiments in which they implanted ovary, lung, and kidney tissue into the thighs of mice. They then injected the mice with melanoma cancer cells. The melanoma cells grew in the ovary and lung tissue, but not the kidney tissue.[316] The seeds needed the proper soil. The subsequent explosion of molecular science has allowed scientists studying both the seeds and the soil to formulate new theories to answer Paget's puzzle, yet his century-old analogy remains often referenced.

The seeds are obviously the cancer cells themselves. In some settings, each single cell functions as an autonomous unit capable of reproducing the cancer. In the laboratory, leukemia cells grown in a nutrient-rich broth are an example. A single leukemic cell in a lab flask can reproduce and eventually its progeny will fill the whole bottle and exhaust the nutrients. This experience supports the idea that a single seed can reproduce a cancer at a distant site and explains the phrase "if even one cell gets out, the patient is in trouble." Scientists have identified characteristics of individual cancer cells which make them more likely to succeed as seeds. These include the ability to grow, dissolve the structures around them, escape into the blood or lymph channels, and attach to their desired new home. These properties of the cancer cell have become targets for treatment.

For many solid cancers, the process may be more complex. The seed may not be a single cell, but rather a clump of cells. Contained within this clump may be both Paget's seeds (tumor cells) but also some old soil from the site of origin of the cancer. The old soil includes supporting cells called stromal cells which may promote the growth of the metastatic cancer at the new site. Scientists, including Fidler, have shown that these clumps of cells form metastasis more efficiently than single cells. Furthermore, since the individual tumor cells in the primary cancer may not be uniform, the seed may contain tumor cells with various properties. This more complex process strains Paget's image, but it also potentially reveals more potential targets for treatment.[317]

The sowing of the seeds may also affect the pattern of spread. For some cancers, there are anatomic reasons which explain the distribution of seeds to specific organs. Consider the difference between colon and rectal cancer. The blood leaving the colon travels through veins which lead to the liver while the blood leaving the rectum passes via a different set of veins which may skip the liver and go to the lung. Colon cancers are therefore more likely to spread to the liver alone, while rectal cancers are more likely to also spread into the lung. Another example of the importance of anatomy is ovarian cancer, where the cancer cells have easy access to the abdominal cavity and tend to spread there, finding fertile soil on the outside of the intestines and other organs.

A fascinating aspect of cancer metastasis is the interaction between the seed and the soil. Although the early theories of Paget's time that cancer cells spread and then recruited normal cells to become cancerous are not generally correct, the seeds do influence the soil. The normal mechanisms that maintain the environment of the soil can be perverted to suit the growth of the cancer. An example of this occurs when cancer cells metastasize into the bones. The normal bone is constantly remodeled by cells which dissolve existing bone (osteoclasts) and cells which make new bone (osteoblasts). Cancer cells can direct the osteoclasts to dissolve bone and thus make niches for their own growth. Treatments which strengthen the bone by inhibiting osteoclasts are used regularly.

The soil can also fight back. Scientists have observed the normal properties of the soil can often resist the spread of the cancer, resulting in dormant metastasis. The immune system in the soil can eliminate the seed. Indeed, promoting immune recognition of metastasis and preventing their growth when they are small is a goal of cancer treatment. The new immune therapies now used for advanced cancers may soon make this a reality.

Stephen Paget wrote that "he who turns over the records of cases of cancer is only a ploughman, but his observations of the properties of the soil may also be useful." Paget's life trained him for modesty as his father was Sir James Paget, the brilliant British surgeon and pathologist after whom several diseases are named, most notably Paget's disease of the bone. Yet Stephen Paget's description of cancer metastasis has provided scientists and patients an image which has served for over a century, a testament to the talents of this ploughman. [318]

"Well, it's more like weeds in the garden, if you ask me," concluded Denise. "But we have to make the best of it. What now? More surgery?"

"No," replied Dr. Matthews. "There are too many small spots on your lung for surgery. We need to give you a treatment for the whole body—"

"Chemo?" interrupted Bud. "They say that's like weed killer."

"No," replied Dr. Matthews. "Chemotherapy does not generally work on kidney cancers. Scientists have found some of the abnormalities in the cancers and have made medicines which block the problem. We call it 'targeted' therapy."

"How do you know the right target?" asked Denise.

"It's an interesting story, at least to oncologists," answered Dr. Matthews. "Scientists figured it out from studying families with inherited kidney cancers . . ."

TARGETING KIDNEY CANCER.

Inherited gene mutations may lead to specific cancers. These genes are often not involved when the same type of cancer occurs in a person who did not inherit the mutation. In medical terms, the "inherited" cancer has a different molecular basis than the "non-inherited" or "sporadic" cancer. For example, women carriers of *BRCA* gene mutations are prone to breast cancer. For most women with breast cancer, the *BRCA* gene is not involved. In some cancers, the genes involved in inherited cancers play a modest role in the non-inherited cancers. An example in this category comes from families who have an inherited mutation in the *FAP* (Familial Adenomatous Polyposis) gene and develop hundreds of colon polyps which lead to cancer. For people who develop sporadic (non-inherited) colon cancer, the *FAP* gene is normal at birth. As the cancer progresses, the *FAP* gene can become mutated within the cancerous cells of some patients. In these situations, studying the inherited cancer can produce information which will be useful in the wider population.

In a few cancers, inherited gene mutations have provided information useful for almost everyone with that cancer. Kidney cancer is a remarkable example of the inherited cancer leading to discoveries useful for the treatment of sporadic cancer. The story begins with the von Hippel-Lindau (VHL) syndrome, a rare genetic condition found in about one out of every thirty-six thousand people. VHL results in unusual benign growths, often of the blood vessels, with names such as hemangioblastoma of the nervous system and angioma of the retina. It may also result in some cancers like pheochromocytoma (adrenal gland cancer) and kidney cancer (also called renal cell cancer). The syndrome was described in pieces, the first being when German ophthalmologist von Hippel found a familial cluster of retinal angiomas (blood vessel tumors) and the second when Lindau added a nervous system blood vessel tumor. Knowing that a family has VHL syndrome allows them to undergo screening for kidney cancer (and the other tumors) which can save lives.[319]

An important clue about the cause of the VHL syndrome came in 1979 with the report of an Italian-American family in which ten members of three generations had kidney cancer. Those who developed kidney cancers were born with a genetic abnormality; parts of chromosome 3 and 8 were switched in a "translocation" in all the cells of their body. [320] The theory was that one of the two copies of the gene responsible for VHL was damaged by this translocation, leaving the affected family members with only one normal *VHL* gene. Later in life, the second normal *VHL* gene would be damaged in the kidney cells, leading to the kidney cancer. This process of cancer development is known as the "two-hit model" and had been proposed earlier in the decade by geneticist Alfred Knudson for the rare cancer retinoblastoma. The theory also meant that the *VHL* gene is located at the site of the translocation on either chromosome 3 or 8. The report signaled the start of the race to find the *VHL* gene in labs across the world.

When this family donated their blood in the 1970s, the ability to look at chromosomes had only recently developed. On her kitchen table, scientist Janet Rowley was about to discover the translocation of chromosomes 9 and 22 which are the hallmark of chronic myelogenous leukemia (CML).[321] Over the next fifteen years, the revolution in molecular biology which allowed scientists to locate, sequence, understand, and manipulate individual genes uncovered the story of the *VHL* gene, which ended up being on chromosome 3. The first portion of the race, describing the location and sequence of the *VHL* gene, was won in 1993 by Farida Latif and other scientists at the NIH. Since not all families with VHL had dramatic translocations visible by studying the chromosomes, Latif's discovery allowed the identification of many families with small deletions or mutations in the *VHL* gene—a tremendous service to those families. Her discovery also began the start of the second portion of the race: to understand and manipulate the VHL system.[322]

The *VHL* gene has turned out to be an incredibly complex regulator of many systems within the cell. The VHL protein targets other proteins in the cell for destruction in the garbage disposals of the cell, called proteasomes. VHL thus controls the levels of many key proteins involved in cell division and activity, including the growth of blood vessels. When the *VHL* gene is mutated, these systems become overactive, leading to excessive cell activity and growth, a ripe environment for cancer. Remarkably, the VHL system was also found to be deranged in many kidney cancers which developed in patients without the inherited von Hippel-Lindau syndrome—the non-inherited or sporadic kidney cancers. In fact, the most common subtype of kidney cancer, called "clear cell cancer," often had damage to the VHL system. This molecular knowledge explains some of the features of kidney cancer, such as their tendency to bleed due to fragile new blood vessels in the tumor, and led to the development of treatments targeted at the specific abnormalities.

At the beginning of the twenty-first century, the treatment of kidney cancer was simple. If the cancer was confined to the kidney, either the whole kidney or the cancerous part was removed. If the cancer had spread, there was chemotherapy, which rarely worked, and immune treatments with interferon or interleukin, which worked occasionally. This century has seen the development of both "targeted treatments" and less toxic and more effective immune treatments for kidney cancer. The targeted treatments for kidney cancer are molecules that block the various proteins which build up when the VHL system is damaged. The first target of these new treatments was one of the proteins called VGEFR-2 (Vascular Endothelial Growth Factor Receptor 2) which causes the growth of blood vessels in the cancer. Sunitinib, brand name Sutent, is a drug which blocks the action of the VGEFR-2 proteins and deprives the cancer of the blood vessels it needs for nourishment. Sunitinib did not cure the cancers, but it could control them, sometimes for years.

In the 1990s, scientists Axel Ullrich at the Max Planck Institute in Munich and Joseph Schlesinger of New York University developed sunitinib. At the time, the full link between the VHL system and kidney cancer was being worked out, and the line of research which lead to sunitinib was developed somewhat independently. In 1991, these men formed the spin-off company SUGEN, named by taking their initials and combining them with GEN for genetics. If this story is familiar, it is because Ullrich was previously a leading scientist with the pioneering pharmaceutical biotechnology firm Genentech, itself named by the combination of Genetics and Technology. In addition to his science, Ullrich mastered the Genentech model of building biotech firms as he also spun-off several other companies. In keeping with this model, SUGEN was sold to the giant company Pfizer, who made sunitinib into a blockbuster drug introduced in 2006, with some of the profits returning to fund the Max Planck Institute.[323]

Sunitinib was the first in a series of targeted therapies which block different proteins increased in kidney cancers, usually because of the abnormal VHL system. Although these drugs had side effects, some occasionally severe, they were a new method of treating kidney cancers. Understanding their actions came from the combined efforts of families and their doctors interested in inherited kidney cancer, the new era of molecular biology, and the modern pharmaceutical industry.

"That doesn't mean my children or grandchildren will get this, does it?" asked Denise.

"No. Your family does not have a history of cancer," answered Dr. Matthews. "Why this happened to you is not known."

"As we used to say at work, 'above our pay scale,' right doc?" concluded Bud.

"Above our pay scale," agreed Dr. Matthews.

The orange Sutent pills arrived in a FedEx truck the next week, along with an array of paperwork which Bud read.

"Gosh, there are a lot of side effects to this pill. Are we sure you should take this?" he asked Denise.

"Dr. Matthews thinks it the best thing and my nurse Rebecca told me everything I need to know. She said I could call her anytime. So, I'm starting," she replied.

Denise's main side effect of the sunitinib was mild fatigue, until about the third week when a skin rash appeared on her legs and arms. Blotches, she called them. Rebecca had her come in for a check.

"I can manage it," Denise said after Dr. Matthews and Rebecca had examined her.

"I know you can, but we don't want it to get worse. So, you are going to take a break for a week; then we will lower your dose," he replied.

"You really have a remarkable outlook," commented Rebecca.

"She sure does," agreed Bud. "I'm lucky to be married to an optimist."

The optimism paid off. The adjustment of the dose allowed Denise to take the medication. After three months, her CT scans showed the spots in her lungs had shrunk. After six months, they remained unchanged. More milestones passed. Sophia graduated from college, Caroline left to start, and Claire kept melting Bud's heart as she moved through school.

"I tried helping her with her homework once, but she kept correcting me. So now I just drive her and her friends around," he updated Dr. Matthews.

As the sunitinib controlled her cancer, Denise's gallstones gradually became more of a problem. Every few weeks brought episodes of dull aching in her belly, which she minimized. Finally, Bud took action.

"These gallstones are killing both of us," he announced to Dr. Matthews. "We've been on this low-fat diet trying to avoid the attacks. Although she won't admit it, she's miserable. And I'm dying of starvation. We have to get them out."

Denise shook her head, resigned.

"Sometimes it's hard to be married to an optimist," Bud pointed out. "They never complain. It makes you look bad to be around them."

Denise's gallbladder came out. Another year on sunitinib brought more milestones.

"My children gave me this for my seventy-fifth birthday," Denise said proudly, showing Dr. Matthews her new iPad.

Claire, now nine, burst into laughter, quickly joined by Bud.

"What's so funny about an iPad?" Dr. Matthews asked Claire.

"Grandma unwrapped it, then said, 'It's beautiful, thank you so much, what is it?' " she gasped, doubling over with laughter as she and Bud hugged.

Denise nodded, smiling. "Claire has taught me how to use it," she added proudly.

The end of sunitinib came later in the year of the iPad. The medication had worked for three years.

"Your scans have shown that there has been some growth of the cancer," Dr. Matthews reported. "Not much, but enough to know it is no longer working."

"Why did it stop working? Did her body get used to it?" asked Bud.

"Not her body," answered Dr. Matthews. "The sunitinib caused those cancer cells that needed what it blocks to die or remain quiet. Over time, cancer cells that used other ways to grow took over."

Bud nodded. "Sounds like survival of the fittest. Claire's been teaching me about that in the car."

Denise's next choice was axitinib, brand name Inlyta, another targeted blocker of the molecules the cancer cells needed to grow. Her body liked this one. If she drank extra water to flush her remaining kidney, there were almost no side effects. After three months, her CT scan improved again.

"We had our fiftieth anniversary this week!" she reported. "All the children and grandchildren were there. And our friends. It was really beautiful."

"I felt bad for her," remarked Bud. "After fifty years with me, you'd think the poor thing could see the finish line."

Axitinib brought more milestones. Sophia found a good job in Boston. Caroline graduated from college and began graduate school in engineering. Bud still drove Claire, but now it was to middle school. After just over a year, however, there was an ending to that medication, too. Denise still felt well, but her scans had worsened.

"This one didn't work as long," noted Bud, worried. "What's next? More pills?"

"No," replied Dr. Matthews. "Now we have a new treatment which allows the immune system to attack the cancer. It's an antibody infusion."

IMMUNE TREATMENTS FOR KIDNEY CANCER.

"Spontaneous regression" of a cancer means shrinkage without apparent reason or treatment; patients often say miracle. Proving spontaneous regressions of cancers or miracles is tricky. Stories of patients near death who survived circulate in every community, including poorly documented medical histories which evolve with time and repeated dramatic telling to resemble reports of UFOs. Yet carefully documented spontaneous remissions do happen. They are well-known in patients with low-grade lymphomas but rare in other cancers. In 1981, Dr. DJ Fairlamb from the Department of Radiotherapy and Oncology at the Churchill Hospital in Oxford described two cases of spontaneous regression of metastasis of kidney cancer, including one patient who had the disappearance of lung metastasis after a large cancer deposit in her groin was treated with radiation. Dr. Fairlamb compiled a list of sixty-five cases of spontaneous remissions of various cancers and suggested they were caused by the immune system.[324] His article joined earlier reports of patients with widespread kidney cancer in whom the cancer disappeared after removal of the involved kidney. These cases suggested the primary cancer in the kidney might secrete factors which stimulated the metastasis and led to speculation about the role of the immune system in fighting cancer.

Other lines of evidence pointed to a role for the immune system in kidney cancers. Physicians had long known that the behavior of kidney cancers was often unpredictable. Some patients with widespread kidney cancer would have stable disease for extended periods, even if they did not experience a spontaneous remission. Generations of medical students had learned that kidney cancers could produce mysterious findings in patients, including the release of various hormones and symptoms like fever. Scientists identified lymph cells in some kidney cancers, just as was seen in melanomas. As immune treatments began with interferon and interleukin, kidney cancers, along with melanoma, became a natural target.[325]

In the 1980s and 1990s, the first immune treatments excited scientists, physicians, patients, and the new biotech industry. In a small percentage of patients with widespread kidney cancer, the intensive immune treatment interleukin-2 (IL-2) produced long remissions and even a few cures. Interferon, less toxic but still challenging, also occasionally controlled the cancer. Unfortunately, lower doses of these immune treatments did not work well and, since kidney cancer usually occurs in older patients who cannot tolerate higher doses, very few benefited. Interestingly, these immune treatments often worked better if the cancer in the kidney was first removed, again leading to speculation that the tumor in the kidney was releasing growth factors which stimulated the metastases or suppressed the immune system.[326] In sum, while early immune treatments helped only a limited number of patients, the idea remained an attractive one.

As the twenty-first century opened, advances in the treatment of widespread kidney cancer began with the introduction of targeted treatments like sunitinib directed at specific abnormalities in the cancer cells. At the same time, immune therapy was also advancing as scientists had uncovered the pathways which some cancers cells used to hide from the immune system. New antibodies called "checkpoint inhibitors" could unmask the cancer and unleash an immune attack. With the history of immune treatments having some success in kidney cancer, this therapy was a logical choice. One of the first, named nivolumab (brand name Opdivo) produced shrinkage or stabilization in some patients with widespread kidney cancer. The dramatic responses seen with IL-2 were not common with these medicines, but they were much better tolerated. The results with these immune treatments are not always predictable. At times the tumors can grow before stabilizing. Some patients have seen generalized improvement after they have received radiation to a spot, recalling the 1981 experience of Dr. Fairlamb's patient who had a spontaneous regression in the lung after radiation to the hip. Predicting who will benefit and combining these immune treatments with other therapies are challenges for the future.[327]

"Do you think this will help me?" Denise asked Rebecca during her first infusion.

"What did Dr. Matthews say?" she asked.

"He seemed to think there is a good chance it will," replied Denise.

"Why did you ask?" probed Rebecca. "Are you worried?"

"Not for me. Not even for Bud. It's the grandchildren. They've never lost anyone, thank God. Their parents and other grandparents are all living. So, I want to prepare them if it's my time," she answered.

"I doubt anyone really knows for sure," said Rebecca. "The results from immune treatments are hard to predict."

Denise's first CT scan looked better in some spots, worse in others. The second scan was about the same as the first. Each time, Bud had the last word.

"It's just above our pay scale."

Today Mrs. Flint was feeling well. The treatment was not giving her any side effects.

"Where is your husband today? Is everything okay?" asked Dr. Matthews as he finished examining her. Claire had watched his every move carefully.

"Bud's working in the garden. I made him plant bulbs for next spring. After all," she paused, smiling, "he's married to an optimist."

"**G**otta go, my doctor's here. He gets very annoyed when I don't hang up right away." Her staccato delivery finished, Rachael Simon turned off her cell phone and placed it in her handbag. Her fashionable outfit befitted the leading realtor in the region. Her face was familiar; it adorned signs in every development. Her personality was dynamic and, in the words of a competitor, Rachael Simon could suck the oxygen out of any room. Sitting nearby was her husband Ken, comfortable in old jeans and a well-worn sweater.

Dr. Matthews sat down. He had just seen her a month ago. She had been feeling well, and her exam, mammogram, and blood work had been normal.

"What's going on?" he asked.

"I want a PET scan."

Four years ago, sixty-three-year-old Rachael Simon had gone for her routine mammogram in the morning. Dr. Stacy Gold called that same evening.

"Rachael, this is Stacy Gold."

"Finally. It's about time you gave up that tiny home I sold you fifteen years ago. That was one of my first sales. I have the perfect place for you."

"No. I'm calling about your mammogram . . . It has an abnormality on it, and you need a biopsy."

"Is it cancer?" In the second before she reasserted control, Rachael's voice betrayed anxiety.

"I'm not sure, but that is possible. We need to get a biopsy," Dr. Gold replied.

The biopsy was done in the mammogram unit the next day. The radiologist had also been a client.

"Remember," she reminded him, "I got you quite a deal on that place, so I expect a good result."

Dr. Arnold Hickson laughed. "It's a great house . . . and we all hope this is benign."

The procedure was painless, and the pathology report was available two days later.

"Rachael, this is Stacy Gold again. Are you in a place you can talk now?"

The biopsy had revealed breast cancer. Rachael would need to see a surgeon.

"Shit . . . okay . . . I'll call Ken, and he'll arrange it in Boston. When do you want to see your new place?"

Dr. Gold laughed softly. "You are amazing. I want you to take care of yourself and let me know if you need any help."

Rachael's next call was to her husband, a well-known fiction writer. They had married young and raised a daughter and son in the Newton suburb of Boston, where Rachael had been a successful realtor. Fifteen years ago, as new empty nesters, they had passed through Saratoga Springs and fallen in love with the Victorian downtown, Skidmore College, and the arts community. They moved, and Rachael Simon made her mark. Saratoga was her new town. She bought and sold it.

That was their public story. The business reality was that Rachael had seen trouble develop in Boston's precarious housing market. In the late 1990s, there were simply not enough available units as the economy was sluggish, builders stymied by a maze of regulations, and home prices rose dramatically. When the millennium arrived, the supply problem improved, but the availability of easy mortgages kept demand and prices high. Rachael saw the bubble develop and knew when prices fell those unqualified owners living on the edge would face ruin. One quiet Sunday morning, as she and Ken had a lazy breakfast with the *Boston Globe* spread out over the coffee table, she made her prediction.

"This market is going to crash. Maybe not as bad as other parts of the country, but it is going down."

"Markets go up and down. You've been through that before. What's different about this one?" he asked, putting down the sports section, where the main topic was the Yawkey's pending sale of the Red Sox to a new syndicate.

"There are people who have no business getting these mortgages who will be owners. When the prices fall, and their mortgage rates rise, they will be in trouble. I don't know when it will happen . . . in three years, five years or ten . . . but it will. And it will be miserable for everyone, including those of us who sold to them."

Ken paused, thoughtful.

"So, what do you want to do?" he asked, knowing she always had a plan. Her proposal was a move to Saratoga Springs. They enjoyed the place, and Rachael knew that the unique community had a housing market which would withstand the bubble's eventual burst. The Saratoga economy was diverse and growing steadily, housing demand was increasing but supply was roughly in balance, and the local lenders were conservative. She could make a mark there.

There was also a personal reason for the move: Rachael's worsening panic attacks. Her condition had started with the birth of her daughter, Kari. A month before the due date, a routine visit had revealed placental insufficiency which led to an unexpected hospital admission. A sudden change in the baby's heart rate triggered her obstetrician's palpable anxiety and a rushed cesarean section. Perhaps because she was premature, Kari cried uncontrollably for six long months. All night. Once she started, the only way to console the child was to hold her facing outward and walk. Ken tried to take as many turns as possible, knowing that despite her remarkable energy, Rachael had always needed sleep to perform well. Still, it often fell to Rachael to walk the nights, carrying Kari. Rachael had always needed control. In the postpartum world of screaming, nursing, and sleep deprivation, that was gone.

The attacks started when Rachael had awakened one night, startled by a rare moment of quiet. Next to her, Ken was sleeping softly. She listened. No crying. Something was wrong, she thought. Something with Kari. The image of her tiny baby was followed by a feeling of impending doom. Her heart raced uncontrollably, she began sweating and became short of breath as she rushed to the crib. Kari was fine, sleeping on her own.

Rachael was not fine. The episodes came again and again, the feeling of doom and anxiety followed by the palpitations and sweating. Sometimes just a visit to the crib was enough to set off the storm. Soon she could not bear to have her daughter out of sight. As sleep became difficult, the reactions became longer. Ken brought her first to the obstetrician, then the cardiologist, and finally a psychologist who specialized in stress management.

STRESS AND CANCER.

Stress is understood by everyone but does not have the same meaning for any two people. The scientific concept of stress was popularized in the 1930s by Dr. Hans Selye, an endocrinologist (a physician who studies the glands and hormones of the body) at McGill University in Montreal. This time was exciting for endocrinologists who began to understand the chemistry and action of hormones. Seyle was a brilliant scientist who studied the effects of various stimuli on animals and first reported them in a brief letter to the prestigious magazine *Nature* entitled "A syndrome produced by diverse nocuous agents."[328] Seyle later expanded his work from the laboratory studies of animals into detailed descriptions of the human condition. His seminal work, *The Stress of Life*, was published in 1956 and updated in 1975 to reflect his lifetime of study and observations.[329]

Selye's basic concept was that various stimuli can produce a reaction which he called the General Adaption Syndrome. The first part, which Seyle called the "alarm reaction," is popularly known as "flight or fight" and results from the rapid release of hormones, primarily from the adrenal gland, which cause a rise in heart rate and blood pressure. The fight or flight reaction had been well documented in 1915 by Harvard scientist Walter Cannon in his book *Bodily Changes in Pain, Hunger, Fear and Rage*. Cannon started with the observation that "fear, rage and pain, and the pangs of hunger are all primitive experiences which human beings share with the lower animals" and described the effects of this reaction on the body, noting "danger makes us feel more alive."[330] Seyle expanded on Cannon's work with a description of the hormonal release and physiologic changes during this event. He also noted that different individuals can respond with a fight or flight reaction to different stimuli—triggers in one person may be different than triggers in another. In some circumstances, the flight or fight reaction can occur without an obvious stress or from a stress which would not normally warrant that response—these are "panic attacks."[331]

Repeated fight or flight reactions produce profound chronic changes in the body, many of which mimic accelerated aging. Selye called these the stages of "resistance" and "exhaustion."[332] For example, chronic stress produces elevated blood pressure which may lead to vascular damage (resistance) and stroke (exhaustion). Repeated fight or flight reactions may also result in behavioral changes to avoid the dreaded stimulus. An example is the fear of being late for a party causing a panic reaction which then leads to social isolation. On the other hand, Selye also made the important observation that some stress is necessary for success in life. In a later philosophical phase of his career, Selye sought to define the balance between useful and destructive stress. He diagnosed the effects of stress in various occupations and prescribed remedies. For physicians, he particularly cautioned about the dangers of excess stress leading to drug addiction, mental illness, and suicide.[333] As a workaholic himself, Selye was probably under chronic self-imposed stress. Near the end of his career, Selye became a spokesman for the tobacco industry as it faced its legal challenges in the 1970s. He argued that the benefits of cigarettes as an effective form of stress reduction offset their overstated potential harms. Clearly even the "father of stress" was not immune to its many effects as it distorted his reality.

Selye's work has been continued by many scientists, physicians, psychologists, and therapists interested in both understanding stress and treating its destructive consequences. Many questions remain unanswered, including one often asked by patients: does stress cause cancer? The World Health Organization's International Agency for Research on Cancer has listed ten characteristics of agents which can potentially cause cancer. Some of these are obvious, such as chemicals which damage DNA. Others are less obvious, such as agents which cause chronic inflammation and lead to stimulation of cells, either directly or indirectly via the activity of the immune system.[334] The theory is that cell stimulation might lead to more activity and a higher chance of errors within the cells which in turn lead to cancer. This sequence occurs in some chronic viral infections, such as hepatitis C, in which a small percentage of patients develop liver cancer. This theoretical sequence also raises concern that chronic inflammation seen with our nation's obesity epidemic might somewhat raise the risk of cancer. It may explain why some anti-inflammatories like aspirin can slightly lower the risk of some cancers.[335] The question of whether psychological stressors which cause Selye's General Adaption Syndrome could also lead to cellular stimulation and a greater risk of cancer is provocative, but not definitively answered. Even if stress raises the risk for a cancer, proving it caused a cancer in an individual will be impossible.

Rachael's anxiety resulted from her paradox; the same intense adrenaline drive and energy which allowed her to swim with the sharks in

Boston's ultra-competitive real estate market could, at times, drive her wild. Over the years, Rachael controlled the attacks. A few periods had been rough, including the children's first days of school, Ken's auto accident, the early days of her children's driving and, of course, college applications. But these stresses were expected, managed with relaxation techniques and some extra medication. This time was different. Their empty nest gave her quiet time while the real estate bubble gave her a real but undefined worry over the future, pushing her system into a constant flight or fight state. Ken agreed that a new environment with less pressure might help. For his part, he could write anywhere.

"I guess if the Yawkeys can sell the Red Sox, we can move to Saratoga Springs . . . Although I think that area is mostly Yankee country," he mused.

The move had worked. The pace was slower, Rachael's panic attacks had abated, and her business had done well even when the housing collapse she predicted took place in 2008. Although she had not foreseen the national financial upheaval, Rachael's belief that Saratoga would experience only a modest slowdown was correct. Ken was also pleased with the region and the easy three-hour drive to their friends in Boston. Life was good.

Living in Saratoga was fine, but treating cancer in their adopted small town was another matter. That still belonged in Boston. After the diagnosis, Ken had arranged a visit to the Breast Center at Dana Farber. Another mammogram and breast MRI preceded a lumpectomy and sentinel lymph node biopsy. Dr. Ann Pearl had then explained the situation.

"Your cancer was small, 1.8 centimeters, or just under an inch in size. It did not spread to the lymph nodes. The cancer was ER/PR positive, meaning it was stimulated by estrogen. That is common in post-menopausal women. The unusual thing about your cancer is that it was also Her-2-neu positive. This is found in about 25 percent of breast cancers. As you probably know, it means the cancers are rapidly growing and tend to spread, but are also very sensitive to treatment with chemotherapy and a drug called Herceptin."

"Bad news, good news," replied Rachael.

"Exactly," nodded Dr. Pearl. "Herceptin is regarded as the wonder drug in breast cancer. It is what we call a targeted therapy."

HERCEPTIN: A NEW WAY TO TREAT BREAST CANCER.

Most cancers are complex, with multiple abnormal genes and cellular machinery which is broken on many levels. It is not clear what is "driving" these cancerous cell. A few cancers have a single dominant abnormality which largely dictates their behavior: the "driver" of the cancer. If that driver abnormality can be corrected, the cancer cells may be controlled. The best example is chronic myelogenous leukemia, where a break on chromosomes 9 and 22 causes the leukemia and the medication imatinib (Gleevec) can reverse the process. For some women with breast cancer, the dominant driver can be extra *Her-2-neu* genes.

In normal breast cells, the *Her-2-neu* gene produces a Her-2-neu protein which sticks out of the cell. The Her-2-neu protein is a "receptor" to which various molecules called "growth factors" attach. When these growth factors attach to the Her-2-neu protein, the portion inside the cell stimulates growth. This inner portion of Her-2-neu protein is called a tyrosine kinase—an activator enzyme. In effect, the Her-2-neu protein takes signals from outside the cell (the growth factors) and translates them into action within the cell (via the tyrosine kinase enzyme). The Her-2-neu protein is an important example of the "growth factor receptor" system which cells use to control growth and activity in response to changes in their environment. Of course, the system is very complicated, and there are many receptors related to the Her-2-neu protein which link together in combinations to stimulate the cells in multiple different ways. Studying growth factor receptors has consumed the careers of our brightest researchers and will occupy bright minds yet to come.

In about 25 percent of breast cancers, duplication of the *Her-2-neu* gene occurs. It is not yet clear why this happens, but the extra *Her-2-neu* genes produce excessive Her-2-neu protein on the outside of the cell. This extra Her-2-neu protein means more activation signals and a rapidly growing cancer with more potential for spread.

Trastuzumab (brand name Herceptin) is an antibody which attaches to the Her-2-neu protein. The immune cells called B-lymphocytes normally produce antibodies to fight infection. Antibodies have two ends. One end attaches to a specific target such as a protein on the outside of an invader or, in the case of trastuzumab, to the Her-2-neu protein. The opposite end can then attract other immune cells to attack and destroy the enemy. In the 1970s, scientists used mice to make antibodies directed against desired targets. In the late 1980s, mouse antibodies against the Her-2-neu protein were developed which caused cancer cells to die or become much more sensitive to chemotherapy. In the 1990s, the humanized form of the antibody, named trastuzumab, produced tremendous benefit when given to patients. When the cancers had spread, trastuzumab and chemotherapy could often shrink and control the metastasis, sometimes for years. When given with chemotherapy at diagnosis, trastuzumab resulted in more cures. A previously devastating form of breast cancer became paradoxically more treatable.

The development of trastuzumab took place at Genentech, the first of the Pharma biotech firms.[336] In 1973, Drs. Stan Cohen of Stanford and Herbert Boyer of University of California at San Francisco developed "cloning," the ability to cut and paste DNA fragments and insert them into bacteria to produce large quantities of a protein. While Cohen stayed in academics, Boyer entered a partnership with Robert Swanson, a venture capitalist who wanted his own company, to form Genentech: Genetic Engineering Technology. Genentech first cloned the hormone somatostatin, which allowed them to reap publicity and additional investment funds. After recruiting more minds, they cloned insulin. Genentech's next success, human growth hormone, become a $2 billion drug. As the excitement peaked, Genentech stock went public, and the rapid rise in price made multimillionaires of the cloners.

Genentech symbolized the biotech industry during the Reagan boom years. The exciting science of the era was given tremendous commercial energy in 1980 when Senators Birch Bayh (D-Ind) and Robert Dole (R-Kans) collaborated on a law which enabled universities and small businesses to patent discoveries and grant exclusive licenses to drug companies. The Stevenson-Wydler Act allowed the National Institute of Health to license drugs discovered in their labs to pharmaceutical companies. These changes encouraged unprecedented collaboration between academia and industry or, depending on one's view, the unprecedented control of academia by industry.[337] Genentech's success encouraged academic institutions or their faculty to spin off biotech firms and collaborate with drug companies, securing their royalties and own place in the commercial world. Genentech's image as a freewheeling biotech company appealed to a new generation of scientists who skipped traditional academic careers to become scientific entrepreneurs. One scientist Swanson persuaded to leave UCSF and join Genentech was Axel Ullrich. In 1985, he cloned the *Her-2-neu gene*.[338] Ullrich then teamed with Dr. Dennis Slamon, an oncologist at UCLA who collected and studied various tumor specimens to show that the Her-2-neu protein was overexpressed in some aggressive breast cancers. In 1987, Genentech scientists produced the precursor mouse antibody of trastuzumab which could attach to the Her-2-neu protein on the cancer cell.

Developing trastuzumab was challenging. One initial problem was that the broader medical community did not expect antibodies like trastuzumab to succeed. The 1980s and early 1990s were the time of peak enthusiasm for new chemotherapy drugs, often used in complex combinations and including high-dose chemotherapy with bone marrow or stem cell transplants. While targeted approaches to cancer were generating interest, antibodies were seen by many as large, clunky molecules which would probably have little clinical effect.[339] Internal issues within Genentech were another problem. Following its early successes, Genentech had turned its attention to interferon, a drug which failed as a cure for viral illnesses in the 1960s but revived in the 1970s as an anticancer drug. After interferon's clinical trials in oncology in the 1980s also largely failed and cost Genentech substantial money, cancer treatment and thus the Her-2-neu protein were not high priorities.[340]

Enter Lilly Tartikoff, whose role in trastuzumab was reported by NBC News' Robert Bazell in *Her 2: The Making of Herceptin, a Revolutionary Treatment for Breast Cancer*. As Dr. Slamon continued his career at UCLA, he treated Brandon Tarikoff, NBC's head of entertainment, for a recurrence of Hodgkin's lymphoma. Tartikoff's wife Lilly, described as a force of nature, became Slamon's benefactor and recruited wealthy businessman Ronald Perelman, owner of Max Factor and Revlon, to the cause. They began the well-known Los Angeles Fire and Ice Ball fundraiser, raising money and launching Lilly Tartikoff as a prominent breast cancer advocate. Slamon used their financial support to help start critical human testing of the mouse antibody, showing that it attached to the cancer cells in patients. Bazell notes that some claim trastuzumab would not have been developed without Lilly Tartikoff's work during this period.[341] Her presence certainly added a dramatic and colorful dimension to the drug's development.

In the late 1980s, Genentech's corporate enthusiasm for trastuzumab rose thanks to Slamon's results, interest from a vice president whose mother was struggling with breast cancer, and company scientists who produced the human version of the antibody.[342] Testing trastuzumab in patients proved to be a complex scientific and sociopolitical undertaking which occurred as the pharmaceutical company Roche purchased majority ownership of Genentech, mixing the freewheeling biotech culture with a more traditional pharmaceutical company.[343] Testing trastuzumab would begin in women with widespread breast cancer who had few other treatment options and a short life expectancy; "little to lose" is a common and brutal description. If it were successful, trastuzumab would then be tested in women with earlier stages of breast cancer where it might increase the cure rate. In this setting, it would be very important to know the side effects since these women might already be cured and "have a lot to lose." The studies would be done in phases:

phase I to determine the best dose, phase II to test the drug in a variety of ways, and phase III to compare it with standard treatment.

Almost everything else about testing trastuzumab was contentious. From a medical viewpoint, there was disagreement about whether to use trastuzumab alone or combine it with chemotherapy. In Dr. Slamon's lab studies the drug worked best when combined with cisplatin, a drug not often used to treat breast cancer because of its limited effectiveness and severe side effects.[344] He advocated the use of cisplatin while other oncology leaders preferred either no partner or chemotherapy drugs more typically used for breast cancer. A forceful clash of medical personalities led to the phase I and II studies being done with trastuzumab alone or with cisplatin while the key phase III study used paclitaxel (Taxol) as the main partner. Initially, the studies did not draw much enthusiasm, and Genentech turned to patient advocacy groups for help in recruitment and expanded study sites to other countries. As promising results emerged, a different problem rapidly arose—patients wanted the drug even if they were not in a clinical trial. Following the example of HIV groups, breast cancer advocates and patients publicly protested Genentech's reluctance to release trastuzumab for compassionate use.[345] These forces ultimately required an alliance of Genentech, breast cancer scientists, and patient advocacy groups to proceed with the clinical testing.[346] Despite the turmoil, the key phase III trial for trastuzumab began in 1995 and ended in 1997. The results were that women with widespread Her-2-neu positive breast cancer treated with trastuzumab in addition to their chemotherapy lived several months longer. This work led to the 1998 approval of trastuzumab for use in women with widespread Her-2-neu positive breast cancer.[347] Although this improvement was overall modest, when trastuzumab was used more widely in the community, a small percentage of women had remarkable responses. During this time, Genetech also helped to standardized testing for the Her-2-neu protein, the target for their treatment.

The next phase of trastuzumab testing attempted to improve cure rates in women with early stage breast cancer. Before trastuzumab, women who had undergone surgery to remove a Her-2-neu positive breast cancer would typically take preventative (adjuvant) chemotherapy, yet often the cancers would recur. The hope was that adding trastuzumab would cure more women. The main concern was that trastuzumab could produce heart damage. Thus, the risk of heart damage needed to be small and the benefit of the drug great. The trials began in 2000. Some physicians offered their highest risk patients trastuzumab before the studies were complete, but most waited for the results.

Trastuzumab exceeded expectations. One large study showed disease free rates increased from 67 percent to 85 percent at the four-year mark, a remarkable improvement by oncology standards which revolutionized the treatment of Her-2-neu positive breast cancer.[348] The rate of heart damage was low. In 2006, the FDA approved trastuzumab for use with chemotherapy in women with early stage (Her-2-neu positive) breast cancer.

Success with trastuzumab led to other treatments directed against Her-2-neu. The molecule lapatinib (Tykerb) was developed to block the activating end of Her-2-neu inside the cell while the antibody pertuzumab (Perjeta) would attach to a different region on the outside. In addition, the discovery that some stomach cancers had high levels of the Her-2-neu protein and responded to trastuzumab challenged physicians to think about cancers in molecular terms rather than the usual tissue classifications. These result with trastuzumab also encouraged the development of other antibodies like cetuximab (Erbitux), used in colon and head and neck cancers. Most importantly, while the targeted treatment imatinib (Gleevec) used for chronic myelogenous leukemia (CML) had shown the potential of modern molecular science in a rare cancer, trastuzumab had proven it in a common one. It is no exaggeration to say trastuzumab launched the modern age of cancer medicine in the general oncology unit.

"Herceptin needs to be combined with chemotherapy. There have been two chemotherapy treatments typically used. We recommend four treatments of Adriamycin and Cytoxan, followed by four treatments of Taxol every two weeks. The Herceptin is given weekly during the time you take the Taxol and then by itself to make a full year."

"That can cause heart damage, right?" Rachael asked.

"Yes, it has to be—" began Dr. Pearl.

"I don't want that one. I want the one that doesn't do that," announced Rachael.

"The second choice is six treatments of two drugs called Taxotere and Carboplatin given every three weeks with the Herceptin. This is also followed by the Herceptin alone to make a year," continued Dr. Pearl.

"That's it," announced Rachael. "I looked them up, and that's the one I liked. It's the best deal. Equal cure and less heart damage."

"Do you want to hear more about the choices?"

"No. Thank you."

Dr. Pearl looked at Ken, who shrugged. "It's how she makes decisions. Houses, deals, chemo, husband. She's usually right, too."

Rachael returned to Saratoga Springs where Dr. Matthews reviewed her history and the plan.

"So, if I take this treatment of the chemo and Herceptin for a year, I'll be cured?" asked Rachael.

"Probably, although there is still a small chance the cancer could return," he replied.

"And this was all figured out in the last ten years?"

"Yes."

"Glad I'm the youngest in my family then." Ken nodded his agreement.

"Do you have any other questions?" asked Dr. Matthews.

"No, but I want the genetic test for breast cancer. The *BRCA* test."

"Well, only about 5 percent of breast cancers are caused by an inherited *BRCA* gene mutation," replied Dr. Matthews. "*BRCA* mutations are usually found in patients diagnosed at a young age who have a family history of breast or ovarian cancer. Jewish families are at more risk. You do not fit into those categories."

"I know all that stuff. I still want the test. You know Lorraine Jones, you did it for her."

"I can't talk about other patients."

"I know that. But she had it and found out she was Jewish. Turns out her father's mother had been from Germany. Who knew? I told her it shouldn't have been a surprise. I mean, she's always winning at mahjong."

"Your insurance will probably not pay for the test."

"It did for Lorraine."

"I cannot talk about her. But they will only pay if you are diagnosed at an early age or have a strong family history."

"I'm not worried, you'll find a way."

Rachael's treatment consisted of the chemotherapy drugs Taxotere and carboplatin with the Herceptin in a four-hour intravenous treatment. At her teaching session, nurse Karen Lange reviewed the medications and their side effects. Karen had also bought a home from Rachael and knew her style.

"You are not to do any business after we start the medications. Do you understand me? If I see or hear any business being done, I will take away your phone. These medicines make you unable to think clearly, and I do not want to find City Hall has been sold," Karen announced.

Ken laughed while Rachael looked mildly annoyed. The day after treatment, Rachael would return for a shot of Neulasta.

"The shot is to boost your white cells and keep you from getting an infection," Karen said. "It may cause your bones to ache for a few days."

"I saw their ad on television," replied Rachael. "A woman talking about how her sister needed the shot to fight her cancer. At first, I thought it was an ad for a dementia medicine. The one with the cancer looked brain dead. Don't let that happen to me. I read on the internet Claritin may help with the bone pain."

"Some people say it does; most don't. Why not wait and see if it is a problem?"

Rachael's first infusion went smoothly. As agreed, she did not transact any business, but by the end of the four hours, she had extracted life stories from every patient in the treatment area except one.

"That fellow down there at the end, Denton he said his name was. He's a little scary. I think I'll leave him alone."

"He's okay once you get to know him," reassured Karen.

"I think he has been in some dark places. I doubt he's a future home sale."

The week after her treatment, Rachael visited with Angela Pagano, the nurse practitioner.

"I was sick. But I had a busy week. We had a party the night I got my chemo. I didn't tell anyone here, of course, or I would be in chemo jail. Anyway, the company had rented a cruise boat on Lake George, and I couldn't miss it. I didn't drink, though. But the motion made me sick. Thankfully, someone had some marijuana brownies, so I ate one of those and felt better until I got dizzy. I think I was stoned."

"Why didn't you take your anti-nausea medication?" asked Angela.

"The brownie looked so good."

Two weeks later Rachael returned for her second treatment in a perfectly matched wig. As Dr. Matthews entered the room, he heard the end of her phone conversation.

". . . Tell him it's my last offer. I'm getting my chemo now, and he better take it, cause I'll be a raging bitch tomorrow."

After a quick exam, Dr. Matthews handed the chart to Karen.

"I think she is ready for her second treatment," he added. "Although it is a bit hard to tell sometimes."

"I know she thinks she is ready," replied Karen. "She called me on her cell from the exam room while she was waiting for you and told me to get everything mixing. 'Rush, rush, rush,' she said."

Dr. Matthews looked up. "What did you say?" he asked.
"I told her she wasn't flying this plane."

❖ ❖ ❖

SAFETY IN MEDICAL CARE.
On a snowy January 13, 1982, Air Florida Flight 90 took off from Washington National Airport. Heavily laden with ice, it crashed into the 14th Street bridge and fell into the Potomac River, killing seventy-eight people, including passengers, crew, and passing motorists. Four passengers and one flight attendant survived. This scene of great horror was also one of great bravery. Overhead a United States Park Police helicopter piloted by Donald W. Usher and manned by paramedic Melvin E. Windsor risked their own crash to pull survivors to shore. Beneath them, Lenny Skutnik jumped into the freezing waters to help. Passenger Arland Williams repeatedly handed the rescue rope to others and thus himself drowned. Williams was memorialized then and years later by President Ronald Reagan when he said in times of crises "our fellow man and yes, I believe our Maker—are waiting to see if we will pass the rope."[349]

The specific cause of the Air Florida crash was a series of pilot and copilot errors: failure to recognize the conditions, failure to delay for proper de-icing, ignoring instrument readings, and, perhaps most glaringly, failing to activate engine anti-ice equipment. When the copilot expressed some concerns, they were ignored by the pilot. Both died.

More broadly, the cause of the crash was a cockpit and flight culture derived from wartime where fighter pilots were deities who made the decisive single-person decisions needed to succeed in battle. The horrific crash of Air Florida Flight 90 is credited with changing the culture of the aviation industry to a system which emphasized communication within the flight team. The industry has become a model for system safety. The results were seen in 2005 at Logan International Airport when a copilot of a US Airways jet recognized an impending crash at takeoff and aborted the flight, saving the plane, and earning the praise of the pilot.[350]

Medical culture has been slowly undergoing the same changes. The image of the decisive surgeon quickly operating to save a dying person dominated health care culture in the same way the image of the fighter pilot with absolute control of the plane dominated the aviation system. In 2000, the National Academy of Medicine challenged this culture with its famous report *To Err is Human*. The Academy reported that between forty-four thousand and ninety-eight thousand Americans died each year from medical complications in hospitals—a widely publicized number used to drive safety improvements.[351]

The number is not precise. The Academy of Medicine did not examine the records of all hospitalized patients; no one could. Instead, they relied on two studies which reviewed a sampling of records to estimate the average rates of adverse events, including those causing death. This rate was then multiplied by the number of hospital admissions to produce the final number. One general problem with this methodology is that the number of hospital admissions in the United States is very large: thirty-three million six hundred thousand at the time of the studies. Even a small change in the rate of adverse events will produce a large change in the number of possible deaths when multiplied by thirty-three million six hundred thousand. Identifying adverse events and determining if they caused death is not easy, and any bias in either direction on the part of the reviewers is magnified greatly. A second issue was the imprecise use of the word "error." These first studies examined "adverse events" which could be the result of medical actions with or without negligence. Only a quarter of the adverse events involved negligence, meaning most adverse events were not errors in the common understanding of the word.[352] The word error was often equated with an adverse event. Finally, although the studies noted that elderly and sick patients with complex illnesses were more likely to have these adverse events, the Academy figures were often reported as if they applied equally to all patients.

Regardless of the imprecision inherent in the Academy's number, the recognition of the problem resulted in multiple efforts to improve patient safety. Many changes have been modeled after the airline industry: checklists, enhanced technology, standardized protocols and, most importantly, attempts to build a culture which encourages all members of the team to speak up when anything seems amiss. Some of the issues in aviation and health care are similar, such as the need to deliver complex, high-volume, high-risk services in an environment with time and financial constraints while dealing with the pressures of the public. Experts such as Captain Chesley "Sully" Sullenberger, the pilot who famously landed his damaged plane on the Hudson River in 2009 and saved the lives of the passengers and crew, have contributed to this effort. A whole new industry in medical safety has developed with its own terminology, statistical analysis, and techniques. Medicare and insurance companies are applying financial pressure to providers by refusing to pay for some preventable adverse effects.[353]

In oncology, chemotherapy administration has historically been an area of great concern because of the complexity of the drugs and the high risk they pose even when used correctly. Adverse events are common even when drugs are used properly without medical errors. When true medical errors with chemotherapy do occur, they can be devastating. Several years before *To Err is Human* was published, one such error occurred when thirty-nine-year-old *Boston Globe* health reporter Betsy Lehman died after being given an overdose of chemotherapy at the Dana Farber Cancer Institute.[354] The Dana Farber responded by instituting many changes in how it delivered chemotherapy to patients and has developed standards used in many other programs.

Progress like that seen at the Dana Farber has been made elsewhere in our medical system. Yet it was reported in 2016 that medical errors are the third leading cause of death in the United States, emphasizing the work still to be done.[355] Medical success itself is making the challenge more difficult. As frontline physicians or nurses know, hospitalized patients are sicker now than even ten years ago and therefore at much more risk for adverse events. The bewildering array of new high-tech procedures and medications which may lengthen or improve life also mean more risk in the hospital. Most analyses do not examine the risk of medical errors in offices or at home, where the increasing complexity of medications and care pose additional dangers even as they offer potential rewards.

Medicine is not air flight, and the differences help demonstrate why medical adverse events are particularly difficult to reduce. Medical care of the individual is complex, and many conditions and patients do not have either clear destinations or flight plans. Medical crashes do not always leave obvious wreckage. Medical errors are often difficult to identify, the consequences uncertain, and the record is usually not as definitive as a plane's black box. When errors occur, there is no National Transportation Safety Board to investigate. In fact, there are powerful legal incentives not to fully examine all errors—physicians and hospitals fear lawsuits. Finally, medicine also has two other key differences from the airline industry. Medicine can't ground its many planes which should not be flying; it is the job of doctors, nurses, and hospitals to get wrecks airborne. And once airborne, many patients choose to pilot their own course.

Three weeks later, Rachael was back for treatment number three. This time she did not call Karen as she waited for Dr. Matthews in the exam room.

"I did better the second time. It was the water from Lourdes," she preemptively declared as Dr. Matthews entered the exam room.

"Lourdes?" he asked, puzzled.

"You know your patient Joan Prince?"

"You know I can't talk about other patients," replied Dr. Matthews.

"But you do know Joan Prince. She told me so, so don't worry about telling me. Anyway, she has a niece with terrible breast cancer.

You don't know her. There isn't much hope for the poor thing, and she's only forty. They were doing a fund raiser for her at the Home Show, and I met them there. I told her I was going through chemo too and how sick I was the first time. They had gone to Lourdes to get some of the healing water, and she gave me some, so I drank it the night after chemo."

"That's nice," replied Dr. Matthews.

"Don't worry. I saved enough for the other four treatments, too."

Two weeks later, Dr. Matthews was surprised to find the results of Rachael's *BRCA* test on his desk. She did not have a mutation. He stopped by the office of his office manager, Patricia Wright.

"Pat, how did you get coverage?" he asked, holding the paper. "She really did not meet the medical criteria."

Pat laughed. "Well, Rachael has AHP for insurance. I called Sandy, their benefits manager, to check on her coverage. Turns out, she knew Rachael. I guess Rachael was involved in the sale of Sandy's house. How did Sandy put it? It's not worth saving $3000 to have everyone in the region hear we denied her . . . It would probably cost them $300,000 in ads to make it up if that tiger got mad." She paused. "Or is it tigress?"

"I'm not sure," Dr. Matthews replied. "I always thought the female was tigress, but then we learned about 'tiger moms,' so now I'm not sure. Anyway, the tigress will be pleased the test was negative."

On her fourth treatment, Rachael sat next to Ben Smith, an older man with a mischievous look who was also getting an infusion.

"What do you have?" she asked him.

"I have breast cancer," he replied. "That's very rare in men, you know."

"I bet," she answered. "Are you getting Herceptin, too. That's what I get."

"Nah," he laughed. "That's only for girls . . ."

"For girls? What do you mean?" Rachael asked.

"Honey, I get His-ceptin." Ben's cackling echoed throughout the treatment room, punctuated as he slapped his thigh, obviously immensely enjoying his joke. Ken's deep laugh quickly followed. For one treatment, Rachael Simon was quiet.

After the chemotherapy finished, Rachael underwent seven weeks of daily radiation treatments, one each weekday. The radiation produced some redness of her breast but otherwise no symptoms.

"They are pretty fussy over there, too," she reported to Karen. "I tried to get them to let me have a few treatments in Hilton Head, but Dr. Chris gave the same safety lecture as you did . . . No rushing, check, check, check . . . Blah, blah, blah."

Rachael also returned every three weeks for a treatment with Herceptin alone. These visits were not unpleasant, a quick meeting with Dr. Matthews and ninety minutes with the nurses. Although Rachael could have worked during these treatments, much to Karen's surprise her cell phone stayed off. She preferred to talk quietly with Ken and visit with the nurses and other patients who she had come to know.

"This isn't so bad," she remarked to Karen after six months had gone by.

"I think you feel safe here, getting the treatment," remarked Ken. To Karen's surprise, Rachael nodded her agreement.

Rachael's year of Herceptin had been her best year ever for home sales. Genentech, too, had a stellar year.

"Do you know what they charge for this stuff?" she asked Karen, who nodded. "When I saw the bill, I bought stock in the company."

Suddenly, the year was over.

"What now? Do I have a party? How do I know I'm cured?" Rachael demanded.

"The party is up to you. About the cure, we don't know for sure," Dr. Matthews replied. "We know the statistics are that most women in your position are cured, but we cannot guarantee for an individual person—"

"What about a PET scan?" she interrupted.

"That won't tell you if there are a few cancer cells which have survived somewhere in your body. Only time will tell that—"

"Well, how do we catch it before it spreads? Won't the PET scans help do that?"

"No," he answered. "Doctors have tried doing regular scans to check patients. There were several problems with that approach. Often the cancers were discovered in between the scans. Often the scans picked up things that were not cancer, leading to more unneeded tests. In the end, there was no survival improvement with the regular scans. And they exposed women who were probably cured to radiation. So, we do scans only if you have a problem or we find something on exam or your blood work. We can also order scans if someone has a personal reason. The most common is that they are making a life change and need to know everything is fine. Changes like taking a new job or going to Africa for a year. We can also order them if someone is having other medical or psychological issues that make it reasonable to do the scans. I must say, though, that the insurance companies are making these situations very difficult. Often they simply won't pay."

"So, I just wait? I don't think I like this," she replied.

"I don't blame you," replied Dr. Matthews, "but there is no good answer. It really is one of the hardest things about being a survivor. When you start to feel anxious, though, remember your statistics are very good. And call us if you aren't sure or need help. You will see your surgeon in three months, and I will see you in six months."

SEARCHING THE BODY: SCANS AND LABS.

In 1962, Electric and Music Industries (EMI) signed an English band named the Beatles to a contract. Their first recording session at the famous Abbey Road Studio produced "Love Me Do," and the rest is history. The Beatles made EMI so much money that the company could support the work of engineer Godfrey Hounsfield who made the first CT scanner and won a Noble Prize.

Maybe. Like much with the Beatles, it is hard to separate fact from fiction, and the Fab Four's contribution to radiology may belong on the B-side of the CT record.[356] Nevertheless, it is true that the CT scan was developed at EMI. In 1971, the first brain CT scan was done. In 1975, the body was added, and within a decade CT scanning was widely available.

CT stands for computerized tomography. Tomograms are x-rays taken at different angles and had been used for years to give better views of spots, particularly in the lung. The multiple x-rays were hung on a lighted board and radiologists would try to imagine the three-dimensional shape. Housenfield's scanner took many tomograms and fused them into an image using the computer, allowing physicians to see into the body. Over the next twenty years, CT and other scans became widely used in oncology to detect tumors at much smaller sizes than regular x-rays. Scanning followed by anxious waiting became a well-established ritual for cancer patients.

For women who had undergone treatment for breast cancer and were hopefully cured, the initial widespread use of CT and other scans in the 1980s and 1990s was followed by increasing restraint. Regular scans can detect recurrence before a woman has symptoms, but studies showed that treatment results are not improved, and the women do not live longer. Simply put, finding that a woman's breast cancer has spread widely through her body a few months earlier usually does not make any difference in her survival. Regular scans also raised concerns about radiation exposure and the need for additional tests to evaluate noncancerous findings. Ultimately, oncology professional societies issued guidelines limiting the use of scans to situations where women have symptoms or abnormal blood tests suggesting a recurrence of their cancer. These guidelines are used in "choosing wisely" campaigns by groups like the American Society of Clinical Oncology seeking to reduce the use of procedures and tests. Insurance companies have been enthusiastic adopters of guidelines to restrict payment for scans. Since there are individual women who have benefitted from testing, patients and their doctors still struggle to decide when to do the tests.

"Tumor markers" or "cancer blood tests" raise many of the same issues as CT scans. The 1960s saw the introduction of the carcinoembryonic antigen (CEA) test for colon cancer, followed in the 1970s by the PSA for prostate and others like the CA27-29 (or related CA15-3) for breast cancer. Like CT and bone scans, the CA 27-79 test was enthusiastically adopted by many oncologists to watch women after treatment for breast cancer. At times, it can detect a recurrence before a woman has symptoms. Like the situation with scans, when the CA27-29 finds recurrent cancer, it is usually widespread, and the outcome is often not changed by early detection. The CA27-29 also produces elevated readings not due to cancer which lead to more tests and anxiety. Studies have not shown any benefit for the CA27-29 test in groups of women, and professional guidelines discourage the use of the test. Since some individual women have benefitted, many oncologists are reluctant to completely abandon the test.

Tumor markers like the CEA, PSA, and CA27-29 rely on a relatively old process called an immunoassay to detect the specific proteins. More specific and sensitive techniques which can be used to detect cancer cells. One example is the polymerase chain reaction (PCR) used in chronic myelogenous leukemia (CML). This rare cancer of the white blood cells is caused by damage which reverses parts of chromosomes 9 and 22, producing an abnormal growth protein which drives the leukemia. CML can be cured by variations of imatinib (Gleevec), the exciting example of targeted cancer therapy introduced in the late 1990s. When patients are treated for CML, their routine blood tests can become normal, yet they can still have the disease. The PCR test was developed in the mid-1980s and is now used to check the results of CML treatment. If the PCR test shows the treatment is not working, the drug will be changed long before the person would otherwise ever be aware of the failure. In patients with CML, modern PCR testing guides treatment.

Applying tests like PCR to women after breast cancer treatment is more complex. All these sensitive tests produce "false positives" (other conditions mimicking breast cancer) and "false negatives" (missing breast cancer). In addition, for these tests to be useful it must be certain that the small number of breast cancer cells they detect cause harm. In some women, small numbers of breast cancer cells might not have clinical meaning if they fail to grow or are controlled by the immune system. Finally, and most importantly, these tests must result in a useful change in treatment (as they do in CML). Even a modern breast cancer blood test which could reliably detect a few cancer cells in the body might not be clinically useful without new treatments. Sorting out the results of modern cancer blood tests is challenging.

Understanding this complexity when you are facing cancer is not always easy. At times, we just want to know everything is okay.

Three years ago, near the anniversary of Rachael's second year from diagnosis, the palpitations made another appearance.

"I thought I was going crazy," she explained to Dr. Matthews. "It started with one my clients who had breast cancer, Donna Bright. You treated her. Anyway, we went to Albany for a breast cancer walk. Afterward, we were having a few drinks, and she had a seizure and ended up in the emergency room. Everything was okay, thank God. But they gave her some vitamins in an intravenous, and she said she felt better right away."

"Okay," replied Dr. Matthews, waiting for the conclusion of the story.

"Well," Rachael continued, "I figured the vitamins were a good idea, so I started on vitamin B12 from the nutrition store. Right away my heart rate went up, and I got scared thinking about Donna, so I went to the emergency room. They put me on a beta blocker and sent me to a cardiologist for an exercise test. I passed that but then I got a migraine, and my blood pressure went up. The cardiologist thought I might have something wrong with my adrenal glands, so he sent me to an endocrinologist. She made me stop the beta blocker and collect my urine for twenty-four hours. Let me tell you, carrying that jug around to open houses was no fun."

"What did the endocrinologist say?" asked Dr. Matthews.

"Well, I never made it back to her. When she took me off the beta blocker, my palpitations got so bad again I had to go back to the emergency room. They spoke to her on the phone and found out my urine was okay."

"Did they start you back on the beta blocker?"

"Yeah. I only took it a few days because Ken threw out the vitamin B12 pills and everything went away. Can you believe it?"

"Are you sure those were vitamin B12 pills?" asked Dr. Matthews.

"Who knows. Anyway, I told Ken he saved me. I might have died from a heart attack. Thank goodness they are over, and I can get back to work."

Palpitations gone, Rachael's home sales at the end of the year reached another high.

Two years ago, the palpitations were back. The cardiologist had her wear a month-long monitor and found no problems with her heart.

"He thinks I'm crazy, which is true. Says I have too much stress, which is also true. Work is tough; they're animals out there—even in Saratoga, which isn't so quiet anymore. You have ten good years, but have to prove yourself all over again on number eleven. And now I am stressed about my parents. They are three hours away, near Boston, and won't listen to me. I keep telling them they need to move into assisted living before something happens. No way, my father tells me. How about a nice ranch, at least? I even found them the perfect place, but he won't hear of it. He insists they are staying in their home; two floors and a basement. Every time I try to help, he undoes it. He has a shop in his basement, and the lights on the stairs going down were so dim I thought he would fall and kill himself. So, I had them changed.

At least that way the stairs were bright. I went back a few weeks later, and he had changed them all back."

"Did he say why?" asked Dr. Matthews, curious.

"He doesn't like bright light in the basement. And that's the way it is."

A referral to a psychiatrist brought Rachael additional anti-anxiety medication and behavioral modification sessions.

"She is a remarkable woman," reported Dr. Issel, the psychiatrist. "She has amazing energy which allows her to succeed in business but can trigger repeated anxiety attacks when she gets under extreme pressure. She has the pressures of trying to stay on top of her game at work and dealing with her parents, particularly her father who sounds just as independent as Rachael. Plus, she also has her cancer history and is scared. She knows so many people, so of course she knows a number who have recurred. And she is taking all their stories to heart. Under her aggressive side, Rachael does care for people. I have her seeing our psychologist, Michelle Brooks, who is very experienced with these issues."

"Good," replied Dr. Matthews. "As you know, it's common for pressures to build like this in survivors, particularly after they have been out a few years. They hear about other patients and get anxious. Even if statistically her chances of a recurrence are getting smaller, the thoughts of going back into our world often get worse. Anyway, I'm glad she has your team. I guess we will see where this all goes . . ."

"Right now, she is still running in the red zone, but hopefully things will calm down."

They did, although the stress of Rachael's parents did not change.

"Mom was in the hospital with pneumonia, and they sent her home with oxygen. I arranged for a monitoring company to come in. They would hook her up with a lifeline and an oxygen thingy to measure her oxygen. They could even put in motion sensors and a camera so I can make sure they are safe. The insurance company was willing to pay for some of it. Part of their plan to keep people safe at home. You know what Daddy did?"

Dr. Matthews shook his head.

"Sent them home. Told the guys he'd be damned if anyone was getting into his house to put in a spy camera for the insurance company or government. And he's still driving. He refuses to go to the doctor anymore in case they try to talk him out of it."

Ken looked up, "He has that same drive that I love about his daughter, too."

Rachael looked at him, mostly lovingly. "Be quiet," she said. Thankfully, once again the attacks faded.

A year ago, the attacks recurred when John Evans, Rachael's longtime tennis coach, announced he was no longer teaching. Although Evans was a private man, Rachael learned that he had pancreatic cancer. The news had rocked her.

"But he looked so good when I saw him. I mean, that guy could run circles around all of us," she reported to Dr. Matthews. "So, when you tell me I look good it doesn't really mean much, does it?"

"Well, it means something, but it does not guarantee there is no active cancer," replied Dr. Matthews.

"And the blood work? That's not very useful either, is it?"

"It is not perfect either," he agreed.

"Maybe I should have a PET scan."

"Is there any reason to think Rachael has pancreatic cancer?" asked Ken.

"No," answered Dr. Matthews. He turned to Rachael. "I know it is hard, but you will meet many people with different cancers, particularly with the number of people you know. You can't get a PET scan every time something happens, no matter how sad or upsetting the situation. That would be bad for you. We need to send you for a scan only if you are having a problem."

Rachael nodded. "I understand. Keep waiting."

The second crisis came six months later. Renee Hampton, a young woman diagnosed with breast cancer shortly after Rachael and with whom she had shared chemotherapy sessions, had a recurrence of her cancer and was restarting chemotherapy.

"It's in her hip and spine. I heard she didn't even have any pain; they found it by accident on a bone density test."

"I can't talk about her—"

"I feel terrible for her. What about me? How do I know it's not it's not in my bones? I think I want that PET scan now."

"Are you having any pain or other symptoms?" asked Dr. Matthews.

"No. Isn't my anxiety enough?" she responded.

"Before we do any tests other than your regular labs, I want you to go back to Dr. Issel and work on your anxiety."

Dr. Issel called a month later.

"Rachael has been doing better. After her friend had the recurrence of her breast cancer, Rachael realized she needed to make changes to survive mentally. She has cut back on work and found a way to step out of the direct competition for sales. Her father is quieter, too. Her sister moved near her parents and has taken over most of the responsibility while Rachael has been a back-up. Her meds are balanced, and Michelle Brooks has her on a regular schedule of visits. She still struggles with thinking there is cancer lurking in her body and that can trigger a panic attack. But for now, she is okay."

"So, we don't need to send her for scans," replied Dr. Matthews.

"Today is good. She will let us know if life changes."

Today's visit came after Rachael had learned Renee Hampton's cancer had worsened.

"I'll tell you why I want a PET scan. Poor Renee . . . She had the same thing as me . . . a small breast cancer. We took our treatments together . . . All that chemo and now she has cancer everywhere . . . And she's going to die soon, right?"

"I'm sorry. You know I can't talk about her condition. What about you? Are you having any new symptoms?"

"I can't tell. I think about Renee all the time. And John Evans. I heard his cancer is growing and he'll be dead soon, too. My heart races and I can't sit still . . . I know my cancer is back."

Ken nodded. "She really is having a hard time. The cancer is consuming her thoughts and setting off the panic attacks. This is the worst I've ever seen her."

Rachael continued. "So, I need a PET scan. I want to be sure I don't have cancer spread throughout me."

"Okay, but—" began Dr. Matthews.

"I know," she interrupted, her words rapid. "I read all about how they are putting pressure on you doctors not to order these scans. Some doctors even lose money when they do."

"That's not the problem here," he continued. "I do not have a financial stake one way or the other."

"What is the problem then?" she demanded.

"Your insurance company will have hired a group of doctors to review your records. They will likely conclude that there is no clear physical reason for the scan. They will say it does not fit into their guidelines. I will argue with them, but it is most likely they will refuse to pay for the test."

Rachael stood up. "I need it . . . and I know you will find a way, just like you did for the genetic test."

Carol Feinman 6: Breast cancer (Boston, 1992)

Almost three years had passed since Carol's chemotherapy. She and Nancy Pyle had finished exercising in the sweaty gym where Carol now felt strangely at home among the muscular body builders, martial artists, and serious weight lifters. Nancy pointed out a popular protein supplement sold behind the counter.

"Most of that stuff is garbage," she pronounced. "But this is all natural, and I think it will help you repair muscle."

Carol decided to check with Dr. Carl, who had become well known for his studies on the use of alternative medicine and remained a good natured and compassionate touchstone. He carefully read the label.

"I can't see how anything here would be harmful to you and it certainly provides a good amount of protein," he answered. "As part of your exercise program, I think it is a fine addition. Let's just do a baseline set of lab tests to check the liver and kidney function. After you have used it for a few months, we can repeat them just to be sure. You are doing a wonderful job, Carol."

"Thanks. I feel great."

Carol went directly to the main lab. The waiting room contained a few healthy looking middle-aged people, one mother with a nervous looking preteen daughter, and an old man in obvious good humor dressed in a dated three-piece suit and carrying a hat. Different from my usual place, she thought. She sat across from the old man.

"The doctor says I need my sugar checked," he announced to Carol. "Sugar, shumugger. When you are my age, do you really care about sugar?"

"You should," replied Carol instinctively.

"Why?" he asked. "I've had a good life. My parents brought me here from Austria as a child. I remember the boat ride. Such waves. I lived through the depression, survived the War, raised my family, and have seen my grandchildren grow. I'm an old man. Why should my doctor check my sugar? If it is high, he will take away my Babka in the morning. It shall not be so . . ."

Just as he was warming to the subject, the phlebotomist approached, a large black man who obviously knew him.

"You take me away from this beautiful young woman to draw my blood . . . There is no justice," the old man moaned dramatically.

"No justice this morning, Henry. Not from us vampires."

"Oy vey. Good luck, my dear," he told Carol, bowed, and walked slowly off.

It's nice to be outside the Oncology Unit, she thought. On the other hand, it has been exciting to see what is happening in the breast cancer world. The fund-raising, runs, and pink ribbons. Two weeks ago, she and Nancy had marched in Boston Commons to support the cause.

BREAST CANCER AND THE BIRTH OF PINK.

In 1990, the federal government spent a pitiful $77 million on breast cancer.[357] By 1993, it was $443 million, an increase attributable to the breast cancer advocacy movement which that year petitioned President Clinton to expand funding with over 2.6 million signatures.[358] Despite this success, breast cancer remained well behind HIV in the race for government dollars. In 1990, the allocation for the virus had been $1.6 billion, greater than the entire cancer budget.[359] Why was HIV so successful and breast cancer so neglected?

The discovery of HIV as the cause of AIDS in 1984 came after the illness had spread through the gay community and among intravenous drug users. Initially unknown and undetectable, by 1987 the virus had killed twenty thousand people in the United States alone, and it seemed the gay community would be decimated. Yet that year also brought the rise of the AIDS Coalition to Unleash Power (ACT UP), the aggressive group which would change how America set health care priorities and made funding decisions. Although AIDS activism was a complex social process with many players, the defining moment is often credited to ACT UP founder Larry Kramer, an outspoken author and playwright, who issued his famous call to fight or die.[360] ACT UP challenged all aspects of the political, medical, and biotech structure and fought for HIV funding using dramatic public displays and confrontation, following the motto of Malcolm X, "by any means necessary."[361] It was an impressive mobilization of human resources which rapidly produced results and confirmed their slogan "silence equals death."

Breast cancer activism developed more gradually. In the 1940s, socialite Mary Lasker challenged the then stagnant American Cancer Society to become more relevant. In the 1950s, Terese Lasser began the Reach to Recovery program for women who had undergone mastectomy, challenging the surgical establishment.[362] Despite their efforts, breast cancer remained stigmatized, hidden from public view, and ignored in establishment funding processes. In the 1970s and early 1980s, substantive changes began. Well-known women courageously brought their breast cancers into the public spotlight: actress Shirley Temple Black (1972), first lady Betty Ford (1974), Happy Rockefeller (1974). Accompanying this public awareness was activism. Pioneer Rose Kushner, a forty-five-year-old journalist at the time of her diagnosis in 1974, worked to change the surgical approach of the time. She refused, then publically condemned, the "one-step procedure" in which a woman underwent a biopsy then immediately had a mastectomy if cancer was found, waking up unsure if she had lost her breast or not. Kushner served as the public representative on the National Institute of Health (1979), worked with famed surgeon Bernard Fisher to promote the radical concept of "breast conservation" with lumpectomy and radiation, and later helped form the National Alliance of

Breast Cancer Organizations (1986). She died of metastatic breast cancer at age sixty.[363] Other women, including Betty Rollin, an NBC news reporter, and Andre Lorde, a poet and African-American feminist, made personal accounts of their experiences in print and on film.[364]

Modern breast cancer organizations began with the foundation of the Susan G. Komen Breast Cancer Foundation in 1982 by Nancy Brinker, who named it after her sister who died of breast cancer. One year later, the first Race for the Cure in Dallas, Texas, attracted seven hundred women.[365] In 1986, many smaller breast cancer groups joined the umbrella National Alliance of Breast Cancer Organizations, although the Komen Foundation remained independent. By the late 1980s, breast cancer was openly discussed, changing treatment options were promoted by pioneering women breast surgeons like Dr. Susan Love, and multiple grassroots organizations existed across the country. Women's issues were gaining traction, and the National Institute of Health began a "major commitment to research on women's health and illness" called the Women's Health Initiative to study issues like heart disease, female cancers, and osteoporosis.[366]

Despite the advances of the 1980s, funding for breast cancer remained minimal. Beginning in the 1990s, this finally changed as a complex and multi-dimensional breast cancer movement matured. The Komen Foundation expanded its more traditional fundraising and corporate sponsorship strategies. Other groups with a variety of different political viewpoints encompassing feminist and minority outlooks also grew. In 1991, many of these groups formed the National Breast Cancer Coalition (NBCC), a national lobbying organization with a more aggressive, occasionally militant, outlook. Among its many activities, the NBCC worked with President Clinton on a National Action Plan on Breast Cancer and helped develop the Department of Defense Breast Cancer Research Program.[367] As one might expect with a serious disease which strikes all women, the complex breast cancer movement of the 1990s resists easy definition. Its breadth is seen in two iconic images. One is the photo of artist and breast cancer activist Matuschka in which her open dress revealed a mastectomy scar, seen on the cover of the Sunday, August 13, 1993, *New York Times Magazine*. The raw and palpable emotion in Matuschka's self-portrait remains an enduring symbol of the disease and its treatment.[368] The second iconic image from the 1990s is the pink ribbon, a gentler and broadly appealing symbol of hope and resolve worn across the country.

The influence of AIDS activism on the breast cancer movement in the 1990s was profound. The AIDS movement had significantly changed the public and political landscape for disease funding. It also had a significant effect on individuals. "They showed how to get through to the Government," reported activist Shelia Swanson. "They took on an archaic system and turned it around while we were dying."[369] Although in general the breast cancer movement was less confrontational and many of their tactics unique, the direct demonstration of the result of breast cancer in Matuschka's photograph was the type of call to action that ACT UP members would have appreciated. Possibly the best summary came from activist Elenore Prez, who noted that "AIDS has created a terrible, wonderful model for us all."[370]

Which brings us back to the the pink ribbon. In 1991, the Visual AIDS Artists' Caucus in New York created the red ribbon, a six-inch, V-shaped ribbon worn to symbolize AIDS Awareness. They chose red for its "connection to blood and the idea of passion—not only anger, but love."[371] The red ribbon was worn by Jeremy Irons at the 1991 Tony Awards, became an international symbol, appeared on a U.S. postage stamp in 1993, and remains in use today.[372] The profound influence of the AIDS red ribbon led to the immediate use of the pink ribbon for breast cancer, first by the Komen Foundation at their 1991 New York City Race for the Cure. In 1992, the formidable combination of breast cancer survivor Charlotte Hayley, *Self* magazine editor Alexandra Penny, and cosmetic leader Evelyn Lauder began the mass expansion of the pink ribbon as the symbol of breast cancer known today. From the terror of AIDS had come another wonderful model.

The next day, Carol received a phone call from Dr. Carl telling her something called the alkaline phosphatase was elevated.

"It might be nothing," Dr. Carl reported, trying to be reassuring but not entirely succeeding. "But I called Dr. Spiegel, and he wants you to have a CT scan and a bone scan, then meet with him."

Carol and Rose returned to the oncology unit to hear the results.

"I'm sorry, Carol, but the scans show the cancer has recurred," Dr. Spiegel said softly. "You have three spots in your liver. They are small, each about one inch. You also have spots scattered in the bones of your spine, pelvis, and ribs."

"Oh, God," answered Rose. Carol looked dazed.

"None of these areas are immediately threatening to you," he continued after a moment. "But we need to start you on chemotherapy."

Carol nodded, still not sure what he meant. Rose took the lead.

"What chemotherapy?" she asked. Dr. Spiegel outlined the program of Adriamycin and Cytoxan given intravenously every three weeks.

"My cancer is back?" asked Carol after he finished.

He nodded. CJ joined them in the room. She sat on the other side of Carol and held her hand.

"How will we tell mom?" Carol asked Rose, crying.

They told Betty that night. As they walked up the steps of the familiar brownstone, Carol began to smell the ultrasound jelly. She remembered her trip up these stairs four years ago. When I first felt the cancer, I thought I could hide it, she thought. But I couldn't. Now there was no chance, no way for Carol to let her mother down easily. Betty knew as soon as they walked in.

"What's the matter? What has happened?" she asked. They sat in the front living room as Rose spoke and Carol sobbed, the smell of the brownstone and her childhood breaking down her last vestige of control. Betty hugged and rocked her.

"Don't worry, dear. It will be alright."

Carol's chemotherapy program began the next week. A few days before, Carol and Rose met with CJ to review the medications and the side effects, starting with nausea and vomiting. Carol recalled Nancy and Scott, the couple she had met during her first chemotherapy treatments.

"His wife told me he had terrible vomiting and needed to be put into a coma for his chemo. I know this Adriamycin and Cytoxan is much harder than what I had before. Will that happen to me?" Carol asked.

"What she said was true a few years ago, but it's very different now," said CJ. "We have a new medicine . . ."

CHEMOTHERAPY NAUSEA AND VOMITING: THE MIRACLE OF ZOFRAN.

Mice do not vomit when given chemotherapy. They lack the appropriate vomiting zone in their brain stem. The scientists studying chemotherapy in these rodents may have appreciated the clean cages, but their colleagues studying chemotherapy vomiting needed a different species. These researchers turned to ferrets, weasel-like, carnivorous mammals which grow to weigh about two pounds and vomit when given chemotherapy. In 1987, a group of British researchers reported that a compound named GR38032F could prevent vomiting in ferrets given the potent chemotherapy cisplatin. A year later similar results in humans were published. In 1991, the FDA approved the miracle drug ondansetron, brand named Zofran, for chemotherapy induced nausea and vomiting.

The story of ondansetron begins in 1715 in an old London house in Plough Court where Silvanus Bevan opened his apothecary. Bevan was a Quaker, described as "possessed of the reliability and shrewd business acumen [of] so many of that persuasion."[373] His firm prospered, providing medicines to English physicians and those in the colonies. In the 1790s, William Allen assumed control of the firm and with his second wife provided the name Allen & Hanburys.[374] Allen was also a Quaker with a broad range of scientific and philanthropic interests who made Plough Court a remarkable center of scientific and intellectual discourse. In an interesting historical twist, Allen was tutored by John Hodgkin, Sr., the father of Thomas Hodgkin, who later served as Allen's secretary. Although their short relationship ended with Hodgkin's disappointment at being denied an apprenticeship, the work introduced him to Guy's Hospital.[375] It was there Hodgkin later reported on the lymphoma which still bears his name (and for which ondansetron later would be very useful to those undergoing treatment). For the next hundred and fifty years, A & H was a successful pharmaceutical firm.

In 1958, Allen & Hanburys was acquired by Glaxo as the pharmaceutical industry began to consolidate into modern large corporations. A & H initially remained a separate division of Glaxo headed by well-known drug developer David Jack, using their expertise in "receptors" to produce several asthma medications and the stomach acid reducer ranitidine (Zantac). Receptors are cellular "locks" which have "keys," called ligands in scientific terminology. When the key (ligand) reaches the lock (receptor), an action takes place. During the 1970s and 1980s, scientific interest developed in receptors for 5-hydroxy-tryptamine (5-HT), also known as serotonin receptors. Jack's team and others described 5-HT receptors in many different tissues, including the gastrointestinal tract and brain. They also discovered 5-HT receptor blocking agents, which they hoped might treat headaches, mental illness, dementia, and bowel problems like colitis. Although they never realized most of these goals, A& H scientists did develop sumatriptan, which was useful for migraines, and GR38032F, which prevented chemotherapy vomiting in those unfortunate ferrets.[376]

The human studies were impressive. Cisplatin is a powerful chemotherapy which produces immediate debilitating nausea and vomiting. Patients receiving cisplatin were usually hospitalized and placed on high-dose infusions of anti-nausea medications like metoclopramide, which themselves had side effects like uncontrolled twitching or contorted movements and required large doses of diphenhydramine (Benadryl) and sedatives. Once the treatments were over, many patients could never return to the place they were given or even see the doctors or nurses involved for fear of triggering "recall" vomiting. Ondansetron dramatically reduced the nausea and vomiting produced by cisplatin. The importance of ondansetron in cancer treatment is hard to overstate. It allowed the administration of chemotherapy to many patients who would otherwise have been unable to tolerate the vomiting. Oncology treatments moved from the hospital to the outpatient clinic or office.

CJ's second topic was blood counts. Most importantly, low white blood count. Once again, Carol recalled the fear of infection she had with her first treatment.

CJ was once again reassuring. "Well, we have something new for that, too . . ."

NEUPOGEN: NEUTROPHILS TO THE RESCUE.

Growing white blood cells is not easy. Normal bone marrow white cells and even cancerous white cells (leukemia) usually die when placed in a flask in the lab. In the 1960s, separate groups of scientists in Israel and Australia identified substances which would enhance the growth of white blood cells. The group in Israel named theirs "mashran-gm" combining the Hebrew word "to go forth" with "gm" for granulocytes and macrophages (both white cells). The Australian group called their substance CSF for colony stimulating factor.[377] Although both groups are given credit for the discovery, the less poetic term CSF has endured.

Over the next twenty years, various CSFs were laboriously purified and identified in laboratories across the world. In the 1980s, the revolution in molecular biology allowed scientists to clone genes and insert them into bacteria to produce pure recombinant molecules. In 1985, Amgen scientist Larry Souza and Japanese scientist Shigekazu Nagata cloned the gene for G-CSF, which stimulates the production of granulocytes, also called neutrophils, which are white blood cells critical for fighting infections. The biotech firm Amgen in the United States and the brewer Kirin in Japan patented and produced G-CSF, combining new biotechnology with old beer money and fermentation experience. Amgen named their product Neupogen, choosing to use "neutrophil" rather than "granulocyte" in the name.

G-CSF's ability to stimulate the production neutrophils was important. As the use of chemotherapy had expanded in the 1970s and 1980s, physicians quickly realized that these drugs could produce low white blood counts, particularly low neutrophil counts (called neutropenia). Low neutrophil levels made patients vulnerable to overwhelming infections which could be fatal. Physicians had learned that when patients with low neutrophils had a fever, the time-honored approach of searching for an infection while waiting to treat with the proper antibiotic did not work. This dreaded complication of "febrile neutropenia" (fever with a low neutrophil count) demanded immediate treatment with broad spectrum antibiotics. Although this aggressive use of antibiotics reduced the number of deaths, the fear of neutropenia and hospitalization limited the use of many chemotherapy drugs. In 1987, G-CSF was tested at Memorial Sloan Kettering Cancer Center and markedly reduced the risk of infection due to low blood counts in patients receiving intensive chemotherapy. In 1991, the FDA approved G-CSF (Neupogen), which allowed physicians to safely give intensive chemotherapy and, combined with ondansetron to control vomiting, made chemotherapy treatments outside the hospital the norm. These products revolutionized cancer care.[378]

Neupogen also added luster to Amgen, the prototype for a successful modern medical biotech firm. Initially known as <u>A</u>pplied <u>M</u>olecular <u>Ge</u>netics, Amgen was co-founded in 1980 by William Bowes (after he left the pioneering biotech firm Cetus) with CEO George Rathmann, himself known as "Mr. Biotech." Capitalizing on investor excitement produced by companies like Genentech, Rathmann was successful in obtaining initial funding for Amgen's start, which today is recalled as a (possibly romanticized) collection of sneaker wearing, bicycle riding scientists laboring together in a small building in Thousand Oaks, California. Amgen survived lean financial times, partnered with Kirin, developed and marketed both its red cell stimulating drug Epogen then Neupogen, whose combined sales reached the billion-dollar mark in 1992.[379] In the words of its sales force, "neutrophils paid the bills."

"What about hair loss?" asked Carol.

"I'm sorry," answered CJ. "We don't have a good answer yet for that. Some women wear wigs. I can help you with that. Others just wear hats."

"What about those ice packs I saw some women use the first time? Did they help?" asked Carol, referring to an attempt by some women to pack their heads in ice while the chemotherapy was infusing into their body.

Rose looked puzzled. "Ice packs?" she asked.

CJ nodded. "The cold kept the blood flow to the scalp down, so less chemo reached the hair follicles. A few women thought it helped, but then someone reported a patient who had the cancer come back on her scalp. That was the end of that. We haven't seen them in few years."

CJ sat with Carol and Rose for nearly an hour, discussing how to prepare for fatigue, maintain nutrition, and even tell her friends. As they prepared to leave, Rose stopped and put her hand on CJ's arm.

"Carol often mentioned how good you were with her, but I had no idea a nurse could do so much . . ."

ONCOLOGY NURSING.

The Crimean War is high on the list of modern humankind's most confusing savagery. A conflict known to few modern Americans, it was fought from 1853 to 1856 and pitted Russia against the Ottoman Empire (modern Turkey), France, and England, with modest support from Sardinia and Austria. Most of the fighting took place on the Crimean Peninsula in the Black Sea, hence the name, and was for control of the region where Europe, Russia, and the Middle East meet near the modern Turkish city of Istanbul, at the time called Constantinople. The longstanding Ottoman Empire was failing, and Russia sought to fill the void. The War was also partially religious, continuing the struggles between Latin Catholics (French), Orthodox Catholics (Russia) and Muslims (Turkey) for dominance of this area so near the Holy Land. Complex personalities and ambitions of world leaders played a role, including Tsar Nicholas (Russia), Sultan Abdulmecid (Ottoman Empire), Napoleon III (France), and Queen Victoria (England). The Crimean War was one of the first major conflicts fought with exploding shells and modern rifles, advanced weapons which brought new efficiency to the slaughter, although disease still effectively competed to cause suffering. The War was also one of the first -conflicts covered in real time by the news media, notably the *Times* correspondent William Howard Russell who exposed British government mismanagement and fueled public resentment. The outcome was a defeat of Russia and the end of at least two hundred fifty thousand and possibly up to one million lives.

Recent histories of the Crimean War have synthesized these complex historical forces and linked them in fascinating ways to modern global issues,[380] yet the conflict is most commonly associated in the

English-speaking world with images from two famous poems. "The Charge of the Light Brigade" was written in 1854 by England's Poet Laureate Alfred, Lord Tennyson to commemorate the slaughter of a British cavalry unit ordered to attack a Russian artillery position at the end of a long valley. Correspondent Russell's account of the bravery of the unit formed the basis of the poem and its famous stanza,

> "Boldly they rode and well,
> Into the jaws of Death,
> Into the mouth of hell
> Rode the six hundred."

Elsewhere in the poem, Tennyson noted that the order to charge which sent the Light Brigade to its death was a communication error, emphasizing the mismanagement theme.

The second lasting memory of the Crimean War is that amid the savagery a woman from an upper-class British family began to organize care for the wounded. Her name was Florence Nightingale. She, too, was immortalized in verse when Henry Wadsworth Longfellow in 1857 described her as the "Lady with the Lamp" in his poem "Saint Philomena."

> Lo! in that house of misery
> A lady with a lamp I see
> Pass through the glimmering gloom,
> And flit from room to room.

Nightingale was born in 1820 in Firenze (Florence), Italy and raised in Victorian England. As a young woman, she had an interest in nursing, at the time considered a disgraceful profession unless undertaken by a religious order and certainly not suitable for someone of her social standing. Nightingale fought prejudice within her own family to become superintendent of a women's hospital in London, a position which gave her experience to serve in the Crimean War. In the process, Nightingale turned down marriage proposals which she feared might trap her in the life of a "bird in a gilded cage." Struggling against formidable conditions, chauvinistic attitudes, and incompetence, Nightingale used her determination to essentially rebuild military hospitals and devise systems for feeding, clothing, and caring for the wounded. In contrast to the managers of the war, she was beloved by the troops and admired by the British public.[381]

After the Treaty of Paris had ended the fighting, Florence Nightingale returned home to England. It was there she embarked upon an equally remarkable phase of her life. Limited by a mysterious illness, she turned to writing and over the next half century produced thirteen thousand letters and two hundred books and pamphlets.[382] Nightingale covered a wide range of subjects from the role of nurses to health care organization to statistics. She died in 1910 having redefined the profession of nursing.

Five years after the Crimean War ended, the American Civil War (1861-5) joined the list of terrible human destruction, albeit with a less confusing list of antagonists. At least six hundred twenty thousand died as North was pitted against South. This brutal conflict also produced beautiful poetry, such as Julia Ward Howes' "Battle-Hymn of the Republic," sung today with its famous stanza and chorus,

Mine eyes have seen the glory of the coming of the Lord;
He is trampling out the vintage where grapes of wrath are stored;
he hath loosed the fateful lightning of His terrible swift sword,
His truth is marching on.

Glory, Glory Hallelujah, Glory, Glory Hallelujah,
Glory, Glory Hallelujah, His truth is marching on.

As on the Crimean Peninsula, amid the slaughter came a woman to nurse the wounded. Described by Brigade Surgeon James Dunn as the "Angel of the Battlefield," she was named Clara Barton. Born in North Oxford, Massachusetts in 1821, Barton had also been attracted to nursing as a child, first ministering to her brother who became seriously ill after a fall. After traditional physicians nearly bled the boy to death, a follower of the botanist Samuel Thompson is given credit for his recovery, but it is most probable that Clara Barton's nursing saved her brother. Barton went on to become a teacher, established a free school for the poor, and became possibly the federal government's first female employee. Like Nightingale, Barton's passion for her work also dictated that she remained "free of matrimonial ties."[383]

As the Civil War started, the care of the wounded or ill Federal soldier was disjointed. Nightingale's work in the Crimean War had been noted, and President Lincoln authorized the formation of the U.S. Sanitary Commission, a private volunteer organization which sought to supplement the work of army surgeons. The Commission's director of nursing was Dorothea Dix, famous for her work with the mentally ill. Since there were no formal nursing programs in the country, this was on-the-job training. The Commission raised significant funds, obtained supplies, and organized care behind the lines, but had less success in providing front-line battlefield nursing. Barton received permission from the Surgeon General to tend to the wounded soldiers and used her own funds to start a battlefield relief organization. She moved her wagons and nurses to the front lines where she gained fame for her care of the wounded, providing an image of nursing which would attract great public attention. After the war, she devoted herself to discovering the fate of missing soldiers by forming the quaintly titled but effective Office of Correspondence with Friends of the Missing Men of The United States Army.[384]

In 1869, Barton traveled to Europe and met Dr. Louis Appia of the Internal Committee of Geneva, today known as the International Red Cross, which had been founded by Frenchman Henry Dunant five years earlier. Winner of the first Nobel Peace Prize, Dunant had been horrified when he witnessed a battlefield similar to those of Nightingale and Barton in Solferino, Italy. In response, he had organized the Red Cross Treaty, also known as the Geneva Treaty, which would later form the modern rules of warfare known as the Geneva

Convention. The Red Cross name and symbol came from the inverse of the Swiss flag (white cross on red) flying in Geneva. Barton worked with Red Cross volunteers in the Franco-Prussian war before returning to the United States where she promoted the Geneva treaty, ultimately signed by President Chester Arthur in 1882. Barton led the American Red Cross until 1904 and expanded the mission to include providing relief from natural disasters.[385] She died in 1912, her life an example of the Red Cross Nurse's Creed engraved in stone outside the Washington, D.C. headquarters.

> Wherever disaster calls
> there I shall go.
> I ask not for whom,
> but only where I am needed.

Beginning on the battlefields of the nineteenth century, Nightingale, Barton, and other similarly determined women transformed nursing and established its critical role in both the treatment of the individual patient and in the organization of the delivery of care. Over the next hundred years, their pioneering work led to the creation of the formal definition and ethics of the nursing profession which we understand today.

The "War on Cancer" was fought on a less barbaric but complex battlefield. This war brought advances in surgical techniques and radiation which required specialized nurses who understood the intricacies of these specialties, yet it was in the medical oncology inpatient and outpatient units that nurses faced the greatest challenges. The complexities of chemotherapy combined with its tremendous side effects called for a special type of nurse, one who could combine intelligence, technical skill, and compassion while comforting patients fearing death. It rapidly became the responsibility of oncology nurses to use the new supportive treatments like ondansetron (Zofran) for nausea and G-CSF (Neupogen) for low white blood counts. In 1973, the American Cancer Society held the first National Cancer Nursing Conference in Chicago, and a small group proposed an organization specifically for cancer nurses. Starting in 1976 with four hundred eighty-eight nurses, by 2016 the Oncology Nursing Society had thirty-nine thousand members.[386] Oncology nurses changed their battlefield dramatically as chemotherapy treatments moved from the hospital ward to the outpatient unit or office. Patients received complex treatments while living their lives at home, supervised and comforted by these descendants of Nightingale and Barton.

"I'm glad we have all these new medicines, but chemo still sucks," Carol reported to CJ after her first treatment. She had experienced some mild nausea for a few days; saltines seemed to help the most. Her mouth was a little sore, and she was achy, but overall it was not too bad.

The next issue was her hair. At work, Roger organized the team to take Carol to buy a wig, courtesy of Carlton Associates. Mary and Sophia had made preliminary selections, but Roger had reserved a salon owned by a friend on Newberry Street and made the final decisions. Carol sat as he inspected the choices.

"Perfect," he finally announced. "You look magnificent."

"It's very close, but not exactly like my hair," Carol commented, looking at her reflection as Roger stood, arms crossed, obviously pleased.

"Precisely, dear," he smiled, then pointed out the few changes he wanted to the stylist before continuing. "People will know something about you is a little different, but they will not understand what. It will keep them guessing. You need an air of mystery. Now, all we need is a special hat to go with it . . ."

"I've always wanted to get a hat from Harrods," she answered thoughtfully. "You know . . . in London."

Roger looked at Carol, feigning surprise. "I certainly do know Harrods. And some day we shall go. But for now, we will select the best the colonies have to offer."

Once the wig was secured, Nancy Pyle took over.

"You're not waiting for the chemo to make it fall out," she said over the phone. "You have to show you are in charge. I'm coming over to shave it off."

Carol agreed, and Nancy arrived at her apartment the next evening. Her five feet twelve inches and two hundred plus pounds was packed into jeans and a worn gray T-shirt while her own newly shaved head glistened. Behind her came two men from the gym whom Carol recognized, both with long-standing shaved heads. It was more muscle and less hair than Carol had ever seen on three people.

"Nancy, what did you do?" Carol asked, laughing and hugging her friend.

"These two knuckleheads having been daring me to do this for years," she grumbled, pointing her thumb backward over her shoulder.

"I'm Ben, and this is Dan," announced the fractionally larger of the two behemoths, "and we are here to pay off the bet." He set down the three pizzas and two six-packs on Carol's table, obviously prepared to eat and enjoy the show. It's a strange world, thought Carol later that night as she rubbed her sensitive scalp in the mirror and adjusted to her new look.

After three treatments, Carol knew the routine: one hard week, then two which were good. Scans confirmed her cancer had significantly improved. Dr. Spiegel wanted Carol to do three more cycles before the next testing.

After that visit, Rose visited Betty, just like when they were both young, and mother took eldest daughter's report at the end of the day.

"What will happen to Carol now?" asked Betty. "What do the doctors say?"

Rose weighed her words as she thought of Carol's warning to protect Betty.

"They say we will have to keep going and see how the treatment works," she replied evasively.

"What then?" asked Betty.

Rose hesitated.

"Don't protect me, Rose," she continued sadly. "It's not necessary . . ."

Rose nodded. "Hopefully this treatment works, then she gets a break. When the cancer grows back, she takes more chemo . . . until it stops working. Then . . ." She shrugged, almost helplessly, and it was quiet until Betty spoke.

"Then we take care of her, like we did Christine."

They sat together in silence.

2:00 Debra Packard: Breast Cancer

"She's with her husband and son in the big room," reported John Welt. "She said you didn't need to examine her and would just be talking."

"That's true," agreed Dr. Matthews. Debra Packard had been diagnosed with breast cancer three months ago. She had undergone a lumpectomy, recently completed radiation, and was here to discuss the next step in treatment.

John paused for a minute. "She's different. The son seems normal. And I can't figure the husband. Good luck in there."

Sitting in the first chair was Debra, a sixty-eight-year-old woman dressed in a unique combination of a vest, sweater, skirt, and leggings which somehow hung together but would be difficult to categorize. At her feet was a cloth book bag emblazoned with the slogan "Ban Fracking Now." Next was her husband Bud, dressed in plain chinos and a plaid shirt. At the end was her son, Ken, wearing a conservative gray suit. After greeting them, Dr. Matthews settled into his chair.

"How did your radiation go?" he asked Debra.

"There are things that doctors should think about when they send patients for treatments." She sat upright as if to lecture.

Dr. Matthews glanced at Ken, who rolled his eyes.

Debra's cancer was detected on the routine mammogram she had not wanted, a reluctance born from a deep suspicion of radiation, medicine, and most doctors. Fortunately, Debra had long been enamored with Dr. Andrew Weil, a pioneer of "integrative medicine" and found one of his disciples nearby. Dr. Humana Carey was an enthusiastic young woman who had completed four years of medical school followed by three years of family and integrative medicine residency under Dr. Weil at the University of Arizona. Four years ago, after her training finished, she had moved to Albany when her husband was recruited to the new nanotech complex. Dr. Carey had first worked at the Medical College, where she enjoyed teaching but found the grind of seeing twenty patients a day oppressive. After a year, she joined Capital Integrative Medicine, a private suburban group with four other physicians, including experts in Lyme disease and complementary treatments for cancer patients. The office boasted two nurse practitioners, a naturopath, nutritionist, acupuncture, reflexology, massage therapy, compounding pharmacy, infusions, and a psychology practice with expertise in stress management. Dr. Carey saw ten patients daily, four days a week, so there was ample time. Her patients were generally in excellent health, and on the rare occasions they needed hospital services, she could refer them to her former colleagues. Since insurance did not cover most of their services and patients paid, she did feel somewhat guilty that she was not serving the poor. But she enjoyed the work and told herself there would be time for that later in her career.

For Debra, Dr. Carey was worth the forty-five-minute drive. On that day, they had reviewed her general medical health, discussed her diet, exercise routine, stress management, and supplements.

"You are due for your mammogram," reminded Dr. Carey at the end of the visit. "It has been two years."

"I don't want the radiation. It's bad for you. I keep fighting my dentist on it, too."

"Radiation can be bad," agreed Dr. Carey, "but the dose for the mammogram is low, and you do not get much other radiation. Plus, you protect yourself with your lifestyle."

"What about a thermogram?"

"We don't know enough about it yet, so let's do this mammogram. If it is okay, then we can go another two years. Maybe the thermogram will be ready then."

"Well, if you think so. I'll do more juicing ahead of time to protect me. But I'm not happy about it."

The mammogram took place a week later. Debra did not mind the compression of her breasts; physical discomfort had never bothered her. She hated the idea of the x-ray beams entering her body. She had read once they could shred DNA, an image that stayed in her mind. As Debra stood in the cool room, she visualized her body repairing itself. Like restoring a painting, she thought.

In the radiology suite, Debra's mammogram appeared on the screen. The radiologist described the small jagged area in the upper outer portion of her left breast as a suspicious "stellate lesion." Per protocol, the Breast Health Nurse Navigator contacted Debra and had already scheduled a biopsy followed by an appointment with the hospital's breast surgeon. Debra would be efficiently guided through the health care delivery system.

Debra was stunned but reacted instinctively. "I'd like to see Dr. Gannon. I know him."

The Navigator paused, her work undone. "Okay, he's a good general surgeon. I can call his office. If he agrees, we can go ahead with the biopsy, and I will call you with the results as soon as they are ready. Then you can have an appointment with him."

Debra found Bud in the study, reading. After she had given him the news, they sat together. He was good at that, sitting quietly and rubbing her back while her thoughts raced. Shit, why me? I did everything right. I ate right. I juiced. I even visualized all the cells in my body in perfect order. Now this. Now they'll want to give me their damn chemicals. She looked up and saw the picture of Ken and his family. For a moment, she was back in California with Ken as a smiling baby and her first husband, the three of them happy. You can't blame the Bastard for this, said her reasonable self. Sure you can, answered the angry part. Blame him for everything. But even as Bud rubbed her back and she felt gratitude for his love, the evilest psychotic part of her whispered the words she hated the most: The Bastard will never want you back now. Stop it, she thought. You better let Ken know.

For Ken, the call from his mother was one he had long dreaded. Ken was the product of a brief union in the early 1970s between a lovely aspiring art student and a stunningly handsome chemistry major in southern California. A few surviving Polaroids of the happy hippy couple and their baby were evidence that the first Bohemian years of their life together had gone well. While Debra taught painting at the local co-op, her husband's chemical research had led to a method of enhanced synthesis of high fructose sweeteners and a small company well positioned in the world of mass food production. At the start, the corporate life and the extra money was exciting. But as negotiation dinners replaced beach parties and trips to Las Vegas substituted for camping, things changed. Ken's father merely said they had grown apart. Debra was less circumspect, stating the Bastard had traded her for a fashionable Barbie doll who would be pleasing to investors, a damn Bitch.

The divorce had been bitter. Surprisingly, finances were not the issue. Ken's father was not yet wealthy and later had been generous to Debra, who herself never needed much money. One problem had been Ken. In the beginning, Debra had wanted to raise her son alone, but the negotiated agreement sent him to boarding school, a decision she resented. Ken himself was certain the decision was correct. He loved his mother, but they were very different. And there was her depression, which appeared intermittently for several years after the split. Ken admired her for working through that period, teaching and continue to paint. She often said her art got her through those times. When Ken had married, moved east and had children of his own, Debra had agreed to come. The time with Ken's own family had eased her pain about sending him away, and she found Bud.

There was one other reason the divorce had been so bitter, something about which Debra never spoke. She still loved the Bastard. And had for years. In rational moments, she told herself what she loved was a time when they were young, and the future was endless. That was gone, never to return. But in her weakest moments, part of her still dreamed he would take her back. She was never fully free of him, even after she moved across the country. Ken carried his last name, although by design none of his children were named after the Bastard. One bad moment came when Debra found Ken's daughter playing with a Barbie doll who reminded her of her replacement; she wanted to rip the head off the cursed Bitch. That was also the horrifying instant when Debra realized Ken had the name of Barbie's boyfriend. It was too late to change that. The worst moment came after she had fallen in love with Bud and discovered he had the same legal first name as her ex-husband. The Bastard is everywhere, she thought. She hated him. And still loved him.

When the call came, Ken immediately had images of struggles to come. Although Ken knew that Debra would age and eventually develop an illness, his fervent wish had been that his mother's decline would be a rapid one at the end of a long, healthy life. He honestly acknowledged that this hope went beyond her needs to his own. He simply hated dealing with his mother when she was sick. He admitted that since Debra had been with Dr. Carey, she had been more tolerable. But he was still wary, a lesson learned over many years.

"She sees things differently," he told his wife for the thousandth time several years ago when Debra had hurt her back. "She won't listen to reason or the doctors. She has to do it her own way or with the help of some random person who took an online course in some ridiculous subject."

"This isn't news, Ken," his wife had patiently replied. "She does everything her own way, from health to finances to art. Thank goodness she has Bud."

"I know. But it drives me crazy. Every time the doctor suggests something, she reacts against it. I pray to God she never gets anything serious."

"Relax, honey. There is nothing you can do. She is an amazing woman with her own ideas which are always the opposite of yours. You

say left; she says right. You say up; she says down. You're the scientist . . .
What's the rule? For every reaction, there's an opposite reaction."

NEWTON, MODERN MEDICINE, AND THE BEGINNING OF ALTERNATIVES.

Newton's third law of physics states that for every action there is
an equal and opposite reaction. Although strictly speaking the law
describes forces applied to interacting objects, it is widely quoted in
other fields: economists refer to it when discussing monetary policy,
biologists in the systems they study. Physicians quickly learn that their
actions on patients often trigger physiologic reactions.[387] The medical profession itself has also experienced an effect recalling Newton's
third law: standard treatments often encourage the use of alternative
medicine. In 1998, David Eisenberg and his colleagues reported in the
Journal of the American Medical Association that almost 40 percent of
Americans used non-traditional therapies.[388] While the number itself
came as a surprise, equally shocking to many was that the flagship journal of the American Medical Association would publish Eisenberg's
results. This second shock was understandable since the interaction
between traditional medicine and alternative medicine has produced
another force well known in physics: friction.

Modern medical science started in the early nineteenth century.
Before that time, medical theory was so far removed from today's
concepts as to be unrecognizable. Over the first half of that century,
the study of the origin, or pathophysiology, of disease began. Medical
schools expanded and introduced teaching based on scientific principles. This change in medicine followed over a century of advances in
other areas of science. In physics, Newton's 1687 publication of his laws
in the *Mathematical Principles of Natural Philosophy* moved the field from
a mixture of Aristotle's philosophies, the dogma of the Church, and
individual experiences to a set of core concepts and common language

of mathematics still used today. Scientific inquiry in other fields ranging from biology to chemistry to geology broke with the past, often with the formidable risk of challenging the teachings of the Church. As this scientific thinking began in medicine, alternative medical philosophies also emerged which are recognizable today. Two contrasting figures in the early nineteenth century illustrate the differences between traditional and alternative medicine: Richard Bright ("the father of the kidney") and Samuel Thomson ("the father of botany").

Richard Bright was born in 1789 into a prosperous family in Bristol, an English commercial city which owed much of its prosperity to the so-called triangular trade which included African slavery and the New World. Bright's father, also named Richard, was a successful banker who was interested in science and able to afford his family an idyllic home quaintly called "Ham Green House." When Richard (junior) showed an interest in medicine, his father was concerned for the "odium, [the] envy, the narrow-mindedness" of the field.[389] Despite these parental worries, Bright was well educated, first attending boarding schools and ultimately medical school in Edinburgh. In all phases of his education, Bright learned of the revolutionary concepts in geology, chemistry, physics, ethnology (anthropology), politics, and economics.[390] It was common practice for many well-off young men to make a "Grand Tour" of Europe as part of the transition into adulthood. When the war with France precluded a trip, Bright signed on for an exploration of Iceland, where he contributed work in geology, botany, and zoology.[391] Bright later made several visits to the continent and published highly regarded and meticulous observations on Hungary.[392] He toured many medical schools, met leading physicians including Laennec (the discoverer of the stethoscope), and became internationally known.

Bright's medical career was spent at Guy's Hospital in London with Thomas Addison and Thomas Hodgkin, forming the "great triumvirate" at the core of Guy's revolutionary teaching and research facility.[393] Like Hodgkin, Bright was a firm believer in the importance of correlating symptoms of disease with pathology, called "morbid anatomy." Bright studied many diseases and produced detailed case histories and drawings of careful autopsies, often performed by Hodgkin.[394] He is best known for his work on the kidney, an organ hidden in the back of the abdominal cavity which was typically ignored in favor of the heart or liver. Even today, understanding the kidney is a major challenge for medical students and most physicians will readily admit they do not retain much of that knowledge. Bright described the disease state called dropsy, known today as severe fluid retention or anasarca. He observed that dropsy is often associated with kidney disease and described several different appearances of the diseased organ. He pointed out that some cases of dropsy included protein in the urine, which he detected by heating the urine in a spoon over a candle. In so doing, Bright was a pioneer in using chemical techniques to help make a diagnosis.[395] His powers of observation and descriptions so advanced medical science that at his death it was reported that "there has been no English physician . . . who has effected not only so great an advance in the knowledge of particular disease, but also some greater revolution in our habit of thought and methods of investigating morbid phenomenon and tracing the aetiology of disease as the late Dr. Richard Bright."[396]

Bright was honest and extremely hardworking. He possessed an artist's eye for detail and made remarkable drawings of his patients, both in life and on the autopsy table. He married twice, the first time to the daughter of his boss at Guy's, the famous Dr. Benjamin Babington. After his wife's untimely death a year after the wedding, he remarried and raised a full family. Bright was not a charismatic man but gained international recognition. For many years, diseases of the kidney which produced protein in the urine were described by the eponym "Bright's disease."

Bright's work was part of the renaissance in medical science foretold by his family's slogan, *post tenebras lux* (after the darkness, light).[397] Like Newton's laws did for physics, this period established the scientific approach and vocabulary used today. Yet Bright's work did very little to help his patients. His understanding of kidney disease and his brilliant descriptions of gross pathology were milestones in theory and diagnosis, but his treatment options remained very limited. The practicing physician of Bright's day still used bleeding, blistering, purging with harsh emetics, and mercury. Bright himself resisted the use of these treatments, writing a paper on avoiding bloodletting except in select cases and describing the toxicity of mercury, a common treatment for syphilis.[398] Ironically, Bright's cautiousness cost him some patients who wanted aggressive treatment. Despite his contributions, Bright's chosen profession remained barbaric as the advances in anesthesia and germ theory, which would dramatically benefit patients, had yet to come.

As Bright was advancing medical science in London, a Newtonian reaction to the treatments of the medical profession was taking place across the Atlantic in the person of Samuel Thomson. In 1822, Thomson published his *New Guide to Health or Botanic Family Physician*, a work that contained "his complete system of practice on a plan entirely new: with a description of the vegetables made use of and directions for preparing and administering them, to cure disease."[399] The guide was the written culmination of years spent developing and promoting a system of herbal remedies known as Thomsonianism. As some traditional physicians such as Bright were beginning to use the scientific method to advance their field, Thomson drew from his own life experiences. The autobiography which starts his book describes a childhood far different from that of Bright. In the wilderness of New Hampshire, Thompson developed an early fascination with herbs, including his discovery of a plant he called *Lobelia* which produced vomiting when chewed. He enjoyed feeding it to other boys "for sport." He also developed a deep distrust for traditional physicians after witnessing their treatments of his own injuries and sickness within his family. As he matured, Thomson articulated his dissatisfaction with the "fashionable" methods of treatment used by traditional physicians, which he described as large amounts of "medical poisons" like mercury and opium combined with tortures like bleeding, all administered with a healthy dose of arrogance.[400] While in this respect Thompson was unknowingly in agreement with Bright, his response was very different. Thomson turned his interest in botanicals to healing and developed his system of remedies based upon his deductive reasoning that all diseases were caused by bodily cold which could be restored with the production of natural heat.[401] He used six classes of natural medications, including *Lobelia*, cayenne pepper, and witch hazel, which he administered in various forms, including enemas, and combined with vigorous steam baths to produce heat. Thomson marketed his system by emphasizing both its natural ingredients and public fear of the tools of the traditional practitioner.[402] It could be used by those with common sense and little formal education. Thomsonianism had particular appeal in Jacksonian America, where Andrew Jackson's election had ushered in an age of anti-intellectualism, freedom, and economic opportunity mixed with worship of the frontier.[403] Thomson was tremendously successful, and by the late 1830s, an estimated 10–20 percent of the country used his methods, with higher rates in the South and Midwest.[404]

Thomson himself was a man of intense contradictions. He was not well educated in the formal sense, yet was a brilliant marketer who became wealthy. He believed the common man was capable of self-healing, yet was reportedly as arrogant as any university trained traditional practitioner. His system promised to teach families to control their own health care, yet he protected his work even to the point of obtaining patent rights.[405] As his Thomsonianism became popular, its creator ran afoul of traditional practitioners and was arrested several times, briefly incarcerated, and banned from some areas. His system fragmented with his death, yet references still appear to the "father of botany" in modern alternative and herbal publications. Interestingly, for all his work promoting his theories, one of Thompson's greatest contribution to modern healthcare may have occurred indirectly.

In the early 1830s, a follower of Thompson cared for a young man who had fallen during a barn raising and afterward developed a mysterious illness. Traditional physicians had directed his sister to apply leeches to cause bleeding and given up when there was no improvement. Using Thompson's system, the leeches were abandoned, steam baths prescribed, and the patient eventually recovered. The young man was David Barton, and his young nurse throughout the ordeal was his sister, Clara Barton, who would later help revolutionize nursing. The direct beneficial role of Thompson's treatments in Barton's recovery may have been primarily to stop the bleeding and poisoning, but the indirect effect of encouraging Clara Barton to pursue nursing was profound.[406]

The stories of Bright and Thomson illustrate the contrasts between traditional and alternative practitioners which emerged at the beginning of modern medicine in the early nineteenth century. Bright represented the best of establishment medicine of his era: highly educated and scientific in his approach yet with few useful treatment options for patients. Thomson embodied the ideals of Jacksonian America: independent, democratic, and at times anti-intellectual in his approach and infused with common sense, freedom, and a vision tied to nature.[407] Bright's science was primitive by today's standards, but many of his observations remain valid. Although the theory behind Thomson's system would probably not find many modern adherents, his use of deductive reasoning and own experiences combined with reverence for the natural and a suspicion of scientific inquiry pervade current alternative medicine. Bright was loyal to Guy's Hospital and would be at home in our academic centers. Thompson's antiestablishment personality is certainly recognizable in today's alternative practitioners. Bright's measured restraint in the use of the toxic treatments would probably be similar in today's traditional medical world. Thomson's common-sense approach to healing, rejection of unnatural chemicals, and the use of natural herbal products would certainly enjoy widespread support. As modern medicine developed, these differences present in the early nineteenth century between the "father of the kidney" and the "father of botany" would intensify and persist, even until today.

Dr. Gannon's office was plain and the staff efficient. After examining Debra, Dr. Gannon spoke with her, Bud, and Ken.

"It is a cancer. You need it out. It's small, so you don't need a mastectomy, but you will need radiation afterward. The office staff will make you a referral to the radiation oncologist. I'll take a few lymph nodes, too, so they are checked. We will also set up a referral to our medical oncologist, Dr. Matthews, in case you need any chemotherapy or hormonal treatments."

Surprisingly, Debra had no questions and was accepting, almost submissive. Ken approached her afterward.

"Mother, you were very quiet today. Dr. Gannon seems a bit old school and not really your type. Do you want another opinion? You mentioned that the nurse said there is a breast surgeon in town . . . a woman. Do you want to see her?"

Debra shook her head. "He's not my type. But do you remember when Bud was so sick, and no one could figure it out? It was Dr. Gannon who came in at midnight to operate and saved his life. That night I promised myself if I ever needed a surgeon, he would be it."

Bud nodded in agreement. "That was terrible. I had that bowel blockage from all those adhesions. Dr. Gannon came in and did the surgery. Then I got that infection with the c diff. I was so sick all I could do was poop and watch NASCAR all day. By the end of the time in the hospital, I was so crazy I even enjoyed it. NASCAR, I mean. But every morning, between seven and seven thirty, there was Dr. Gannon, waking me up, checking me over. Never said much, but he saved me, no doubt."

"What about the radiation doctor and oncologist?" Ken asked. "Will you go to them as well?"

"I don't like the idea of radiation, but I will go since I don't want to annoy the man operating on me," replied Debra. "But I'm never taking chemotherapy. I'll see what Dr. Carey says."

A week later they entered the Radiation Oncology Unit. Debra first surveyed the art, which included one painting by a local artist she recognized and several by artists unknown to her or Bud. She nodded her approval and proceeded to the check-in window. So far, so good, thought Ken. At least the art made the cut. After the nurse had taken the history and Dr. Chris did his exam, they all met in a conference room. Dr. Chris presented the history of the clinical trials which proved the combination of lumpectomy and radiation were as good as mastectomy. He reviewed the studies that showed without radiation, the risk of the cancer returning in the remaining breast tissue was very high.

"If you choose lumpectomy and do not have a mastectomy, you need radiation," he concluded.

Ken could see his mother begin to dig in and tried to aid Dr. Chris.

"Does the radiation impact the lungs or heart? How do you aim it?" he asked. "Are there any long-term problems?"

Dr. Chris showed them a CT scan with colored lines.

"This is a treatment plan. It shows the target and the doses the tissues of the breast and nearby body receive. Imagine it as a three-dimensional bull's-eye which we have twisted and turned using the computer. You can aim the beams at the target from different angles and shape the beams using the machine. The computer helps us put it all together." His enthusiasm was obvious.

"It's artistic, in a way," commented Ken.

Debra looked at him sharply. "Don't be patronizing. You sound like your father."

Dr. Chris looked puzzled. "Well, we will begin when you have healed from your surgery, usually about four weeks later."

That went well, thought Ken as they left. He had driven Debra and Bud to the appointment and brought them home. Despite being midsummer, the gray, cool day caused Debra and Bud to huddle together in the back of his Toyota van. In the rearview mirror, he saw them laughing and, for a second, they almost looked like his children playing together.

"Fifteen?" offered Bud.

Debra laughed. "No, seventeen," she rejoined.

"What does that mean?" asked Ken.

"Your mother has a rating system for the doctors she meets based on how young they look," explained Bud. "Twelve years old is for the medical students and fifteen for the interns."

"So Dr. Chris looked young. He's very well trained," answered Ken, mildly indignant.

"Don't get huffy, dear," his mother replied. "I'm sure he's a regular Doogie Hoser . . . quite the young scientist."

THE FLEXNER REPORT: MODERN MEDICAL EDUCATION.

By the beginning of the twentieth century, there was a modest chance that a sick patient might physically benefit from an interaction with a physician. New medical science was being developed at leading universities while anesthesia and germ theory had opened the age of surgery. Yet the state of medical education in the United States was dismal. A patchwork medical education system unleashed large numbers of ill-trained physicians onto the public. U.S. medical schools ranged from a few like John Hopkins, which accepted only students with an undergraduate degree and provided high-quality training, to many proprietary schools which accepted students with little education and had few facilities. In response to this situation, the Carnegie Institute commissioned Abraham Flexner to write a report which would change the course of medical education and practice in the United States.

Abraham Flexner was not a physician. With his selection, the benefactors of the Carnegie Foundation clearly indicated that trained educators rather than physicians would reform medical education. Flexner had begun his career as a high school teacher, studied university education in Europe, and wrote the *American College*. Flexner was of German descent and admired that nation's educational system.[408] Although he had little medical experience, Flexner understood the progress made in modern science and believed the training of physicians should be as rigorously standardized as that of engineers. The timing was right as Flexner's commission followed several years of discussion in the American Medical Association about the problems with medical education as well as efforts at improvement in select medical schools.[409] Flexner had the support of many key figures in the educational, medical, and philanthropic communities. In the medical aspects of his work, Flexner was influenced by Drs. William Welch and William Osler, the respective Dean and Chief of Medicine at Hopkins, both advocates of the German medical school system.[410] Flexner's massive project required tremendous energy as he visited every medical school in the country in what must have been a bone wearying journey.

Flexner released his *Medical Education in the United States and Canada: A Report to the Carnegie Foundation for Teaching* in 1910.[411] The Report outlined his ideal medical educational system, described the state of U.S. medical education, and cataloged the facilities and programs of all one hundred fifty-five medical schools and many osteopathic and homeopathic schools. It was a magnificently comprehensive and shockingly bleak assessment. Most of the schools accepted students without proper preparation, lacked faculty, laboratory, and clinical teaching facilities, and had limited access to patients. After calculating the nation's need for physicians, Flexner recommended the closure or merger of most medical schools and a curriculum for the thirty-one survivors. Included in the merger list were some of today's most prestigious schools, such as Harvard and Tufts. Flexner also uniformly rejected osteopathic and homeopathic schools on the grounds they had no scientific basis and poor facilities.

Flexner's advocacy of governmental control over medical education produced the expected opposition from those it criticized, yet the Carnegie Foundation and its supporters vigorously and successfully promoted its recommendations. They established the state licensing of medical education we now take for granted. Although about half of the medical schools remained open, the Flexner Report ended the era of proprietary, for-profit medical schools. For those schools which remained, the Report brought much-needed standardization to physician education. With its European, and particularly German, scientific approach, the Flexner Report marked the beginning of the modern American medical system. Today's medical education with basic science followed by clinical training in a research university supervised by teaching faculty follows the pattern begun at John Hopkins and promoted in Flexner's Report.

The Report was not without its faults. The narrative contains demeaning descriptions of African-Americans as both patients and doctors and was dismissive of women in the profession.[412] Often ignored, these words were a disturbing failure to advance the ethics of the profession and revealed troubling prejudices. These attitudes and the resultant consolidation of medical schools reduced the opportunities for women to enter the profession,[413] while the recruitment of African-American students only began decades later. A more subtle criticism is that Flexner strongly emphasiszed science over humanism. He started with an elitist view of patients, whom he felt had minimal ability to understand scientific medicine or select a good physician. One revealing description of patients came when he advocated that the state use physicians as social instruments to increase the health of the "nation's wage-worker."[414] Flexner's doctor-patient relationship also emphasized the advancement of scientific knowledge through research over care of the individual patient. Flexner's strong bias towards a centralized system shows when he references Elie Metchnikoff, a Russian biologist trained in the German system who equated physician control of childbirth with a more advanced civilization.[415] An additional limitation of the Report was Flexner's use of a war-like model of disease which also tended to favor a less humanistic treatment approach: "The body diseased is like a city besieged."[416] Flexner left little room for freedom within his educational system, stating "control in the social interest inevitably encounters the objection that individualism is thereby impaired. So it is, at that level; so it is intended."[417] Even recognizing the hyperbolic language popular in his time and acknowledging that he modified his thinking later, the reader can imagine the ideal physician of the Flexner Report as a scientifically trained white male general, coolly fighting disease while serving the state, science, and his patients.

During the twentieth century, our powerful, scientifically based, academic system of medical education emerged from the chaos of American medical education. Flexner's defenders rightly give him much credit.[418] Over the same century, the world would witness physicians acting as horrifying scientific social instruments: Germany in World II and the Tuskegee Syphilis Experiment in the United States are obvious examples. Calls began for a more holistic view of medicine, a stronger definition of medical ethics, and a search for balance between science and humanism in the profession. In this debate, Flexner's critics have in part blamed him for the lament of famed bioethicist Edmund Pellegrino that doctors became neutered technicians in the service of science rather than in the service of patients.[419] Yet even as Flexner promoted medical education based on science, another opposite reaction which he probably would never have predicted occurred: patients developed their own ideas.

On the morning of the surgery, Ken worked in his office while his wife accompanied Debra and Bud. He had an important deadline upcoming, but there was more. Ken knew that sitting in the waiting room with his mother while she offered opinions on the health care system and the age of the doctors would have driven him insane. His wife was an expert at distracting Debra in conversation, had almost endless tolerance for her lectures, and relieved Ken of any guilt.

The surgery went well. Dr. Gannon had met them in the recovery area.

"He said it was small and came out easily with a good margin around it. He took the lymph nodes nearby, but they felt normal. He will see Debra again next week," reported Ken's wife.

That evening Ken visited Debra and Bud at their home, a classic looking farm house in nearby Galway filled with an amazing collection of her art. Each time Ken entered the foyer and looked right into the living room, he was struck anew by the brilliant colors filling the walls of the room and creeping onto the floor and ceiling. At one point, Bud had hung a painting of Debra's in the large room, a bright rendition of several people in a style which Ken always thought of as primitive, although his training was limited to a single introductory college art course. After it was hung, Debra had felt the painting was too isolated, and so the entire room had become her canvas. To his left was the living room, containing a much quieter display of her art and occupied by Bud's extensive collection of aquariums. It was in this peaceful place that he found Debra, sitting in a chair and reading.

As they spoke of the surgery, Ken was pleased to hear his mother compliment Dr. Gannon and the surgery center. Maybe I was wrong about her and a serious illness, he thought. Or maybe it's the residual effects of the anesthesia. Whatever the reason, Ken found his mother relaxed and reflective. He enjoyed this rare moment as she reflected on his childhood and their current life. After a few minutes, she paused as if preparing to say more, until Bud entered the room with freshly brewed tea and the moment passed. As he served them and sat down, she changed the subject.

"Here is a book I found about radiation," she reported, holding up *Rad Art: A Journey Through Radiation Treatment* by Sally Loughridge. "It's quite a remarkable collection. The artist is a woman who underwent the same radiation I will get. Each day after her treatments she did a painting and wrote a few lines."

Ken looked through the book and the many different images. "Are you nervous about the radiation?" he asked.

"No. But I hate the idea of something going through my body, cutting up all my DNA and cells."

Bud nodded. "You have had that fear for a long time."

The three of them sat together, sipping their tea. Ken watched his mother lean back and close her eyes. She is still a remarkable, beautiful, and very complex woman, he thought. As she drifted asleep, Debra saw the Bastard, still young and handsome, reaching out to take her hand.

Ken attended the brief post-op check with Dr. Gannon.

"You are healing well. The cancer was small, under two centimeters. The lymph nodes were clear. You should have the radiation. With the surgery and radiation, you are probably cured, but there is a small chance some cells escaped. So, I want you to see Dr. Matthews to discuss whether you need chemotherapy or hormonal treatment. The staff will make you an appointment. I'll check you again in six months."

At the desk, Debra took the appointment card for Dr. Matthews.

"I will go see this Dr. Matthews," she replied, thanking the secretary. Once again, Ken was surprised.

"To make Dr. Gannon happy?" he asked.

"Yes, but I also found out his mother is an artist that I know, so maybe he's not so bad. Anyway, I won't be taking any of his chemotherapy. I have plenty of other options . . ."

SCIENCE, ART, AND OUR PHILOSOPHIES.

After the excitement of receiving their medical degree, new physicians face the anxiety of internship. In this difficult year, they quickly learn medical theory is different from medical practice. Their first call at night reporting a patient has a headache makes their knowledge of the anatomy of the brain and the mechanisms of neurotransmitters seem inadequate. Fortunately, the nurse usually knows what to do and, after a few months, so does the physician. Good physicians ultimately learn to integrate theory and practice, but doing so is the great challenge often described as the melding of the "science" and "art" of medicine. The proper mix of science and art is often viewed differently by alternative practitioners. The debate over this mix often reflects the answer to the classic question of "how do we know what we know?"

At the start of the twentieth century, the rise of science promised to bring traditional medicine's theory and practice closer together. Abraham Flexner certainly thought so when he advocated infusing medical education with scientific training. Physicians would use research to assess treatments and "begin with science and work through the entire medical curriculum consistently, exposing everything to the same sort of test."[420] Although most physicians at the time were not used to scientific rigor, Flexner noted "a new school of practitioners has arisen which . . . seeks to study, rationally and scientifically, the actions of drugs, old and new."[421] For Flexner and his supporters, testable scientific rationale was the basis of the medical model. Alternative models without scientific standards were rejected. Order was imposed.

Not everyone embraced the medical science of the nineteenth and early twentieth centuries. As recounted in James Whorton's *Natures Cures: The History of Alternative Medicine*, the United States has a rich legacy of alternatives to traditional medicine which started with fascinating cult-like groups whose names often suggested the basis of their treatments: herbalism, magnetism, hydropathy, and Christian Science.[422] While many of these early alternative philosophies rose and vanished with the health and fortunes of their pioneers, we still recognize several survivors from this era: osteopathy, chiropractic, homeopathy, and naturopathy. By Flexner's time these practices had long been in political and legal conflict with traditional medicine which they insultingly called "allopathic" medicine, a name coined by the founder of homeopathy and derived from Greek meaning "other than the disease." Given many of the brutal treatments used by traditional doctors, the name was apt and later adopted with equanimity by the medical profession.[423] Regardless of their names, these alternative philosophies all differed from Flexner's new school in that they derived theory from deductive reasoning and personal experience rather than experimental science. As the science of the twentieth century challenged these alternative therapies, they responded in very different ways.

Osteopathic medicine is now mainstream, but it has an alternative origin.[424] Osteopathy was developed in 1874 by Andrew Still, a fascinating man whose autobiography records his adventures as a pioneer child, anti-slavery politician, Civil War veteran, and founder of his medical system and school.[425] Still had a remarkable understanding of anatomy and believed disease resulted from misalignment of the skeletal system (the word os in the name is from the Greek for bone) and pressure on the arteries. He advocated therapeutic manipulation and commonsense, drugless remedies. Still's legacy is paradoxical. His theory of disease was simplistic even by the standards of his day. For example, his analogy of Bright's disease to curdling milk was a far cry from the detailed work done in Guy's Hospital fifty years earlier.[426] Still's work invoked religious appeals to the Creator. He often refused to acknowledge many advances in medical science and called for the "war for the truth under the banner of osteopathy," yet grudgingly accepted surgery if his treatments failed.[427] He had dramatic public disputes with organized traditional medicine while expressing personal admiration for many medical doctors.[428] Nevertheless, Still's writings convey a sense of humanity that seemingly made him a well-liked practitioner.[429] Near the end of Still's life, despite his opposition, osteopathy began the long process of adding the use of surgery, drugs, and medical science to its program. Although friction between osteopathy and traditional medicine took years to overcome, today the D.O. degree is virtually identical to the M.D. degree. Osteopathy embraced the scientific method, even if its founder did not.

Chiropractic has taken a less enthusiastic approach to science. Its founder was Daniel David "D.D." Palmer, a short, bearded man with powerful hands who was a magnetic healer with a personality to match. In 1895, Palmer had a chance encounter with a hearing-impaired man whose spine he manipulated. The story has more than one variation, but Palmer interpreted the subsequent improvement in the man's hearing as resulting from his action. The next year Palmer begin practicing chiropractic, a name meaning "done by hand."[430] Like Still, Palmer's philosophy was not scientific and was derived from his varied experiences. In a massive 1910 text, the *Chiropractor's Adjustor*, Palmer advanced the theory that diseases resulted from the subluxation of the spine which would affect both the nerves and an ill-defined vital force of the body. Unlike the more reflective Still, Palmer was a fiery, dogmatic man who eagerly fought any opposition and aggressively promoted the business side of his field. His work also took on decidedly religious and moral tone. In the *Chiropractor*, he wrote his practice "deals with subjective, ethical religion—the science which treats of the existence, character and attributes of God, the All-pervading Universal Intelligence."[431] Palmer certainly considered himself a prophet. His son, B.J. Palmer, born to the second of his five wives, followed his father into the field and their relationship was a fascinating example of familial rivalry. Whatever their differences, the Palmers and their practitioners were in constant conflict with both traditional medicine and osteopathy. Despite these battles, chiropractors expanded through the 1920s and 1930s, establishing schools and hospitals. With expansion came the need for self-regulation which, to a considerable degree, chiropractic leader John Nugent accomplished in a manner like that used by Flexner with traditional medicine.[432] Over time, chiropractic came to some degree of accommodation with medical science, encouraged by the desire for acceptance by state licensing bodies and insurance payers. Chiropractors even participated in clinical trials testing different treatments for back pain.[433] Eventually, most practitioners modified Palmer's original theories, and the portions of their practice that focused on the mechanics of spinal manipulation and health maintenance became more mainstream.

While osteopathy eventually embraced medical science and chiropractic at least made some accommodation, homeopathy has remained immutably unscientific. It derives from early nineteenth-century ideas of German trained physician Samuel Hahnemann who, perhaps ironically for the German-loving Flexner, believed that drugs which produced symptoms of a disease would treat the disease. Homeopathy thus derived its name from the Greek homoios (like) and pathos (suffering). Hahnemann's philosophy of "like cures like" had one major problem: the patient often got sicker when given the drugs. His results were better when the drugs were massively diluted, and this process became the cornerstone of his treatments. Traditional practitioners were quick to point out the arithmetic of dilutions soon removed any active ingredients and derided homeopathy as unscientific. Yet it is the nonscience of homeopathy which has made it enduringly appealing. Its many defenders articulate the sentiment of Shakespeare's Hamlet when he noted, "There are more things in heaven and earth, Horatio, Than are dreamt of in your philosophy."[434] Homeopathy faded early in the twentieth century, partially under pressure from scientific method, but was reinvigorated in the last quarter. Today, homeopathic treatments are popular, and their theory and use continue to be an irritant to mainstream medical practitioners who call for their regulation and scientific testing.[435]

Naturopathy rejects medical science in favor of all things natural, with the precise definition left to the intuitive feelings of the practitioner. In 1901, (another) German named Benedict Lust opened the American School of Naturopathy in Manhattan. An American immigrant, Lust had contracted tuberculosis but recovered in one of Germany's popular health spas, where he underwent a strict form of natural cure which included hot and cold baths, walks in the snow, and various herbs. To these Lust added components which would be in keeping with his view of nature, ranging from health food to health equipment to health clothing. Naturopathy embraced the concept that disease was a departure from the benevolence of nature and, hence, treatments should embrace nature. From the start, naturopathy disdained conventional science, including drugs, serum therapy, and vaccinations.[436] In the middle of the century, enthusiasm for naturopathy waned, but it was also rejuvenated later in the century. Naturopathy encompasses many other philosophies and is aptly described as therapeutic universalism (minus allopathic medicine). As Whorton notes, "in 1989, the American Association of Naturopathic Physicians formally recognized that naturopathic medicine is ultimately defined 'not by the therapies it uses but by the philosophical principles that guide the practitioner.' Contemporary naturopathic literature still abounds with professions of faith in vitalism, respect for the healing power of the vital force, and the superiority of natural therapeutic agents to artificial ones."[437]

By the middle of the twentieth century, the scientific theory which Flexner embraced seemed poised to transform medical practice. Germ theory and the development of antibiotics revolutionized the treatment of infectious diseases. Treatment for viruses ranging from hepatitis to the common cold was close at hand, as when Flash Gordon used interferon in outer space as a cure for a deadly comic strip infection.[438] Breathtaking surgeries were becoming routine. In cancer medicine, the "Whipple Procedure" was done regularly, a surgical tour-de-force which removed tumors of the pancreas then re-attached the pancreatic and bile ducts back to the small intestine. Hodgkin's lymphoma and some types of leukemia were cured with chemotherapy and it seemed other cancers would soon yield to the right mix of new drugs. Public expectations were high. Yet it rapidly became evident that even this amazing modern medical science could not solve many health problems. Antibiotics did not treat all infections and overuse produced unneeded adverse reactions and bacterial resistance. The common cold struck the pharmacy executives who lined up for inoculations of interferon.[439] Surgeries had complications and chemotherapies terrible side effects. The almost infinite complexity of human beings seemed to defy medical science as advances in theory led to more questions in practice. At the same time, physicians trained in Flexner's model seemed ill-prepared to handle this complexity, some were accused of being distant, too busy, and losing their human touch.[440] Although many medical educators acknowledged these criticisms and included more humanism in physician training, Flexner's scientific method remained the cornerstone of the medical curriculum.

In the 1960s, as promises of John F. Kennedy's New Frontier turned into the rage against the Vietnam War and authority, the dramatic social changes of the time were mirrored in the resurgence of alternative medicines. Vietnam was to be a scientific engagement, coolly undertaken by the disciples of Defense Secretary Robert McNamara who believed that our modern military would overwhelm the enemy—Flexner felt similarly about the war on disease. Yet the North Vietnamese proved resilient—as did the illnesses which refused to be cured by medical science. The weapons of war proved imprecise as agent orange, napalm, and mass bombings made horrific scenes of civilian casualties—medicine saw the toxicities of surgery and chemotherapy. Protests rose against the authorities who wielded power—and the organized medical profession was challenged. The demands for new social values in the Age of Aquarius were echoed in medicine by the promotion of multiple alternative treatments. Steve Jobs, a leader in new technology who delayed his cancer surgery while he attempted alternative treatments, noted that "the sixties produced an anarchic mind-set that is great for imagining a world not yet in existence."[441] The sixties were the era of everything for those promoting alternative medicine. Homeopathy and naturopathy enjoyed renewed popularity. Acupuncture returned to the Western world. Therapeutic touch and bioelectromagnetics joined visualization and both traditional and new world prayer and healing.[442]

During the last quarter of the twentieth century, complex forces competing for the post-Vietnam national identity were at work in both the traditional and alternative medical communities: biomedical science, communication technology, big business and pharmacy, the global economy, environmental awareness, and the changing ethics of individual choice. The plethora of options and philosophies unleashed in the 1960-70s became widely discussed by a public which witnessed the successes of advocacy for HIV/AIDS and later breast cancer. The era of medical debate dominated by elites like Flexner (or chiropractic treatments controlled by the Palmer family) was replaced by an explosion of public information and discussion. In 1991, Congress expanded the public nature of the debate about alternative treatments by forming the Office of Alternative Medicine (OAM) as part of the National Institute of Health—a decision they forced on the NIH.[443] The language of the debate also changed when term "complementary and alternative medicine" (CAM) was proposed to acknowledge that alternative treatments could be used in addition to traditional medicine. This progressed to the proposal to unite the two disparate worlds under the label "integrative medicine." A Department of Integrative Medicine was established at the University of Arizona by Dr. Andrew Weil, a graduate of Harvard Medical School who promoted his own distinctive brand of wellness. As Whorton notes, this cacophony was accompanied by a lessening of the friction between traditional and alternative medicine.[444] It is true by the end of the century Eisenberg's landmark study reporting that almost 40 percent of Americans used non-traditional medicine was published in the *Journal of the American Medical Association*.[445] Yet the truce was at most partial. Fierce debates continued, as when the editors of the *New England Journal of Medicine* called for the end of the scientific free ride given to alternative medicine.[446] As the century closed, traditional and alternative medicine still largely operated in two different worlds.

The twenty-first century has seen attempts to reconcile traditional and alternative medicine by promoting integrative medicine. In contrast to using alternative treatments in place of traditional medicine, integrative medicine is "informed by evidence, and makes use of all appropriate therapies."[447] In oncology, leading cancer centers offer versions of integrative medicine. For community hospitals, the American College of Surgeons certification lists reflexology, massage therapy, and chiropractic care as rehabilitation services which should be available for cancer patients.[448] The for-profit oncology chain Cancer Treatment Centers of America boasts of their naturopaths in public advertising. Integrative medical practices often hire classically trained oncologists to review the treatment plans for patients undergoing chemotherapy so they can provide support.

Despite these programs, collaboration between physicians and alternative practitioners is minimal. On a practical level, most physicians do not have time for detailed discussions of alternative practices. The medical payment system, electronic medical record, and numerous administrative and regulatory burdens already challenge even the most humanistic physician. Alternative practitioners seeking insurance payment for their services will face these same pressures, encouraging many to remain a cash business practiced outside the traditional medical delivery system. On a philosophic level, efforts to demonstrate the effectiveness of alternative practices using scientific techniques have largely failed. The practitioners who endorse alternative treatments are not inclined to perform rigorous testing while serious scientists usually have relatively little interest in these studies. Often the benefits which many of these techniques claim to produce are highly subjective and difficult to document. Thus, studies of alternative treatments are often criticized on one side for lacking scientific methodology and the other for not testing the alternative practice in its correct form. Even if these studies were done more regularly, it is not clear they would produce integration. Science is not a practice in accommodation, but rather an open and argumentative search for answers. The persistent problem remains the differing answers to the question "how do we know what we know?"

The debate over the mix of science and art in medicine, the varied answers to the question of how we acquire knowledge, and the distinct views between traditional and alternative practitioners continue. The paradox of our day is that while science continues to advance exponentially and again promises a new age in medicine, alternatives proliferate. Now the debate is not controlled by cult-like figures or Flexner reports, but occurs in public. In this confusing time of many choices, most patients are pragmatists. For serious illnesses, they seek traditional medical care rooted in science to which they may add other treatments. For less serious illnesses or those with limited effective traditional medical treatments, alternatives and the unscientific yet hopeful comfort they may provide continue to have great appeal. Patients become the designers of their own unique integrative systems. For all patients, one can only hope the last word belongs to Oliver Wendell Holmes, the distinguished American jurist, who wrote in his poem "The Morning Visit,"

> Of all the ills that suffering man endures,
> The largest fraction liberal Nature cures.[449]

Debra was pleased with the art in Dr. Matthew's office, but he was no Dr. Carey. Despite her feelings, she put forth her best effort to engage him in meaningful conversation. During a circuitous interview, Dr. Matthews ascertained that Debra had very few medical problems, so he moved on to the family history. Her parents had both lived into their nineties, longevity she attributed to a life of growing their own food.

"Do you know about those GMOs? They manipulate the genes to make the crops resistant to the pesticides so they can pour more toxic chemicals on them to kill the bugs that are resistant to the toxins they used before. Damn chemists, I can't stand them."

Dr. Matthews inquired about Debra's sister.

"Well, she lives in Arizona and has always been a piece of work. Thinks she knows everything. Going to save the world and all that.

When I told her about my problem, I had to listen to the whole story of her breasts, and how she was worried they might be cancerous. But she never had cancer, if that's what you mean. She did have one interesting medical thing you might care about. She was saved by Ebola."

Debra explained that her sister had been on a missionary trip to West Africa when the epidemic broke out.

"They were all sent home on the next plane. When she walked off the plane, she collapsed. They took her to hospital and found out she had a brain aneurism which was leaking. They operated, and she is fine, still the same piece of work. If she had been in Africa, she would have died. So, that terrible virus saved her."

Dr. Matthews asked if Debra had other children.

"Good heavens, no. And Bud's not Ken's father. That man lives in Silicon Valley, making his millions, a damned chemist. What I ever saw in him I don't know. I was probably in a haze. After all, it was the seventies. And that was before he went corporate. Anyway, thank goodness fate brought me Bud. We met at working at the animal shelter years ago . . ." She paused for breath.

"Do you work in an animal shelter, too?" Dr. Matthews asked, instantly regretting the question.

"Not for long. I tried it. I like the animals, but could never stand the people. They're very demanding. The things they expect, you wouldn't believe it. You would think they wouldn't be so damn picky. Bud worked there before he started his own rescue service. He's very good with the animals. Last year he rescued a seeing eye dog who flunked out of school. He thinks Bud is blind and leads him around." Bud nodded.

"So, is it fair to say there is no history of breast or ovarian cancer in your family?" Dr. Matthews summarized, trying to redirect the conversation.

Ken spoke affirmatively. "There is none in the family."

As Debra changed for an exam, Ken explained further in the hallway.

"My father is a chemist who became CEO of his own company. Mother is, well, mother. I was the product of that short-lived union. Thank God it ended. You cannot imagine two more unsuited people. Fortunately, she found Bud."

"Are you more like your father?" asked Dr. Matthews.

"In some ways, but not all. I am an electrical engineer with no artistic talent. My parents split when I was very young. She lived in California until I was married and moved here, then she followed us for the grandchildren. I've always divided time between them and their two very different worlds. Mother is an amazing painter."

"Sounds like she is lucky to have you here."

"Yeah, well, she is luckier to have my wife and children. Debra is not your typical mother-in-law or grandmother."

After the examination, they regrouped.

"Dr. Gannon removed the cancer and a few of the lymph nodes using the sentinel node biopsy. Since you had the lumpectomy—" Dr. Matthews began.

"I know. I need the radiation. Everyone is afraid I won't take it." She smiled sweetly at Ken. "But I will. Now, what are you going to try to sell me?"

"Well," replied Dr. Matthews. "I will tell you what we know . . ."

REFINING ADJUVANT CHEMOTHERAPY FOR BREAST CANCER: ONCOTYPE TESTING.

"Adjuvant" chemotherapy is given after surgery to eliminate any remaining cancer cells; a concept pioneered in women with breast cancer. The problem with adjuvant treatment is that while some women benefit from the chemicals, many do not, including those cured by the surgery and those who die despite the extra treatment. Whether they benefit or not, all the women may experience side effects. In the most extreme situation, this means that some women already cured by surgery may be permanently damaged or die from this extra treatment. Thus, it is particularly important that the effectiveness of adjuvant chemotherapy be proven in clinical trials.

Clinical trials of adjuvant chemotherapy are carefully designed to measure the benefits and risks. Usually, this involves assigning patients to either a new treatment or the standard treatment in randomized fashion using "flip of the coin." All clinical trials need to be approved by institutional review boards to assure patient rights are respected. The information about patients is collected by data managers and analyzed by statisticians. Finally, the results are reported and made available to critics for review. These important trials often involve hundreds or even thousands of patients at many hospitals. The cost is significant. Enrolling patients adds time and complexity to an already stressful meeting between patient and doctor or nurse. Yet this is the exact type of science Flexner envisioned his new breed of physicians would use to test their treatments.

Adjuvant treatment of breast cancer was first studied in the 1960s with a single dose of chemotherapy given at the time of surgery in the operating room, an approach which did not yield dramatic results. In the 1970s, longer treatments given after surgery produced positive results. Clinical trials done from the 1980s through the first decade of the twenty-first century showed that increasingly intense adjuvant chemotherapies could improve survival and be considered for larger numbers of women. There were limits, however. As the treatments became more intense, each step typically produced progressively smaller statistical improvements. In addition, as more women with lower risk cancers were studied, the improvements also became smaller (since more were cured by surgery alone). Within the profession, arguments began over the magnitude of benefits needed to endorse chemotherapy treatments. For a woman at low risk for a recurrence, did a small improvement in survival seen in a clinical trial justify treatment?

Adding to this debate over adjuvant chemotherapy was a change in thinking about how to best determine a woman's risk from her breast cancer. At the start of this era, in the 1960s and 1970s, the primary factor used to assess the risk of spread of a breast cancer was the "stage," determined by the involvement of the lymph nodes (none is better) and size (smaller is better). Other factors, including growth rates (slower is better) and whether the cancers had the estrogen receptor (and were thus "fed by estrogen" with positive being better) were important but subordinate to the stage. In an obvious way, this made sense: larger cancers which involved the lymph nodes and were thus a higher stage were more likely to have spread.

During the 1980s and 1990s, it became increasingly understood that separating breast cancers into "biologic groups" was as important as staging. This process began with widespread testing of breast cancers for the estrogen receptor (ER). Breast cancers which had the estrogen receptor behaved differently than those without the estrogen receptor, even when they were the same stage. They had a better initial prognosis, chemotherapy was less effective, and studies proved many of these women could be effectively treated with the antiestrogen tamoxifen. In fact, for premenopausal women (still producing estrogen) with ER-positive cancers, some of the benefit of chemotherapy resulted from its action to put them into menopause and thus reduce their estrogen. Later in this era, the discovery of the *Her-2-neu* gene and protein identified breast cancers with the opposite biology—they were aggressive cancers which were better treated with more intensive adjuvant chemotherapies and ultimately targeted treatment with trastuzumab (Herceptin).

For many women with breast cancer during this era, clinical trials provided clear guidance on the use of chemotherapy. On one extreme, younger women with cancers which involved the lymph nodes and were ER-negative could be confident that chemotherapy clearly improved their survival. On the other extreme, older women with small cancers and clear lymph nodes which were ER-positive could forego chemotherapy and use tamoxifen. Unfortunately, many women still struggled with the decision of whether to take chemotherapy or not. For example, younger women with smaller ER-positive cancers which did not involve the lymph nodes faced the difficult decision about whether to add chemotherapy to tamoxifen. Their dilemma was illustrated in a clinical trial done in 1988 by the National Surgical Adjuvant Breast Program (NSABP) called B-20. Over two thousand women with small estrogen-fed breast cancers which did not involve the lymph nodes received the anti-hormone treatment tamoxifen. By "flip of the coin," two-thirds also received one of two possible chemotherapies.[450] Eight years later, 88 percent of the women treated with surgery and tamoxifen were alive.[451] Chemotherapy improved the results by 4 percent. The trial was offered as evidence that more women should receive chemotherapy.[452] Many refused.

The key question was whether the 4 percent of women who benefited from chemotherapy in this study could be identified. In other words, could biologic grouping using modern molecular techniques determine treatment? As part of B-20, the breast cancer samples were sent to Pittsburgh for storage in NSABP Tumor Bank, a collection which now holds over ninety thousand samples from patients with breast and colon cancer.[453] Although during B-20, the Tumor Bank was in its infancy and it was not yet clear how it would be used, data managers, nurses, and secretaries collected over six hundred samples. As they worked, advances in molecular biology allowed the analysis and manipulation of DNA and RNA. The development of the PCR (polymerase chain reaction) allowed the amplification of even the smallest amounts of DNA for research. Shortly after the B-20 study ended in the late 1990s, a variation of this technique called RT-PCR allowed scientists to quantify the tiny amounts of RNA and thus study gene expression. Could this allow identification of the cancers which would benefit or not from chemotherapy?

Scientists used RT-PCR on the samples from the B-20 study to identify genes which might predict the behavior of the cancers. They proposed a gene panel, later called Oncotype DX, which would predict both the aggressiveness of the cancer and the effectiveness of chemotherapy based upon the cancer's gene expression—giving the cancer a "risk score." Testing the Oncotype DX in a study like B-20 would have normally required a decade. However, since the patient outcomes to B-20 were already known, Oncotype DX was rapidly validated on the stored patients' samples. The patients, physicians, nurses, data managers, and secretaries who did the B-20 study and filled the tumor bank for later use had formed a remarkable team which never met.

The Oncotype DX (and other similar tests) dramatically changed the ability to determine which women with early stage ER-positive breast cancers might benefit from chemotherapy. Those whose cancers had low scores could confidently skip the treatments and not worry that they had failed to "do everything." Those with high-risk scores could take treatments knowing the side effects were for a good reason. For those with scores in between, more work would be done. In addition to this practical use, the Oncotype DX emphasized the importance of determining the biology of cancers as well as using the traditional staging of cancer size and spread to the lymph nodes.

Flexner would be pleased.

Two weeks later, Debra's Oncotype DX result was available. Dr. Matthews explained.

"Remember, this test looks at the particular genes which have gone bad in your cancer. It does not test for any gene abnormalities you might have been born with, okay?" Ken nodded while Debra and Bud studied the paper. "The pattern of the expression of these genes can predict how likely it is the cancer has spread and tells us if it might respond to chemotherapy. Cancers where the risk of spread is high and chemotherapy would be statistically useful are called high risk. Cancers where the risk of spread is low and chemotherapy is not useful are called low risk. There is an intermediate group where chemo probably is not useful, but the numbers are not large enough to be sure. Your cancer is in the intermediate group, but close to the low risk, so there is not likely to be any benefit to chemotherapy, although it is possible."

"So, chemo is not needed . . .," concluded Ken.

"I do not recommend chemotherapy, but this data is not seen as conclusive by everyone. There was a study to examine this issue, and we are awaiting the results. Until we have that information, some patients in this situation do elect to take chemotherapy. Also, remember all these patients were treated with antiestrogen therapy. In those days, it was tamoxifen. Now we usually use medications called aromatase inhibitors. The cancer cells are fed by estrogen, and these medications block the production of estrogen in the cells."

"Sounds reasonable . . .," nodded Ken.

"Maybe for you," announced Debra, "but not for me. I don't want any hormones or antihormones or anything like that."

"Since they offer benefit in terms of improving the survival rate and have no serious side effects, they are routinely recommended. Would you consider at least trying them?" Dr. Matthews asked.

"No."

Ken spoke up. "What kind of benefit are we talking about?"

"Well," replied Dr. Matthews, "the cure rate with surgery and radiation alone is about 80 percent and the pill, called an aromatase inhibitor, probably raises that about 5 to 7 percent."

"So not much," concluded Debra.

"It depends on your perspective," replied Dr. Matthews. "We consider it a big benefit for something which is very safe. It is a much greater benefit than for the use of blood pressure medicines or cholesterol medicine."

"I wouldn't take those, either," replied Debra, feelings she confirmed with Dr. Carey at an appointment a week later.

"You wound is healing well," Dr. Carey commented. "Did you use the honey on it?" In a phone conversation after the surgery, she had recommended a honey preparation to promote wound healing.

"I couldn't," Debra replied. "I was afraid to ask Dr. Gannon about it. He's very fussy about his incisions. He's old school."

Dr. Carey laughed. "That's okay. Many of the young surgeons are using it, but it might be too much to ask for an older one."

"I have the radiation next," replied Debra. "I don't want it, but I know Ken will never forgive me and I don't want the cancer to come back. But that's it. I won't take any of their meds. I don't want anything artificial, even if that oncologist says I should. I'm afraid of what it will do to my bones and the rest of me."

"Well, there is evidence that you can improve the prognosis with exercise, diet, and weight loss," Dr. Carey replied. "So, let's work on those." Over the next thirty minutes, they made a comprehensive wellness plan to prepare her for radiation.

The radiation started smoothly. They had a routine. After breakfast and coffee, Bud drove her to the facility. She could have made the thirty-minute drive herself, but he insisted. Each morning she was positioned on the table and received the radiation, a physically painless process but one she found upsetting. She waited for the hum and click which would signal the beam was piercing her body.

"It's creepy," she told Bud. "I hope the herbs and supplements protect my good cells."

"I thought the nurse and Dr. Chris told you not to take them during the treatments."

"Yeah, well, I won't tell them. What they don't know won't hurt them. I hope they work."

By the end of the seven weeks, Debra was tired. Not overwhelmingly exhausted, just tired. Her breast had become sore, the skin peeling. It's ugly, she thought. From deep within she would again hear the annoying little voice telling her the Bastard would never want her that way. When she closed her eyes, she would see him, young and golden blond, playing with little Ken on the beach. Why does that Bastard come? I have Bud, who is so good to me.

This must end, she thought. They were in the study drinking the tea Bud had brewed, sitting together quietly. In the aquariums lining the walls, the fish floated or darted in seemingly random motions, occasionally chasing each other, oblivious to her plight.

"Ken's a good son," she broke the silence.

"Yes, that he is." He waited. Bud was good at that.

"I keep thinking about him when he was young . . . What he was like as a boy and our life then."

Bud nodded and kept waiting. Debra continued.

"I have also found myself thinking about his father. Sometimes I imagine I want to talk to him again. I hope that doesn't upset you. Is that bad?"

"I think it's pretty natural, going through what you are now. The old days when we were young look good right now. We remember our old friends and lovers when they were young, too."

Debra looked down at her cup. It's more than that. You better tell him, announced the psychotic part of her brain, until Bud spoke again.

"You know, I still think of Chichi from time to time," he announced.

"Chichi?" asked Debra, puzzled.

"After Liz and I split, I ended up briefly in Miami. I met a girl named Chichi, and we dated for a few months. She was a hot Cuban dancer. Actually had a show career."

"You never told me this," said Debra. "What happened?"

"After a few months, Chichi started doing the cha-cha with someone else. I was heartbroken and moved away. A few years later, I learned that Chichi died in a car accident. And, you know, I was very sad, almost depressed, even though I knew I would never have seen her again. Yet part of me still wondered . . . But, anyway, sometimes I think of her when I eat refried beans."

"Why didn't you ever tell me this?" asked Debra.

"The truth?" asked Bud.

"Of course," answered Debra.

"Well, I like going to the Cantina with you . . . And I love their refried beans. I didn't want you to feel like we were with Chichi every time I ordered them."

"She must have been a bitch to leave you."

"I'm glad you think so . . ."

Maybe the Bastard isn't such a problem, she thought.

Today, Debra's monologue was surprisingly short.

"I hated the radiation," she started, "but in truth, it wasn't too bad on my body. My skin was a little burned, and I was a little tired. Right, honey?" She turned toward Bud, who nodded.

"You did very well, I thought," he replied softly.

"And the people were nice. The place was clean, and the staff was very professional, as they say on Trip Advisor. In fact, I met one of your old patients there; she works as a volunteer. Do you know who I mean?"

Dr. Matthews shook his head.

"Well, of course I can't tell you because of HIPPA. But she likes you a lot."

Ken groaned. "Mother, you can tell the doctor, he just can't tell you anything."

"It doesn't matter, dear," she replied and turned back to Dr. Matthews. "You know what really bothered me?"

He shook his head again.

"It was the thought that when those beams went through my body, they might be shredding my soul. We don't really know if they do that, do we?"

"I don't," answered Dr. Matthews. The room was silent for a minute. In the background, the low, deep vibration of a passing Amtrak train could be felt.

"Well, I am certainly glad to be done with this cancer . . .," said Debra, after a moment.

"Did you consider if you would take the antihormonal treatment?" asked Dr. Matthews. "The Oncotype test did not show a conclusive benefit for chemotherapy, but there is a statistical improvement in survival if you take the pill."

"I don't want to put anything like that in my body. I'm going to do things naturally, boost my immune system. I'm working with a naturopath, too." She was definitive. Even Ken knew not to argue.

"I understand your wishes," nodded Dr. Matthews. "But will you at least come back and let me keep track of you?"

"Yeah, you have good art work here. And Dr. Gannon said I had to. Particularly since I told him I wasn't taking the pill. He said you would keep after me to take it."

"That's true," nodded Dr. Matthews.

"And I told him I would keep saying no."

"I believe that is true, too."

Ken nodded and rolled his eyes, again.

2:20 Billy Jackson: Esophageal cancer

"Hello, Mr. Jackson," said Dr. Matthews as he entered the examination room and shook hands with the tall, distinguished looking older man who rose from the chair. Arnie Jackson had a weathered face, but a full head of gray hair despite his seventy-eight years. He wore a dated but meticulously pressed suit and held a hat.

"Hello Dr. Matthews," he replied formally. "Do you remember my daughter, Mary? She has come home to help with Madge and Billy." Mary, an attractive woman in her early fifties with similar gray hair, smiled pleasantly as they also shook hands.

"I surely remember Mary. How is Madge?" asked Dr. Matthews as they sat. Three weeks ago, Arnie's wife had suffered a stroke and recently returned home from rehab.

"She is moving much better. She understands everything but her words are still a little jumbled and she gets frustrated."

"I'm glad she is improving," he answered. "And how is Billy doing?"

"That's what we are here to talk about . . ."

Billy Jackson was fifty. He had been born with Down syndrome. Why he was given an extra chromosome 21 was a mystery to everyone but his mother.

"God gives us what He wants. We must love all the children we are blessed to get," Madge Jackson had told Dr. Matthews more than once.

When the blessing that was Billy Jackson arrived in 1967, Arnie and Madge were a young couple in their late twenties with Mary, a bouncy three-year-old. Five years earlier the high school sweethearts had taken over Arnie's family farm in Schuylerville, about ten miles from Saratoga. With a hundred and fifty cows and many pigs, goats, dogs, and cats, it was hard work. At the start, they had help from Arnie's father and younger brother Paul. Shortly after Mary's birth, however, Arnie's father had suffered a massive stroke and needed a nursing home. After the shock, Paul had decided he was taking a job driving long-haul trucks.

"It's too much for me," he had told Arnie one evening as they sat together on the porch while Madge settled Mary. "I'm not built for this like you and Pop. I can't be pinned down on this farm, never able to leave. This is a big country and it's changing. I'm twenty-three. I want to see it, not stay in this place . . . And it's hard work here, too. Every day the same grinding routine. You see what it did to Pop. And for what? He should have been a millionaire the way he worked."

Arnie nodded. He knew Paul was not built for this work.

"Listen to me," Paul said. "Talk it over with Madge, but consider this. Sell the farm, and we could go in together on our own truck. We could split the driving. That way we would each be home half the time and keep the truck going full-time. The fellow who is home could deliver feed and do the winter plowing. It'd be a nice life."

Arnie and Madge discussed the offer.

"It could be a nice life, Arnie," she agreed. "I wouldn't mind seeing you work less. And I worry about how we will handle it when Paul leaves—"

"He's not running out," interrupted Arnie. "He said he'd give us plenty of time to find help. He's a good brother."

"I didn't mean otherwise, dear," she answered patiently. "What I was going to say was that it could be a good life, but only if you're happy with selling the farm. It has been a part of you and the family for years. Grandma used to say there is a lot that goes into a good life. You are different from Paul. You need to think it over and pray on it."

Prayer didn't produce immediate results. Every Sunday after the morning milking, Arnie and Madge attended church, followed by early dinner with her nearby family and a visit to Pop at the nursing home. Despite multiple sermons, Arnie's dilemma remained unresolved until one blisteringly hot and muggy afternoon. He had just dumped a pail of slop in front of the swine and sat down on the overturned bucket to rest. As he drank some water and wiped his brow amidst the grunting of the beasts, buzzing of the flies, and smells of the earth, Arnie craved watermelon. A childhood memory of a similar day with his father, the two them laughing while they ate the juicy fruit, spat the seeds, and threw rinds, provided him the answer. He wanted that for his children.

"We keep it," he told Madge that night. "It's part of me . . . This place, this soil. I want it to raise Mary and any more children we get here."

"I knew that, dear," she said, kissing his forehead. "It will be our labor of love."

Somehow, they had managed. Paul left for his life on the road but kept his word and provided an occasional respite. Their older neighbor and experienced farmer, Roger "ZZ" Denton, became Arnie's mentor.

"For your family farm it's all about size," ZZ told him. "The right size. Too big and the cash flow will always threaten you, too small and you can't weather a storm. Either way, the banks will end up with your land. And we all have storms; it's the nature of our business. Molly and I have had ours. They come out from nowhere."

Arnie and Madge's first storm wasn't farm business; it was the birth of their second baby, Billy.

"He has mongolism," the doctor told Arnie in the waiting room. "He'll never be normal. There's a home for these people in Albany and one up near Lake Placid. I gave your wife a sedative, and when she wakes up, we can tell her before she sees the baby."

There was no reasoning with Madge, sedative or not.

"Bring me my Billy," she told them. "We are going home, Arnie."

"You can't leave now. You just delivered last night. How will you take care of him?" asked the doctor.

"You don't think I know about babies? Besides my own, I've a whole farm full of babies." Her eyes blazed. "You think I would leave him here with people who think he belongs in a warehouse?"

"You're upset. We understand—," tried the doctor in his best calm, authoritative voice.

"You may understand surgery," Madge fired back. "But you don't understand me. God has given us this child, and we are going to raise him, whatever it takes."

A few days later Dr. Benjamin Anthony made a house call. He was young, fresh out of his residency in pediatrics at Albany Medical College and starting a practice. As Arnie would remind him years later, his dark hair was a bit long, he didn't own a tie, and drove an old Volkswagen Beetle. He examined Billy carefully, then sat with them as he held him.

"Well, he does have mongolism. We've learned that means he has an extra chromosome number 21, so three instead of two. I've seen pictures of the chromosomes for these babies. No one knows why it happens."

He paused as Billy squirmed and burped. "Besides their appearance, sometimes these babies have heart or stomach problems, or other physical ailments. I don't find any of those in Billy, but we'll need to watch him. The main problem is in their development. They are retarded, so they do things later than other children and never get to normal. Surprisingly, some of them can function pretty well, others not so much. There is no way to know except see. They don't tend to live as long as most people, but again it is hard to tell."

"He is staying with us," said Madge.

Dr. Anthony smiled. "I heard that from the hospital staff. You are right. Times are changing. Not all these children go into institutions now. There are parents keeping them at home and teaching them to get the most of their lives. I brought you some information about a group in Chicago, so maybe you can write or call them."

Madge read the pamphlet. The Mongoloid Development Council had been formed in Chicago by Kay McGee, who had fought to bring her own baby with Down's syndrome home. A phone call gave Madge the tools she needed.

"Arnie, listen to this," she told him that evening. "Mrs. McGee has a daughter named Tricia with the same condition. They don't call her mongoloid. They say she has Down's syndrome."

"That sounds nicer," agreed Arnie, pleased Madge was happy but not really expecting much more.

"Yes, well that's not all. The best is that their daughter goes to a regular school. With help, of course, but she goes. And they know another person with Down's syndrome who is thirty-five and lives alone. Not in a warehouse, either."

"I'd like that for Billy," said Arnie. "If anyone can do it, you will."

ZZ Denton agreed.

"I don't know much about these types of problems," he said as Arnie struggled to express his worries about Madge and Billy. "But I know about farms. They're good, honest places to work. You and Madge are good folk. And if your child ain't got all the blessing you might wish for him, well, at least there is no better place for him to be than with you here."

Madge and Arnie raised Billy on the farm. It wasn't a normal childhood. Billy was slow to sit, that took a year. He was slow to creep along the floor, that took almost a year and a half. He walked at two years. He was never talkative, but he learned to speak in short sentences. Most importantly, Billy was happy. He loved his parents, adored his sister Mary, and enjoyed his animals, particularly his pigs.

Billy even went to school. The principal, a long-time friend of Dr. Anthony, helped Madge's advocacy. Billy mostly enjoyed school, less so when Madge made him do homework. He was particularly happy when some of the boys encouraged him to run track. He loved his uniform. They even gave him a varsity letter which Madge and Annie framed and hung in the living room. After school, he worked on the farm, except on Mondays and Fridays when he swept the church.

ZZ Denton also had a son, Will. Shortly after Billy was born, the draft sent Will to Vietnam. Arnie witnessed his friend's agony.

"I know he has to go, just like I did in the Second War. He's no coward running off to Canada. He's no Cassius Clay, neither. He loves his country. But I hate to see it, knowing what he might face and seeing Molly suffer. I just pray they know what they are doing over there . . ."

Arnie told Madge the news that night. "For once, I was almost thankful for Billy's condition, knowing he would never have to go. Then I felt guilty."

"You can't win with any of those feelings, dear," Madge replied. "All you can do is your best with what the Lord gives you and . . ."

"I know," he smiled, continuing, "and milk the cows each morning." It was their private joke. No matter what, you had to milk the cows each morning.

Will had survived the war, but barely. The upright young man who left Schuylerville came back different, dark and brooding. Will never said much, but the stories of what he did in those tunnels in hell provided the explanation. Armed with only a pistol and a knife, he had been lowered into the steamy darkness to confront unspeakable terrors and enemies. His mind never completely cleared of those visions and his return was marked by horrible dreams and rage which caused father and son to fight.

"I don't know him," a distraught ZZ told Arnie. "My own son, he's gone, and this man I don't know is here. He goes into rages and won't work. I get so mad with him. I know it's not his fault . . . But how can I keep him here?"

Arnie had no answer. The tension between ZZ and his son built until it seemed something would explode. Arnie always remembered the afternoon ZZ's daughter Karen came running to the field to find him.

"Mr. Jackson, please come quick. Daddy collapsed, and Will's trying to help him. Please hurry."

Arnie ran, trying to keep up with Karen until they reached the Denton's kitchen. In the distance, he could hear the siren begin wailing, calling the volunteer fire and rescue squad into action. ZZ lay unconscious on the floor as Will did CPR. Arnie knew the ambulance would never arrive in time, the squad was scattered at their jobs.

"Give me the keys to the truck," he told Karen. He backed the flatbed up to the door. They hoisted ZZ into the back and Arnie drove while Karen held her father and Will continued his CPR. It was a twenty-five-minute ride to the hospital, but Will never missed a beat.

"He was a machine," Karen said later. "You've never seen anyone so determined in your life. He would not let Daddy die."

ZZ survived. The doctors said it was a miracle. Will said nothing. To Karen or Molly's knowledge, father and son never spoke of that day, though it changed them both. ZZ found patience and Will some measure of peace. After ZZ's discharge from the hospital, the two were inseparable, usually just walking together in silence.

Despite the equilibrium he found, Will never was able to lead a normal life. He could not marry or have children; the demons were always nearby. He still had bleak moments. Yet no matter how bad he felt, Will could never resist Billy. For some reason, Billy could make Will Denton feel at ease.

Arnie remembered another hot afternoon when he had taken Billy, then about seven, to repair the fence around the pig pen. As they finished, ZZ and Will stopped by after one of their long walks, the father strengthening his heart and the son escaping his demons. They had brought a large watermelon which Will sliced effortlessly. As the foursome ate the runny fruit, Billy threw a rind at the pigs, but hit Will instead. The million-to-one shot left the curved rind stuck perfectly to Will's head. At the sight, Billy fell backward, laughing so hard his father was briefly afraid he might have hurt himself. It was contagious. ZZ joined in, then Arnie. Finally, to Arnie's amazement, Will Denton laughed too. For five minutes, as rinds, seeds, and laughter filled the air and even the pigs seemed silenced by the spectacle, it did not matter how many chromosomes you had or where you had gone to war.

Of course, not everyone was supportive. Madge remembered the strange looks and occasional taunts when she walked with her son. Most of the time she ignored it, even though it hurt. The worst came when Billy was about ten, at the A & P Supermarket.

"Hey, watch out retard," said a big, unkempt man, probably about thirty, as he elbowed Billy aside to reach into the cooler. Billy and Madge had been waiting at the meat counter as the butcher had gone in back to get their order.

"Where'd a cute thing like you get a runt like this?" asked his partner, a skinny redhead. "Some defective father probably? Hah, hah, hah. Want a real man?" It was a mean, boozy laugh.

Madge had pulled Billy close, angry and fearful at the same time. Before she could answer, Jimmy, the store's elderly attendant, had come around the corner, sweeping.

"Hey, leave them alone, you two," he said angrily.

"Shut up, old man or I'll stick that broom up your ass. Oh, I get it. You got a thing for retards?" sneered skinny.

Only the arrival of the butcher, carrying Madge's order and a meat cleaver, ended the exchange.

Jimmy, who worked with Billy at church, was distraught. "I'm so sorry, Mrs. Jackson. They are idiots. Please don't let them upset you . . ."

He could see Billy was scared, so Jimmy sat him in his chair near the register with some ice cream while Madge finished their shopping. As they left the market and entered the parking lot, the two men again approached. Billy shrank.

"Get away from us," Madge yelled. "I'll call the police."

The big man stopped about ten feet away and held up his hands.

"Ma'am, we made a terrible mistake in there," he said. "We were wrong. Please let us help you take your groceries to the car."

Madge moved the cart away from them. "Get away from us," she warned again. "I swear I'll call the police."

"Please ma'am," the big man persisted. "You don't understand . . . We are sorry. And if we don't help you, we are going to be dead, too."

Madge stopped. "You're crazy, get away."

"Please, lady," begged the skinny one, looking as if he was about to cry. "That guy will kill us dead if he don't see us helping you . . .

please." He nodded toward the other end of parking lot. Madge looked and saw a small, thin man leaning casually against a landscaping truck. Even though his face was in the shadow of a work cap, she knew it was Will Denton. For some reason which she could never quite explain, he looked very dangerous. Madge paused for a moment, letting the two men squirm.

"You're right," she said finally. "You idiots had better help me. Or you both will certainly be dead."

About five years later, Billy paid his friend back. Over the course of that winter and spring, ZZ's heart had weakened. By summer, the father and son hikes became walks to the end of the road in the cool of the evening. Billy watched his friend help his father down the drive and home again. Finally, in August, ZZ had died, and the walks were no more. It was a quiet evening a few weeks later when Madge noticed Billy putting on his shoes, an unusual action. He always kept to his rituals. After dinner came bath, television, ice cream, then bed.

"What's the matter, Billy? Why are you putting on shoes?" she asked, puzzled.

"Walk with Will," he replied. And over the remainder of that summer and fall, each evening Billy walked with Will down the road and back.

"It really helped get Will going again. He could never turn Billy down," Karen said later.

Arnie missed ZZ, too.

"He was a good man," he often said to himself as he worked.

To Madge, he was more explicit. "ZZ helped us to keep this farm. He helped a lot of people in the area, too, just like us. He was a good father to Will and Karen and had a good marriage to Molly. I think that was the most important thing."

Madge agreed. "Grandma said the key to a good life was a good marriage. 'Pick a good one and hope you get lucky,' she used to say. So, I did." She hugged him.

The subsequent years of their own good life had passed to the rhythm of the seasons. As Paul had said years before, they were built for the farm. When they reached their early sixties, they both knew they needed to plan.

"I'm Dad's age when he had his stroke," Arnie told Madge. "I feel good, but what if something happens? What will you and Billy do?"

"Do you want to sell, honey?" she asked. "The horse people are offering quite a bit for farms like ours."

He shook his head. "This is a farm. We feed people. I hate to see it end up a hobby for some rich person. After Funny Cide, all those fellows with money think they can be like the McMahon's. Just buy land and start raising thoroughbreds. When they get bored and move on to something else, we'll have lost the farmland forever."

Karen Denton provided the answer. After ZZ's death, the Dentons had faced the same problem of having a family farm which would not be taken over by the next generation, yet which they did not want to give up to development. Karen, a lawyer in Saratoga, had worked with a land trust which helped family farms stay in service. She made the same arrangement for the Jacksons. Arnie and Madge would stay as long as they wished, then their property would be transitioned to a new family to work. The farmland would stay intact. Mary, now married and living in Albany, promised Billy could live with her when the time came.

"You won't be rich this way," Karen had warned them before they signed the papers. "You could make more money selling to a developer."

Annie nodded. "On this farm, I always felt rich . . . even when we had no money."

Over the last fifteen years, they had all grown older. Arnie and Madge had slowed. Despite the help they hired, the cows and crops had dwindled. Billy, too, had aged. The pigs remained his specialty, though they were fewer in number. He still swept the church, but only once a week. His friend Will visited regularly, now fighting another battle in his hard life, this time against multiple myeloma. Still, as the seasons passed, they were content.

The storm had come one day when Billy had been eating lunch and gagged on a piece of meat. His face turned red.

"Arnie, Billy's choking," yelled Madge.

As Arnie turned to help him, it became clear Billy was not choking. The food was painfully lodged lower down, in the middle of his chest.

"Hurt me, here," he held his fist over his heart.

Arnie managed to get Billy to drink some milk and wash the meat down. Some ice cream for dessert calmed him.

"Have you ever seen him do that before?" he asked Madge later.

"Never," she replied.

After Arnie had thought for a bit, he continued.

"Well, I'd like to take him to the clinic. I remember years ago Doc Ben saying he could have problems with his digestive system."

The young Physician's Assistant at the Health Clinic checked Billy over.

"He seems fine," she said. "But if you want him seen by a GI doctor, we can arrange it."

Billy enjoyed Dr. Nancy Hinson, a Jamaican gastroenterologist with a beautiful lilting voice.

"I terrific," he announced as she finished her exam.

"You are terrific, Billy," she agreed. Turning to Madge and Arnie, she added, "I doubt he has anything seriously wrong, but because he might not be able to tell us exactly what he is feeling, I think I should do an endoscopy and look inside his stomach. I don't want to miss anything."

Madge and Arnie had worried that Billy might have trouble with the hospital and anesthesia, but Dr. Hinson's report made those anxieties insignificant.

"I found a blockage at the end of his esophagus near the stomach," she said before Billy awoke. "It is where his food was getting stuck. It looks like a cancer, but we won't know for sure until the biopsy report comes back in two days."

Madge paled.

"What now?" Arnie asked.

"You need to see an oncologist. They will want a PET scan, so we will make those arrangements," Dr. Hinson replied.

"We know Dr. Matthews," replied Arnie. "He takes care of our neighbor Will."

ESOPHAGEAL CANCER: COMPLEX SURGERY.
The esophagus is commonly known as the tube which allows food to pass from the throat to the stomach, a simple description which belies its complexity and fails to explain the difficulty of esophageal surgery. In fact, the esophagus is a remarkable muscular organ which passes through the chest near many critical structures, including the bronchial tubes, major blood vessels, and the vagus nerve. Its muscular action is under the control of an extensive set of nerves which cause it to both contract to propel food and close tightly to resist the intrusion of acid from the stomach. The esophagus is lined with cells like those of the throat, called squamous cells, and thus differs from the lining of the stomach, which contains many gland cells which secrete acid. In daily life, we feel the esophagus only when acid from the stomach reaches it, causing heartburn or acid reflux.

Cancers of the esophagus develop in the lining cells. Roughly half of these cancers resemble the original esophageal lining cells and are "squamous cell cancers," while the remainder resemble the lining of the stomach and are "adenocarcinomas," meaning gland-like cancers. Squamous cell cancers of the esophagus are often caused by tobacco and alcohol use and have been declining in frequency while adenocarcinomas have become more common. Some adenocarcinomas result when chronic acid reflux damages the lower squamous lining of the esophagus and causes it to change into a more gland-like appearance, a condition called "Barrett's esophagus." Gastroenterologists now attempt to diagnose Barrett's esophagus, begin antacid treatment, and watch carefully with regular endoscopies to reduce the risk of these adenocarcinomas. Once cancers develop in the lining of the esophagus, they tend to invade through the muscle and then spread in the lymph and blood systems. Unfortunately, this spread or metastasis has often taken place by the time the cancer has caused symptoms like food blockage or pain.

While the obvious treatment for esophageal cancer is removal, the surgery has proven extremely difficult. Consider that while the age of modern surgery began with the discovery of anesthesia by Morton in 1846 and the removal of a portion of the stomach took place in 1881 by famed German surgeon Billroth, esophageal surgery did not become routine until the 1940s. Several obstacles caused this dramatic difference. Entering the chest was very difficult since the lung on the side of the incision would collapse; the loss of oxygen and pressure on the nearby blood vessels required the surgeon to work very rapidly or risk disaster. In addition, surgeons learned that any contact with the vagus nerve near the esophagus could result in a fatal slowing of the heart. Finally, even if the surgeon could work rapidly, avoid the vagal nerve, and remove the cancerous portion of the esophagus, sewing a new connection within the chest was risky. The pressure within the esophagus produced by swallowing would often burst sutures and result in a fatal leak of fluids into the chest. The first famously successful removal of the midportion of the esophagus for cancer was done in 1913 by Franz Torek,[454] an American of German descent described after his death in 1938 as one of the country's greatest surgeons.[455] Torek operated at the German Hospital in New York, later renamed Lennox Hill, on a sixty-seven-year-old woman with a cancer in the middle of her esophagus. He removed the woman's esophagus and substituted an external rubber tube outside her chest which allowed her to swallow food and have it travel into the stomach. His patient lived for twelve years before dying of pneumonia at age seventy-nine, and her story has survived in generations of surgical textbooks.

Torek's famous surgery aside, routine operations to remove cancer and reconstruct the esophagus required the development of endotracheal intubation (inserting a tube into the main airways of the lung) in the 1930s. The tube allowed inflation of the lungs using positive pressure, avoiding the uncontrolled collapse of the lung after an incision in the chest and giving surgeons more time to work. The tube also revolutionized anesthesia. Before this time, chloroform or ether was dripped onto a mask over the patient's face. The patient's own breathing would regulate the anesthesia: more breathing, more drug, more sedation, then less breathing and less drug in a cycle. The tube made the use of constant deep anesthesia possible since the anesthesiologist could now control the patient's breathing.[456] Japanese surgeons were pioneers in aggressive esophageal cancer surgery, using three incisions in the abdomen, chest, and neck. A common Western variation still in use today was introduced in 1946 by Welsh surgeon Ivor Lewis who made both an abdominal and right chest incision to remove the esophagus. Lewis lived from 1895 to 1982 and spent the peak of his career in London, where he partnered with his wife, anesthesiologist Dr. Nancy Faux, in both their surgical and family life.[457] His operation is still called the Lewis esophagectomy. Variations of the surgery exist, including those using minimally invasive techniques. Whatever the procedure, the anatomic obstacles mean the operation is complex, requiring an expert surgeon and an otherwise healthy patient.

Once removal of the esophageal cancers and reconstruction became routine, another problem emerged. Despite Torek's first success, surgery cured only about one-quarter of patients. The cancer would typically recur either in the nearby lymph nodes within the chest or in other parts of the body. The grim reality is that before esophageal cancer is detected, it has usually spread via the lymph system or blood stream. Since the lymph nodes near the esophagus are highly interconnected, that spread is hard to predict. In the 1980s, radiation and chemotherapy treatments were introduced in an attempt to increase cure rates. In theory, radiation can cover a larger area and potentially sterilize more lymph nodes than a surgeon can remove while chemotherapy might kill cancer cells which have spread outside the area. Over the years, numerous studies have been done treating patients with various combinations of radiation, surgery, and chemotherapy. None of the results have been ideal. Combining these treatments requires a healthy patient and experienced team. The combination of radiation (usually about six or seven weeks) with chemotherapy (often given weekly) results in tremendous irritation of the esophagus. Patients usually need a feeding tube inserted into the stomach and careful nutritional management, particularly if surgery is to follow. The result has been that when the cancers are in an early stage, surgery is first. If the cancers are larger or the lymph nodes are involved, radiation and chemotherapy are done first and, depending on the outcome, surgery considered later.

The visit to Dr. Matthews followed the PET/CT scan. Mary joined them.

"Will comes here," Billy announced as Dr. Matthews entered the room.

"Yes, he does," answered Dr. Matthews. "He told me you were his friend."

"I Will's friend," agreed Billy.

Dr. Matthews explained Billy's situation with a picture.

"There is a cancer near the bottom of Billy's esophagus, the tube which carries food from the throat to the stomach. It is called an adenocarcinoma. From the PET/CT scan, we did not see any spread of the cancer."

"Thank God," Madge replied as Arnie nodded. Dr. Matthews briefly reviewed the options of surgery or beginning with chemotherapy and radiation.

"You cut it out," Billy announced, nodding and pointing at the drawing.

"That's a good choice, Billy," replied Dr. Matthews. "We can also give you some treatments to shrink it down first."

"Okay. Terrific."

"Come on, Billy, let's go visit Will," suggested Mary. After they had left, Dr. Matthews explained the combined radiation and chemotherapy program in detail.

"Do you think he can do it?" asked Arnie.

"You know him the best," answered Dr. Matthews. "What do you think about his ability to follow the instructions, hold still during the radiation, and endure the side effects? Can he get through it with your help?"

"God gave us Billy," answered Madge, in a tone which took Arnie back to the day of Billy's birth. "And we are going to the best for him, whatever you say it is."

Before Billy started treatment, he had a visit with the surgeon at Albany Med. Billy was nervous visiting the large hospital, but Dr. Bruce Saul was a friendly man who put him at ease.

"I agree with Dr. Matthews that the best plan is to start with the chemo-radiation, then do the surgery. Billy will not be able to eat with the radiation, so I will put a feeding tube into his stomach. You can give him nutrition that way. I'll take it out when I do the surgery. Is that, okay, Billy?" he concluded.

"You cut it out," answered Billy.

"I cut it out," smiled Dr. Saul.

"Terrific," answered Billy.

Billy's treatment consisted of radiation each day and chemotherapy once a week. The radiation treatments were straightforward; the whole process took about fifteen minutes. Billy was scheduled in the late morning, so as not to interfere with the milking of the remaining cows. He bonded quickly with Dr. Chris and the staff at the center.

"No hurt," he reported after the first treatment. "I terrific."

The chemotherapy treatments were longer, about three hours. Billy typically fell asleep after the anti-nausea medications. As his first treatment infused, Angela Pagano, the Nurse Practitioner, saw Madge watching Billy closely and sat beside her.

"You take good care of him," she said.

Madge nodded. "When he was born, they wanted to put him in a facility. Arnie and I wouldn't let them. He's been a good son, and I hate to see him suffer."

Angela nodded, and they sat quietly for a few minutes, then Madge continued.

"You know, I read in a magazine how they test for this Down's syndrome now. Most of the women who get a positive test are told to have abortions. One of the companies that sells the test even put a picture of a girl who was like Billy on the advertisement. Her family was really upset." She stood up, fixed his blanket, and kissed his forehead. Billy stirred softly.

"I had to fight to bring my baby home. Now some mothers have to fight to keep their babies."

"It's a complicated world," Angela agreed, not exactly sure what to say.

By the fourth week of his treatment, Billy was beginning to feel pain in his lower chest and was unable to swallow. Madge kept close track of his input through the feeding tube, regularly checking with the nurses.

"You are doing a great job. You could have been a nurse," complimented Angela.

Madge's storm came without warning as Billy entered his last two weeks of treatment. Madge and Arnie had been sitting together having coffee and some pie, as he later explained.

"I could see she was having some trouble. She dropped her fork and started slurring her words. The rescue squad brought her to the hospital where they said she was having a stroke and gave her medications to break up the blood clot right away. Then they took her to Albany Med by helicopter, and the doctors there worked on her. Thank God they did, too. I remember what happened to Pop years ago. Back then there was nothing to do, so they just put him in bed, and he never recovered. It's so different now. She was in a special intensive care. And they say she'll get better. She can move and understands but is having some trouble speaking. She'll be in rehab after they discharge her, but they think she'll come home."

Father and son finished the treatments.

"How is Billy doing with his nutrition?" Angela asked Arnie as Billy slept.

"He misses his mother, but we are getting six cans in every day. He's been a real trooper," Arnie replied. "Madge would be proud of him."

Angela nodded. "You two have done a great job with Billy. I'm sure it wasn't always easy."

Arnie thought for a moment. "Not much in life is easy," he answered. "When Madge and I were first married, we weren't sure we'd be able to keep the farm. But we did. I had grown up on that farm and wanted to share it with my children, like my father did with me. And you know what?"

Angela shook her head. "What?" she asked.

"With Billy, I got to share the farm more than I ever would have dreamed. You know, he loves pigs . . . and watermelon."

A month after the treatment finished, Dr. Hinson did a repeat endoscopy which showed the tumor was gone. A CT scan was also clear. Dr. Chris met with Arnie and Billy.

"The radiation and chemotherapy have worked beautifully. You can consider skipping the surgery," he stated. "The studies in this situation are not clear, and many people do not feel the surgery helps. It will be a real stress on Billy."

Dr. Saul disagreed.

"The surgery is the best approach. This is Billy's best chance."

The choice led to today's visit.

"I'm not sure what to do," continued Mr. Jackson. "Do I send Billy for the surgery or not?"

"Do you think he can do it?" Dr. Matthews asked them both. "He will need to be in the hospital for several days at least."

Mary answered, "I think he can do it. I can be with him, and Dad can stay with Mom."

"From the first day, Billy said we were going to cut it out," mused Dr. Matthews.

"He still does," answered his father.

"Then I believe that's your answer."

66 "Tell me she's okay. Tell me," burst out the older of the two women as Dr. Matthews entered. One was sixty-five and the other forty. Except for the differences caused by twenty-five years of aging, they could have been identical twins.

"Mom, wait. Let him sit," interrupted the younger woman, her daughter.

Daughter and mother had been together on this journey for seven years. It had started when Sarah Taylor's Pap test was markedly abnormal—she had cervical cancer.

THE PAP SMEAR.

On October 13, 1913, a young Greek couple arrived in New York. They spoke no English and had little money, so she labored as a seamstress while he worked for a Greek newspaper and played the violin at a restaurant. Their new life was different. In Greece, she had been raised in a famous military family while he was an accomplished physician. Yet George Papanicolaou and Andromache Mavroyeni (Mary) succeeded in America and made an enduring contribution to women's health.[458] Together, they developed the Pap smear to detect cervical cancer.

The concept that cancer cells could be identified in bodily fluids belongs to Dr. Walter Hayle Walshe, a British physician and prolific author who noted in his 1843 work *Diseases of the Lung* that the sputum of patients with lung cancer could contain "microscopical characters of that product."[459] Walshe was a professor of morbid anatomy at London's University Hospital as the medical profession was beginning the long and difficult process of incorporating science into practice, hoping understanding would produce better treatments. Walshe reported the rocky start, noting that "When morbid anatomy was first seriously cultivated, the effects on medical practice were deeply depressing . . . but . . . the conviction has gradually been forced upon observers, that many diseases . . . are mitigable by treatment."[460] Given the difficulties faced in understanding basic illnesses, it is not surprising cancer posed even greater challenges. In 1844, Walshe's comprehensive work *Anatomy, Physiology, Pathology and Treatment of Cancer*, classified cancers using taxonomy like that of botanists of his era, relying on the visual appearance, feel, and locations of tumors as described by various physicians. The book is a fascinating example of the early struggle to define cancer.[461]

In the new world of scientific medicine of the 1800s, the microscope became an important tool. The diagnosis of cancer is commonly made by examining a piece of tissue (a biopsy) under the microscope but can also be made by examining small numbers of cells found individually or in clumps, the field we know today as "diagnostic cytology." While tissue samples from biopsies allow the pathologist to see cancer cells invading normal tissues, cytology relies on the features of the cells independent of any surrounding tissue. Johannes Muller in Berlin made the first smears from cancers in 1838, and other investigators soon followed. At the end of the nineteenth century, examining cells in the urine was an accepted method for the diagnosis of bladder cancer.[462]

During the 1920s, George and Mary Papanicolaou had found work at New York University and Cornell Medical School. He was a pathologist and she a technician studying reproductive cycles. It was here that he discovered cervical cancers could be detected by examining vaginal swabs, the foundation of the Pap smear. During the same period, Romanian physician Aurel Babes collected cells from the cervix and receives partial credit for the test in his native land.[463] In the 1930s and 1940s, Papanicolaou joined with gynecologist Herbert Traut to test, publish, and promote his technique. By the 1960s, the Pap smear had been endorsed by the American Cancer Society, use became widespread, and deaths from cervical cancer declined. As it saved lives, the Pap smear demonstrated the power of early detection and the potential for screening large populations, lessons for cancer control which continue to the present. The Pap smear also profoundly advanced the understanding of cancer among medical professionals and the public. As they taught and disseminated their technique, Papanicolaou and Traut also gave a course in cancer development, describing the changes seen from normal to premalignant to malignant cells.[464]

George Papanicolaou became famous for his discovery, yet Mary played a key role in developing the Pap smear. She was an excellent technician and teacher in the lab. In addition, she provided numerous (daily?) vaginal smear samples, earning one biographer's description as the "most over-tested woman of all-time," the American Cancer Society's description as "Companion to Greatness," and her husband's label as "my wife and my victim."[465]

The problem with Pap testing is that you must go to the doctor. And that takes money, which Sarah, who in 2009 was a single thirty-two-year-old mother with a four-year-old daughter, did not have, even working full-time as an office temp and using her mom for child care. Health insurance? That had been gone years earlier. Sure, there were programs, but who had the time to sign up? And Sienna needed things.

They made a big fuss on March 23, 2010, when President Obama signed the Affordable Care Act. Sarah had been too busy working and feeding her girl to notice, but Mom had paid attention.

"They say it's going to give health insurance to many people who can't afford it. Maybe it will help you," she said. Mom had always liked to listen to President Obama. He was such a good communicator.

"Sure, Mom," Sarah answered. "You always liked him anyway. But don't cross that Michele. She's tough. I bet she'll be President herself one day."

"Really, dear. I believe him. But don't tell your father. Anyway, I'm going to check on it for you."

"Sure, Mom. Thanks. Gotta get to work. I packed Sienna's lunch already." As she waited for the bus on that cold morning, Sarah thought about health insurance. It would be nice. But since when did the government ever care about me. I make too much for Medicaid, but I'll never get enough for real insurance.

Mom was right. Her good-looking President kept his word, and the next year Sarah had insurance. She even occasionally listened to the debates. So what if the government has to pump up the system? At least I got coverage. Now I can get a doctor, she thought. I hear that Dr. Gold is good.

Julia Roberts, the Nurse Practitioner in Dr. Gold's office, asked Sarah about her daughter.

"Is the father involved?" she asked. "Do you have any help raising her?"

Sarah nodded. "I have help. We live near my parents. Dad is older and has some back problems, so he doesn't do much, but Mom is great. They both love her."

"That's very good. Her father isn't around?"

Sarah shook her head. "No, he would have been . . . but he died before she was born. He had depression and . . . well, when he couldn't take it anymore . . ."

Julia patted her hand. "You've had a tough life, and you deserve credit for getting through it. I'll have the nurse come in and get you set up. Then I'll check you over and do your Pap smear and HPV testing."

As she waited in the stirrups, Sarah remembered those days. Could it be that five years had gone by? Sometimes it seemed like yesterday, other times it was hard to even see his face. He had been a nice guy, boy really, when they first met in high school, and she had a crush on him from afar. Sensitive and artistic, she had thought. They had gone their separate ways, she to work and he to college. She smiled as she remembered the day they met almost ten years later. He was shopping for a gift for his mother, and she was behind the counter. She never thought he would recognize her, but he did. After a few awkward moments, he left with perfume and her number. For a year, it had been wonderful. He told her of his problem with depression, but until it hit she could never have imagined the power of those chemical forces within his wonderfully creative brain. They were so strong nothing could relieve his pain. Not the doctors, not their medicines, not his mother, not Sarah, not even their love. A bottle of pills ended his suffering when they stopped his heart, just as their baby's heart had started to beat within her.

She had gone around and round. He was weak to do that, to take his own life. It was selfish. She and their baby were his victims. His mother, too. No, he fought it. He tried so hard, for so long, so many times. Blame the disease, she was told. Blame society. Blame yourself for loving him. Blame the doctors for not locking him up. Blame God. Go back to blaming him. But he tried so hard and was so sweet. I loved him. There was no good answer. The thinking was tiring. Soon there was Sienna, who needed to be fed and changed and paid for.

Her sad reverie ended with the exam.

"It was very nice to meet you," Julia said after finishing the exam. "I think everything is fine. I did find a small sore area on your cervix; it looked like a small irritation. So, I want you to come back and see Dr. Gold in a few weeks to be sure it has healed." Sarah left the office feeling pleased, until they called her back in. As she had heard, Dr. Gold was very good. The news was not.

"Your Pap smear shows you have a cancer of the cervix. I think it is in an early stage, but it needs treatment."

TREATMENT OF CERVICAL CANCER.

Some cervical cancers are found by Pap testing and are not visible on an exam. These can often be cured using surgery to remove the lining of the cervix, although some women will opt to have removal of the uterus and cervix, called a "simple hysterectomy." When cervical cancers are visible but small, the favored treatment is surgery called a "radical hysterectomy." This surgery removes the uterus and cervix, some portion of the vagina and usually the ovaries. The lymph nodes in the pelvis are also removed. For some young women who desire to preserve the option to have children, the operation can be modified to save some of the uterus and ovaries. If the cancers are large when discovered, radiation treatment is used, typically with chemotherapy. The radiation treatments can cover a wider area than the surgeon could easily remove.

The decision regarding which treatment to use requires experience and judgment. The decision is difficult because there is no precise way to tell exactly how large or deep the cancer is before surgery. If at surgery the cancer is found to be more extensive than initially thought, patients receive additional radiation and chemotherapy.

The results of treatment depend upon the degree to which the cancer has grown and spread. Cancers visible only under the microscope are almost always cured. Smaller visible cancers treated with radical hysterectomy have a higher cure rate (over 90 percent) than larger cancers needing radiation and chemotherapy (70 percent). Early detection saves lives.

Sarah's memory of the next six months was a blur of tests, surgery, chemo, and radiation all jumbled with images of Sienna and Mom. Her memory of Dr. Valerie Ivanov was crystal clear, however. The strict Russian gynecologist in her black top and white lab coat never left any doubt where Sarah stood.

"You must have surgery," Dr. Ivanov told her on their first meeting. "Depending on pathology, maybe radiation and chemo, maybe nothing. We cannot know now. I remove everything unless you plan to try for more children."

"More children?" asked Sarah, momentarily puzzled.

"Yes. If you want more children, I remove only cervix and part of uterus. It is not guaranteed, but may be possible. If cancer is more extensive, it will not be possible." Dr. Ivanov explained that leaving a portion of the uterus might allow for pregnancy, one that would be more complex and require surgical delivery since the cervix would be gone.

"Which is better?" asked Mom.

"This depends what you want," replied Dr. Ivanov.

Mom answered. "I think that's too risky. You shouldn't take any chances."

Sarah selected the complete surgery, knowing she did not want more children. She did not have a man in her life and could not see one anytime soon. Raising Sienna was hard enough without the complication. Plus, there was Mom and Dad. And now this.

Her memory of the operation also faded with time, but Dr. Ivanov's report afterward was one she would never forget.

"The pathologists found the cancer was more advanced than we thought. It was deeper, and there were cancer cells in one lymph node. This means you have treatment with radiation and chemotherapy. You will go to Dr. Matthews in Saratoga."

Dr. Matthews reviewed the plan.

"Dr. Ivanov probably removed all the cancer, but we cannot be completely sure. You are young and healthy, so we would like you to have radiation treatment daily for about six weeks and once each week you will have an infusion of a chemotherapy called cisplatin."

Dr. Chris at the radiation oncology unit was enthusiastic.

"We can treat the rest of the area so that if there are any cancerous cells left, they will be eliminated."

At her first radiation treatment, as the heavy lead doors closed and she lay on the table, Sarah had another thought.

Why me?

CAUSES OF CERVICAL CANCER.

In 1944, Dr. Joseph Meigs, professor of gynecology at Harvard Medical School, wrote a review article for the *New England Journal of Medicine* on cervical cancer, at the time a common and devastating cancer. Dr. Meigs described the treatments of the day and correctly predicted the regular use of the Pap smear would offer early detection, yet he was puzzled as to the cause of cervical cancer, noting "there is no known etiologic factor . . . but childbearing, lacerations, infections, syphilis, hormones and hereditary all play a part. A tendency to cancer must be present, and some other factor must be the spark that starts the fire."[466] Thirty years later, pioneering cancer epidemiologist Dr. Valerie Beral hypothesized that the spark for cervical cancer was a sexually transmitted infection. As opposed to clinicians who treat individual patients, epidemiologists study disease patterns in populations. Dr. Beral had examined rates of cervical cancer in successive generations of women from England, Wales, and Scotland. She found the risk was related to an earlier age at first intercourse and increasing number of sexual partners of a woman and her husband.[467]

The first infection suspected as a cause of cervical cancer was herpes simplex type 2, the virus which produces genital herpes. When this link could not be proven, the focus in the 1980s turned to human papilloma virus (HPV). Interestingly, the complexity of HPV infection frustrated epidemiologists, and it fell to laboratory scientists to make the connection.[468] Pathologists knew that HPV could cause wart-like growths and found the viral DNA in a range of precancerous changes and cancers.[469] In 1983, German virologist Dr. Harald zur Hausen identified high-risk subtypes of HPV, first type number 16 then 18, in cervical cancer and was awarded the 2008 Nobel Prize in Medicine.[470] His work combined the descriptions of the cytology (cellular appearance) of cervical cancer made by Papanicolaou and Traut with modern molecular techniques to establish the role of HPV. When epidemiological studies confirmed the findings, it was clear that HPV was the "spark that started the fire" of cervical cancer.

HPV will infect 80 percent of men and women in the United States, although most will never have any adverse consequences. For a few women, the HPV infection will start a chain of events in the cells lining the cervix. In these women, the DNA of the virus can become part of the normal cellular DNA and direct changes in the cell. This process is referred to as transformation by scientists and is visible in Pap smears or biopsies. It may lead to precancerous changes, called cervical intraepithelial neoplasia (CIN), which can progress to cancer. There are about forty subtypes of the HPV virus, and some are more likely to cause transformation, particularly types 16 and 18. Women with weakened immune systems or other infections may be more vulnerable.

The discovery of HPV as the cause of almost all cervical cancer occurred during the time immediately following the sexual revolution. This change in social mores might have further raised the rate of cervical cancer, but screening programs based on the Pap smear were in place which reduced the risk in the U.S. and developed countries. The discovery of HPV as the cause of cervical cancer also raised an exciting possibility beyond screening: the prevention of the cancer by vaccination.

The following week, Sarah asked Karen Lange the same question.

"I don't know for sure," the nurse replied. "I don't think anyone can give you an answer as to why you got it. We know the HPV starts it all off, but why in you? Why not in everyone? Most everyone has HPV. Other genes? Other viruses? God? Luck?"

"I wasn't with many men . . . I read that causes it."

Karen nodded. "Well, if you have more sexual partners, you have more chances to get one of the more dangerous HPV strains. But women with very few partners get this cancer, and most with many do not. So, don't feel that you did anything wrong to cause this cancer. Cancer doesn't care."

The weekly chemotherapy treatment cisplatin required anti-nausea medication and several hours of intravenous fluid to avoid kidney damage. Mom often came with Sarah for these treatments.

"You look so young," commented office secretary Anna Budney to Mom. "I always heard people say you could be Sarah's sister."

"People always do say Mom looks young," agreed Sarah.

"Mostly people say that when I'm with her father," replied Mom. "Of course, that's the good of marrying a man fifteen years older. The bad is now I can see what's coming. And I don't like it. Hearing aids, new knees, back surgery."

"I did the same thing," agreed Anna. "My husband is older than me, too. He's falling apart. What a mess. But he knows it and just laughs. Doesn't let anything bother him. He already donated his body to Albany Medical College. That way I won't have to worry about funeral expenses, as long as he dies within a hundred miles of the College. When we go away he always tells me if he looks bad, just put him in the car and drive like heck toward Albany. 'Get within a hundred miles,' he says."

Sarah laughed. "Dad's not like that. He's worried about everything. Constantly checking the weather, making sure Mom has stocked up on food, and always has flashlights with batteries. Those FOX News Alerts that sound like the world is ending are killing him. And he keeps Mom running."

Mom nodded in agreement.

Sarah drove herself to most of the daily radiation treatments where she became friendly with an older woman having treatment for a throat cancer. As the days went by, Sarah became concerned by progressing redness of the woman's neck and mouth, yet her friend sat stoically.

"How do you manage?" asked Sarah. "My treatment makes sitting and peeing a little uncomfortable, but at least I can eat. You never complain."

Her granddaughter, a concerned looking woman in her mid-thirties, nodded agreement.

"You do what you must, dear," replied the old woman. "I was a young girl in London during the War, and my mother brought me to work with her at the burn hospital. I learned there I must never complain."

As the woman went for her treatment, Sarah waited with her granddaughter.

"She remarkable, particularly for her age," Sarah remarked.

"Dr. Chris didn't want to treat her, but she insisted. She told him she wasn't ninety yet and she could take it." She paused. "My parents were killed in an accident when we were young, so Grandma raised us—myself, my sister, and brother. And that's not all. She adopted another boy a year younger than my brother so it would be even. She raised four of us."

Eventually, the treatment ended and life resumed. Work needed her. Sienna started grade school and really needed her. Mom helped, but also needed her. Dad needed everyone. There was hardly time to get it all done and pay the bills. Sure, once in while she worried about the cancer. But mostly she was just too busy and too tired.

She would have liked to find another man. Jessica, one of her old friends, had asked her about that on one of the rare times they were able to get away.

"I wouldn't say no," Sarah had answered. "But it's a little hard to see that right now. I'm not the neatest package—single with a child, the cancer stuff, and pretty tight with my parents. That'll scare off most men."

Jessica nodded, "How are your parents?"

"Mom is good, but worries about me and Sienna. Dad is getting older, he's seventy now. His back is bad and is in pain, so he's home most of the time. He's a worrier, too."

"About you?"

"About everything. The economy. If he had money, his house would be full of gold or silver. The world, terrorists, you name it. And the weather. He fits up Mom's car with studded snow tires. I don't even know where he gets them, but you can hear her coming a mile away." She paused. "But underneath it, he's a good man. And he loves Sienna."

Sienna had blossomed at Lake Avenue School. The principal, Dr. Williams, had learned of Sarah's struggles and kept a special watch on the child.

"I've always thought she had her father's creativity," Sarah had told Dr. Williams. "But I've been scared she might have his depression, too."

"We haven't seen any sign of it," answered Dr. Williams. "Her teachers and our psychologist say she is totally normal in that regard. That's what I see, too. And she has some special talents."

"Thank you. I could not bear to think of her with that pain."

It was in 2014, three years after Sarah's treatment, that her own pain hit—a sudden, excruciating stabbing in her back. After twenty minutes it was gone, then back, wave after wave, so bad she vomited, again and again. Finally, Mom said enough and brought her to the emergency room.

"You have blood in your urine. I'm pretty sure it's a kidney stone," said the Physician Assistant, a woman about Sarah's age. "We should get a CT scan."

Sure enough, the stone was there, not far from the bladder.

"You should pass it soon. We will give you intravenous fluids and pain medication."

The passing of the stone produced relief, but the other news did not.

"There are some swollen lymph nodes in your abdomen. Did you know you had those?" asked the Physician Assistant.

Sarah shook her head, drowsy from the pain medication. Lymph nodes, she thought. She hadn't heard about lymph nodes since after her cancer surgery.

The lymph nodes lead to a PET scan and an appointment with Dr. Matthews.

"There are three mildly enlarged nodes in your upper abdomen. The PET scan shows some activity in these nodes—"

"Are they cancer?" interrupted Mom.

Sarah patted her mother on the leg. "Mom, let him finish." Her mother nodded.

"We don't know if they are cancer," answered Dr. Matthews. "It is possible they are an inflammation of some sort, not cancerous at all."

"How do we tell?" asked Mom anxiously.

"We have two choices," replied Dr. Matthews. "One is to watch and repeat a CT scan in six weeks—"

"I don't like that waiting," interrupted Mom. She turned to Sarah. "I know, let Doctor finish."

"The other choice is to do a biopsy. It would require an operation. I do not think we could risk a needle biopsy due to the location of these lymph nodes."

Mother and daughter looked at each other.

"Of course, it's your choice," began Mother. "But if you want my opinion—"

"Have the operation," concluded the daughter knowingly.

Dr. Ivanov agreed with Mom. "You must know. I will do the surgery next week."

The surgery went smoothly, but Dr. Ivanov also saw other small growths scattered in the pelvis. The biopsies confirmed that both these and the lymph nodes were cervical cancer. The cancer had sown its seeds four years ago and some, having been outside the radiation beam and surviving the chemotherapy, were growing.

"You take chemotherapy now," said Dr. Ivanov. "You fight more."

The chemotherapy was every three weeks; two standard drugs named carboplatin and paclitaxel plus an antibody named bevacizumab, designed to prevent the cancers from making their own blood vessels.

"The idea is that the chemotherapy will kill the cancer cells and the bevacizumab will keep them from regrowing," explained Dr. Matthews. "If we can get good shrinkage, we can stop the chemotherapy and just continue the bevacizumab alone. That usually has much fewer side effects."

Mom had stopped Dr. Matthews alone later in the hall.

"You have to save her. I can't raise my granddaughter. I'm too old, and my husband is fifteen years older. Sienna needs her mother."

Jessica had picked her up after the second treatment. Her news was not good, either.

"Bastard of a husband left me," she reported. "Ran off with some bimbo. Now I'm screwed. I'll never get child support from that piece of crap. Here I am, pushing forty and I got three kids and no husband. Thank God, I got my mother. I feel bad complaining to you, though. You have cancer."

"One kid, no husband, and cancer for me. Three kids, no husband for you. And only one head of hair between us," summarized Sarah. "Haven't we done well?"

Except for her hair loss, Sarah did do well with the chemotherapy. After four months, she and Mom met with Dr. Matthews.

"Your PET scan is now normal," he reported. "We cannot find any evidence of any cancer activity. Now—"

"It's over?" asked Mom.

"Let him speak," cautioned Sarah.

"What this means is that we cannot see anything, but there are still some cancer cells," continued Dr. Matthews. "And we would like to try to control them for as long as possible using the bevacizumab without the chemotherapy. You should still come every three weeks for the infusion, and we will do another PET scan in about four months."

Anna Budney was happy to make the new schedule. "I'm glad you finished your chemo treatments. You really look good. How's Dad?"

"He's sore, but okay," answered Mom. "How's your husband."

"Still going," smiled Anna. "Every morning he wakes up and says the same thing. 'Honey, I didn't see any white light last night, and I'm still on the right side of the grass. Guess I get another day.' "

Sarah came every three weeks for the bevacizumab. She felt well, her hair regrew, and her PET scans stayed clear. In the summer of 2016, Sienna turned eleven and Sarah took her to the Peerless pool with Jessica and her children. Sarah updated Jessica on her last scans and plans to continue treatment.

"So, I'm good, for now," she concluded. "How are things with your ex?"

"He's a bastard, but at least he's paying," answered Jessica. "He's still holed up with that bimbo. She has a few kids of her own and is stuck here, so I guess he'll stay around. That's good for me in terms of the money."

"But it's hard seeing him," continued Sarah.

"Yeah, but I guess it's better for the kids." She paused. "It is a man's world, though. You know, I have this neighbor who raises Alpacas. She was telling me one of her males got out of line and started biting. Know how she fixed it?"

Sarah shook her head.

"Alpaca sausage," announced Jessica.

"Well, I don't know about that," laughed Sarah. "But maybe things will get better. I know Sienna won't get what I have. She got her vaccination last week."

CERVICAL CANCER VACCINES.

Developing viral vaccines is difficult. To produce the desired effect, either the whole virus (inactivated or modified to prevent it from being dangerous) or a specific part of the virus must be given to the person to stimulate the immune system to produce antibodies ("elicit an immune response" in medical jargon). To be protective, these antibodies must neutralize the virus when it later infects the person. Designing the vaccine is often technically difficult since the antibodies may not be protective (a common problem in HIV vaccines) or the virus can mutate (the seasonal influenza virus).

Developing a vaccination against HPV had special challenges. One problem was that HPV does not grow in the lab, so producing the vaccine from the virus itself would be very difficult. A second problem was that the antibodies the immune system produced would need to reach the surface of the cervix. Since the anti-HPV antibodies would circulate in the blood stream, enough would need to be made to slip out from the blood vessels. Once the antibody reached the surface of the cervix, it would need to neutralize the virus. If all this took place, then the prevention of HPV cervical cancer might be possible. Of course, testing the vaccine, obtaining governmental approval, and gaining public support would be entirely separate matters.

The science was brilliant. HPV is a package composed of viral DNA surrounded by a protein capsule. In the late 1990s, scientists produced variations of these capsular proteins which would assemble into empty virus-like particles.[471] These virus-like particles produced a tremendous immune response, enough to allow the antibodies to block viral infection of the cervical cells. Since the capsules were empty, there was no risk of infection. Although the vaccine work was done by many scientists, most the credit is given to Drs. Ian Frazer of Australia and Dr. Jian Zhou (who sadly died in 1999 at age forty-two from the consequences of viral hepatitis).[472]

The proof the vaccine would work came in 2002 in the *New England Journal of Medicine*. About two thousand four hundred young women received either a placebo or a vaccine against HPV subtype 16, the selection done by random chance. For those not infected at the start, the vaccine was completely protective. Most importantly, the women who received the vaccine did not develop the precursor changes described by George and Mary Papanicolaou a century ago which could lead to cancer.[473] When further studies confirmed the vaccine's effectiveness, it was clear that Dr. Meig's spark which started the fire of cervical cancer, identified as a sexually transmitted disease by Dr. Beral and HPV by Dr. zur Hausen, could be squelched by Drs. Frazer and Zhou's virus-like particles.

HPV vaccines received approval for use in the United States in 2006. They should be administered at ages eleven or twelve, before sexual activity begins and when the antibody response is best. Experts recommend vaccination of both girls and boys, both to reduce transmission and because HPV also causes cancers of the head and neck and penis. Despite the science, in 2014 only about 40 percent of girls and 20 percent of boys in the United States received the HPV vaccination.[474] Nearly a hundred years of dedicated work met the realities which hamper public health vaccination programs: cost, fears of side effects, and lack of clear strategies to incorporate recommendations. The HPV vaccination also faced the added burden of requiring a discussion of sexual activity, not usually a favorite parental conversation.[475]

For two and a half years, the bevacizumab worked. Then one night the pain returned. Shit, Sarah thought, not those kidney stones again. Thirty minutes later she knew it was not the stones. This was different, worse. She knew this meant something serious. Jessica took Sienna while Mom took her to the ER.

"Her abdomen is rigid," reported Dr. Newcomb, the emergency room physician, to Dr. Cannon, the surgeon on call. "And her CT scan shows free air."

To Sarah and Mom, Dr. Newcomb explained in more detail.

"Somewhere in your gastrointestinal system, there is a hole which is leaking. We can see the air on the CT scan. Dr. Cannon is on his way in. He needs to operate to find and repair it."

"Dr. Ivanov is her surgeon," said Mom.

"I don't think she can wait for a transfer to Albany," answered Dr. Newcomb. "She needs this surgery right away."

After examining Sarah, Dr. Gannon agreed. "From the CT scan, I believe you have a hole in your stomach. I spoke with Dr. Matthews about your treatment. He tells me that this can occur with the medicine you are getting, most commonly in the area where the radiation was, the pelvis. Either way, I need to find and repair the damage. You cannot wait."

Thankfully, it was a small hole in the stomach which had only leaked into a confined area. Dr. Gannon was able to sew it closed. A hole in the colon would have probably meant several operations and the possibility of a colostomy and infection. Sarah awoke in the ICU, Mom by her side. Her recovery was rapid, and they met with Dr. Matthews before discharge.

"We cannot use the bevacizumab anymore," he said. "Now we watch."

"I don't like that. What happens if the cancer grows?" asked Mom.

"We have many choices. If it grows, we can use more chemotherapy. Or we can send her to a major center for a discussion of targeted options which might be specific to her cancer."

PERSONALIZED "PRECISION" CANCER MEDICINE.
The promise of "personalized and precision" cancer medicine is that individual patients will have their tumors tested for DNA mutations and be prescribed treatments targeted at their specific abnormalities. The late 1990s saw this approach work in chronic myelogenous leukemia (CML), where identification of the DNA abnormality led to remarkable success with the use of the targeted treatment imatinib (Gleevec). A leukemia which had previously been devastating was cured in most people. Although CML is a relatively rare cancer with

one main DNA problem, the hope was that this strategy would work for more common and complex cancers with multiple, unpredictable mutations.

Precision medicine requires the ability to find DNA mutations and give treatments which target the abnormalities. The ability to sequence DNA, which began in the 1970s and improved in the 1990s with the Human Genome Project, has reached the point where "high-throughput genomic testing" allows routine sequencing of large numbers of samples. Several labs now offer DNA sequencing of cancer specimens which can identify many mutations. Although the DNA mutations cannot yet be corrected, some produce effects which targeted treatments can reverse. The powerful combination of academia, biotech, and the pharmaceutical industry has produced an understanding of the role of these DNA abnormalities in different cancers and a variety of treatments. Personalized and precision medicine is ongoing as tumors are tested, mutations found, and targeted treatments prescribed to patients.

Does it work? In 2016, Drs. Ian Tannock and John Hickman in the *New England Journal of Medicine* noted that "the concept of personalized medicine is so appealing that seemingly only curmudgeons could criticize it."[476] Yet they did offer an important critique. From a scientific viewpoint, they noted several potential problems with this approach. Most cancers are not uniform and the DNA analysis may vary depending upon the location biopsied. Mutations may change over time and analysis of a single biopsy at one point in time may not be useful. Many DNA mutations may not "drive" the cancer; they are so-called irrelevant "passenger" mutations. Even if it is successful, personalized treatments will likely result in more resistant cancer cells with other mutations. They point out that there has been no evidence that this approach works for most patients. Despite these cautions, research goes on while individual patients and their doctors try.

In the spring of 2017, Sarah's PET scan had shown more activity in the lymph nodes. Dr. Matthews had reviewed the choices.

"We can reuse the same treatment. It was very successful. Or we could send you to a major cancer center where they could do another biopsy and analyze the DNA of cancer. That might tell us if other targeted treatments could be used or you are eligible for any protocols they might have. The advantage is that we can always use the standard chemotherapy later. We are in good health otherwise and, if they have a protocol, they would be interested in you."

"I don't think she should be a guinea pig," began Mom.

"Mom, wait. I would like to go and hear what they say. Jessica can go with me, while you and Dad watch Sienna."

After a lecture by Dad about how to handle a terrorist attack, Sarah and Jessica rode the train to Memorial Sloan Kettering Cancer Center for a needle biopsy of the lymph nodes. The pathologist confirmed this was a recurrence of the cervical cancer and the specimen was sent for "next generation sequencing." In this procedure, the DNA of the cancerous cells was analyzed for mutations or alterations in hundreds of key genes.

Two weeks later Dr. Susan Jenkins, the gynecologic oncologist at MSKCC, met with Sarah and Jessica. She was a serious woman in her late thirties, obviously brilliant.

"Your cancer has two mutations, one in the *KRAS* gene and the other in *NF1*. This means that we can try some different treatments. We do not have any clinical trial for you here, but Dr. Matthews can give you temsirolimus, letrozole, and metformin at home. I will call him."

Dr. Matthews explained more.

"The mutation found in this *NF1* gene means that a drug we use in kidney cancer called temsirolimus might be effective. The other two seem to help it."

Sarah began a program of a weekly intravenous treatment with temsirolimus and the daily pill letrozole. After a few weeks, they added the metformin pill.

"It is used to treat diabetes," Karen Lange said. "For some reason, it can also make these treatments work better."

The pills were easy, but the intravenous treatments were hard. After three months, Sarah felt tired. Still, she thought, I can do this. It beats the chemo. As she was half asleep on the table for the forty-five minutes of the PET scan, she saw faces. Sienna. The man she had loved. Jessica. Dad. Mom. Her cute ex-President and his wife. It was okay, since for once they were all smiling.

Today's visit was for the results.

"The PET scan shows no change," answered Dr. Matthews. "Everything is stable, and there is nothing new."

"Thank God. You can keep going," announced Mom, hugging her daughter.

Sarah shrugged. "Well, I guess that's the plan. Come on Mom."

As they rose to leave, Sarah looked at Dr. Matthews.

"We have to stay on time today. Dad wants her to get the studded tires put on her car. In case there is an early snow." She laughed. "We've got the newest of the new for cancer and the oldest of the old for the car."

Carol Feinman 7: Breast cancer (Boston, 1992–1993)

It was spring when Carol and Rose met Dr. Spiegel. After six cycles of treatment, her CT scan had shown the spots in the liver were gone. The bone scan showed her bones were healing.

"We have a choice," concluded Dr. Spiegel. "You can continue on with treatment or take a break. If you keep going, it is possible more chemo might keep the cancer away longer, but your body will get worn down. If you stop, you can enjoy feeling good for a while, but you may be back on chemo sooner. The general rule is to treat to the maximum response, then stop. Although it is hard to be sure, I think you are there and should take a break."

"I'd like to take a break over the summer," replied Carol.

"What happens if it starts to grow again?" asked Rose.

"Party pooper," Carol answered and stuck her tongue out at Rose.

"It depends on the length of the break. If the cancer stays away for more than six months, we would probably go back to the same treatment, although in a weekly format. If it comes back sooner, we will try something different."

The summer of 1992 brought surprisingly cool weather to Massachusetts. In Boston, the Red Sox were even colder, destined to finish last in the Division as even the normally steady Wade Boggs had a bad year. The political world was warmer as Bill Clinton challenged President Bush while Ross Perot made his famous sucking sound, imitating the nation's job loss under NAFTA. For Carol, it was a magical time, almost as if she never had cancer. The routine of her family, coworkers, and friends brought back her former life. She even took the bus to New York City to visit her brother Steven. One morning they went to nearby Christopher Park to see George Segal's Gay Liberation statue which Mayor Dinkins had recently dedicated. As they sat near the stark white figures of two standing men and two seated women which memorialized the 1969 police raid on the gay Stonewall Inn, Carol found it surprisingly peaceful. She found herself thinking about Roger and his struggles in Boston. She imagined her brother's life as a slight, thoughtful, gay, Jewish boy in New York City.

"You've haven't had it easy, have you?" she asked him.

"You should talk," he answered, with the sense of irony which she loved.

"I guess," she agreed. "You know, I found this cancer walking in the park near the duck sculpture." He knew where she meant. "I always thought it was odd, finding something serious near a duck sculpture. It probably should have been here . . ."

Steven thought for a moment. "I don't think your cancer should be found here or anywhere, but clearly it's not my call. This stuff is complicated. The ducks at least I understand."

There were a few reminders of reality. Carol still had very little hair. CJ had told her it would take months to regrow, but she had secretly hoped it would be faster. She avoided her favorite actress since Meryl Streep's new movie was *Death Becomes Her*. And looking at her scarred breast still hurt. Even so, the wonderful months flew by.

As summer ended, Carol joined Roger and Allen in Provincetown for the week following Labor Day. She had spent the holiday itself with Betty, Rose, and her family, after which her sister had returned to work while Cynthia and Alisa went back to school. The weather on the Cape was beautiful, and the departure of the crowds meant the streets and harbor were quiet. Allen was a fine cook while Roger set an elegant table and selected unique wines. The ocean view from their home was spectacular. Carol could watch the waves roll in and almost imagine she was born in a different era, her life revolving around the rhythm of the sea.

Except that her bones hurt. Carol had noticed it a few weeks earlier and tried to convince herself it was just muscle aching. Everyone in Boston had heard about Roger Clemens' pulled groin. Maybe that's what I have, she rationalized. Maybe I'll trade in Dr. Spiegel for Dr. Pappas, she told herself. But deep inside, she knew what it meant.

"I don't want to go back," she told Roger as they sat on the deck watching the day's light gently fade, listening to George Michaels and Elton John sing "Don't Let the Sun Go Down on Me."

"I don't blame you," he replied, assuming she was referring to the music.

"No, Roger. I mean treatment. They're going to tell me I need more chemo again. I don't want it. I had a good summer; my hair is just starting back." She took off her hat and rubbed the short growth. "I can't go back to that taste and smell."

"I'm sorry, dear," he replied, took her hand, and they sipped their wine as the darkness engulfed them.

Carol was right. The news from radiology was bad. The cancer had grown again in her liver and bones. By then it was early October. The foliage had burst into color and fallen, leaving only a few depleted stragglers. Carol, too, was drained as the pain in her back and pelvis had become present most of the day. While she still went to work, her team was careful not to send her on field trips. Nancy made her stop exercising, coming by in the evenings for a short walk instead of the gym.

"You need to be back on treatment," said Dr. Spiegel. "The cancer is growing again. If there are any spots which are particularly painful, we can give radiation to them."

"There's nothing like that," she replied tiredly. "I just feel weak and sore all over my body."

"What's the treatment?" asked Rose.

"There is a new chemotherapy drug named Taxol," answered Dr. Spiegel. "It has been successful in women who have ovarian cancer and some with breast cancer. The Dana Farber is starting clinical trials next month in women with breast cancer. I think you should enroll."

TESTING TAXOL.

In 1962, a young botanist named Arthur Barclay from the U.S. Department of Agriculture harvested the bark of a Pacific yew tree near Mount St. Helens in Washington for the drug discovery program sponsored by the National Cancer Institute (NCI). After about five years of work, scientists Monroe Wall and Mansuki Wani isolated a drug from the bark which they named Taxol (generic name paclitaxel). Since the molecule was large and complex, it took until 1971 to work out the structure. Although it was soon evident that paclitaxel killed cancer cells in the lab with amazing power, it took eight more years and a brilliant researcher from Albert Einstein named Susan Horwitz to discover that it worked by damaging the microtubules which form the scaffolding of cells. Despite the excitement in the laboratory, paclitaxel could not be used in people because it would not dissolve in water, requiring further work from NCI scientists. It was not until 1984, after twenty-two years of work, that human testing began.

The results of the first clinical trials were dramatic by oncology standards. When women with advanced ovarian cancer treated with many other drugs received paclitaxel, it shrank the cancer in 30 percent.[477] The major problem was getting a supply of the drug. Stripping the bark from the yew trees was not a good solution since it would take the bark of an entire tree to give about one dose for one patient. The first answer was a semisynthetic paclitaxel obtained from the needles of a yew shrub. The better answer came when the Florida State University lab of Dr. Robert Holton developed a synthetic paclitaxel. Within a few years, paclitaxel was the leading oncology drug in the world, helping thousands of patients with breast and ovarian cancer live longer. Shortly after the publication of the results of the first clinical trials, the NCI awarded the rights to paclitaxel to Bristol-Myers, a highly controversial decision given the profits the company realized.

The early clinical studies of paclitaxel were also controversial, particularly when the drug was in short supply. The enthusiasm of many well-meaning scientists, physicians, and advocates had led to tremendous hope and expectations. Many researchers wanted to test paclitaxel in small clinical trials designed to maximize knowledge by giving it over various infusion times and in combination with other drugs. Patients and advocacy groups, encouraged by the preliminary reports, wanted it made widely available to those suffering from advanced breast cancer. The National Cancer Institute compromised by opening a clinical trial for two hundred fifty patients at hospitals across the country, a number far greater than typical for such early studies.

In early October, Carol met Dr. Lynn Weber, the pleasant young oncologist in charge of the trial, who agreed she was a good candidate for the study. Carol would be admitted to the Dana Farber Cancer Center for a twenty-four-hour infusion of the drug. Dr. Weber reviewed the side effects, and Carol signed the consent forms. Treatment would begin in the second week in November.

As they left, Carol thanked her.

"I'm glad you have this study for me."

Rose had a different view.

"Don't stop with this," she commanded Dr. Weber. "You better find something else."

The month was long. Each day, Carol felt more tired and in more pain. At work, Roger noticed her struggle and spoke to her privately.

"Why don't you take a few days off, Carol? You're having a tough time."

"I don't want to let you down," she answered. "Even though I know I haven't been much use outside the office lately. I'm also afraid if I stay home my sister or mother will think something is wrong."

They compromised with Roger finding work for her at home two days a week. Nancy, too, had seen the changes and helped by doing her food shopping, stopping over in the evening and putting her through some gentle stretches. Two weeks before the Taxol was to start, Steven came for a visit. As they sat alone in her apartment before meeting the rest of the family at Betty's for dinner, Steven was surprised to see how hard it was for Carol to move.

"I'm sorry, Carol. I didn't realize how tough it was for you."

"It's really been the last two weeks that I've had trouble walking," she answered. "I've been trying to hang in there until the Taxol starts. And I don't want Rose and Mom to see me like this . . . It serves no purpose. I can't get the treatment any faster since the study just won't be opened for two more weeks. Thankfully, the girls are so busy that they have Rose and Mom distracted."

"They'll see you tonight," he warned.

"That's what I have this for." She held up a small medicine bottle as Steven raised an eyebrow. "Liquid morphine, liquid gold . . . Just tell them I had a few drinks. They'll believe that."

Carol leaned heavily on Steven as she climbed the stairs to Betty's brownstone. Fortunately, Betty was distracted preparing Carol's favorite vegetable soup and roast, and they arrived before Rose. The dinner went surprisingly well, with Cynthia and Alisa providing entertainment centered on teasing their Uncle Steven.

"How long will you stay, Steven?" asked Rose after the dinner was over and they had coffee.

"I'm between projects, so I have a few weeks off. I thought I might stay with Carol until she starts her new treatment." Carol nodded as if she knew, thrilled with Steven's announcement. Betty and Rose were also pleased.

"But I am tired," he continued, sensing that the effects of the morphine were wearing off his sister. "So maybe we can go soon, Carol, if that's okay with you." She nodded gratefully.

As Steven drove, she asked him about his decision.

"You don't have time off, do you?" she asked.

"I have time," he answered, "and it's nice being with you."

She decided not to press him. Just enjoy him and be grateful, she thought. The waiting was certainly easier with Steven. He fit in well with her life.

"You never told me you had such a gorgeous brother. If only I wasn't taken . . .," announced Roger.

Nancy also approved. "He's tiny, but quite the Ju-Jitsu man. He certainly could surprise a person."

Rose and Betty were also relieved that Steven was home.

"The girls are keeping me so busy. Truthfully, I am relieved that Steven is here and watching over Carol," Rose told Betty.

"They think alike," agreed Betty. "He's so good with her. I wish . . ."

"That he would move back," finished Rose.

Most importantly, Steven kept Carol calm. As it became harder to move each day, she could feel life leaving her. The pains seemed to travel. One hour it was her lower back, then her side, then hips. It made no sense. Maybe this is what it is like to die by inches, she thought. Where is that Taxol? Why do I have to wait? I'm sure it is in the hospital. She imagined a vial sitting in a locked shelf in that big hospital building. Put it in me, she begged.

By the time Carol entered the Dana Farber Cancer Institute, Steven had brought her in by wheelchair. Her room on the clinical trials unit of the sixth floor was spacious, with a window that looked out over Brookline Avenue and the Au Bon Pain restaurant. The nurse started her IV, then stuck EKG leads onto her chest and attached the wires to the small box hanging on the bed.

"What are those for?" asked Steven.

"This Taxol produces a lot of irregular heartbeats. They don't seem to be serious, but we monitor them to be sure. You can walk around the ward, just bring this Walkman with you." She held up the box, showing Carol how to remove it. A few minutes later, flowers arrived. Steven looked puzzled.

"Roger," Carol said.

He nodded, instantly understanding. "Of course."

Dr. Weber came with her team, two even younger looking women physicians and two medical students, both men. They examined Carol and reviewed the plans once again.

"I'm more than ready," Carol concluded. "Just hook me up."

As the group left, one young woman remained behind.

"I'm Cathy Johnson. I'm a research fellow here now. I met you years ago when I was a medical student with Dr. Spiegel. I remember your mom and sister were with you then. I'm sorry to see you having to do more treatment." Steven introduced himself, and they chatted for a few minutes before she left.

"They all seem very nice here," commented Steven. "Very dedicated."

Carol nodded and closed her eyes. "You know, I thought I was going to do something special, like her. I figured I'd work for a few years doing fun stuff and then write a play or something. I thought I might base it off my job. It could be a comedy, you know. But after this past month, I don't think I'll never have the energy, even if this stuff works."

Steven held her hand as she opened her eyes.

"I think you need to focus on a short-term goal, like getting better," he said softly. "After that, the future will take care of itself."

A soft knock on the door interrupted her reply. It was Roger, making his typical visit before any family was likely to be present.

"Am I intruding?" he asked softly.

"Never," Carol replied. "I can't imagine two people I would want more to be around me. Steven was just cheering me up in a moment of self-pity."

"We all need that," Roger replied.

"Steven tells me I need a short-term goal and seeing you has given me the inspiration for mine," she replied, as Steven looked puzzled.

Roger sat down opposite Steven. "Well, I'm delighted to be useful. What, my dear, is our goal?"

"I'm taking this Taxol," she announced. "And when it makes me better, and my hair is gone, I am taking the two of you and Nancy to Harrods to buy a hat."

When Steven continued to look puzzled, Roger explained.

"Carol has a beautiful hat face, even when her hair is gone. We are not sure there is anything on this continent that does her justice, so we have been considering a visit to London."

"I'm in," answered Steven.

The Taxol made her better. Not right away, but slowly. The twenty-four hours in the hospital were no fun, although the infusions themselves went smoothly once the nurses and doctors learned to ignore the irregularities in her heart beats. She had almost no nausea. Still, she always felt grimy and sweaty when she left, even though the rooms were immaculately clean and temperature controlled. She looked forward to her first shower, which always made her think of washing away the smell of that ultrasound jelly. As she dried herself, she would see her baldness and misshapen breast reflected in the mirror. Ignore it, she thought. After makeup and a blouse, I still clean up nicely. And I'm getting that hat.

Steven had to wheel her out of Dana Farber following the first infusion, but three weeks later Carol walked in, a little uncomfortably, but on her own. A week after that treatment, Nancy had been able to take her for a few walks and practice some stretching. Steven saw her through the second treatment, then returned to New York after promising to return soon. Rose and Betty, too, were happy to see her improvement.

USING TAXOL.

The results with Taxol (paclitaxel) in women with advanced breast cancer were reported in 1995. These women were in difficult circumstances, having already had many other chemotherapies. Most patients received four cycles of paclitaxel. The main side effect was low white blood count which often required hospitalization but was then treated with G-CSF (Neupogen). The response rate was 23 percent, meaning the women had significant shrinkage of the disease. The average time the responses lasted was five months, and their typical survival was about ten months. No patient was cured.[478]

The adjective used to describe these results depended upon perspective. For scientists and research physicians, "impressive" was a common choice. Paclitaxel had caused shrinkage of cancers which were resistant to adriamycin, the best drug at the time. Paclitaxel could now be tested in combination with other drugs and in early stage breast cancer, where it might increase the cure rate. Pharmaceutical representatives were effusive, "groundbreaking" was their common word. Treating physicians and nurses were usually more circumspect, the word "useful" combined with the phrase "some good responses" sought to balance hope with reality. In the media, adjectives ranging from "exciting" to "disappointing" appeared as the hype of Taxol met the study results. For individual patients, the adjective could change daily.

London was forty degrees and rainy that winter week in early 1993. As the big jet landed, Carol could have cared less. She felt good. With Steven, Roger, and Nancy, she saw the changing of the guards at Buckingham Palace, Big Ben, the London Museum, and Abbey Road. Cancer could never take this trip away. When she bought the perfect hat at Harrods, her smile said it all.

June 13, 1993
Dear Roger,
I missed the chance to say a real goodbye last week. After Carol's death, every-thing was so hectic that I never felt like there was a moment for me to put my thoughts together. Even now, part of me doesn't understand that she is gone

while part of me is relieved and part of me is numb. But even in this sorry state, I know there is a debt we all owe to you that can never be repaid.

Although we knew the Taxol would not work forever, we were all shocked when Carol had the seizure, and we learned the cancer had spread to her brain. After that, she was never again herself. I shared some of your doubts about the radiation but felt the need to try. Once she went into the coma, I also wished she could have been at home rather than having two months of extra life in the hospital which she could not appreciate. I know neither of us would have given her the chemotherapy into her brain. It was never going to help. But Rose and my mother had to fight to the very end. During our lives together, I have forced them to face some things they did not want to hear, but this time I could not. Maybe I was a coward. Maybe I didn't want to face it myself. And part of me rationalizes that Carol wanted them to make the decisions, so they would at least have the peace of having done everything. I hope that is true and, if not, that she forgives me.

You were wonderful to Carol. I remember when she was first diagnosed and told me how you made her feel like she was still alive, still part of work and life. Your trip to the Caribbean before she started her radiation was a special gift. During her chemo, she could always count on you to make her laugh. And whenever she was in the hospital, you brought her in a little bit of home. You may not realize how much that meant. I will never forget out trip to Harrods. It never would have happened without you. It gave her joy and gave me memories that I will keep for my life. As I write this letter, I see her beautiful smile under that hat.

Carol loved you. All our family owes you thanks, even those who can't see through their grief to say it yet.

I hope to see you when I return to Boston, or you visit New York.

All my love to you and Allen,

Steven

3:00 Joseph Lawrence: Glioblastoma

"How is Joseph?" asked Dr. Matthews as he sat down across from Julia Lawrence, a well-dressed fifty-seven-year-old woman who looked tired.

"Well, his children finally agreed with hospice," she replied. "I never thought they would."

"Is he more settled now?"

She nodded.

"You took good care of him," he continued. "And still are."

"Yeah, I guess . . .," she trailed off. "You know, I didn't plan on this. It's such a damn shame."

Julia Lawrence had the intake meeting with hospice a month ago.

"How did you meet?" asked Joan Williams, the hospice nurse. Joseph Lawrence was asleep in the study, now converted into a first-floor bedroom, as Julia and Joan sat in the nearby living room.

"At our thirtieth college reunion, five years ago. He was standing there, and I asked him to dance. I remember Stevie Nicks and Tom Petty's 'Stop Draggin' My Heart Around' around was playing." Julia smiled wistfully. They had both been fifty-two.

"Had you known each other before?" asked Joan.

"We had met as seniors in college and liked each other, but we were both in relationships. Graduation came, and we went our separate ways. We would see each other occasionally at reunions, but both had our lives. I married a big-time stockbroker in the City and had two sons and a house in Westchester, the whole deal. Of course, once the boys left, I was yesterday's news and traded for his trophy wife." She paused and sipped her coffee. "Joseph had gone to medical school, moved to New Jersey, and become a general surgeon. He and his wife had two sons and a daughter. At some point, he became so severely allergic to latex that he had to stop operating and take an administrative job. About a year before we met, his wife had died of breast cancer. Joseph told me it was one of the aggressive types; she had only been diagnosed about two years before."

"Did you start to date then?" asked Joan.

"Yeah," Julia answered. "Although his children were upset. They were all out of the house, but they wanted to remember Mom and Dad as they were. I didn't fit into that picture. I think they figured it wouldn't last long. When he proposed about a year later, they were furious."

"How did you handle it?'"

"Well, we tried to make them understand. The boys were okay. Gregory eventually gave us his blessing and Mitchell was at least civil. But Caroline never forgave me. We had a small, quiet wedding and when Joseph took a job for an insurance company in Albany, we moved to Saratoga. That was four years ago."

"Did his children visit?"

"Gregory visited fairly often. He was married, no kids, lived in New York City, and had his own life. Mitchell had moved to Philadelphia and rarely came. Caroline still lived near their old home and always resented me, no matter what Joseph said. At first, he tried to explain and include her, but finally, he just gave up, hoping she would come around when she was older. Still, for two years we were happy . . . very happy."

"What happened?"

Julia was quiet, the memory still fresh. Two years ago, almost to the day, Joseph had awoken with a bad headache. Two hours later, he collapsed on the floor. An ambulance ride to the ER, a CT scan, another ride to Albany Med, emergency brain surgery. Brain bleeding, they said. Into a cancer. A brain cancer, something called glioblastoma multiforme.

CLASSIFICATION OF BRAIN CANCER.

Cancers in the brain are frequently metastasis which originated elsewhere in the body, such as the lung or breast. These are usually known to the treating physicians from the patient's history and easily identified by the pathologist who recognizes the cancer is formed of cells not normally found in the brain. In contrast, true "brain cancers" start from the cells of the brain.

Understanding brain cancers require knowledge of the normal brain, a daunting challenge for the owners of even the most brilliant of these two- to three-pound organs. In a gross simplification, the normal brain can be divided into three parts: the cerebrum (the outer portion responsible for thinking, voluntary movements, hearing and vision), the brainstem (the inner stalk which controls basic functions like breathing), and the cerebellum (located in the back which controls balance and coordination). Most brain cancers in adults develop in the cerebrum, that large outer portion of the brain which controls the activities which define our lives.

One of the striking visual aspects of the cerebrum is its many folds. These allow for much more brain surface area and many more neuronal connections. A dead cerebrum has a gray outer layer ("gray matter") and a white inner portion ("white matter"), but in life this outer layer appears a darker pinkish color due to blood flow. The cerebrum has three lobes, named from front to back as the frontal (obvious), parietal, and occipital. Inside the brain are spaces called ventricles filled with spinal fluid. Early scientists like Leonardo da Vinci were fascinated by these spaces and thought much of the brain's activities took place in them rather than the solid tissue.

Under the microscope, the outer gray matter of the cerebrum is seen to contain many cell bodies while the inner white matter has many fewer cell bodies and is made up of projections from the cells (the wires of the brain). The most glamorous of the brain's cells are the neurons, which receive and transmit information and somehow link together to give us thought. The care and feeding of the neurons are the responsibility of the glial cells, also called macroglia. These caretaker cells, which surround and outnumber the neurons about ten to one, come in four types. Astrocytes are the largest, named because they have a star shape. Oligodendrocytes are the most common, named because they have few branches. Ependymal cells line the ventricles and produce spinal fluid, while microglia are the immune cells.

Most adult brain cancers start from glial cells, the caretaker cells. The modern description of brain cancer began in 1926 when Harvey Cushing and Percival Bailey published the formidably titled book *A Classification of the Tumors of the Glioma Group on Histogenetic Basis with a Correlated Study of Prognosis*. At the time, Cushing and Bailey published their work, primary brain cancers were generally all termed gliomas, although they could have very different behaviors in patients. Bailey examined over four hundred of Cushing's samples in a three-year effort to better describe the cancers using their cellular appearance and determine their prognosis.[479] The authors were an interesting pairing.

Dr. Harvey Cushing (1869-1939) was one of the giants of American medicine and the "father of modern neurosurgery." Born the youngest of ten children, Cushing came from a family of medical practitioners which included his father, with whom he was very close. He attended Yale and Harvard Medical School, then studied at Johns Hopkins. There he met William Halsted, the famous surgeon known for developing the mastectomy and the modern demanding surgical training program, and Dr. William Osler, the "father of modern medicine."[480] At Hopkins, Cushing became one of the world's premier neurosurgeons. His pioneering work allowed the age of surgery, which began after the discoveries of anesthesia and antisepsis in the mid-1800s, to include the brain as he steadily "opened the closed box" of the skull.[481] Cushing also contributed to the adoption of the Johns Hopkins model of medical education and elevation of American surgery to a leadership position in the world.[482] In 1912, Cushing returned to Boston to participate in the expansion of Harvard Medical School and its new hospital endowed by the gift of Peter Brent Brigham. In addition to his many surgical contributions, Cushing was a trauma surgeon in France in World War I and a prolific writer who won a Pulitzer Prize for his biography of Osler. This legendary man was also a complex figure. Deeply committed to his patients, at times he was also a hard and erratic taskmaster, unkind husband, and discriminated against women and minorities.[483]

Dr. Percival Bailey (1892-1973) had humbler roots. He was born and raised up in the "barren clay hills of southern Illinois (which) did not produce good corn or hogs, but . . . superb men."[484] Leaving his abusive father at fourteen, Bailey attended the University of Chicago, where he developed an interest in neuroanatomy, and medical school at Northwestern University. After his internship, Bailey joined Cushing at the Peter Bent Brigham Hospital in Boston (now the Brigham and Women's Hospital). In almost a decade together, Cushing and Bailey revolutionized the classification of brain tumors, yet their relationship was not always smooth. Bailey left on several occasions, upset with the domineering Cushing's behavior. For example, when Cushing learned Bailey planned to marry, he visited the young woman's uncles in New York City, telling them this marriage would ruin Bailey's career by distracting him from his work. The family was reportedly so impressed with Cushing's description of Bailey that they blessed the union, which lasted happily until his death in 1973.[485] After leaving Boston and Cushing in 1928, Bailey returned to University of Chicago and Northwestern University where he had a distinguished career in many areas of neurological science, including psychiatry, earning the title of "Mr. Neurology."[486] He was beloved by his family and many students.

The work of these two different but highly influential men began a classification of brain cancers which remains in place today. Modern pathologists use grading systems based on Bailey and Cushing's work combined with genetic studies to describe these cancers. The worst is glioblastoma multiforme. As the name implies, these cancer cells start from the glial cells but take multiple forms under the microscope. It is a highly aggressive cancer which infiltrates the normal brain tissue, resists treatments, and has a poor prognosis.

It had been a long day. Joseph was brought out of the operating room that evening and into the neurosurgical ICU. Dr. Jacob King, the neurosurgeon on call, was also tired, but kind.

"I found the tumor and the bleeding and was able to remove the cancer," he told Julia. "It will take several days for him to wake up and for us to see how he recovers. We should have a pathology report in a few days."

The ICU nurse tried to get Julia to go home. "We will keep him sedated tonight while he is intubated, at least until tomorrow."

"No," she replied. "I would like to stay with him tonight. His children will be here tomorrow, and I don't want him alone." She stroked his bandaged head.

The next day, Gregory and Mitchell arrived first. Julia went home to shower and rest. When she returned, Caroline was there, holding Joseph's hand.

"Hello Caroline," she tried. "I'm sorry you had to come for this . . ."

Caroline nodded but said nothing. After a few minutes, she got up to leave. "If only he had stayed in New Jersey, where he belonged," was her parting shot.

Gregory apologized. "I'm sorry, Julia. She's just upset."

"It's natural," agreed Mitchell.

Julia just nodded. I'm upset, too, she thought. Bite your tongue, swallow blood. Joseph had always told her how much he appreciated that whenever Caroline was around.

For three endless days, she waited. Watching her husband, hoping for a recovery. Watching his daughter, hoping to avoid an explosion. Watching his sons, hoping for some help. Finally, they all met again with the neurosurgeon.

"The cancer was in the right frontal part of the brain and had started bleeding. I removed all the cancer that I could without damaging the normal brain. This is called maximal debulking surgery. The pathology report showed this cancer was a glioblastoma, an aggressive brain cancer."

"Does that mean you got it all?" asked Caroline. "Will my father be okay?"

"I got all that I could easily remove, but this type of cancer has finger-like growths which extend into the normal brain tissue. I could not remove them without damaging too much of his brain."

"What about the rest? How do we get rid of that?" pressed Caroline.

"Dr. Book will come by tomorrow. She is our neuro-oncologist and will give you more information, but it will be radiation and chemotherapy when he recovers."

Julia was alone in the ICU that night. The unit was quiet, just the sound of the breathing machine, in and out, in and out. Joseph was motionless, his head wrapped in a bandage, a tube in his mouth connecting him to the ventilator, and multiple IV lines. Above him, the display of blood pressure, heart rate, and blood oxygen pulsated. God, I hope you are in there, she thought as she held his now swollen hand.

"Hopefully, he will come out of his coma soon," commented the ICU nurse as she made her rounds.

"Coma? He's in a coma? From the cancer?" asked Julia, surprised. Later she would mark this as the moment which ended her innocence.

"Not from the cancer itself," answered the nurse. "He had bleeding into the cancer, and the blood pressed on the rest of the brain, causing swelling. That will take several more days to go down. Then he will wake up."

The meeting with neuro-oncologist, Dr. Sharon Book, was the next day. She reviewed the events and the treatment plan.

"After this surgery, he should have radiation and a chemotherapy pill called temozolomide. This can all be done as an outpatient. Usually, it is well tolerated. We will begin in a few weeks. After he wakes up and goes home."

TREATMENT OF GLIOBLASTOMA: PART 1.

Surgery is the first treatment for most "solid tumors." Radiation can be used to destroy nearby cancer cells left behind after the operation. Cancer cells elsewhere need to be killed by "systemic therapy," commonly chemotherapy, targeted treatments, or immune therapy.

Glioblastomas multiforme are difficult to remove with surgery. Since the normal glial cells surround and nourish the neurons, glial cancers like glioblastoma intermingle with the neurons. Completely removing all a glioblastoma would also result in the loss of large sections of the normal brain. Neurosurgeons remove as much cancer as possible without producing extra damage, a difficult judgment. If there is time, sophisticated brain mapping techniques may guide the operation. When successful, this surgery is called "maximal debulking."

Since surgery alone rarely cures glioblastomas, radiation is given afterward to attempt to destroy the remaining cancer cells. Unfortunately, glioblastomas are resistant to radiation while the normal brain tissue can tolerate only a relatively low dose. The radiation beam kills cells by slicing their DNA and glioblastomas appear to contain "cancer stem cells" which can efficiently repair DNA and cause the cancer to regrow.[487] The concept that within rapidly growing cancers like glioblastomas there are slower growing stem cells which resist treatment and then regrow the cancer is important. Scientists are working to understand these cells.[488]

Adding chemotherapy to the radiation modestly helps, although the "blood-brain barrier" prevents many chemotherapy drugs from entering the brain. This barrier is a tight seal between the cells of the blood vessels in the brain, designed to keep toxins in the blood out of the brain tissue. The chemotherapy most commonly used is temozolomide, synthesized in England in the 1980s. It was developed in a team effort, combining funding from the British government, university academic work, and clinical testing by a pharmaceutical company. The work was methodical and the "emergence of temozolomide into the clinical spotlight (was) neither a triumph of rational drug design nor (did) it result from any outstanding biological insights. Rather, it (was) the product of a fruitful collaboration between chemists, pharmacologists, pharmacists and clinicians, all of whom served their apprenticeships well."[489] Temozolomide damages the DNA of cancer cells and thus augments the effects of radiation. In the key studies, the use of temozolomide during radiation and then by itself after surgery increased the survival rate from 10 percent to 27 percent at two years.[490] The FDA approved it in 2005.[491] We know that temozolomide works better in cancers which do not repair DNA well, called MGMT methylated cancers (MGMT is the repair gene, methylated means the gene is inactivated). Unfortunately, even in these sensitive cancers, the cancer stem cells can usually repair the damage from temozolomide and keep growing.

As described in the classic textbook *Adams and Victor's Principles of Neurology*, this is "a bleak but vitally important chapter of neurologic medicine."[492]

A few days later, Julia noticed the first sign of Joseph's awakening. The breathing machine had been removed, and the sedatives cut back, but Joseph had remained in his coma.

"Look, he crossed his legs," she pointed out, excitedly.

"So what?" asked Caroline dismissively.

"That's what he does when he's lying in bed," explained Julia, undaunted.

"I never saw that," replied Caroline. "It must be something new. There's a lot of that now." She left the room, indignant.

Julia was right, the crossing of Joseph's legs had been the start. Over the next two days, he opened his eyes, responded to instructions, and eventually smiled and spoke. Two days later he was walking. Before discharged, they met again with the neurosurgeon, Dr. King. Joseph seemed to understand what had happened.

"Thank you for saving me," Joseph told Dr. King, demonstrating his usual politeness.

"You're welcome," answered Dr. King. "You have a good team here."

"Dad will do everything he needs to," announced Caroline. "He's going to beat this."

"Well," replied Dr. King. "I'm sure getting home will be a good start."

Home was a mixed start. In the beginning, the children hovered. After a few days, Gregory left. Julia was sorry to lose him. Mitchell stayed a few days longer. Julia was neutral about his departure. Caroline was the challenge. She spent the days with her father but refused to sleep at their house. Julia hated their tense truce, interrupted by false gaiety when a few local friends or colleagues visited. It was a relief after another week when Caroline left, finally satisfied her father could walk and carry on a conversation.

Except Joseph was not normal. Julia had seen hints, but it was when they were alone that she felt the full impact. Something was missing. If you didn't know him well, you could miss it. He would respond to questions accurately, but not offer answers. He understood, but wouldn't plan. What was in that part of your brain they took out?

A visit from one of Joseph's old medical school friends gave Julia clarity, but not comfort. Frank Levine was also a general surgeon who practiced in rural Maine. Julia fondly remembered her first visit to

Frank and his wife, Sally, at their sprawling farmhouse. It had been early in her marriage to Joseph, and the Levines had warmly welcomed her into their medical fraternity. During the week in the hospital, she had called Frank regularly for his advice.

On this day, Frank sat with his old friend before the three of them ate Chinese food. Frank had remembered it was Julia's favorite, a simple act with value for her fatigued body and ego. After dinner, Joseph needed to sleep, so Frank and Julia sat for coffee.

"What did his doctors say?" Frank asked.

"The neurosurgeon said he got what he could, but there was probably some left behind. The oncologist said he should get radiation and chemo," she replied. After a moment of quiet, she continued.

"How did I miss this? Is there something I should have noticed? He was working and seemed tired, but normal. We were doing everything. I was annoyed with him for not cleaning out the gutters last weekend, all silly stuff."

"You didn't miss anything, Julia," replied Frank.

"You know him as well as anyone. How does he seem to you?"

Frank looked sad, but directly at her.

"Like a person who has lost an important part of his frontal lobe," he began.

ANATOMY OF THE BRAIN: THE FRONTAL LOBE.

During a series of meetings of the French Anthropological Society in 1861, a debate took place between physicians Paul Broca and Ernest Aubertin. Broca had been discussing the relationship between the size of brain and intelligence.[493] Aubertin reported that he and his father-in-law, Jean-Baptiste Boullaud, had localized the speech center to a region in the frontal region of the cerebrum of the brain (the cerebrum, the thinking portion of the brain, is divided into three lobes called the frontal, parietal, and occipital). At the time, this was a radical assertion since the accepted dogma was that the brain functioned as a single unit. Broca had recently met a patient who might counter Aubertin's assertion. "Tan" was a fifty-one-year-old man admitted to the hospital with a severe infection of the right leg which would likely cause his death. The poor fellow was known to have lost his ability to speak at a young age and was only able to say the word tan, hence his name. Broca challenged Aubertin to examine Tan, confirm the findings, and agree that if his theory were correct, they would find a lesion in the frontal region of the man's brain. After Aubertin did his examination and agreed, the obliging Tan died, and Broca conducted the autopsy.[494] The oldest damage to Tan's brain was where Aubertin predicted.[495] Although Broca acknowledged that Aubertin was correct in Tan's case, he did not immediately accept that specific areas of the brain controlled specific functions until he examined many other patients (and their brains). Damage to the region of the frontal lobe that produces a loss of speech is referred to as Broca's aphasia (loss of speech), depriving Aubertin, his father-in-law, and Tan of medical immortality.[496]

In the years since Aubertin's theory, Tan's sacrifice, and Broca's report, many different functions have been localized to specific regions of the brain. Since the brain is symmetric, each region has a similar region on the opposite side. For some functions, the pathways and relationships between the two sides are well described. For example, the motor strip in the back of each side of the frontal lobe controls voluntary movements. The right-side motor strip controls the left side of the body and vice versa. This anatomy explains why a person with damage (like a stroke) to the right motor strip could lose the ability to move the left side of the body. Other processes require the combined activities of multiple areas of the brain, and the relationship between the two opposite sides is complex. Among the most mysterious regions of the brain is the forward part of the frontal lobes, which generations of medical students have learned by studying the unusual case of Mr. Phineas P. Gage.

In a December 13, 1848 letter to the *Boston Medical and Surgical Journal* (today the *New England Journal of Medicine*), Dr. J.M. Harlow of Cavendish, Vermont reported a "very severe, singular, and, so far as the result is taken into account, hitherto unparalleled case, of that class of (brain) injuries, which has recently fallen under my care."[497] Harlow's exuberant prose was needlessly restrained given the standards of his day and the story. His patient was Phineas Gage, a vigorous twenty-five-year-old foreman of a road building crew described as energetic, respectful, and well liked. On September 13, 1848, Gage was tamping blasting powder into a hole when he became distracted. The iron rod he was using struck a rock and caused an explosion which propelled the rod into the left side of Gage's face, up through the left eye, and backward through the left frontal lobe of his brain. The rod weighed just over thirteen pounds, was three and one-half feet long, and the pointed end struck Gage. The poor man is reported to have fallen backward and convulsed but was able to walk with the help of his men. Remarkably, Gage survived his wound, and Harlow's notes detail a fascinating mix of prudent emergency surgical care followed by remarkable recovery despite a post-injury infection and the medical treatments of the day. Harlow concluded the case would be "exceedingly interesting to the enlightened physiologist and intellectual philosopher."

Harlow was correct that Gage would become (medically) famous. Twenty years later, Harlow provided an update on his knowledge of Gage's life after the accident, noting that his patient had changed. "Previous to his injury, though untrained in the schools, he possessed a well-balanced mind, and was looked upon by those who knew him as a shrewd, smart business man, very energetic and persistent in executing all his plans of operation. In this regard, his mind was radically changed, so decidedly that his friends and acquaintances said he was 'no longer Gage.'"[498] The general historical consensus taught to students is that Gage became distracted, irritable, and less responsible, although it is difficult to confirm these impressions. By contacting the family, Harlow obtained Gage's skull, allowing the study of the damage by multiple investigators, including recent images with modern computer reconstructions.[499] The result has been an understanding of the frontal lobe which Mr. Gage's accident has illustrated to thousands of medical students.

The frontal lobe is now understood to be a "new part" of the brain which has evolved to control "executive" functions such as reason, behavior, and abstract thought. Scientists have discovered that different "tracts" (groups of neurons) within the lobe have specific roles within these broad categories. Damage to these tracts, particularly in the front part of the frontal lobe may lead to a variety of symptoms ranging from apathy to aggressive disinhibition to the appearance of primitive behaviors, called "frontal lobe release." Famous neurologist Oliver Sack's description of a man who killed his girlfriend while under the influence of PCP illustrates the complexity of the frontal lobe. The man had repressed the memory of the murder until he had a frontal lobe injury in an accident. The man's frontal lobe release unleashed vivid memories which prompted a suicide attempt.[500] Modern studies of Phineas Gages' injury have shown that it damaged an "extended network of areas that are commonly activated during the performance of decision-making, emotion processing, and reward tasks."[501]

The front of the frontal lobe helps makes us . . . us.

"I always hated that term executive function," continued Frank. "But I guess it is as good as any. Joseph has damage to the part of the brain that gives a person drive and organization, the will to succeed. He won't be the same. He seems to be that gentle man we all loved, but the punch he also carried is gone."

"Will it come back?" asked Julia, crying.

"No," said Frank. "That much damage cannot be repaired."

"What will happen to him?"

"The truth is that the radiation and chemo will hold it off for about a year, give or take a few months. Then it will be back. It always is with glioblastomas."

"Is there anything else we can do?"

"They are trying many new approaches, but nothing is much good yet."

"What do I do?"

"The best you can. I know it won't be easy."

Explaining what had happened to Joseph wasn't going to be easy either, but Julia wanted to try before the children returned. Frank agreed to help, and the three of them had breakfast on the porch, their favorite spot.

Frank had summarized the events. "You're pretty lucky that Julia moved as quickly as she did," he said. "You certainly owe her one." Joseph laughed and held her hand.

"Everything I remember about glioblastomas is bad," Joseph said.

"It still is, my friend," answered Frank. "I wish the news was better, but at least the surgeon was able to remove the bulk of the tumor. Hopefully, the radiation and chemo can hold off the rest."

Joseph thought for a minute. "I'm glad we had sausage and eggs for breakfast. I think I'll skip the vitamins. Sounds like I won't be needing them."

Frank spent the rest of the day with his friend, allowing Julia to run errands. When Frank left late that afternoon, Julia walked him to his car.

"He's quite a guy," Frank said as they parted. "You know, he wanted to see his MRI, so we loaded it on the computer, and I showed him. He looked at his own brain with that big hole in it. And you know what he said?"

Julia shook her.

"It's amazing how little you use as a doctor." Frank laughed ruefully. "Even in medical school he was like that, dry and ironic. I'm glad he still has that."

"Please come back soon," Julia pleaded.

"I will. He made me promise to come back. Said he needed me to help drink all his good wine."

The meeting the next week with Dr. King was brief, the neurosurgeon's office quiet. Dr. Book's appointment was a different matter. Her crowded office contained obviously sick people, many disabled, bald, and with swollen faces. Some were in wheelchairs. As they chatted and laughed, Gregory, Mitchell, and Caroline looked unconcerned, oblivious to Julia's growing horror as she imagined Joseph in that state. Dr. Book was about an hour late, but it was hard to fault her given the patients. She was pleased with Joseph's neurologic exam.

"You seem to be doing very well," she commented.

"He is," answered Caroline. "We have our Dad back; now we want to cure him."

Dr. Book outlined the plan for radiation and the oral chemotherapy. Caroline had a list of questions: Avastin? Gene therapy? Vaccines? Duke? Mass General? Dr. Book patiently answered each as Joseph drifted off and Julia felt helpless. Finally, Caroline reached the Optune device, a cap worn by patients which produced alternating electrical fields to help control the cancer.

"The cap is fairly controversial," explained Dr. Book. "It fits on your head, which must be kept shaved. It is worn all day except for an hour or two and produces an electrical current which is supposed to disrupt the cancer cells. The studies are debated, and it is a great deal of work, so we usually reserve it for later. But you could use it after the radiation."

Joseph looked up. "I don't want to wear that."

"But Daddy, it might help fight the cancer," pleaded Caroline.

Joseph turned to her and said gently. "No, honey. I won't wear it. Not that thing."

Thank God, thought Julia.

The daily radiation treatments made Joseph tired and the pills nauseous, but it was livable. Julia drove him most days, a few friends occasionally substituted. Frank and Sally visited for a week and were a great help with organizing life.

"What are you going to do about work?" Frank asked as they sat on the porch, sipping one of Joseph's best wines.

"I'm not sure. We don't need the money, but I don't like quitting," answered Joseph. Frank recognized his friend's difficulty making the decision.

"I think you should pack it in," replied Frank. "Spend your time with this beautiful woman." He gestured to Julia.

Joseph nodded. "Okay." He paused. "Can I cancel my colonoscopy, too?"

Frank laughed. "Yeah, pack that in, too. And come visit us in Maine."

The radiation finished near the end of 2016. The chemotherapy continued with pills for five days each month. Since they produced only modest nausea, spring and summer that year brought a taste of something resembling normalcy. Each morning, Joseph and Julia had breakfast together and walked the garden. They filled their days with events in town or nothing at all. A June visit to Maine was wonderful, two weeks during which Julia almost forgot about glioblastoma. The children had calmed down. Gregory and Mitchell called regularly and made occasional short, pleasant visits. Caroline was less predictable, and Julia still found her calls intrusive and visits tormenting. In late summer, she announced her first pregnancy to Joseph, while barely accepting Julia's congratulations. Most importantly, although Joseph was still not quite himself, he was kind and funny. Life was good.

Almost to the year, the headaches started. At first, they would go away with one or two ibuprofens; soon it took more. Getting up in the morning became harder, breakfast later, and walks shorter. Then Joseph's memory worsened. Within two weeks he had lost interest in everything. Julia remembered Frank's words. One year is over, she thought. As she sat with Joseph in the exam room after an MRI, part of her hoped Dr. King was delayed. Maybe he'll be called to an emergency, she thought. If he doesn't come, then I can't get the news I know is coming. She looked at Joseph who sat quietly, his damaged brain evidently unperturbed.

"The MRI shows the cancer has regrown in the area it was before," Dr. King reported.

"What now?" asked Julia.

"More surgery is possible. I can remove the area," he answered.

Caroline was furious. "I knew he should have worn the Optune," she snapped when they had all gathered again. Joseph was sleeping, and his children and Julia sat in their living room.

"It was his choice, Caroline," answered Gregory. "You heard him."

"But why? Why wouldn't he? It makes no sense," she continued. "He'll never know his grandchildren now." For a minute, seeing her pregnancy and distress, Julia felt pity.

"I want him to go to Boston. To Dana Farber," she announced, as astonishment replaced Julia's pity. "They will help him there."

"Sure," agreed Mitchell. "That's a good idea."

Maybe for you, thought Julia, but not for Joseph. And not for me. Who is going to get him there? Manage all his things? Bite your tongue, she thought. Swallow more blood. Remember, he appreciated that.

Somehow, she did it. When they entered the Brigham and Women's Hospital, Julia was struck by its speed and energy. Joseph looked around, but without the interest she knew he should have felt. The neurosurgical chief, Dr. Gray, was a dignified man in his early sixties.

"I understand you were a general surgeon," he addressed Joseph.

"Not for many years, now," Joseph replied. "I was . . . something happened."

"Your allergy, Daddy," interrupted Caroline. "He had a latex allergy."

After completing his examination, Dr. Gray addressed them all.

"The cancer has grown back near the edges of where it was removed," he pointed to the MRI. While Julia felt dismayed seeing the hole in his brain, the children seemed unconcerned. "I will need to remove this area to remove this growth." Dr. Gray pointed to the scan.

"Will he be himself afterward?" asked Julia. Joseph gazed at her, smiling sadly.

"He will lose some more function," he replied. "We cannot help that. We will try to minimize it. Without surgery, he will also continue to lose function as the cancer grows."

"What are the other choices?" asked Julia calmly.

"Some people do opt for comfort care only, hospice."

Caroline would hear none of it. On a phone call to her husband later, she made no effort to keep her voice down, not caring that Julia heard her words.

"I can't understand what he ever saw in her. She's a soulless bitch."

Julia had her own phone call with Frank.

"It's what was special about him I'm afraid for," she told him. "How do we know what we are doing to him is right? How do we know more surgery is better? His daughter says I'm a soulless bitch, but what about his soul? Are we destroying that?"

FINDING THE SOUL.

On March 11, 1907, the *New York Times* reported that Dr. Ducan Macdougall, "a reputable physician of Haverhill," had measured the weight of the soul at between one-half and a full ounce. Macdougall had placed six dying patients on a specially constructed scale. In five of the patients, the weight of the body diminished at exactly the time of death. In one man (the third tested), there was a short delay in the loss of weight, attributed to the poor fellow being "a phlegmatic man slow of thought and action."[502] Since three-quarters of an ounce are twenty-one grams, this metric determination of the weight of the soul has appeared in several references, including a film of the same name. In modern times, Macdougall's attempt to scientifically measure such a historically elusive concept was repeatedly debunked. During his own life, is not clear how much credence was given to his discovery— the *Times* report appeared above two other articles: one noting the celebration of the one-hundred-twenty-fifth-anniversary of the birth of

Irish rebel Robert Emmett, and the second announcing a night school for butchers.

Macdougall has not been alone in his quest to measure and define the soul. In ancient Egypt, the heart recorded the essence of life. After death, the organ was weighed, and a heavy heart filled with sin would not be allowed into the afterlife, but rather consumed by Ammit, a part lion, hippopotamus, and crocodile monster.[503] Hebrew scholars variously located the soul in the nose or abdomen.[504] Plato (428–348 BCE) split the soul into three parts, the intellectual soul in the head, the sensitive part in the chest, and the vegetative part in the liver. His student Aristotle (384–322 BCE) placed the location in the warm heart rather than the cold brain. Other ancient Greeks began the transition of the anatomic location of the soul to the brain, including famous anatomists Herophilus and Erasistratus (circa 290 BCE) of the Alexandria Medical School.[505] The Roman physician Galen confirmed this belief, probably in part because of his experience with the destruction of the nervous system as surgeon to the gladiators (130–200). In the repressive medieval ages controlled by the Church, St. Augustine (354–430) proclaimed the location of the soul was in the ventricles of the brain, the hollow spaces filled with fluid.[506] The Renaissance saw Leonardo da Vinci (1452–1519) produce detailed drawings of the human body, including the brain, which also localized the soul to the ventricles. The father of modern philosophy Renee Descartes (1596–1650) concluded the pineal gland, a small nut shaped organ in the center of the brain, was the source.[507] These attempts to localize the soul were confounded by a lack of understanding of anatomy and brain function. The microscopic descriptions of neurons by Czech anatomist Johann Evangelist Purkinje (1787–1869) and the work of Paul Broca (1824–1880) in localizing the speech area began our modern age of understanding of the brain and thought.

When Macdougall weighed the souls of his dying patients, the consensus among *Times* readers almost certainly would have been that the soul was distinct from the body and thus his experiment was not completely irrational. This belief derived from Western religious experience and thinkers like Descartes who asserted the working of the mind is separate from the body. This concept is often referred to as mind-body dualism, recognizing that mind and soul have been used somewhat interchangeably. In 1949, philosopher Gilbert Ryle ridiculed this notion of a separate soul, describing it with his famous phrase "a ghost in the machine," picked up in the 1960s by controversial essayist Arthur Koestler in a book of the same name and musically by the Police in their 1981 album. This debate over the existence, substance, and location of the soul as well as the nature of the mind has continued even as molecular science has brought a better understanding of the anatomy, cellular and genetic structure, and organization of the nervous system. We now believe there are approximately eighty-six billion neurons in the human brain, making an extraordinary number of connections. Do thought and the soul require a certain number?

"I don't know" replied Frank. "We used to talk about this kind of thing in medical school and residency. Joseph always had the final answer. 'It's good to be a general surgeon,' he would say. 'We just worry about the plumbing. Remember that even the best philosophers need their bowels to function.' I loved his irony." He sounded wistful.

"But you probably have no choice," Frank continued. "You need to push on for the children. I do not think they will accept the death of their father without another try. I'm sure Joseph would do that, too. He would often say that we sometimes treat people to benefit the survivors. It might be different if it were just you two alone."

The second surgery was both familiar and different. This time it was elective, and since Joseph had not had bleeding and compression of his brain, the recovery was quicker. Dr. Gray seemed pleased that his deficits were not much worse. As Julia wheeled Joseph out of the hospital, she overheard Caroline pointedly comment how good her father looked.

During the year after the first surgery, Julia had moments when she could convince herself life was almost normal. Not now. When Frank and Sally visited, she shared her concerns.

"He's not here," she said. "It's still his voice, still his answers to questions, but it's not him."

To Sally, Julia privately added more.

"The first time, although he lost interest in sex, sometimes it would come back. It was never like before, but that was okay because I knew he still loved me. Now, I'm not sure. He says yes if I ask him if he loves me, but everything else is gone," she cried.

Sally put her arm around her, not sure what to say.

"I just want him to say he loves me without me asking, like he would before. It's just a little thing . . ."

For her part, Caroline wanted more time.

TREATMENT OF GLIOBLASTOMA: PART 2.

As bleak as the reputation of glioblastoma multiforme has been, advances in this vital work are ongoing. The classification system originally developed by Harvey Cushing and Percival Bailey has been modified to include modern molecular understanding, and new treatment strategies have emerged.[508] Targeting specific pathways associated with the DNA mutations found in glioblastomas is one approach, but unfortunately, there is no single dominant abnormality such as seen in cancers like CML (chronic myelogenous leukemia). Glioblastomas have many different abnormalities. Finding and targeting the glioblastoma stem cells is another approach, also very challenging. The immune treatment used in lung and other cancers, as well as vaccines are under study. While the brain had long been considered a site of relatively little immune activity, some reports suggest this strategy may be possible. Many patients receive antibodies to block the growth of new blood vessels which feed the cancers.

An interesting approach to the treatment of glioblastoma multiforme is the use of "tumor-treating electric fields," a strategy based on the electrical conductivity of the body. Electrical impulses which produce muscle or nerve activity in the body are well known, but there are also small electrical fields within cells. These electrical fields allow polar molecules (named because they have a charge) to enter, leave, or move within the cell and contribute to important cellular activities. In the lab, applying alternating electrical currents of the proper frequency to cancer cells disrupts activities, including cell division. Placing electrodes on humans with brain cancer slowed the cancerous growth.[509] In 2015, investigators in Switzerland reported a study in which patients with glioblastomas who had undergone surgery followed by radiation and temozolomide had either more temozolomide alone or also wore an electric field device. The patients assigned to the device wore the electrodes attached to their shaved scalps continuously, interrupted only for short breaks for "personal needs." Wearing the device produced almost no medical side effects and patients lived longer (twenty-one versus sixteen months).[510]

Treating glioblastomas with electrical currents has been controversial. The method of action is not well understood, raising doubts about the concept among some physicians. There are scientific criticisms of the trial, particularly because everyone knew who was wearing the device. This type of problem in clinical trials can lead those who are getting the treatment to feel better and push on longer, a variation of the placebo effect.[511] Despite these concerns, the device was approved by the FDA for progressing glioblastoma in 2011 and as initial treatment in 2015.[512] Further work will go on.

Even as science produces more effective treatments for glioblastomas, patients and their families will continue to struggle with the damage already done. It is not clear how that problem will ever be solved.

Wearing the Optune headpiece for twenty-two hours a day was irritating to his scalp, but nothing much bothered Joseph anymore. For Julia, it was upsetting. She knew him as a proud, private man. The cap meant they could not leave the house without attracting stares. Dr. Book had been ambivalent about using it, but Caroline had pushed her into admitting it might help. An MRI four months later showed worsening of the cancer.

Caroline still wanted more. In front of Gregory and Mitchell, she challenged Joseph and Julia. She had called Dana Farber and found a clinical trial for him.

"You can't give up, Daddy. Don't you want to see your grandchild? Please. Let's make another trip to Boston."

Joseph had nodded. "Okay, honey . . . whatever you say."

"It was a trap," Julia explained later to Frank and Sally. "She knew he would agree with her. He agrees with anything now. He's not himself. He would never have wanted to live like this."

"It's hard to get everyone to agree to the right limits, particularly when the patient can't make the decision," agreed Frank. "It's something we all struggle with."

"This is my limit," said Julia. "I will bring him to Boston one more time to try their clinical trial. Then he comes home. If there is something we can do here, fine. If not, that's it. I won't see him dragged around the country. I am his wife and health care proxy. If Caroline doesn't like it, too bad."

Julia found the trip difficult. The physical aspects of the journey were burdensome since Joseph could walk only short distances. A greater challenge was in her mind. They had visited Boston several times before his illness and Julia found herself haunted by her memories of his jokes as they paddled on the pond in the Commons and walked the Paul Revere trail. Their eyes might both see the same thing, but only her mind recalled what they thought of it, how it had struck them as funny or sad or ironic. The dirty April sky over the Charles River only made it worse.

Inside the Dana Farber, it was bright and the atmosphere serious but determinedly hopeful. Dr. Quinn, the neuro-oncologist, was generous with his time, explaining the purpose of the study was to determine whether blocking something called the "epidermal growth factor receptor" would shrink the cancer. Joseph would receive a weekly one-hour infusion of an antibody. Gregory accompanied them to the visit. Caroline, now almost to her due date, attended on Skype. They signed the formidable paperwork listing all the possible side effects and made an appointment to begin in two weeks.

Returning home to Saratoga Springs was also sad. Joseph was physically tired, not wanting to do anything beyond eating and sitting on the porch. One afternoon as he napped, Julia had washed his clothes and was putting them away when she opened his closet. Lined up were all his suits, neatly pressed. They smelled of him. She remembered how good he looked in them, so like a doctor. He'll never wear them again, she thought. The tears came with the next thoughts. They won't fit his sons. What will I do with them when he dies? As she sat in the closet and cried, she was so alone.

Gregory came with them to Dana Farber for the first infusion. Thank God, she thought, I don't want to be alone. As soon as they began the medication, Joseph's face turned red, his breathing became short, and his blood pressure dropped. The terrified look in his eyes said it all.

"We can try altering his medications," mused Dr. Quinn after Joseph had recovered. "Although that was a pretty serious reaction."

"No," answered Julia. "We are done." She turned to Gregory. "You need to explain this to Caroline so she understands. We will not put him through this again." He agreed.

Dr. Quinn and Dr. Book conferred and recommended the drug bevacizumab, an antibody designed to help stop the growth of blood vessels feeding the cancer.

"He can get it every three weeks with Dr. Matthews in Saratoga," reported Dr. Book. "It usually has very few side effects."

That was four months ago. Every three weeks, Julia brought Joseph to the office for the infusion. As advertised, it had very few side effects. Shortly after the first infusion, Caroline gave birth to her baby boy, also named Joseph. Julia had driven her husband to New Jersey for a visit and watched as he held his grandson.

"He looks like you, Daddy," gushed Caroline. "And I see some of Mom in him, too."

Joseph smiled. Julia swallowed more blood.

Over the next three months, Joseph's decline was steady. Julia saw it at home. Mornings stretched into lunch hour. Dinner and bedtime came earlier. The television was on endlessly, as the back and forth between President Trump and his haters reached a fevered pitch which drove Julia to distraction. Joseph watched unimpressed. Eventually, she realized he did not even understand.

Tracy Callahan, the Nurse Practitioner, had also noticed the change.

"Do you want to keep bringing him here to do this?" she asked Julia a month ago as Joseph slept in the lounge chair and received the infusion.

Julia looked surprised. "I don't know. I guess I'm doing it out of routine . . . and fear." She explained about the children. "I'm not sure what else to do."

Tracy answered. "It is time for hospice."

HOSPICE AND PALLIATIVE CARE.
In 1948, a forty-year-old man named David Tamsa was dying of cancer in Archway Hospital in London. A Jewish refugee from the Warsaw

Ghetto, Mr. Tamsa's life had been bleak. Yet this young man made a tremendous contribution by establishing a friendship with a social worker on the ward, Cicely Saunders. The two discussed the idea of a dedicated place for the end of life. Mr. Tasma left Ms. Saunders his modest savings and the thought that he would be "a window in your home." Through his death and her subsequent life, hospice was born.[513]

After the conclusion of World War II, the focus of modern medicine was on cure. The next two decades combined scientific optimism with new antibiotics, advanced surgeries, and chemotherapies. As the limits of modern science and medicine became apparent, they were often difficult for practitioners to acknowledge. This was particularly true in end-of-life care. Patients with terminal illnesses were often admitted to hospitals for pointless testing and aggressive treatments or cared for at home with little support. Pain control and other symptom management measures were not well understood. Perhaps most importantly, death was a failure and not to be discussed with patients. Medical school textbooks of the time admonished against end-of-life conversations, reporting they would cause loss of hope.

Cicely Saunders' experience with David Tasma's death, combined with the loss of her father and a religious conversion, gave her own life its mission to comfort the dying. After being advised that she would best achieve her goals as a physician, Saunders graduated from medical school at St. Thomas' Hospital in her late thirties and immediately began her work. In the late 1950s, she started planning for a dedicated facility and, after almost a decade, opened St. Christopher's Hospice in London in 1967. The practical aspects of her program included aggressive management of physical pain using regular doses of oral morphine, a revolutionary concept at the time. Many physicians believed narcotics would produce tolerance and addiction, failing to recognize the difference in their use at the end of life. Another radical concept was to study medications in dying patients. St. Christopher's originally used heroin to control pain, but demonstrated in a randomized study that morphine was equally effective.[514] Saunders and her colleagues also studied depression, spiritual and social needs, bereavement, grief, and home care. In addition to her immensely important specific contributions, Saunders articulated a broad vision of end-of-life care which laid the foundation for the modern hospice movement. She was beloved and highly decorated for her work. Her early research fellow and colleague Dr. Robert Twycross summarized her beliefs in a tribute at her death in 2005 by noting that, "she conveyed a message to those she cared for: 'You matter because you are you, and you matter to the end of your life. We will do all we can not only to help you die peacefully, but also to live until you die.' "[515]

Saunders shared her vision with partners across the world. Florence Wald, the Dean of the Yale School of Nursing, invited Saunders to lecture. Profoundly impressed, Wald visited and worked at St. Christopher's before forming a group in 1971 to develop an American version called Connecticut Hospice. The philosophy of Wald's organization resembled St. Christopher's in its humanity, yet had differences in areas of nursing control (more), patient privacy and autonomy (more), and religious overtones (less) which gave it an American style. A critically important difference was the Americans' decision to start with outpatient care while attempting to integrate hospice into the complex health care system, rather than remain independent as St. Christopher's had done. Navigating state and federal regulations was a formidable undertaking, and it took until 1978 to secure licensing for the Connecticut Hospice inpatient program. Then came the even more arduous national legislative process of obtaining hospice benefits recognized by insurers, including Medicare in the mid-1980s. The political and legislative ordeal was bewildering, yet by 1993 in the United States, hospice was "an accepted part of the health care continuum."[516] By 1998, there were three thousand hospice programs in the United States,[517] a number that had risen to six thousand one hundred in 2104. The most common places of hospice care are the home (36 percent), followed by a hospice facility (32 percent), nursing home (15 percent), residential facility (9 percent), or hospital (9 percent).[518]

Their broad range of services included specialized nursing care, pain and symptom management, psychosocial and spiritual support, supplies, and bereavement counseling.

Discussions of the end of life, such as those by psychiatrist Dr. Elizabeth Kubler-Ross's 1969 book *On Death and Dying*, aided public acceptance of hospice. Based on over five hundred interviews of dying people, Dr. Ross outlined stages of dealing with death and stimulated a public dialogue on dying. Dr. Ross lectured, testified in numerous meetings, and educated physicians.[519] These discussions altered the physician-patient relationship as it related to death, particularly the notion of not providing patients with information. As Florence Wald noted, the hospice movement developed "in the 1960s, when the idea of questioning authority was everywhere, including the authority of physicians. This led to an opening up of the roles physician and patient played."[520]

Despite the growth of hospice care, integration into the medical systems in the United States and England has been incomplete. From the start, payments to hospice were low compared with high-technology care while regulatory hurdles have been formidable.[521] Physicians and hospitals have often been reluctant to give up authority. Hospice work is specialized, hard, and emotionally draining. Most importantly for patients, benefits are often only available for the last six months of life. In addition, patients must forego intensive treatment which, in the words of Florence Ward, "cut right through the principle that hospice care should be an alternative available to the patient from the beginning of the illness and throughout."[522] For many patients with cancer, this means treatment with surgery, chemotherapy, and radiation continues even when the benefits are unclear. When treatment becomes obviously futile, the patient enters hospice care in a drastic break, usually with death in sight. Patients, families, and providers almost universally regard hospice programs as wonderful, but dread this abrupt transition.

"Palliative care" programs have attempted to address these issues by promoting the concept of palliative care along the continuum of serious illness and exploring different financing methods and structures. In the public arena, palliative care organizations have taken an active role in the political, payment, and regulatory discussions regarding end-of-life care. In hospitals, these programs often serve patients as they undergo the most technological and costly care, including in ICU settings. They have helped promote education and quality-of-life research, including certification of physicians and programs. From a practical standpoint, the challenge remains to blend these programs, which often have an inpatient hospital focus, with largely outpatient hospice programs. A myriad of details remains to be solved to incorporate palliative and hospice care together into the medical system.[523] As these programs become more institutionalized, palliative care also confronts the philosophic challenge posed by Dr. Twycross in his tribute to Cicely Saunders.

> "The question for us today is: Is palliative care in danger of moving from the creative and disruptive influence of charisma to the cosy ambience of routinization? I hope not.
>
> Palliative care services, even in Britain, generally have not yet reached their full holistic potential. But movements tend to become monuments. So the best tribute we can give to Cicely is to make sure that hospice, that palliative care, remains a movement with momentum, and maintains an ongoing creative tension between charisma and routinization."[524]

Modern molecular treatments for cancer have added to the challenge of providing palliative and hospice care by further blurring the transition between aggressive therapy and end-of-life care. Many of these treatments have much less toxicity than traditional chemotherapy. For individual patients, it often takes considerable time to determine whether they are effective and the testing results are often difficult to interpret. Control of the cancer may be the result. The traditional transition from active treatment to hospice care becomes even more difficult as patients and families do not wish to stop a relatively non-toxic treatment. The tremendous cost of these treatments means they cannot be in a hospice budget. For patients with advanced cancers, the era of molecular science means it is more important than ever that palliative care and hospice is available while these treatments are still ongoing, another challenge.

Regardless of the technology and organizational challenges, the enduring goals for palliative and hospice care remain those recorded in the memorial for Cicely Saunders by her colleague Dr. Sam Klagsbrun, when he quoted her own words:

> "I have tried to sum up the demands of this work . . . in the words 'Watch with me.' Our most important foundation for St Christopher's is the hope that in watching, we should learn not only how to free patients from pain and distress, how to understand them and never let them down . . . but also how to be silent, how to listen and how to just be there."[525]

At the hospice intake meeting, Joan had listened carefully to Julia's story.

"I understand," she answered. "I think we can help you to keep your husband at home. We have some good people who can meet with his children and hopefully help them to understand as well."

When Dr. Matthews met with the family, even Caroline agreed it was time to stop the treatments. Once the medical facts were accepted, the social worker, chaplain, and Joan each took their turns. The details of death needed organization, their patient comforted, and the survivors supported.

Tracy had summed it up. "As best you can, you need to celebrate his life and comfort him."

Today, Julia and Dr. Matthews sat quietly together for a few minutes.

"Is there anything else we can do?" asked Dr. Matthews, breaking the silence.

"No. The hospice nurse says it won't be too much longer. His sons are both there all the time. His daughter and her husband are staying in a hotel with the baby. Even she seems okay. She was actually almost nice to me this week."

"You did a good job with them," replied Dr. Matthews. "I know it wasn't easy."

"Thank you." She stood up to leave. "You know, after he dies, I'll never see them again. What will I do with all these memories?"

For that, there was no answer.

3:20 Glen Waters: Lymphoma

Glen Waters, a handsome sixty-eight-year-old man, was seated in a chair with his crutches nearby.

"I feel good, really no complaints," he announced, raising himself slowly from the chair to the exam table. He moved smoothly despite his disability.

"Any changes I should know about?" asked Dr. Matthews as he examined him, paying close attention to his lymph nodes.

"Nothing with me," he paused and looked reflective. "Just my mother . . ."

It was in October 2001 that the pick-up truck hit Glen Waters from behind, never even slowing for the red light. At least, that's what they told him.

"I remember leaving for work that morning. One minute I was probably sitting in the car, sipping coffee at the red light and listening to Gershwin. The next thing I know, I am in the ICU at Albany Med, tubes everywhere. I don't remember anything, the firemen, helicopter ride, none of it."

Glen had a ruptured spleen and multiple fractures, including ribs, right arm near the shoulder, both legs, and spine. Surgeons removed his spleen, pinned and set his bones, and watched his bruised kidneys and liver heal.

"It was my version of the Twin Towers. An ordinary day which changed everything," he recalled.

Glen had rebuilt what he could. In months of rehab, he learned to stand again and to walk short distances with crutches. He could lift his right arm, almost to his head. It was enough to do activities of daily living, but not to work. Not as the conductor of the regional orchestra, where he was in his prime at fifty-two.

Glen learned some other things, too. He had always loved his wife, Diane, but had not always remembered how much. Months of her nursing had reprised the refrain they had used when the children were young, "more than the sun and the moon." He learned more about music, too. He had always loved it, but now it sustained him through the pain and the work of recovery.

There was one more thing Glen learned. When the trauma surgeons had his abdomen open to remove his spleen and stop the bleeding, they noticed some swollen lymph glands. Several had ended up under the microscope in the pathology lab.

"You have a low-grade lymphoma," reported Dr. Matthews after Glen had recovered enough to hear the news. "This is a cancer of the lymph cells and is widespread throughout your body. The good news is that they generally grow very slowly and sometimes even shrink on their own. We do not treat them unless they grow rapidly or start to bother you in some way. The treatments are chemotherapy, but are usually mild. The bad news is that we cannot get rid of them completely without very intensive chemotherapy and a bone marrow or stem cell transplant from another person, something we would prefer not to do. So, we will be likely managing this for a long time."

"Considering everything else, that doesn't sound so bad," answered Glen.

"At some point, you will likely need some treatment. Only time will tell. We never really know the future with these lymphomas," concluded Dr. Matthews.

"Well," replied Glen, "none of us really know our future. We sure learned that this year."

CLASSIFYING LYMPHOMAS.

Lymphomas are cancers of the lymphocytes, among the most complex and mysterious cells of the body. In the broadest sense, lymphocytes are the police officers of the immune system, patrolling for outsiders. There are a variety of lymphocytes: B-cells which make antibodies, T-cells which regulate the immune system, killer cells which attack invaders, and subtypes of each. These various lymphocytes can be found circulating in the lymph nodes, blood, or the tissues. Since any of these lymphocytes can turn cancerous, there are a bewildering array of different lymphomas with complex names which are often incomprehensible to patients and most physicians. To make the classification even more confusing, some lymphomas appear primarily in the blood and are grouped with leukemia. The first description of a lymphoma is often credited to Thomas Hodgkin in 1832 when he wrote his famous paper, "On Some Morbid Appearances of the Absorbant Glands and Spleen."[526] Hodgkin's work lay buried in the archives of Guy's Hospital in London until brought to attention by Samuel Wilks in the 1860s. It then took another hundred years until the development of a rational classification system of lymphomas.

What took so long? Why are lymphomas so hard to understand? Physicians like Hodgkin and Wilks working in the mid-nineteenth century faced several challenges. Most of the enlarged lymph nodes they examined resulted from infections like tuberculosis or syphilis rather than lymphoma. In their era, diagnoses were made by "gross" examination of the tissue using touch and visual inspection. It was not until the second half of the nineteenth century that the microscope became widely used. Even with the microscope, lymph cells were hard to identify until proper stains were invented. For example, it took until about 1900 that the "Reed-Sternberg cell," the hallmark of Hodgkin's lymphoma, was described by Dorothy Reed and Carl Sternberg. Dr. Reed deserves a special note since, in addition to the complexity of lymphoma, she faced the challenge of being a brilliant woman in a man's world. Born in Columbus, Ohio in 1874, she studied chemistry and physics at Massachusetts Institute of Technology, graduated from Smith College and Johns Hopkins University School of Medicine. After making her enduring description of Hodgkin's disease, Reed experienced the longstanding struggle of the woman physician balancing work and family life, facing criticism from several now forgotten male colleagues about her productivity. Despite this environment, Reed continued her career and made many important additional contributions to women's health.[527]

Nineteenth century physicians of both sexes studying lymphoma faced another problem: no one really understood cellular biology or cancer. "Morbid growth" is probably the term which best characterizes their understanding of cancer. One visionary who provided a modern description of cancer in 1838 was the German scientist Johannes Muller. He was an early adopter of the microscope who noted that cancers are cells which resemble the tissues from which they arise.[528] Muller's definition was not immediately embraced. An example of the extant confusion is the reporting of the first cases of leukemia (cancers of the white blood cells) in the 1840s by Dr. John Hughes Bennet in Edinburgh, Dr. Rudolph Virchow in Berlin, and French physician Alfred Donne.[529] Regardless of which of this trio is credited, their descriptions focused on the very basic idea the disease was accompanied by excess white blood cells with little consensus as to their significance.[530] Virchow, a prominent German physician and Muller's student, later advanced key concepts about morbid growths in his book *Cellular Pathology*, a medical classic which gained him fame as "Hippocrates with the microscope." Yet even Virchow had significant misunderstandings, such as believing that all cancers started from connective tissue.[531] The modern understanding that cancers result from uncontrolled cellular growth did not develop until well into the twentieth century.

The classification of lymphomas began with Hodgkin's lymphoma, resulting in the grouping of all the others as non-Hodgkin lymphoma (NHL). It soon became evident that the NHLs are very diverse and difficult to subclassify, a problem reflected in the bewildering names from the early twentieth century such as lymphosarcoma, pseudoleu-kaemia, and reticulum-cell sarcoma. Beginning in the 1950s, patholo-gists developed complex systems for classifying NHL based on their cellular origins. Although these systems were a first step, they guide treatment. As the successful use of chemotherapy began in the 1960s and 1970s, both physicians and patients were often left wondering "what will happen and what do I need to do?"

For treating physicians and patients, the 1980s brought a use-ful classification of NHL called the Working Formulation, the name reflecting its development by clinicians and pathologists.[532] Although soon replaced, the system's concepts remain a useful way for the non-specialist to think about lymphomas and are often still used to com-municate with patients. The Working Formulation divided NHL into three groups: high-grade, intermediate, and low-grade. The "high-grade lymphomas" were very rapidly growing and fatal within days or weeks unless treated. These patients were usually very sick and needed intensive chemotherapy given in the hospital, but occasionally could be cured. The "intermediate-grade lymphomas" were quickly grow-ing, fatal within weeks or months without treatment. Patients could be either sick or well, needed outpatient chemotherapy, and were often cured. "Low-grade lymphomas" were (and still are) the most mysteri-ous. Patients were usually not ill and might even have a long history of lymph nodes which had swollen and then shrunk. Chemotherapy could control low-grade lymphomas, but rarely produced cures. Lymphomas were also classified as beginning from B-cells (the antibody producing cells) or T-cells (controlling cells raised in the thymus). The B-cell lymphomas are much more common, while the T-cells lymphomas are both less frequent and predictable. The Working Formulation group-ing gave patients and treating physicians an idea what to expect.

Modern classifications of lymphoma use the concept of "clini-cal-pathologic-molecular" subtyping to form groups. This approach relies on the appearance of the cells under the microscope, special stains, flow cytometry to examine cell surface proteins, chromosomal studies, and molecular genetic analysis. The classifications allow the division of NHL into many different groups which have specific behaviors and treatments. As new technologies and treatments emerge, the groupings change. The same patient in the 1980s who had an "intermediate-grade large cell lymphoma" might today be diagnosed with a "double-hit diffuse large B-cell lymphoma with *c-MYC* and *BLC-2* translocation," resulting in treatment based on the molecular findings. While this subtyping can help select specific treatments, for patients the vocabulary may seem as confusing as the descriptions of the 1800s. The questions answered by the Working Formulation still resonate: "what will happen without treatment and what do I need to do?"

After the accident came Glen's realization that he would no longer conduct, something he had done since ninth grade. He had long loved the combination of music and physicality brought together in the conductor. In his high school, the football and hockey players were the premier athletes and the coddled playboys of adolescence. As he watched from behind his piano, he had always been a little jealous of their prowess and power. Then one day in orchestra old Mr. Snead had challenged the football team's offensive line to stand behind him and pretend to conduct Tchaikovsky's *1812 Overture*. When the almost fifteen minutes had ended and the recorded cannons fired, only one lineman had finished, his heavy arms quivering. As he saw the gray-haired teacher hold out his own hands rock steady despite the exertion, Glen knew he wanted to lead an orchestra. Mr. Snead was not easy. It had taken two years of practice before he was even allowed to rehearse. He would never forget his first performance as senior when he conducted his classmates in Tchaikovsky's *Marche Slave*.

With his body shattered and conducting impossible, Glen felt himself sinking into depression. His wife hoped music would rescue him. He had always done some arranging. At her urging, he began composing and teaching, uncertain where it would lead.

THE COMPLEXITIES OF LOW-GRADE LYMPHOMAS.
Low-grade lymphomas are mysterious. Patients are usually not ill. Their lymph nodes may swell then shrink without causing other symptoms and are often found by accident. Even when untreated, these lymphomas can occasionally "spontaneously regress" (vanish) for periods of time. Under the microscope, the cells appear as nearly normal small lymphocytes, often forming patterns seen in the normal lymph node called follicles. Hence, the most common type of low-grade lymphoma is named "follicular lymphoma." Since normal lymphocytes circulate like police officers on patrol, usually these lymphomas are widespread. Only rarely are they localized to one area and cured with radiation.

Beginning in the 1950s, chemotherapy treatments were used to shrink and control low-grade lymphomas. Simple treatments would often work for years, but rarely produced cures. Over the next thirty years, experimentation with more intensive chemotherapy programs did not produce much better results. In young patients, intensive high-dose chemotherapy with a stem cell transplant from another person could result in a cure but was a risky procedure. For older patients, controlling a low-grade lymphoma might be enough to allow other health problems to cause death, a bittersweet success for the oncologist. For middle-aged patients, these extremes were often both unsatisfactory. Given these choices, the general rule developed in the 1980s and 1990s which still applies today is "watch and wait." Patients are treated with chemotherapy only when necessary, usually when the lymph nodes become uncomfortably large or the lymphoma grows within the bone marrow and lowers the blood counts. The effects of several months of chemotherapy may last for years, but eventually the lymphoma will reappear and the discussion repeated. At times, some part of the low-grade lymphoma may "transform" into a more aggressive "intermediate or high-grade lymphomas." Intensive chemotherapy may eliminate the transformed lymphoma, but the stubborn low-grade lymphoma often recurs.

Patients with low-grade lymphomas often feel they are unique among cancer patients. For patients with cancers of the breast, lung, or colon, early detection and prompt treatment can save lives. In patients with low-grade lymphomas, the workup and diagnosis may produce the same anxiety as with these better-known cancers, yet the plan may be observation with no treatment. While "watching and waiting" can bring the relief of avoiding chemotherapy for the moment, it has other stresses. Patients often struggle with the concept that the lymphoma is incurable. Knowing that treatment will likely be needed but not knowing the timing is unsettling. After treatment, it is not clear how long the lymphoma will remain controlled. For patients trying to plan their lives, low-grade lymphomas are described as a confusing "long walk in gray weather."

Adding to the hope, but also the confusion, in this gray landscape, is the rapidly changing technology.

Glen had taught many students the structure of the symphony is in four movements. It begins with the sonata, which contains its parts called the exposition, development, recapitulation, and an optional coda. Following the sonata are three movements, often called the adagio, minuet, and allegro. Glen imagined his lymphoma as a symphony. The opening sonata in this strange composition started with the exposition as they first met with Dr. Matthews and learned of the diagnosis. The development and the recapitulation came in a trip to the Dana Farber Cancer Institute and Dr. Robert Wightman.

"We cannot tell you when you might need treatment," began Dr. Wightman, reviewing the issues Glen had already learned but developing some new themes about ongoing research, including his own. His final recapitulation covered the reasons for treatment and choices. To this point, Glen had found it an interesting but not surprising visit. The tone changed when he asked about survival in his situation. Expecting to hear a vague generality, he was surprised when Dr. Wightman added a disturbing coda to the end of the sonata.

"Well, as I said, it is hard to tell. I think you probably have eight to ten years."

That night as Diane slept and Glen sat alone in the piano room, his emotions swirled. Could there be such a defined limit to my life? I thought my injuries were the problem. Did I work so hard to overcome them so this lymphoma will kill me? Why go on? The thoughts came so rapidly he needed to drive them out. He chose a recording of Mussorgsky's *Night on Bald Mountain*, performed by the Dallas Symphony Orchestra and conducted by Eduardo Mata, one of his favorite conductors. Somehow it was fitting, both the tumultuous music and Mata's unexpected death in a 1995 plane crash. Don't give up. We do not know our futures, he repeated. We have learned that lesson this year.

"Darn right we did," said his wife the next morning at breakfast. "You have come too far to give up. You need to work on your music and teaching. Stop imagining your death." She was right, of course, in her definitive way. He had always loved that about her, the clarity of her thoughts.

"And one more thing," she added. "If you are going to be thinking of this damn illness as some kind of symphony, make sure Mahler wrote it. I don't want this ending soon."

Mahler would be good, he agreed. Perhaps Symphony No. 3.

Glen's next two years were quiet from the lymphoma viewpoint. He continued to compose small pieces and teach privately. Family life was good. Their son and daughter were both married. He walked his daughter down the aisle, slowly and carefully, but without a cane. His mother was happy in her new assisted living. In the strange lymphoma symphony of his mind, he thought of this period as the second movement, a slow and peaceful adagio.

The music changed in late 2003 with a blood test.

"Your kidney function is slightly abnormal," reported Dr. Matthews. "Not enough to be dangerous but we need to find out why." An ultrasound showed Glen's lymph nodes had enlarged and were obstructing the flow of urine from the kidneys to the bladder; a back-up called hydronephrosis (hydro meaning water, nephrosis meaning kidney disease). A CT scan showed many more enlarged lymph nodes. The lymphoma was active and threatening.

"We need to start treatment. You have two options . . ."

❖   ❖   ❖

RITUXAN: DAWN OF A NEW ERA.

A dramatic change in the therapy of low-grade lymphomas occurred in 1997 with the approval of the antibody rituximab (Rituxan). This story began in 1975 when Drs. Cesar Milstein and Georges Kohler produced monoclonal antibodies, a discovery which won them the 1984 Noble Prize. Their technology meant that antibodies against various targets could be made in large enough quantities to use in patients. Antibodies were touted as "magic bullets" against cancer, but obstacles quickly emerged. Antibodies were not easy to make, struck unintended targets which caused them to either be used up or damage the wrong cells, or simply did not have any effect even when they hit the right target. A fascinating example of these difficulties was encountered in 1980 when scientists at the Sidney Farber Cancer Institute (so named before it became the Dana Farber Cancer Institute) administered an antibody made to target the lymphoma cells of a patient, identified by his initials N.B. In the lab, this personalized antibody attached to an antigen on the N.B.'s lymphoma cells and destroyed them, while avoiding his normal cells. Unfortunately, when given to N.B., the antibody did kill some lymphoma cells but was prevented from reaching many others by fragments of the antigen (the target) circulating in the blood. The conclusion of the report was that this technology was not toxic, but had "significant challenges." [533]

The challenges of using antibodies caused many scientists and investors in the late 1970s and 1980s to abandon them in favor of searching for new chemotherapies or targeted drugs. One scientist convinced of the utility of antibodies was Dr. Ronald Levy of Stanford, who started IDEC Pharmaceuticals in 1985. Dr. Levy had initially hoped to create antibodies unique to each person's lymphoma, the ultimate in personalized medicine. Yet IDEC's success came by making antibodies against a common target called CD20, a target found on both normal B-cells and many B-cell lymphomas. The obvious concern with this approach was that an antibody which attacks both cancer and normal cells would be harmful. But when IDEC scientists gave the antibody to monkeys, the depletion of the normal B-cells did not seem to produce serious side effects.[534] In 1993 IDEC began testing its antibody, called rituximab (brand name Rituxan), in patients. Four years later, in 1997, rituximab became the first monoclonal antibody approved for a cancer. By 2002, sales topped the $1 billion mark. An interesting side note is that IDEC faced financial difficulties as it began clinical testing. Despite a stock offering and the success of the early clinical trials, the company did not have the money to proceed with the final testing and marketing. In 1995, rituximab was saved by an agreement with Genentech, although the eventual cost to IDEC was steep. For $60 million dollars and its regulatory guidance, Genentech would earn billions of IDEC's potential profit.[535]

Rituximab's initial use was in low-grade lymphoma, either by itself or with chemotherapy. Although rituximab did not cure, for many patients it allowed longer control of the disease and could be used as a maintenance treatment to extend remission. In more aggressive lymphomas, rituximab had relatively little effect by itself but raised cure rates when combined with chemotherapy. Although an occasional patient could have a severe allergic reaction during the infusion, rituximab had relatively few immediate side effects. Since rituximab attacks both lymphoma cells and the normal B-cells which make antibodies needed to fight infection, whether long-term side effects would develop was a major concern. In the testing phase, monkeys did not seem to have ill effects from losing their B-cells, but it was not clear whether humans would react in the same fashion, particularly as more patients with weakened immune systems received the drug for longer periods. Some patients developed reactivation of viral hepatitis, so checking for these infections before starting rituximab became routine. While a rare patient did have other serious viral illnesses, for the most part, the depletion of the normal B-cells was well tolerated. In fact, the ability to deplete B-cells safely with rituximab led to its use to control some disorders where the activity of the B-cells was a problem, such as immune thrombocytopenia (also called ITP—a condition of low platelets due to destruction by the immune system) and other autoimmune conditions.

Other monoclonal antibodies used in various diseases soon joined rituximab: trastuzumab (Herceptin) for breast cancer (1998), Cetuximab (Erbitux) for colorectal cancer (2004), infliximab (Remicade) and etanercept (Enbrel) for immune disorders (both 1998). By the end of 2014, there were forty-seven monoclonal antibodies approved for use with sales approaching $60 billion dollars.[536] The era of the "magic bullet" predicted in 1975 when Drs. Milstein and Kohler developed their technology had finally arrived. More monoclonal antibodies will be forthcoming from many labs, while other scientists continue to work toward Dr. Levy's original goal of making a specific antibody-based treatment for each patient.

"The two options are to use Rituxan by itself or with chemotherapy. By itself, the Rituxan has less chance of working, but you avoid the side effects of chemotherapy. The downside of this approach is that if it does not work, you might end up with a longer treatment if we need to add the chemo later."

"Is there any difference over the long term?" asked Glen.

"We do not know for sure," replied Dr. Matthews. "This is a pretty new idea, but we do not think so."

Glen opted for the Rituxan by itself. Nurse Karen Lange placed his intravenous line and began the infusion. The first two hours were boring. When the rate increased, Glen felt a vague sense of danger. He ignored the sensation until it worsened, becoming accompanied by faint discordant notes of music he could not place. He looked up.

"What wrong, Glen?" asked Diane. Karen heard her words and was instantly at their side.

He could not answer. He wanted to speak, but only gibberish came out. His face flushed and his vision grew dark as the music played louder. He recognized the composition, adding to his anxiety.

Karen turned the infusion off, put an oxygen mask over his face, and administered more diphenhydramine and dexamethasone. As Glen's vision returned, he saw Dr. Matthews over him.

"You had a reaction to the Rituxan. It should pass soon but can be very upsetting. Try to relax," he said.

Glen nodded. "It's getting better," he mumbled, able to speak again.

When the reaction had cleared, Karen reviewed the plans.

"We see these every so often, and they are scary," she began. "Some patients have a feeling of doom."

"I heard music," Glen replied. "It took me a minute to figure out it was *Danse Macabre*, a piece done by a French composer named Camille Saint-Saëns in the late 1800s. It's a song about death. It has some unusual chords and uses the xylophone, which makes a sound like rattling bones. I think the beeping of all the machines fit right in. Anyway, there you are."

"I've never heard that before. It must have been really scary," Karen agreed. "Usually the reactions come as we try to raise the infusion rate, like it did with you. We can restart again tomorrow, but we will finish with the rate low. You will be here with us longer than you thought."

"Longer looks good right now," he mused.

The next day, the rest of the Rituxan infused easily, and Glen returned for three other weeks of treatment. Another ultrasound and CT scan showed improvement: the lymph nodes were smaller and the kidneys back to normal.

Over the next two years, they repeated the Rituxan weekly for four weeks every six months; a plan called maintenance treatment. During those hours, the nurses made him their teacher, starting with a simple question.

"I don't know much about classical music, I'm afraid to say," began Karen. "Where should I start? What should I listen to first?"

Glen nodded. "You don't need to know anything, just listen. Begin with Sergei Rachmaninoff's Piano Concerto Number 2. It has three separate parts, called movements. In each, you will hear something you will recognize or feel from somewhere else."

Each week, it was a new assignment to be discussed as the antibody infused.

"I won't give you those works which are extremely well known," he warned. "Like Beethoven's *Fifth* or Pachelbel's *Cannon*. I want you to experience music you don't know which covers a wide range of emotions."

Their curriculum went on for two years, four lessons every six months, sixteen in all. After Rachmaninoff in the first block came Chopin, Bach, and Grieg, a surprise with *In the Hall of the Mountain King*.

"That one will get us working after lunch," commented Anna, the secretary, who also liked to listen.

Four years after the accident, in 2005, they were done. The sixteen lessons and maintenance treatments concluded.

"Now, I have a question for you," Glen said to Karen. "What is your favorite?"

There was no hesitation. "*Carmina Burana*," she replied.

"Why?"

"It's all of life in one piece," she answered. "Like a day here."

Dr. Matthews met with Glen and Diane to regroup.

"Now we watch again," he noted. "We know that this lymphoma will be back, but we do not know when or where. We do not want to do any unnecessary CT scans. We should avoid exposing any quiet lymphoma cells to radiation which might cause a mutation and anger them, so we will check you with exams and lab work."

Glen considered this time of Rituxan the third movement of the symphony of his lymphoma, the minuet. It had been a formalized, classical dance. After the Rituxan, two more years went by with more compositions, more teaching, and his first grandchild, a beautiful boy born in early 2007 to his daughter. Glen watched as his mother held her first great-grandchild.

The change happened later in 2007, while he was showering. The hot water always felt good on his battered body. He had learned after the accident that what his grandmother had said about feeling the cold in your bones was true. He liked watching the water in his shower, too. He enjoyed seeing the drops on the glass door work their way down, forming rivulets. Their direction seemed random, yet they connected. Like our lives, he often thought, and our futures. On that day, as he had washed under his arm, his fingers slipped over a lump, a lymph node. I know what this means, he thought. More lymphoma.

"It's probably more of the same," reported Dr. Matthews. "Since it is so easily accessible, I would like to do a biopsy to be sure."

There was no change in the appearance of the cells under the microscope, the flow cytometry which tested the markers on the cell surface, or the genetic tests. It was still a low-grade follicular lymphoma.

"It's the same lymphoma," Dr. Matthews told them. "We can simply re-try the Rituxan again, or go on to more add mild chemotherapy. I would prefer to use the Rituxan alone. It worked well last time. You could also return to Dana Farber and see if they have any new protocols or thoughts."

"Having the same enemy is not such a bad thing," Glen replied. "I have been reading about the Native Americans. They did just fine skirmishing among themselves. It was when they got a new enemy that they really had problems."

"Well, I never quite heard it put that way," replied Dr. Matthews. "But today yours is the same old enemy."

Another two years of Rituxan, four weeks every six months for two years. Sixteen more lessons for the nurses, starting with the three Bs: Beethoven, Bach, and Brahms.

"They're like the Rat Pack," announced Anna. "All similar, but a little different."

He finished in 2009, the same year he turned sixty. Glen had dreaded this birthday for years since it marked the age of his father's death. One minute his father was well, the next dead on the garage floor from a burst brain aneurysm. It was his time, they said. Glen and his younger brother had both been tested with brain MRIs and knew this was not their fate. Still, he had always wanted to bypass sixty and reach sixty-one. *What about me now? Where am I with this lymphoma? Is this the fourth movement, the rondo? Or still the third, the minuet?*

"Stop it," answered Diane. "Enough with your father. You are not him. You do not know your future, except that you will be sorry if you waste any of it dwelling on what you cannot control. And no more of this cancer symphony nonsense now. Start writing your symphony."

My symphony? It was the right thought at the right time. *More than the sun and the moon, I love her.* He started at the beginning of 2010, uncertain how long it would take. Mozart completed his symphonies in days, Beethoven took years.

"Don't be like Brahms," encouraged Diane. "I recall that one spent over a decade on his first symphony."

The next year, 2011, was different. He was now sixty-one and past the danger of his father. That's when the swelling under the other arm came, overnight. And it ached.

"Are you having any other symptoms?" asked Dr. Matthews. "Any fevers or chills? Night sweats."

"No'" replied Glen. "I feel fine."

"Good. I still want to do a biopsy. We will ask Dr. Gannon to remove that node."

Glen and Diane returned two weeks later to hear the news.

"The biopsy showed your lymphoma has changed. It has become more aggressive, what we call a diffuse large cell lymphoma. This lymphoma is different from your low-grade lymphoma. We need to treat this with intensive chemotherapy."

CURING DIFFUSE LARGE CELL LYMPHOMA WITH CHOP.
In the 1929 "Graduate Course in Cancer" published in the *New England Journal of Medicine*, Dr. Henry Jackson noted that the term malignant lymphoma described a wide range of conditions "leading eventually to death in practically all cases."[537] Although physicians of Dr. Jackson's era did not yet have the tools to classify most lymphomas, "diffuse large cell lymphoma" would have fit his description. The "diffuse" means the complete obliteration of the normal structure of the lymph node, while "large" referred to the microscopic appearance of the lymphoma cells. These large, rapidly growing lymphoma cells spread quickly. In the 1980s Working Formula classification, these were considered intermediate-grade lymphomas, meaning the patients would die within a few months unless successfully treated. Unlike low-grade lymphomas, "watch and wait" is not a good option for patients with this disease.

In 1975, the first cures in patients with diffuse large cell lymphoma were reported using multi-agent chemotherapy programs. For patients with a disease which had previously been uniformly fatal, the treatments were a beacon of hope. For "chemotherapy faithful" physicians it was a vindication of their efforts to use these chemicals for cure.[538]

The most successful early program was called CHOP, named by using letters from three of the four ingredients (cyclophosphamide, doxorubicin, vincristine (brand name Oncovin), and prednisone) and borrowing the "H" from the chemical structure of doxorubicin. CHOP was an intravenous treatment given once every three weeks over four months and produced a "complete remission," meaning all the tests went back to normal, in half of the patients. About 35 percent were cured.

During the 1980s, major cancer centers sought to improve cure rates in large cell lymphoma by adding more chemotherapy drugs to CHOP. Brilliant laboratory work suggested that combining drugs which worked differently from each other would produce better results. Intuitively the concept made sense, "empty the clip" was the image given to patients. For the chemotherapy faithful, these treatment programs were a chance to push their mastery of this new technology for the benefit of their patients. Progressively more complex and toxic programs with abbreviations like ProMACE-CytaBOM and MACOP-B brought higher cure rates, some approaching 75 percent. Rivalry among the major centers led to heated debates over the best choice, but all agreed this was a great triumph, a "near conquest of diffuse large cell lymphoma" by combination chemotherapy.[539]

To settle the issue of which chemotherapy program was superior, the National Cancer Institute sponsored a study comparing three of the "alphabet soup" recipes and CHOP. Some oncologists objected to the inclusion of CHOP, fearing their patients might receive this obviously inferior treatment. From 1988 to 1993 almost nine hundred patients were randomized to receive one of the four treatments. The eagerly awaited results sent shock waves through the cancer world: all the treatments produced the same results, even the simpler CHOP program.[540]

In addition to restating the painful lesson learned by generations of clinicians that we are never as smart as we think, the study produced several important effects. CHOP became the most commonly used treatment for these lymphomas. Physicians across the world were reminded that the direct comparison of treatments is required to know which one is superior. The better results reported by the major cancer centers with more complex chemotherapy had largely been due to the selection of healthier patients for these treatments. Using newer molecular techniques, scientists dissecting the results did identify patients who might benefit from the complex combinations. Perhaps most importantly, the study provided evidence that further improvements with traditional chemotherapy were likely to be modest and new approaches were needed. This "passing of the baton" occurred as the results of the CHOP study were presented at the American Society of Clinical Oncology and followed shortly after by reports using the new antibody rituximab (Rituxan).

The CHOP and Rituxan were real treatment, not fun. Every three weeks Glen spent all day with the nurses, receiving the intravenous Rituxan and Cytoxan from bags and the red Adriamycin and clear vincristine from a syringe administered by the nurse who watched him carefully. The next day he came back for a shot of Neulasta to keep his white blood cells from going too low and started four days of prednisone pills.

The first few nights after chemotherapy, Glen had insomnia but could not do anything useful. His feeling of being hyper but exhausted was from the prednisone, the nurses told him. When that finished, he crashed and ached. His bones hurt. That was the Neulasta, the nurses told him. The second week was fatigue and some mouth sores. The third week he felt better, almost himself. This would be his pattern, the nurses told him. Round and round it would go, six times. Although he would not tell Diane, this was the final rondo movement in the forbidden symphony of his lymphoma. The climax was nearing. If it worked, he had a future. If not . . .

"Stop worrying about what you cannot change," reminded Diane at the start of that third week. "You are doing everything you can. These good weeks are the time for you to finish your symphony. You've always needed a timeline to meet your goals. Finish it when you finish this treatment."

She was right. Each third week he would write the themes developed during the preceding two, pulling together thoughts and notes written on little scraps of paper. With each cycle, he had less good time to work. The nurses told him that was normal, too.

Then it was over. Glen finished the six cycles of CHOP with Rituxan and the symphony. The results of the chemotherapy were known first.

"The PET scan shows a complete remission," reported Dr. Matthews. "Now we keep watching."

Several months later, Glen's orchestra played his symphony at Procter's Theater in nearby Schenectady. He sat with Diane in the center front row as his music washed over them. Afterward, they called him to the stage, and he stood in front of his colleagues who had played, his friends and family who had listened, and his nurses who had studied.

"What were you thinking up there?" asked Diane, in her usual blunt fashion.

"Nothing can take this away from us," he replied. "No matter what the future holds."

MODERN LYMPHOMA TREATMENTS.
Future treatments for lymphoma will combine the best of the chemotherapy era with exciting new molecular science. Development of traditional drugs continues, as does the revision of classification systems

to improve the ability to predict which are most effective. Massive doses of chemotherapy with "autologous (the patient's own) stem cell support" remain an option for some patients. The riskier but effective "allogeneic (from another person) stem cell transplant" can be used with increasing safety. While these strategies optimize the concepts developed during the last half of the twentieth century, the introduction of antibodies like rituximab near the end of the century announced the arrival of many different modern molecular treatments with fascinating methods of action.

Targeting key growth pathways which are deranged in lymphomas is one new treatment strategy. An example is the oral medication ibrutinib (brand name Imbruvica) which blocks the action of an enzyme called Bruton's tyrosine kinase, an important regulator of normal lymph cell activities which is overactive in some lymphomas. Ibrutinib comes with an interesting story.

In 1952, Marine Corps pediatrician Col. Ogden C. Bruton at Walter Reed Army Hospital published a report of the case of eight-year-old Joseph Holtoner, who had nineteen episodes of severe infections over the preceding four years. Joseph was referred to as a "frequent flier" on the inpatient ward, an apt description given his father was the US Air Force Major General and pilot J. Stanley Horner.[541] Dr. Bruton examined Joseph's serum and found a complete lack of normal antibodies, a condition called agammaglobulinemia (agammaglobulin meaning no antibodies, emia meaning blood). He administered monthly injections of immune globulin to the boy with marked improvement in his infections.[542] Dr. Burton surveyed other pediatric programs at medical schools across the country and found no similar cases. His landmark article reported the first congenital defect of the immune system, now known as X-linked agammaglobulinemia (XLA). Children with the condition do not make antibodies because they have a mutation in the *XLA* gene, found on the X-chromosome. Boys with the mutation will develop XLA since they have only one X-chromosome (and therefore only one *XLA* gene) while girls would be very unlikely to have the condition since they have two X-chromosomes (and thus would need mutations in both *XLA* genes). About one-half of the mutations are inherited, while one-half are new and not found in the family. Since boys with XLA still get some antibodies from their mother until birth, it may take a few months to years for the infections to begin. Joseph, for example, developed serious infections around age four.[543] Dr. Bruton's report and the subsequent age of molecular biology led to the 1993 discovery of the *XLA* gene and the enzyme it produced, named Bruton tyrosine kinase (Bkt) in his honor. This enzyme has an important role in B-cell development and antibody production. Since the absence of Bkt in XLA results in no B-cells in boys like Joseph, the question arose as to whether it might be a useful target for treatment of B-cell lymphomas. Inhibitors of Bkt like ibrutinib (Imbruvica) proved effective in low-grade lymphomas, particularly the condition chronic lymphocytic leukemia/small lymphocytic lymphoma.[544] Ibrutinib is an example of the shift "from a chemotherapy based approach to treatments aimed at the underlying biologic mechanisms of disease occurrence and progression."[545]

Vaccines for lymphoma are an almost unbearably attractive strategy. In theory, patients vaccinated with a protein found uniquely on the cancer cell could have their own immune system recognize and attack the cancer, sending it the way of polio or diphtheria. Selecting the proper target can be difficult. In addition, the immune system needed for the attack is often impaired by the cancer. Successful vaccinations require the proteins in the injection to be formally presented to the person's immune system by cells called antigen-presenting cells (APCs). It has become evident that cancers impair this process. The strategy of creating APCs outside the body and reinfusing them is called "immunotransplantation."[546]

Immune treatments used in other cancers, named "checkpoint inhibition" are part of modern lymphoma treatments. As part of the complex process of recognizing "self" and preventing immune attacks on the normal body, checkpoint molecules act as control switches to suppress the activation of T-cells. Cancer cells may (inappropriately) activate these checkpoint controls and thus escape immune attack. Ipilimumab was the first antibody against one checkpoint called CTL-4. Nivolumab was the second, targeting a different checkpoint called "programmed death-1" (or PD-1). Others are following.

Enhancing the effects of antibodies like rituximab is another strategy. Immunoconjugates are antibodies linked with a lethal payload, such as a toxin, radioactive molecule or drug, which they deliver to the cancer cell. Designing and testing these smart bombs is a complicated but promising approach.[547] Another exciting antibody class has the name "bispecific T-cell engager (BiTE)."[548] For this treatment an antibody is made which attaches to a target on a cancer cell and then links it to a T-cell, handcuffing the villain to the policeman. Even more complex is the engineering of T-cells to express receptors directed against an antigen on the cancer cell. In essence, this is programming the T-cell to attack the cancer and is called "CAR-T cells."[549]

The most radical concept in modern treatment is to either edit or control the malfunctioning genes of the cancer cell. Scientists have found that primitive bacterial cells have a defensive mechanism to identify and destroy viral DNA, named the Crispr/Cas system (for "clustered regularly spaced short palindromic repeat," named after the DNA segments which control the system). Scientists have developed Crispr systems which can be used in human cells and offer the potential to block or edit abnormal gene expression. While there are significant obstacles, there seems little doubt this technology will be utilized to attempt to correct the fundamental defects in cancer cells.[550]

It is quite a future.

The past and the future came together for Glen at today's visit.

"Mom died last month. She was one hundred and three and still sharp as a tack. She knew I've been anxious about this lymphoma for the last fifteen years. Know what she told me?"

Dr. Matthews shook his head.

"The first hundred years are the hardest. After that, you don't worry so much."

3:40 Alisa Cohen: Genetic testing

John Welt brought the chart to Dr. Matthews.

"She's in room three with her boyfriend," he reported.

"Do you mind letting Tracy know?" Dr. Matthews asked, looking up from his computer. "She did the consultation and is going to meet with them."

"Sure. Then we can all end this day."

Three weeks ago, Alisa Cohen and her fiancé Gabriel had met Nurse Practitioner Tracy Callahan for *BRCA* genetic testing. Alisa was a thirty-three-year-old theater professor at Skidmore College referred by her gynecologist, Dr. Stacey Gold.

"My mother has a *BRCA* mutation," began Alisa. "I have known about this since I left home for college. About ten years ago, when I was in grad school in the City, I met with a genetics counselor at Memorial Sloan Kettering. I decided not to do the test, just watch carefully. We moved here two years ago, and Dr. Gold has been doing my exams and ordering my mammograms and MRIs. Now I want to be tested."

Alisa was in perfect health with no children of her own. Tracy drew the family tree, learning both sides were Jewish from Germany.

"My Dad is healthy, and his family has no cancer," Alisa reported as Tracy recorded the names and ages of her father, his parents, two sisters, and their children.

"Dad's side is clear," agreed Tracy. "Now I'm ready for Mom's side."

"Mom had one sister and one brother. Mom's sister, my aunt, died in her thirties of breast cancer. I was young when she died. Mom's brother, my uncle, is fine. He's a great guy and has no children. My Mom's mother, my grandmother, had breast cancer in her thirties but is still alive in her nineties. Feisty, too. Grandma's sister died of ovary cancer."

"Did your mother ever have cancer?" asked Tracy.

"No. After my aunt died, my mother had both her breasts and ovaries removed. She wouldn't take any chances. They didn't have testing in those days."

"That must have been a tough decision," remarked Tracy.

"I think it was, but my mother is a very definitive person," Alisa replied as Gabriel nodded knowingly. "And she saw what happened to the other women in her family."

CLONING THE BRCA GENES.

For many years it has been known that women in some families develop breast and ovarian cancer at young ages. Even in eras when discussions of cancer were taboo, these families were often aware of the danger and known to their doctors. As the age of molecular science started, major academic institutions collected blood and tissue samples from these families in hopes that researchers might someday unlock their dangerous secret. When technological advances in the 1970s and 1980s allowed the study of DNA, scientists began a highly-publicized race to locate the genes responsible for these so-called "familial breast and ovarian cancers." In 1990, a specific region of chromosome 17 was found to contain one of the genes, named *BRCA-1* (BR for breast and CA for cancer).[551] The gene was located using samples from families with strong histories of breast cancer and correlating them with markers known to be on different chromosomes, a technique called linkage analysis.

Knowing that the *BRCA-1* gene was on chromosome 17 started the final sprint to find the exact location and clone the gene, which means to list its DNA sequence. The challenge was searching through the vast amount of DNA in that region. Human cells have roughly six billion "base pairs" of DNA (recall DNA is two strings of bases, so the "pair" refers to a base on one strand and its opposite base on the other strand) broken up into forty-six chromosomes, each containing fifty million to three hundred million base pairs. Only about 2 percent of this DNA is genes; the rest is "empty space" which may serve other functions. A typical gene is made of a few thousand base pairs grouped in multiple short stretches (called exons) separated by stretches of non-gene DNA (called introns). In this area of chromosome 17 there were several million base pairs and many genes, so the search for *BRCA-1* was likened to walking across the country to find a specific small town. In the early 1990s, working with small pieces of DNA was routine, but examining and sequencing large regions was still exceedingly difficult. From 1990 to 1994, the oft repeated goal was to find *BRCA-1* "by Christmas."[552]

Before Christmas of 1994, the *BRCA-1* gene was located and cloned by scientists led by Mark Skolnick of the University of Utah and the biotech firm Myriad Genetics. The finish of the race was reported on the NBC Nightly News, a quaint reminder of evening television's once dominant role as a source of public information. Skolnick's team found *BRCA-1* using an elegant combination of technologies available at the time, including further detailed analyses of samples from families with breast and ovary cancers.[553] Shortly thereafter, the *BRCA-2* gene was found on chromosome 13 and cloned in similar fashion. The techniques used to clone the *BRCA* genes were soon replaced by "brute force" high-output sequencing of DNA and analysis of the RNA which made similar searches for other genes easier.

After the *BRCA* genes were cloned, the cataloging of mutations began. Samples from families with breast and ovarian cancer syndromes, some saved for years, were analyzed to identify mutations and distinguish them from normal variants called polymorphisms. There are approximately one thousand eight hundred mutations in each gene.[554] With a few exceptions, a woman who carries a mutation is at high risk to develop breast cancer (60–85 percent over her life) or ovarian cancer (20–40 percent over her life).

"Basically," Alisa continued, "my mother saw her mother survive breast cancer by having her breasts removed and a hysterectomy. Mom then saw her aunt die, followed by her sister. She felt it was her destiny to have the same thing and she wasn't going to wait."

"So, your mother was tested later?" asked Tracy.

"Yes. When testing became available, Mom was positive. She knows her decision to have the preventative surgery saved her life."

BRCA TESTING.

In the fall of 1994, the *BRCA-1* gene was cloned. In the December 1, 1994, issue of the *New England Journal of Medicine*, breast cancer researcher Dr. Barbara Weber described the accomplishment and the considerable work to be done before testing would be ready for "everyday medical practice."[555] Shortly after that, the first advertisements for *BRCA* testing appeared.

In theory, *BRCA* testing made sense. Once a specific family mutation was known, women who did not yet have cancer could find out if they were carriers. If they had a mutation, they could be watched closely or even have their breasts and ovaries removed before cancer developed. If they were not carriers, they would not be at high risk.

In everyday medical practice, *BRCA* testing is not straightforward. The mutations are found only in about one in every five hundred people, so testing the general population is not worthwhile. Since *BRCA* mutations cause only 5 percent of breast cancers, even testing most women with breast cancer is not helpful. Selecting women with breast cancer diagnosed at a young age (under 40-45), ovarian cancer (particularly at a young age), breast cancer in both breasts, and those in Ashkenazi Jewish families (from eastern Europe) raises the chances of finding a mutation. Men with breast cancer should also consider testing. Yet many families have complicated or limited trees, uncertain ethnic backgrounds, or unavailable family members.

After testing, the results must be interpreted. When a *BRCA* mutation is found ("positive test") in a woman diagnosed with breast cancer, bilateral mastectomies may become part of her treatment plan. When a *BRCA* mutation is found ("positive test") in a woman without breast cancer, she can consider intensive mammogram and MRI breast screening or preventative mastectomies, and salpingo-oophorectomy (removal of the ovaries and tubes). A negative *BRCA* test may be harder to interpret. The most accurate information from testing comes when a family mutation has already been identified in another family member with cancer. In these families, women who test negative are relieved (this negative test is called a "true negative"). If a family mutation is not known, a negative test can be falsely reassuring since not all mutations can be detected (this negative result is often called an "uninformative negative test"). Since knowing if there is a family mutation is so important, genetic testing is done first in family members with cancer to see "if the test works." If all the members of a family with cancer have died or are unwilling to participate, it may be impossible to determine if there is a family mutation.

Understanding other issues is important before testing. Payment for testing and any subsequent treatment, potential insurance discrimination, communication of results to family members, and psychological stresses all require careful discussion. Since 1994, geneticists, genetics counselors, physicians, nurses, ethicists, and various public groups have worked to provide guidelines for patients undergoing *BRCA* testing. Dr. Weber's plea to wait was ignored, but her goals were not as these programs are available across the country.

Alisa had her mother's 2001 report from Myriad Genetics which revealed the *BRCA-1* mutation called "del185AG," meaning a deletion (del) of the 185th (Adenine) and 186th (Guanine) DNA base pairs. When these base pairs are missing, the protein produced by the gene is dysfunctional. The "del185AG" mutation is often found in Ashkenazi Jewish families.

FOUNDER MUTATIONS: FASCINATING STORIES, SIMILAR ENDINGS.

Some ethnic groups have relatively specific *BRCA* mutations, called "founder mutations." These mutations either began in one member of the group or were imported and became concentrated, usually by a combination of breeding within the group, geographical isolation, or a reduction in population. Ashkenazi Jews (those from eastern Europe) have three founder mutations, designated "del185AG" and "5382insC" on *BRCA-1*, and "6147delT" on *BRCA-2*.[556] About one in forty Ashkenazi Jews carries one of these mutations, a considerable concentration compared with the general population in which one in five hundred people have a mutation.[557]

The study of *BRCA* founder mutations is a fascinating fusion of science and history. By analyzing various populations for both these mutations and DNA markers located near the *BRCA* gene, scientists can speculate on the origin and spread of the mutations over time. Initial analysis of the del185AG gene mutation in Ashkenazi Jewish families implied that it began in about the year 1200 CE.[558] When additional work found the mutation in other non-Ashkenazi Jews, the origin was moved back to before the Jewish dispersion after the destruction of the second temple in Jerusalem by the Romans in 70 CE.[559] This earlier time course suggested additional later historical forces may have helped concentrate the mutation in Ashkenazi Jews as they moved into eastern Europe. The second founder mutations, called 5382insC (meaning an extra Cytosine is inserted at position 5382), did not originate in the Jewish population but rather began in either Scandinavia or northern Russia in the years around 200–500 CE. It entered the Jewish population in Poland in about 500–600 CE and may have been distributed across Europe by Vikings as they raided and pillaged, although further work unifying the science with this history is needed.[560]

Founder mutations have produced some remarkable historical surprises, such the discovery of the del185AG mutation in Hispanic Catholics in San Luis, Colorado. This story dates to the middles ages when Jews were welcomed into the region of modern day Spain by its Muslim rulers. As Catholics gradually reconquered the region and began to persecute Jews, some converted (called conversos) while others continued to practice in secret (called crypto-Jews). In 1492, the Alhambra Decree by Ferdinand and Isabella expelled those Spanish Jews who had not converted to Catholicism, resulting in suffering and death remembered even today.[561] Some of these Jews appear to have ultimately reached the area of the southwest United States and Mexico. There has been an ongoing debate over whether traditions seen in those areas represent relics of the crypto-Jews and the finding of the Jewish del185AG *BRCA* founder mutation supports that interpretation.[562]

Regardless of their origin and spread, these mutations all result in the production of an abnormal BRCA protein. The normal BRCA proteins repair damage to DNA which regularly occurs from exposure to toxins, radiation, or during normal cellular activities. The BRCA proteins remove damaged DNA and replace it with the correct sequence, a procedure called homologous recombination. Although there are other DNA repair mechanisms, *BRCA-1* and *BRCA-2* are particularly important for breast and ovary cells. Thus, *BRCA* mutations mean breast and ovary cells may not properly repair their DNA, accumulate damage, and become cancerous. How long the process might take, or even if it will happen at all, is not predictable in an individual.

"When I turned eighteen, my mother told me she was a mutation carrier and I could be tested," Alisa continued. She became momentarily quiet as she recalled her mother's brilliant explanation, remembering thinking how good she must be in the courtroom.

"What do you think I should do?" Alisa had asked at the conclusion.

"You should be tested. The question is when. My doctor says it should be five to ten years before the age of diagnosis of the youngest person with cancer in the family. That would be your aunt. She was diagnosed at twenty-seven with her breast cancer, so you should be tested in the next four years. At the latest when you finish college."

Remembering her aunt had been sobering. Alisa had been ten when she died, the blurred memories powerfully sad.

But genetic testing wasn't happening then. College at NYU was next. Her mother had been mildly upset with Alisa's decision to leave Boston and her reach, but Alisa loved the pulse of Manhattan. Uncle Steven, a filmmaker, was nearby. He would help her into the theater, which she already knew was her major. Genes were something for later, maybe.

BRCA resurfaced two years later when Alisa's sister was tested. Cynthia was two years older, had graduated from Harvard and entered its medical school, preparing to be a neurosurgeon.

"If I need mastectomies, this is a good time," she told Alisa. "I will do them before I start my clinical work. I don't want any disruptions."

Cynthia's plan came as no surprise. Alisa's sister was all business, just like her mother. While the sisters had a good relationship, Alisa found Cynthia was always trying to mold her, make her fit in with their mother and even their grandmother. I am different, Alisa thought, more like my uncle.

Cynthia's test was negative. That palpable relief sustained their mother for a short period, but gradually her attention turned toward Alisa. When college ended, the pressure mounted.

"You need to do this, Alisa. It's a simple test. You need the answer," came her plea.

For Alisa, *BRCA* testing was not simple. She knew that if she tested positive, her mother would not rest until she had preventative mastectomies. She could not bear that drumbeat call for the disfiguration of her body. I don't want to deal with it, she had concluded. I just don't want to lose my breasts.

The compromise between mother and daughter was a visit to Memorial Sloan Kettering Cancer Center for genetic counseling. The breast surgeon was particularly helpful.

"You don't have to be tested yet as long as you have mammograms and ultrasounds alternating with MRIs every six months," she reported. "You can pretend you are negative for at least a few more years until you do feel ready for testing."

The truce afforded mother and daughter by this plan was broken in 2013 when Angelia Jolie made public her *BRCA* gene mutation and prophylactic mastectomies. Alisa's mother had attended a symposium of Jewish physicians and legal scholars discussing the issue.

"This Harvard cancer doctor discussed testing, and the conclusion of the rabbinical legal scholars was it is mandatory under Jewish law to save lives. Dear, you have to do it."

PREVENTIVE SURGERY.
In the 1980s and 1990s, women with breast cancer were increasingly offered alternatives to mastectomy. The choice of lumpectomy and

radiation meant the diagnosis no longer inevitably lead to the loss of a woman's breast. Even the removal of the lymph nodes became progressively less extensive, first with limited axillary dissection, then the sentinel node biopsy. The breast cancer advocacy movement and their pink revolution publicized these options and worked to overcome the reluctance of some surgeons and women to embrace this lesser but equally effective surgery. Given this progress, it seemed ironic that *BRCA* testing might cause twenty-first-century women without cancer to choose to have their breasts removed.

As *BRCA* testing began in the late 1990s, the most obvious question was what a woman with a mutation could do to protect herself from the 60–85 percent lifetime risk of breast cancer. At the start, the benefit of a "prophylactic mastectomy" was not certain.[563] The danger posed by the small amount of breast tissue left behind was an initial concern, but it soon became clear that the procedure was effective—a 90 percent reduction of the risk. For women who elect not to undergo surgery, the advent of MRI allowed earlier detection and thus a low risk of death from the cancer, although often with more biopsies and anxiety. Unfortunately, there is no good method to prevent breast cancer in women with *BRCA* mutations. Tamoxifen or removal of the ovaries may somewhat reduce the risk, yet neither are effective enough to be considered sufficient. Although many women with *BRCA* mutations opt for regular mammograms, ultrasounds and MRIs, over time more have chosen mastectomy.[564] Angelina Jolie's writing in the *New York Times* about her decision to undergo surgery created public discussion and reinforced the benefits in a very personal way.[565]

Many women who undergo mastectomy opt for reconstruction. With a prophylactic mastectomy, less tissue is removed than in a cancer operation and often the nipple and much skin can be saved. Plastic surgeons can recreate the breast using either an implant (filled with saline or silicone) or tissue from another part of the women's body (usually the fat from the abdomen). Improvements in surgical techniques have led to better results, but the reconstructed breasts are never normal and do not have normal sensation. The process can require several operations and risk infection requiring removal of the implant. Understanding the options, selecting a reconstructive surgeon, and preparing for surgery is a major undertaking.

BRCA mutations also raise a woman's risk of ovary cancer to 20–40 percent, a scary prospect given this cancer is difficult to detect, usually widespread, and treated with aggressive surgery and chemotherapy. As with preventative breast surgery, it was not initially clear if "prophylactic salpingo-oophorectomy" (removal of the fallopian tubes and ovaries) would be successful. The concern was that as the ovaries are formed in the embryo and move to their final location, they leave behind cells which cannot be seen or removed but can become cancerous, a condition called peritoneal carcinomatosis. Fortunately, this is a relatively uncommon and the prophylactic salpingo-oophorectomy reduces the risk of ovary cancer by 80 percent.[566] Laparoscopic techniques also made the surgery easier; it is usually done as an outpatient. The recovery from the operation is quick, but if a woman is premenopausal, menopause will immediately result—with all its possible symptoms.

For women who choose preventative surgery, deciding when to have the operations can be difficult. Predicting when an individual woman with a *BRCA* mutation might develop a cancer is imprecise. Breast cancers caused by *BRCA* mutations generally occur at earlier ages than ovarian cancers, but some women with mutations may never develop either cancer. Using the age of diagnosis of other family members is tempting, but offers no guarantees. There is also the worrying phenomenon called genetic drift, which means the age of cancer diagnosis in families may get younger in successive generations. Breast cancers can be detected early by careful watching, allowing for more time to decide about that surgery. Ovarian cancer cannot be detected early, yet removal of the ovaries ends the option for normal child bearing and brings menopause. Hormone replacement after the surgery can relieve the menopause symptoms, but many women are afraid to use this option for long if they still have breast tissue. Given all these issues, the standard medical recommendations are that a woman with a *BRCA* mutation have careful breast screening with mammogram and MRI unless she has had a prophylactic mastectomy and that removal of her ovaries should be done when child bearing is complete.

Women with *BRCA* mutations also have another option which can be considered preventive surgery—genetic selection to prevent their children from carrying the mutation. After an egg is fertilized and grows to the eight-cell stage, one cell can be removed without obvious harm to the eventual baby. The DNA from that removed cell can be analyzed, including for *BRCA* mutations. So, a woman can undergo *in vitro* fertilization, meaning her eggs are removed and fertilized with sperm in the lab. The embryos are checked at the eight-cell stage and only those free of *BRCA* mutations implanted in her body. The procedure is used to "select out" genetic abnormalities and raises many ethical issues. Statistics regarding the frequency of this procedure are not readily available.

Genetic counseling programs for women considering *BRCA* testing explain these issues and mandate time for thought before a sample of blood or saliva is obtained for DNA analysis. After they understand these issues, some young women fear that finding they carry a *BRCA* mutation might cause them to change the trajectory of their lives. They may choose to wait until they have established their personal and professional lives before testing. Others push ahead.

Alisa summarized for Tracy.

"After Cynthia was negative, that left me. For years, Mom has been pushing me to get my testing done. Every time I say later, she tells me I'm just like my aunt . . . Her sister who died."

"So why now?" asked Tracy.

"Well, Mom has been putting more pressure on me now that I am the age her sister was when she died of breast cancer. I know she is getting more anxious." She turned and held Gabriel's hand. "And I have Gabriel now."

Alisa paused, thinking back five years ago to when she had first told Gabriel. Although she had dated other men before, a few even semiseriously, she had never shared the secret, never felt ready. They had been together for about nine months. He was a graduate student from France, handsome and kind. She knew she loved him deeply and thought he felt the same for her, but this would be their first challenge. They had been sitting together on a quiet Sunday morning, doing nothing.

"I need to tell you something about my family," she began. She explained the cancers in her family and her mother's test slowly, hoping he understood. Gabriel's English was very good, but the subject complex.

"I have heard of this," he answered. "You must decide if you are to be tested."

Alisa nodded.

"And if you do test, what will happen?" he asked.

"If I test negative, I'm free of this." She paused. "But if I test positive, I will need to have my breast removed, and later my ovaries."

"That would be sad for you," he answered seriously. "Your breasts are very nice."

"And you?" she asked. "How would you feel about me?"

"I would be sad, too," he said.

"Would you still love me?" she persisted.

"Would you love me if I lost my arm?" he asked. When she nodded emphatically, he continued. "Then why would I feel differently about your breast? La même chose."

"There is more," she warned. She explained that if her test were positive, any of her children would have a fifty-fifty chance of carrying the mutation. She told him it was possible to do *in vitro* fertilization and select the embryos that did not carry the mutation for implantation into the woman.

"That makes no sense to me," he replied.

"I understand it's a strange idea," Alisa answered, thinking of the mechanics of sperm donation, fertilization, and implantation.

"It has not to do with strange. It makes no sense," he answered firmly. "If this technology had been available for your parents, it would have, how would you say, unselect the woman I love."

That had seemed like enough for one day. Although they had discussed it again later, Gabriel had never wavered.

Alisa smiled at the memory before returning to the moment with Tracy.

"Gabriel and I are going to be married next year. He told me it didn't matter to him, but now I think we should know since it will affect his life, too."

Alisa's testing was straightforward. Since her mother had the del185AG gene mutation, there was a fifty-fifty chance Alisa had inherited the same mutation. To exclude any surprises from her father's side, the lab would also check for the other two Ashkenazi Jewish mutations. If Alisa's test were negative, she would be free of the family curse. If Alisa tested positive, she would have a very high chance of breast and ovarian cancer. Tracy completed the counseling by reviewing her options.

After the visit, Tracy had summarized for Dr. Matthews. "She's a lovely thirty-three-year-old Jewish woman whose mother has a known *BRCA-1* mutation, the del185AG. She is in excellent health, never any breast or gynecologic issues, has regular mammograms, breast MRIs, and exams with Dr. Gold. She has one sister, already negative, and no children. Her mother has been pushing her for years to get tested, and now she wants it before she gets married. I've done all the counseling."

Dr. Matthews introduced himself and was quickly satisfied Alisa had no other questions, so Tracy drew her blood and placed it in the package to be sent to an outside lab.

OWNING BRCA.

Once the *BRCA* genes were cloned, the technology to detect mutations was available in many labs, several of which began commercial testing—until Myriad Genetics stopped them. In 1997, the small biotech company in Utah was granted patents for *BRCA-1* and *BRCA-2* and shortly thereafter it issued a "cease and desist" order. Myriad's ownership of these genes and its use of patent protection was one of the controversies unleashed by this new era of genetic testing.

Myriad Genetics was founded in 1991 by Mark Skolnick, the leader of the team which eventually cloned the *BRCA* genes. Skolnick had been instrumental in the establishment of Utah Population Database (UPDB), which combined records of the Utah Cancer Registry with genealogical records from the Church of Jesus Christ of Latter-day Saints (informally called the Mormon Church) and death certificates. The Mormon Church's records dated to the first ten thousand pioneers who were led to Salt Lake Valley in 1847 by Brigham Young. Interestingly, from a genetic viewpoint, this group was diverse and represented many (white) ethnic backgrounds found in the United States, making it a particularly valuable resource. At the time of the BRCA searches in the mid-1990s, the database had information on over one million people.[567] Skolnick's work helped Myriad obtain financial support, including from Eli Lilly, and the resources of the UPDB helped the cloning of the *BRCA* genes.

After cloning the *BRCA* genes, Myriad applied for patents. With *BRCA-1* they faced competing applications from OncorMed, whose patents they acquired. With *BRCA-2* they faced criticism for submitting their application the day before a British coalition also reported sequencing the gene. Despite these initial disputes, by the late 1990s, Myriad was the sole proprietor of the *BRCA* testing in the U.S. and most of the world. As Myriad rolled out testing, the combination of scientific and clinical excitement with the promise of financial reward produced a fascinating struggle.[568]

Myriad's sole possession of *BRCA* produced benefits. The company offered high-quality laboratory work, obviously an important first step as genetic testing for a common cancer was introduced. Myriad offered its testing through physicians, experimenting only later with "direct to consumer" marketing in a few areas. Their educational material helped both clinicians and patients. Since Myriad was the only source of testing, their complete database allowed a more rapid characterization of *BRCA* abnormalities as either mutations or normal variants. This database also meant that when patients were unsure if they had undergone testing or as the testing technology changed, it was easy to find results. Multiple companies doing testing would have made this initial process of characterizing abnormalities and tracking results more fragmented. Had Myriad been a government or academic program, it would have been judged a success for achieving these results.[569]

Not everyone was pleased with this arrangement. Myriad's cease and desist order infuriated many scientists who believed that once genes were discovered, they should be available for research. Although the company eventually made clear the order did not apply to research testing, the resentment (possibly mixed with some jealousy) persisted.[570] As guidelines for testing were developed, many regarded Myriad's marketing with suspicion. In the academic medical community, debate arose over who should control testing and counsel patients. Geneticists and genetics counselors asserted their expertise but were few. Oncologists, breast surgeons, and oncology nurses felt they were well positioned to understand the issues while obstetricians/gynecologists and primary care physicians were already involved in women's cancer screening. Ethicists had their viewpoints. State governments established advisory groups and organized guidelines.[571] Health insurance companies and administrators also weighed in on the proper use and cost of this testing. Life and disability insurers affirmed their rights to use testing in evaluations for policies.[572] Patient advocacy groups sought to make appropriate testing widely available while promoting protection against discrimination. All these constituencies typically had little experience with patent law or sympathy for Myriad's corporate goals, so criticism of the company often became a starting point for consensus.

The fundamental nature of Myriad's business required that it set a price to maximize (or at least produce) profit based upon predicted use, a decision for which there was no precedent. The company then had to promote testing within the ill-defined bounds of proper use of the new technology. Although *BRCA* testing comprised only a minuscule portion of health care expenditures and was insignificant compared with new drugs, the importance of breast cancer prompted considerable public interest in the price. At about $3500 for a complete test, the price was commonly viewed as high. In addition, Myriad's promotion of testing was often termed aggressive. For example, the company supplied clinicians a method to estimate the risk of a positive test which encouraged testing in some lower risk groups, although it may have underestimated the positives in the higher risk groups. This could be viewed as either a scientific difference of opinion or a strategy to sell tests to the more numerous low-risk women.[573] In the final analysis, Myriad's customers often viewed it as a reliable company while it was sharply criticized by its numerous public detractors, including the author Michael Crichton who wrote the book *Next* about an evil biotech company. Crichton included an essay in his book specifically denouncing Myriad's ownership of *BRCA* testing as part of a discussion of patent protection in the biotech world. In the financial world, the opinion was that Myriad's investors should win a "Nobel Prize for patience" since it took until 2008 for the company make a profit on $500 million dollars of investment.[574]

Regardless of Myriad's pricing and presentation of the technology, it was inevitable that the company's control of *BRCA* would face legal challenge—owning the rights to a gene was unacceptable to many groups. In 2009, the ACLU and Public Patent Foundation sued Myriad, the University of Utah Research Foundation, and the U.S. Patent and Trademark Office. After several years of twists and turns in the legal system, on April 15, 2013, the case reached the Supreme Court as *Association for Molecular Pathology et al. v. Myriad Genetics, Inc. et al.* The basic question was whether a gene could be patented by its discoverers. On June 13, 2103, the Court resoundingly answered "no," and Myriad lost its patent protection. The opinion, written by Justice Thomas and joined by Justices Roberts, Kennedy, Ginsburg, Breyer, Alito, Sotomayor and Kagan, began with a remarkable explanation of molecular science and concluded with the finding that naturally occurring DNA, including the *BRCA* genes, could not be patented. Justice Scalia concurred in the judgment but, in his immitigable style, refused to endorse the scientific explanations since he was "unable to affirm those details on my own knowledge or even my own belief."[575] Most of the public probably agreed with him on all counts.

Predictably, Myriad's loss of the *BRCA* patents produced more competition. Several labs offer the testing, now often combined with analysis of other genes. Prices have declined as competition and new advertising has increased. Combined with greater experience in genetic counseling, this has further pushed *BRCA* testing into the "everyday medical care" envisioned when the genes were first cloned. More patients anxiously await their results.

Alisa and Gabriel were holding hands as Tracy entered the room, sat opposite them, and went right to the point.

"You do not have the mutation," she said. "The test was negative."

As Alisa smiled, Gabriel looked relieved. She kissed him then turned to Tracy.

"I'm very glad. Thank you for doing the test and being so supportive," she said.

"What now? Is there anything else we must do?" asked Gabriel, still processing the information.

Alisa answered. "No, my dear. We can tell my mother that I will not be like Aunt Carol. It all ends here."

Acknowledgments

My thanks to those who shaped my professional life starts with two outstanding physicians: my late father, Xavier (Sam) Mastrianni, and his brother, Anthony Mastrianni. Even before I considered this career, these two sons of Italian immigrants taught me what it meant to be a "doctor's doctor" as they bore witness to the American dream. My premedical career began in the Saratoga Springs City Schools, where my mathematics teacher, Peter Kurto, thought I had potential and organized his fellow teachers to push me along—an example of what the public-school system can accomplish when good teachers have freedom. The Department of History at Princeton University taught me to write. My medical training started at Albany Medical College, where the faculty combined highly technical academic work with an apprenticeship in a remarkably personal manner. My advisor, the late Dr. Orlando Hines, prescribed the details of my training in his gruff voice, which always conveyed great humanism to his patients but did not encourage course options for his students. He insisted I study the basic foundations of medicine and surgery, and I remain grateful. My fellow students also contributed to my education in thousands of ways—they are a remarkable group. My medical residency was at the George Washington University in Washington, D.C., where I saw first-hand the ravages of HIV/AIDS and the medical and political struggles of that plague. Once again, I met a remarkable faculty dedicated to their patients and medical education. A chance discussion with one professor over lunch about emerging molecular science led me to study cancer medicine.

My hematology/oncology training program at Beth Israel Medical Center/ Harvard Medical School in Boston was breathtaking. The program directors, Dr. Lowell Schnipper and the late Dr. Stephen Robinson, assembled an oncology dream-team whose stars included Drs. Lawrence Shulman, Steven Come, J. Paul Eder, and the late Roger Lange. Along with many other faculty members and a remarkable nursing staff, they were on the cutting edge of the "age of chemotherapy." After clinical training, I entered the lab of Dr. Daniel Tenen, where I learned of both the molecular techniques which would change our world and the passion of brilliant scientists. Most of those who contributed to my professional education cannot be listed; they are too numerous. But I hope this incomplete list reinforces that medical education, of all types and at all levels, is the underpinning of our healthcare system.

After six years in Boston, I returned to Saratoga Springs as an oncologist to begin my clinical career and repay my teaching debt to Albany Medical College. In starting an oncology practice, I relied on two outstanding radiation oncology colleagues, Drs. Lance Hellman and Alex Frank. They and countless others, including physicians, nurses, and office staff made it a success.

Acknowledging those in my personal life is a pleasure. My father and mother, Beverley Mastrianni, provided my siblings and me with remarkable childhood. My children (Angela, Francesca, and Sam), in-laws (Dolores and Angelo), and extended family bless my adult life. At the center of it all is Lucille Albergo, an oncology nurse practitioner, mother, and my partner. Together, we raised our family and began the practice in Saratoga Springs. Her work influenced every patient who entered the office and is on every page in this book.

The final acknowledgment goes to my patients. As my father said, "when patients come to us for treatment, they are trusting us not only with care of their illness, but in a broader sense they are trusting us with their lives. They share with us their views of themselves, their families and their world. The more vulnerable they are, the greater care we must take, not only to respect the power of their illness but their individual strengths and uniqueness. When they leave here, they should not only feel better about their illness, but better about themselves. In other words, their illness should never be treated at the expense of their humanity." I am grateful for what my patients have shared and in awe of their courage and humanity.

References

CAROL FEINMAN 1: BREAST CANCER

1. Chapter One "Introduction to the History of Breast Cancer" by William Donegan in <u>Cancer of the Breast</u> edited by William Donegan and John S. Spratt, Fourth Edition, W.B. Saunders Company, Philadelphia, 1995. This is an excellent starting point.

2. The *New England Journal of Medicine* is the premier medical journal in the United States. In 2012, the *Journal* published a series of articles to celebrate its 200th anniversary. These articles are a fascinating course in the history of medicine. The article reviewing surgery is: Gawande A. Two Hundred Years of Surgery. N Engl J Med; 336:1716-23, 2012.

3. Worboys M. Joseph Lister and the Performance of Antiseptic Surgery. Notes and Records of the Royal Society of London 67(3):199–209, 2013. This reviews Lister's struggles.

4. <u>The Cambridge History of Medicine</u> edited by Roy Porter, Cambridge University Press, Cambridge, 2006. This period is covered in Chapter 6 by Roy Porter, titled "Hospitals and Surgery." See page 199.

5. The debate over the extent of the mastectomy required to treat breast cancer extended over many years and involved many famous medical figures. Chapter One "Introduction to the History of Breast Cancer" by William Donegan in <u>Cancer of the Breast</u> edited by William Donegan and John S. Spratt, Fourth Edition, W.B. Saunders Company, Philadelphia, 1995, is an excellent review.

6. Chapter One "Introduction to the History of Breast Cancer" by William Donegan in <u>Cancer of the Breast</u> edited by William

Donegan and John S. Spratt, Fourth Edition, W.B. Saunders Company, Philadelphia, 1995, describes these procedures.

7. Harris JR, Lippman ME, Veronesi U et al. Breast Cancer. N Engl J Med; 327:390-398, 1992.

HAROLD CRIMONS: SMALL CELL LUNG CANCER

8. From the World Health Organization. http://www.who.int/mediacentre/factsheets/fs297/en/. Accessed 2/17.

9. The Cigarette Century by Allan M. Brandt, Basic Books, New York, 2007. Chapter 1. This history of tobacco should be read by anyone interested in public health or medicine.

10. Forces of Habit: Drugs and the Making of the Modern World by David T. Courtwright. Harvard University Press, Cambridge, 2001. Page 70.

11. Forces of Habit: Drugs and the Making of the Modern World by David T. Courtwright. Harvard University Press, Cambridge, 2001. Pages 14-18 review this early history.

12. The Cigarette Century by Allan M. Brandt, Basic Books, New York, 2007. Page 25.

13. Forces of Habit: Drugs and the Making of the Modern World by David T. Courtwright. Harvard University Press, Cambridge, 2001. Pages 112-122 review this period.

14. The Cigarette Century by Allan M. Brandt, Basic Books, New York, 2007. Chapter 2.

15. As told to the author.

16. <u>The Merck Manual</u>, Eighth Edition, Merck & Co, Inc., Rahway, NJ, 1950. Page 1284.

17. <u>The Emperor of All Maladies</u> by Siddhartha Mukherjee, Scribner, New York, 2010. The struggles of the Surgeon General and his Committee begins on page 258.

18. <u>The Cigarette Century</u> by Allan M. Brandt, Basic Books, New York, 2007. Chapter 7 and 8.

19. <u>The Cigarette Century</u> by Allan M. Brandt, Basic Books, New York, 2007. Chapter 11 and 12.

20. <u>The Cigarette Century</u> by Allan M. Brandt, Basic Books, New York, 2007. Chapter 11 and 12.

21. <u>The Biology of Cancer</u> by Robert A. Weinberg, Garland Science, New York, 2014. This comprehensive text, written by one of the leaders in molecular biology, covers this process in detail.

22. Haggard HW and Smith GM. Johannes Muller and the Modern Conception of Cancer. Yale J of Biol and Med; 10(5):419-436, 1938.

23. <u>The Biology of Cancer</u> by Robert A. Weinberg, Garland Science, New York, 2014. Page 468.

24. <u>The Biology of Cancer</u> by Robert A. Weinberg, Garland Science, New York, 2014. Page 2.

25. Smith BD, Haffty BG, Wilson TJ et al. The Future of Radiation Oncology in the United States From 2010 to 2020: Will Supply Keep Pace With Demand? J Clin Oncol; 28(35):5160-5165, 2010.

26. <u>Strange Glow: The Story of Radiation</u> by Timothy J. Jorgensen, Princeton University Press, Princeton, NJ, 2016. See chapter 1, page 25 and chapter 6, page 120.

27. "Medical linear accelerator celebrates 50 years of treating cancer." by Mitzi Baker in Stanford Report, April 18, 2007.http://news. stanford.edu/news/2007/april18/med-accelerator-041807.html. Accessed 12/16.

28. See Chapter 21 "Principles of Radiation Oncology" by Theodore S. Lawrence, Randall K. Ten Haken and Amato Giacca in Cancer: <u>Principles and Practice of Oncology, 8th Edition</u> by Vincent DeVita, Theodore Lawrence and Steven Rosenberg, Lippincott Williams & Wilkens, Phildelphia, 2008.

29. Woywodt A and Matteson EL. Wegener's granulomatosis—probing the untold past of the man behind the eponym. Rheumatology; 45:1303–1306, 2006.

30. The Holocaust Museum, Washington, D.C. 4/16.

31. Topaz M, Shafran-Topaz L, Bowles KH. ICD-9 to ICD-10: Evolution, Revolution, and Current Debates in the United States. Perspectives in Health Information Management / AHIMA, American Health Information Management Association; 10(Spring): 1-8, 2013.

32. Green A, Humphrey E, Close H et al. Alkylating Agents in Bronchogenic Carcinoma. Am J Med; 46:516-525, 1969.

33. Ihde D. Chemotherapy of Lung Cancer. N Engl J Med; 327(20): 1434-1441, 1992.

KATHY MULVANEY: HODGKIN'S LYMPHOMA

34. Hodgkin's lymphoma is also written as Hodgkin lymphoma and Hodgkins lymphoma.

35. The chapter contains a reference to Dr. J Maxwell Chamberlain. The information comes from Sloan H. J Maxwell Chamberlain, 1906-1968. Ann Thorac Surg; 32:109-110, 1981.

36. The details of Hodgkin's life come primarily from two works: Perfecting the World: The Life and Times of Dr. Thomas Hodgkin 1789-1866 by Amalia and Edward Kass, Harcourt Brace Jovanovich, Orlando, 1988. This is a detailed and wonderfully written account of Hodgkin's life. Edward Kass was an internationally known expert in infectious diseases who established Harvard's Channing Lab (among his many accomplishments). Amalia Kass is a well-known historian. Both were honored with named Professorships at Harvard. Thomas Hodgkin: Morbid Anatomist, Social Activist by Louis Rosenfeld, Madison Books, Lanham, Maryland, 1993, is another enjoyable work with a slightly different perspective on Hodgkin's life. A third brief overview and perspective about Hodgkin's life in the context of modern cancer care is provided by a well-known pioneer in cancer medicine, Dr. Samuel Hellman: Hellman S. Thomas Hodgkin and Hodgkin's Disease: Two Paradigms Appropriate to Medicine Today. JAMA; 265:1007-1010, 1991.

37. Richard Bright 1789-1858 Physician in the Age of Reform by Diana Berry and Campbell Mackenzie, Dorset Press, Dorchester, 1992. Chapter 2 covers the same era.

38. Thomas Hodgkin: Morbid Anatomist, Social Activist by Louis Rosenfeld, Madison Books, Lanham, Maryland, 1993. Page 131. The added comment is the author's.

39. The Cambridge History of Medicine edited by Roy Porter, Cambridge University Press, New York, NY, 2006. This covers the history of this period. See page 153.

40. The Cambridge History of Medicine edited by Roy Porter, Cambridge University Press, New York, NY, 2006. Covered in Chapter 6, "Hospitals and Surgery" by Roy Porter.

41. The Cambridge History of Medicine edited by Roy Porter, Cambridge University Press, New York, 2006. Page 197.

42. Perfecting the World: The Life and Times of Dr. Thomas Hodgkin 1789-1866 by Amalia and Edward Kass, Harcourt Brace Jovanovich, Orlando, 1988. This provides an introduction to the Quakers in Chapter 1.

43. Perfecting the World: The Life and Times of Dr. Thomas Hodgkin 1789-1866 by Amalia and Edward Kass, Harcourt Brace Jovanovich, Orlando, 1988. Page 7.

44. Thomas Hodgkin: Morbid Anatomist, Social Activist by Louis Rosenfeld, Madison Books, Lanham, Maryland, 1993. Page 9.

45. Perfecting the World: The Life and Times of Dr. Thomas Hodgkin 1789-1866 by Amalia and Edward Kass, Harcourt Brace Jovanovich, Orlando, 1988. Page 17-27.

46. A Brief History of Disease, Science and Medicine by Michael T. Kennedy, Asklepiad Press, Mission Viejo, CA, 2004. Page 126.

47. This history is well covered in both Perfecting the World: The Life and Times of Dr. Thomas Hodgkin 1789-1866 by Amalia and Edward Kass, Harcourt Brace Jovanovich, Orlando, 1988 and

Thomas Hodgkin: Morbid Anatomist, Social Activist by Louis Rosenfeld, Madison Books, Lanham, Maryland, 1993.

48. This history is covered in both _Perfecting the World: The Life and Times of Dr. Thomas Hodgkin 1789-1866_ by Amalia and Edward Kass, Harcourt Brace Jovanovich, Orlando, 1988 and _Thomas Hodgkin: Morbid Anatomist, Social Activist_ by Louis Rosenfeld, Madison Books, Lanham, Maryland, 1993.

49. _A Biographical History of Guy's Hospital_ by Samuel Wilks and George Thomas Bettany, Ward, Lock, Bowden & Co, London, 1892. Page 384. Wilks provides a first-hand account of the issue.

50. _Perfecting the World: The Life and Times of Dr. Thomas Hodgkin 1789-1866_ by Amalia and Edward Kass, Harcourt Brace Jovanovich, Orlando, 1988. Chapter 18, page 273. _Thomas Hodgkin: Morbid Anatomist, Social Activist_ by Louis Rosenfeld, Madison Books, Lanham, Maryland, 1993. Page 162.

51. _Perfecting the World: The Life and Times of Dr. Thomas Hodgkin 1789-1866_ by Amalia and Edward Kass, Harcourt Brace Jovanovich, Orlando, 1988. Chapter 32, page 499.

52. Hodgkin, T. On some marked appearances of absorbent glands and spleen. Medico-Chirurg. Tr. London; 17:68-114, 1832.

53. Banerjee AK. Sir Samuel Wilks: a foundering father of clinical science. J Roy Soc Med; 84: 44-45, 1991. Describes Wilks and his contributions to medicine.

54. Wilks, S. Cases of enlargement of lymphatic glands and spleen (or, Hodgkin's disease). Guy's Hosp Rep: 11:56-67, 1865.

55. Bonadonna G. Historical Review of Hodgkin's Disease. Brit J Haem; 110:504-511, 2000.

56. Rosenfeld C. Hodgkin's Disease: Origin of an Eponym—And One That Got Away. Bull NY Acad Med; 65(5):618-632, 1989.

57. DeVita V, Chu E. A History of Cancer Chemotherapy. Cancer Research; 68:8643-8653, 2008. Dr. Vincent DeVita, a pioneer in the use of chemotherapy, captures the excitement and disappointments of these early efforts.

58. DeVita V, Chu E. A History of Cancer Chemotherapy. Cancer Research; 68:8643-8653, 2008.

59. The Emperor of All Maladies by Siddhartha Mukherjee, Scribner, New York, 2010.

60. DeVita V, Chu E. A History of Cancer Chemotherapy. Cancer Research; 68:8643-8653, 2008.

61. The history of the Lasker Awards and a set of photographs of the winners is on the Lasker Foundation website (www.laskerfoundation.org). Accessed 1/17.

62. The Mary Lasker Papers. Profiles in Science. U.S. National Library of Medicine. https://profiles.nlm.nih.gov/ps/retrieve/Narrative/TL/p-nid/199. Accessed 2/17.

63. The Emperor of All Maladies by Siddhartha Mukherjee, Scribner, New York, 2010. See pages 111-114.

64. Mary Lasker's oral history is available from Columbia University Libraries Oral History Research Office of Notable New Yorkers.

http://www.columbia.edu/cu/lweb/digital/collections/nny/laskerm/. Accessed 1/17.

65. From the World Health Organization. http://www.who.int/mediacentre/factsheets/fs297/en/ Accessed 2/17.

66. Greenfield WS. Specimens illustrative of pathology of lymphadenoma and leucocythoemia. Tr. Path. Soc. London; 29:272-304, 1878. His description appears on page 303.

67. Jackson H, Parker F. Hodgkin's Disease. N Engl J Med; 230(1):1-8, 1944.

68. Burkitt DP. The Discovery of Burkitt's Lymphoma. Cancer; 51:1 777-1786, 1983. This is a very descriptive account of the discovery.

69. Epstein A. Burkitt lymphoma and the discovery of Epstein-Barr virus. Brit J Haem; 156:777-779, 2012.

70. Epstein A. Burkitt lymphoma and the discovery of Epstein-Barr virus. Brit J Haem; 156:777-779, 2012.

71. Burkitt DP. The Discovery of Burkitt's Lymphoma. Cancer; 51:1777-1786, 1983.

72. Henle G, Henle W and Diehl V. Relation of Burkitt's tumor-associated herpes-type virus to infectious mononucleosis. Proc Natl Acad Sci USA; 59(1):94–101, 1968.

MARK LUCIANO: CHRONIC MYELOGENOUS LEUKEMIA

73. The description of the growth of CML as "leisurely" was made in the classic textbook <u>Blood: A Textbook of Hematology</u> by James H. Jandl, Little, Brown and Company, Boston, 1987. Dr. Jandl was

a well-known hematologist who wrote an entire textbook himself. Since in the modern age of medicine most textbooks are written by multiple authors, this was a singular accomplishment. His writing often includes highly personalized and poetic descriptions of blood disorders.

74. Kamada N and Uchino H. Chronologic Sequence in Appearance of Clinical and Laboratory Findings Characteristic of Chronic Myelogenous Leukemia. Blood; 51(5):843-850, 1978.

75. Drucker B. Translation of the Philadelphia chromosome into therapy for CML. Blood; 112:4808-4817, 2008. Dr. Drucker pioneered the treatment of CML with imatinib, and his article is a complete review.

76. Drucker B. Translation of the Philadelphia chromosome into therapy for CML. Blood; 112:4808-4817, 2008.

77. Chandra HS, Heistekamp NC, Hungerford A et al.: Philadelphia Chromosome Symposium: commemoration of the 50th anniversary of the discovery of the Ph chromosome. Cancer Genetics; 204(4):171-179, 2011. This article provides some personal aspects of the discovery.

78. Chandra HS, Heistekamp NC, Hungerford A et al.: Philadelphia Chromosome Symposium: commemoration of the 50th anniversary of the discovery of the Ph chromosome. Cancer Genetics; 204(4):171-179, 2011.

79. Chandra HS, Heistekamp NC, Hungerford A et al.: Philadelphia Chromosome Symposium: commemoration of the 50th anniversary of the discovery of the Ph chromosome. Cancer Genetics; 204(4):171-179, 2011.

80. Institute of Medicine (US) Immunization Safety Review Committee; Stratton K, Almario DA, McCormick MC, editors. Immunization Safety Review: SV40 Contamination of Polio Vaccine and Cancer. Washington (DC): National Academies Press (US); 2002. Available from: https://www.ncbi.nlm.nih.gov/books/NBK221113/ doi: 10.17226/10534. Accessed 12/16.

81. Berg P and Singer M. The Recombinant DNA controversy: Twenty years later. Natl Acad Sci USA; 92:9011-9013, 1995.

82. Berg P and Singer M. The Recombinant DNA controversy: Twenty years later. Natl Acad Sci USA; 92:9011-9013, 1995.

83. The NIH Recombinant DNA Guidelines: Brief History and Current Status. Issue Brief Number IB82057 by Judith A. Johnson, 1982. https://digital.library.unt.edu/ark:/67531/.../IB82057_1982 Jul07.pdf. This is a summary of the events.

84. The Recombinant DNA Controversy. A Memoir. Science, Politics and the Public Interest 1974-1981 by Donald S. Frederickson, ASM Press, Washington, DC, 2001. Dr. Frederickson was director of the NIH, and his memoirs provide an interesting view of the issues.

85. Chandra HS, Heistekamp NC, Hungerford A et al.: Philadelphia Chromosome Symposium: commemoration of the 50th anniversary of the discovery of the Ph chromosome. Cancer Genetics; 204(4):171-179, 2011.

86. Daley GQ, Van Etten RA, Baltimore D. Induction of chronic myelogenous leukemia in mice by the P210bcr/abl gene of the Philadelphia chromosome. Science; 247:824–830, 1990.

87. The Emperor of All Maladies by Siddhartha Mukherjee, Scribner, New York, 2010. The discussion of this chemistry is beautifully detailed on pages 431-433.

88. Drucker B. Translation of the Philadelphia chromosome into therapy for CML. Blood; 112:4808-4817, 2008.

89. Radich JP. How I monitor residual disease in chronic myeloid leukemia. Blood; 114:3376-3381, 2009.

90. Windows into the Earth: The Geologic Story of Yellowstone and The Grand Teton National Parks by Robert B. Smith and Lee J. Siegel, The Oxford Press, Oxford, 2000. This is an excellent history of the park and its geology for the non-geologist. Much of the history which follows comes from this text.

91. Brock T. The Value of Basic Research: Discovery of Thermus Aquaticus and Other Extreme Thermophiles. Genetics; 146:1207-1210, 1997.

92. Making PCR: A Story of Biotechnology by Paul Rabinow, The University of Chicago Press, Chicago, 1996. This is a history of Cetus which describes the development of the PCR in the context of the upheaval of the time and the personalities of those involved. It includes some interesting interviews with the key figures.

93. Making PCR: A Story of Biotechnology by Paul Rabinow, The University of Chicago Press, Chicago, 1996. Page 47.

94. Making PCR: A Story of Biotechnology by Paul Rabinow, The University of Chicago Press, 1996. Page 62.

95. Making PCR: A Story of Biotechnology by Paul Rabinow, The University of Chicago Press, Chicago, 1996. Page 93.

96. Making PCR: A Story of Biotechnology by Paul Rabinow, The University of Chicago Press, Chicago, 1996. Page 128.

97. Making PCR: A Story of Biotechnology by Paul Rabinow, The University of Chicago Press, Chicago, 1996. Page 159-164.

CAROL FEINMAN 2: BREAST CANCER

98. Fisher B, Ravdin RG, Ausman RK et al. Surgical adjuvant chemotherapy in cancer of the breast: Results of a decade of cooperative investigation. Ann Surg; 168:337-356, 1968.

99. Two trials began the era of adjuvant chemotherapy treatments for breast cancer: Fisher B, Carbone P, Economou SG et al. L-phenylalanine mustard (L-PAM) in the management of primary breast cancer: A report of early findings. N Engl J Med; 292:117-122, 1975. Bonadonna G, Brusamolino E, Valagussa P et al. Combination chemotherapy as an adjuvant treatment in operable breast cancer. N Engl J Med; 294:405-410, 1976.

100. The era of adjuvant chemotherapy for breast cancer in the United States began with "CMF," a combination of oral cyclophosphamide with intravenous methotrexate and 5-FU given for twelve months. Later, it was found that six months were equally effective. As described in this chapter, a comparison of six months of CMF with three months of the more intensive combination "AC" (doxorubicin (Adriamycin) and cyclophosphamide (Cytoxan)), given intravenously every three weeks, produced the same results. Because AC was shorter, it was preferred by most physicians and patients. AC was the base program to which the drug paclitaxel (Taxol) was added in the 1990s. The new program, "AC-T," modestly improved the cure rate. Physicians at Memorial Sloan Kettering Cancer Center in New York then shortened the period between the treatments from three weeks to two weeks, further

improving the cure rate. The new program became "dose-dense AC-T" used today.

SANDRA WARREN: BREAST CANCER

101. Warner E. Breast Cancer Screening. N Engl J Med; 365:1025-1032, 2011. This is an example of an academic discussion about mammograms using a case study.

102. The USPSTF website is worth reviewing. http://www.uspreventiveservicestaskforce.org. Accessed 8/16.

103. Oeffinger, KC, Fontham ETH, Etzioni R, et al. Breast Cancer Screening for Women at Average Risk: 2015 Guideline Update From the American Cancer Society. JAMA; 314(15):1599-1614, 2015.

104. Rosen PP, Lesser M, Kinne DW et al. Discontinuous or "Skip" Metastases in Breast Carcinoma. Ann Surg; 197(3):276-283, 1983.

105. Borgstein PJ, Pijpers R, Comans EF et al. Sentinel lymph node biopsy in breast cancer: guidelines and pitfalls of lymphoscintigraphy and gamma probe detection. J Am Coll Surg; 186(3):275-283, 1998.

106. Giuliano AE, McCall L, Beitsch P et al. Locoregional recurrence after sentinel lymph node dissection with or without axillary dissection in patients with sentinel lymph node metastasis: the American College of Surgeons Oncology Group Z0011 randomized trial. Ann Surg; 252(3):426-432, 2010.

107. Fisher B, Ravdin RG, Ausman RK et al. Surgical adjuvant chemotherapy in cancer of the breast: Results of a decade of cooperative investigation. Ann Surg; 168:337-356, 1968.

108. Fisher B, Slack N, Katrych D et al. Ten Year Follow-up of Patients with Carcinoma of the Breast in a Co-operative Clinical Trial Evaluating Surgical Adjuvant Chemotherapy. Surgery, Gynecology & Obstetrics; 140:528-534, 1975.

109. These two trials began the era of adjuvant chemotherapy treatments:

Fisher B, Carbone P, Economou SG et al. L-phenylalanine mustard (L-PAM) in the management of primary breast cancer: A report of early findings. N Engl J Med; 292:117-122, 1975.

Bonadonna G, Brusamolino E, Valagussa P et al. Combination chemotherapy as an adjuvant treatment in operable breast cancer. N Engl J Med; 294:405-410, 1976.

110. Velez-Garcia E, Moore M, Vogel CL et al. Postmastectomy adjuvant chemotherapy with or without radiation therapy in women with operable breast cancer and positive axillary lymph nodes: the Southeastern Cancer Study Group experience. Breast Cancer Res Treat; 3 Suppl: S49-60, 1983.

111. Fisher B, Brown AM, Dimitrov N et al. Two months of doxorubicin-cyclophosphamide with and without reinduction therapy compared with 6 months of cyclophosphamide, methotrexate, and fluorouracil in nodes positive breast cancer patients with tamoxifen non-responsive tumors: Results from the National Surgical Adjuvant Breast and Bowel Project B-15. J Clin Oncol; 8: 1483-1496, 1990.

112. Wood WC, Budman DR, Korzun AH et al. Dose and Dose Intensity of Adjuvant Chemotherapy for Stage II, Node-positive Breast Carcinoma. N Engl J Med; 330:1253-1259, 1994.

113. False Hope: Bone Marrow Transplantation for Breast Cancer by Richard Rettig, Peter Jacobson, Cynthia Farquhar and Wade Aubry, Oxford University Press, New York, 2007. The book documents rise and fall of bone marrow transplant, albeit through a lens of hindsight.

114. Antman KH, Rowlings PA, Vaughan WP et al. High-dose Chemotherapy with Autologous Hematopoietic Stem-Cell Support for Breast Cancer in North America. J Clin Oncol; 15:1870-1879, 1997.

115. Antman KH, Rowlings PA, Vaughan WP et al. High-dose Chemotherapy with Autologous Hematopoietic Stem-Cell Support for Breast Cancer in North America. J Clin Oncol; 15:1870-1879, 1997.

116. Hendersen IC, Berry DA, Demetri GD et al. Improved outcomes from adding sequential Paclitaxel but not from escalating Doxorubicin dose in adjuvant chemotherapy regimen for patients with node-positive primary breast cancer. J Clin Oncol; 21(6):976-983, 2003.

117. Citron ML, Berry DA, Cirrincione C, et al. Randomized trial of dose-dense versus conventionally scheduled and sequential versus concurrent combination chemotherapy as postoperative adjuvant treatment of node-positive primary breast cancer: first report of Intergroup Trial C9741/Cancer and Leukemia Group B Trial 9741. J Clin Oncol; 21(8):1431-1439, 2003.

JOHN EVANS: PANCREATIC CANCER

118. Merchant N. Eat When You Can, Sleep When You Can, and Don't Mess with the Pancreas. Sur Oncol Clin; 25(2):xv-xvi, 2016.

119. Whipple AO, Parsons WB, Mullins CR. Treatment of Carcinoma of the Ampulla of Vater. Annal Surg; 102(4):763-779, 1935.

120. Christy NP. Allen Oldfather Whipple 1881-1963. The Journal of the College of Physicians and Surgeons of Columbia University. www.cumc.columbia.edu/psjournal/archive/archives/jour_v18no3/faculty.html. Accessed 12/16.

121. Whipple AO. The Training of the Surgeon. J Natl Med Assoc; 49(5):295-304, 1959.

122. Cancer: Principles and Practice of Oncology by Vincent T. DeVita, Samuel Hellman and Steven A. Rosenberg, Lippincott Williams & Wilkins, Philadelphia, 2005. Pages 375-379.

123. "Oxaliplatin Approved for Advanced Colorectal Cancer" in Oncology Times; 24(9):31, September 2002.

FRANK JAMES: NON-SMALL CELL LUNG CANCER

124. In 1834, The Royal College of Surgeons had 200 fellows and 8000 licentiates. Most were apothecaries who had taken the examinations. In contrast, there were only 113 Fellows and 275 licentiates of The Royal College of Physicians, figures reported Richard Bright 1789-1858 Physician in an Age of Revolution and Reform by Diana Berry and Campbell Mackenzie, Royal Society of Medicine, London 1992. Page 115.

125. Burroughs, Welcome and Co.: Knowledge, Trust, Profit and the Transformation of the British Pharmaceutical Industry 1880-1940 by Roy Church and E.M. Tansey, Crucible Books, Lancaster, 2007. This work describes the start of the company.

126. Burroughs, Welcome and Co.: Knowledge, Trust, Profit and the Transformation of the British Pharmaceutical Industry 1880-1940 by Roy Church and E.M. Tansey, Crucible Books, Lancaster, 2007. Page 182.

127. "A Rising Drug Industry" by Arthur Daemmrich and Mary Ellen Bowden in *Chemical and Engineering News*, June 20, 2005. This article provides a useful outline of the rise of the pharmaceutical industry and is available at http://cen.acs.org/articles/83/i25/ RISING-DRUG-INDUSTRY.html.

128. Experiment Eleven: Deceit and Betrayal in the Discovery of the Cure for Tuberculosis by Peter Pringle, Bloomsbury, London, 2012. This book documents the poor treatment of Albert Schatz, the PhD student working for Professor Waksman.

129. Pharmcopolitics: Drug Regulation in the United States and Germany by Arthur A. Daemmrich, The University of North Carolina Press, Chapel Hill and London, 2004, Page 55.

130. Charles Heidelberger and Robert Duschinsky patented 5-FU and their application details the synthesis process (US2885396).

131. Corfield PJ. Poison Peddlers to Civic Worthies: The Reputation of Apothecaries in Georgian England. Soc Hist Med; 22(1):1-21, 2009.

132. Reputation and Power: Organization, Image and Pharmaceutical Regulation at the FDA by Daniel Carpenter, Princeton University Press, Princeton and Oxford, 2010. This is an exhaustive history of the FDA.

133. Pharmcopolitics: Drug Regulation in the United States and Germany by Arthur A. Daemmrich, The University of North Carolina Press, Chapel Hill and London, 2004, Page 23.

134. Pharmcopolitics: Drug Regulation in the United States and Germany by Arthur A. Daemmrich, The University of North Carolina Press, Chapel Hill and London, 2004. Page 23-24.

Reputation and Power: Organization, Image and Pharmaceutical Regulation at the FDA by Daniel Carpenter, Princeton University Press, Princeton and Oxford, 2010. Page 73. This chapter gives a detailed description of the creation and passage of the Act.

135. Pharmcopolitics: Drug Regulation in the United States and Germany by Arthur A. Daemmrich, The University of North Carolina Press, Chapel Hill and London, 2004, p 61. These U.S. cases were the result of Merrell's enrolling thousands of U.S. doctors to act as clinical testers of the medicine, a common practice in that era which ended as modern clinical trials became standard.

136. Dr. Kelsey's recollections are available on the FDA website. https://www.fda.gov/downloads/AboutFDA/WhatWeDo/History/OralHistories/SelectedOralHistoryTranscripts/UCM406132.pdf. Accessed 3/17.

137. The FDA has an excellent history. https://www.fda.gov/newsevents/speeches/ucm324214.htm. Accessed 3/17.

138. The report of the use of thalidomide in the medical literature is:

Singhal S, Mehta J, Desikan R et al. Antitumor Activity of Thalidomide in Refractory Multiple Myeloma. N Engl J Med; 341:1565-1571, 1999.

In the lay press: "Thalidomide Found to Slow a Bone Cancer" by Sheryl Gay Stolberg in The New York Times, November 18, 1999.

139. "FDA and Clinical Drug Trials: A Short History" by Suzanne White Junod, available on the FDA website www.fda.gov, covers many of these issues with a history of selected clinical trials.

140. <u>Reputation and Power: Organization, Image and Pharmaceutical Regulation at the FDA</u> by Daniel Carpenter, Princeton University Press, Princeton and Oxford, 2010. Page 401 begins an interesting discussion of these battles.

141. <u>Reputation and Power: Organization, Image and Pharmaceutical Regulation at the FDA</u> by Daniel Carpenter, Princeton University Press, Princeton and Oxford, 2010. Page 410.

142. Although underappreciated in today's world, the curse of diphtheria is well documented in many sources. The *Wikipedia* articles on the illness and the death of Princess Alice are useful starting points.

143. http://www.historyofvaccines.org/content/articles/passive-immunization. The Philadelphia College of Physicians website has an excellent history of vaccines and the controversies over vaccinations. Accessed 3/17.

144. http://www.lister-institute.org.uk/about-us/our-heritage/ includes a photograph of Tom. Accessed 3/17.

145. <u>Burroughs, Welcome and Co.: Knowledge, Trust, Profit and the Transformation of the British Pharmaceutical Industry 1880-1940</u> by Roy Church and E.M. Tansey, Crucible Books, Lancaster, 2007. Page 203.

146. In New York State, the Wadsworth lab is an example which can be found at: https://www.wadsworth.org/search/results/diphtheria. Accessed 3/17.

147. From <u>The Truth About the Drug Companies</u> by Marcia Angell, Random House, NY, 2004.

148. Genentech: The Beginnings of Biotech by Sally Smith Hughes, The University of Chicago Press, Chicago, 2011. This book details the rise of the company and forms much of the basis of this section.

149. Genentech: The Beginnings of Biotech by Sally Smith Hughes, The University of Chicago Press, Chicago, 2011.

150. Genentech: The Beginnings of Biotech by Sally Smith Hughes, The University of Chicago Press, Chicago, 2011. Page 59.

151. Genentech: The Beginnings of Biotech by Sally Smith Hughes, The University of Chicago Press, Chicago, 2011. Chapter 4 beginning on page 75. See also chapter 5, page 126.

152. Genentech: The Beginnings of Biotech by Sally Smith Hughes, The University of Chicago Press, 2011. Beginning page 142.

153. "A Tale of Taxol" by Frank Stephenson on the Florida State University website. www.rinr.fsu.edu/fall2002/taxol.html. Accessed 12/15.

154. "The Discovery of Camptothecin and Taxol." A history by the American Chemical Society at www.acs.org/.../camptothecintaxol/discovery-of-camptothecin-and-taxol-commemorative-booklet.pdf. Accessed 12/15.

155. McGuire WP, Rowinsky EK, Rosenshein NB et al. Taxol: a unique antineoplastic agent with significant activity in advanced ovarian epithelial neoplasms. Ann Intern Med; 111(4):273-279, 1989.

156. "Bristol-Myers Squibb to Pay $670 Million to Settle Numerous Lawsuits" by Melody Petersen in The New York Times, January 8, 2003.

157. The National Cancer Institute website promotes Taxol as a "Success Story." https://dtp.cancer.gov/timeline/flash/success_stories/S2_Taxol.htm. Accessed 12/15.

158. Dr. DeVita makes his views clear in a review of the book <u>The Story of Taxol: Nature and Politics in the Pursuit of an Anti-Cancer Drug</u> by Jordan Goodman and Vivien Walsh, Cambridge University Press, New York, 2001. Dr. DeVita's review appeared in N Engl J Med; 344:1335-1336, 2001.

159. <u>The Truth About the Drug Companies</u> by Marcia Angell, Random House, New York, 2004. Page 58-59.

CAROL FEINMAN 3: BREAST CANCER

160. Randy Shilts' <u>And the Band Played On: Politics, People and the AIDS Epidemic</u>, St. Martin's Press, New York, 1987, was a rallying cry for the gay community. It is highly critical of almost everyone: the gay community, government, and many medical/scientific leaders. Mr. Shilts died of AIDS in 1994. A more traditional historical account of the epidemic is <u>AIDS at 30: A History</u> by Victoria Harden, Potomac Books, Washington, D.C., 2012. Ms. Harden was the founding director of the Office of NIH history and an award winning medical historian.

161. A nice review of the debate is "Researchers Clear 'Patient Zero' from AIDS Origin Story" by Michaeleen Doucleff, NPR, October 26, 2016 at www.npr.org/sections/health-shots/2016/.../mystery-solved-how-hiv-came-to-the-u-s. Accessed 12/16.

162. MMWR; 50(21):430-434, 2001. Available at CDC.gov. Accessed 12/16.

163. "A Brief Chronology of Retrovirology" in <u>Retroviruses</u> by JM Coffin, SH Hughes, HE Varmus, editors, Cold Spring

Harbor Laboratory Press, Cold Spring Harbor, 1997. Available from: http://www.ncbi.nlm.nih.gov/books/NBK19403/. Accessed 3/17.

164. "A Brief Chronology of Retrovirology" in <u>Retroviruses</u> by JM Coffin, SH Hughes, HE Varmus, editors, Cold Spring Harbor Laboratory Press, Cold Spring Harbor, 1997. Available from: http://www.ncbi.nlm.nih.gov/books/NBK19403/. Accessed 3/17.

165. A brief summary of the controversy is found in a profile of Dr. Harold Varmus, a brilliant scientist and NIH director at https://profiles.nlm.nih.gov/ps/retrieve/Narrative/MV/p-nid/190. Accessed 12/16.

166. The FDA timeline is found at www.fda.gov/ForPatients/Illness/HIVAIDS/History/ucm151074.htm. Accessed 12/16.

167. <u>HIV And The Blood Supply: An Analysis Of Crisis Decision-making</u> by Institute of Medicine (US) Committee to Study HIV Transmission Through Blood and Blood Products, LB Leveton, HC Sox, MA Stoto, editors, National Academies Press, Washington, D.C., 1995. See "History of the Controversy." Available from: https://www.ncbi.nlm.nih.gov/books/NBK232419/. Accessed 12/16.

168. An excellent general timeline can be found at https://www.aids.gov/hiv-aids-basics/hiv-aids-101/aids-timeline/. Accessed 12/16.

THOMAS JONES: MELANOMA

169. Mimh M. Why Wallace? Hum Path; 30(5):489-490, 1999.

Farber E. Wallace Henderson Clark, Jr.: An Appreciation. Hum Path; 30(5):498-499, 1999.

170. Breslow also did calculations of the volume of the tumor, but this process has been generally abandoned in favor of his simple depth measurement.

171. Breslow A. Thickness, Cross-Sectional Area and Depth of Invasion in the Prognosis of Cutaneous Melanoma. Ann Surg; 172:902-908, 1970.

172. Balch CM. Measuring Melanoma—A Tribute to Alexander Breslow. J Am Acad Derm; 5(1): 96-97, 1981.

173. Interferon: The science and selling of a miracle drug by Toine Peters, Routledge, London and New York, 2005. This is a complete text on the history of interferon.

    Pieters T. Interferon and its first clinical trial: looking behind the scenes. Med Hist; 37(3):270-95, 1993. This article preceded the book and gives more detail into the initial discovery phase of interferon.

174. Zoonomia; or The Laws of Organic Life, Vol II. by Erasmus Darwin, D. Carlisle, Boston, 1803. Page 208.

175. Merigan TC. Interferons of Mice and Men. N Engl J Med; 276:913-920, 1967.

176. Interferon: The science and selling of a miracle drug by Tione Pieters, Routledge, London and New York, 2005. Page 14.

177. Interferon: The science and selling of a miracle drug by Tione Pieters, Routledge, London and New York, 2005. Page 25.

178. Interferon: The science and selling of a miracle drug by Tione Pieters, Routledge, London and New York, 2005. Page 33.

179. Interferon: The science and selling of a miracle drug by Tione Pieters, Routledge, London and New York, 2005. Page 40. The cartoon is reproduced here.

180. Pieters T. Interferon and its first clinical trial: looking behind the scenes. Med Hist; 37(3):270-95, 1993. Pieters makes this point very clearly in this article and again later in his book.

181. Interferon: The science and selling of a miracle drug by Tione Pieters, Routledge, London and New York, 2005. Page 74.

182. The commentary was titled: Interferon. Br Med J; 2:1612, 1964.

183. Friedman RM. Clinical uses of interferons. British Journal of Clinical Pharmacology, 65:158–162, 2008. This brief article gives a nice summary of the different types of interferons and these biologic issues.

184. Interferon: The science and selling of a miracle drug by Tione Pieters, Routledge, London and New York, 2005. Page 103.

185. Interferon: The science and selling of a miracle drug by Tione Pieters, Routledge, London and New York, 2005. Page 109.

186. "Defecting to Great Scientific Success," by Claudia Davis in The New York Times, July 22, 2103.

187. Vilcek J. Commentary: Fifty Years of Interferon Research: Aiming at a Moving Target. Immunity; 25:343–348, 2006.

188. "Research Scientist Gives $105 Million to N.Y.U." by Richard Perez-Penaaug in The New York Times, August 12, 2005.

189. https://www.youtube.com/watch?v=HpdqrFda7XM. A series of video interviews with Dr. Vilcek give the history of his life.

190. Burnet M. Cancer—A Biologic Approach. III. Viruses Associated with Neoplastic Conditions. Br Med J; 1(5023):841–847, 1957.

191. DeVita, Hellman, and Rosenberg's Cancer: Principles & Practice of Oncology, Tenth Edition, Vincent T. DeVita, Jr., Theodore S. Lawrence, Steven A. Rosenberg, editors, Wolters Kluwer Health, 2015.

192. Interferon: The science and selling of a miracle drug by Tione Pieters, Routledge, London and New York, 2005.

193. Friedman RM. Clinical uses of interferons. British Journal of Clinical Pharmacology, 65:158–162, 2008. This article reports the workshop was on April 1 and comments on the date. Interferon: The science and selling of a miracle drug by Toine Pieters, Routledge, London and New York, 2005. Page 125. Pieters reports the date as May 30.

194. Interferon: The science and selling of a miracle drug by Tione Pieters, Routledge, London and New York, 2005. Page 103.

195. "Leading U.S. Cancer Doctors Agree To Issue Warnings on Interferon." By Victor Cohn. *Washington Post*, June 15, 1980.

196. Interferon: The science and selling of a miracle drug by Tione Pieters, Routledge, London and New York, 2005. Page 158.

197. Interferon: The science and selling of a miracle drug by Tione Pieters, Routledge, London and New York, 2005. Page 132.

198. Friedman RM. Clinical uses of interferons. Brit J Clin Pharm; 65:158–162, 2008.

199. Kirkwood JM, Strawderman MH, Ernstoff MS et al. Interferon alfa-2b adjuvant therapy of high-risk resected cutaneous melanoma: The Eastern Cooperative Oncology Group Trial EST 1684. J Clin Oncol; 14(1):7-17, 1996.

200. Kirkwood JM, Manola J, Ibrahim J et al. A pooled analysis of eastern cooperative oncology group and intergroup trials of adjuvant high-dose interferon for melanoma. Clin Cancer Res; 10(5):1670-1677, 2004.

201. Rosenberg S. IL-2: The First Effective Immunotherapy for Human Cancer. J Immunol; 192:5451-5458, 2014.

202. Oppenheim J. IL-2: More than a T Cell Growth Factor. J Immunol; 179:1413-1414, 2007.

203. Kendall Smith. The Discovery of the IL-2 Molecule. www.kendallsmith.com/molecule.html. Accessed 9/15.

204. "Cetus: A Collision Course with Failure." By Sally Lehrman in *The Scientist*, January 20, 1992.

205. Making PCR: A Story of Biotechnology by Paul Rabinow, The University of Chicago Press, Chicago, 1996. Page 77.

206. The Transformed Cell: Unlocking the Mysteries of Cancer by Steven A. Rosenberg and John M. Barry, G.P. Putnam, New York, 1992. This is an autobiography of Dr. Rosenberg and describes his pursuit of immunotherapy.

207. Leach DR, Krummel M, Allison JP. Enhancement of antitumor immunity by CTLA-4 blockade. Science; 271:1734-36, 1996.

208. Wolchok JD, Hodi FS, Weber JS et al. Development of ipilimumab: a novel immunotherapeutic approach for the treatment of advanced melanoma. Ann NY Acad Sci; 1291:1-13, 2013.

209. FDA News Release "FDA approves Opdivo for advanced melanoma." December 22, 2014. Available at FDA.gov. Accessed 12/16.

CHARLIE PHILLIPS: NON-SMALL CELL LUNG CANCER

210. Sirisinha S. Evolutionary insights into the origin of innate and adaptive immune systems: different shades of grey. Asian Pac J All Immunol; 32(1):3-15, 2014.

211. Muehlenbachs A, Bhatnagar J, Agudelo CA et al. Malignant Transformation of *Hymenolepis nana* in a Human Host. N Engl J Med; 373(19); 1845-1852, 2015.

212. Suntharalingam G, Perry MR, Ward S et al. Cytokine Storm in a Phase 1 Trial of the Anti-CD28 Monoclonal Antibody TGN1412. N Engl J Med; 355:1018-1028, 2006.

213. There were several investigations resulting in differing criticisms, including the dose of the medication, treatment of six patients in a group, and failure to foresee the tragedy.

214. Leach DR, Krummel M, and Allison JP. Enhancement of antitumor immunity by CTLA-4 blockade. Science; 271:1734-36, 1996.

215. Keler T, Halk E, Vitale L et al. Activity and safety of CTLA-4 blockade combined with vaccines in cynomolgus macaques. J Immunol; 171:6251-6259, 2003.

216. Wolchok JD, Hodi FS, Weber JS et al. Development of ipilim-umab: a novel immunotherapeutic approach for the treatment of advanced melanoma. Ann NY Acad Sci; 1291:1-13, 2013. This article nicely reviews the development of the drug.

217. "Approval for Drug that Treats Melanoma" by Andrew Pollack, *The New York Times*, March 25, 2011.

218. FDA News Release "FDA expands approved use of Opdivo to treat lung cancer." March 4, 2015. Available at FDA.gov. Accessed 12/16.

WALTER GRADY: COLON CANCER

219. The effects of the EGFR pathway can be blocked by the drug cetuximab, but that medication will not work if the *k-ras* mutation has permanently "turned on" the pathway.

220. Cantor D. The Frustrations of Families: Henry Lynch, Heredity, and Cancer Control, 1962–1975. Med Hist; 50(3):279–302, 2006.

221. cdnmedhall.org/dr-phil-gold is the Canadian medical Hall of Fame website which includes a description of Dr. Gold and a brief interview with him and his colleagues.

222. Diamandis EP, Bast RC, Gold P et al. Reflection on the discovery of carcinoembryonic antigen, prostate-specific antigen, and can-cer antigens CA125 and CA19-9.

Clin Chem; 59(1):22-31, 2013. This article is an interesting col-lection of reflections by these scientists about the discovery of their tumor markers.

223. Hammarstrom S. The carcinoembryonic antigen (CEA) fam-ily: structures, suggested functions and expression in normal and

malignant tissues. Sem Cancer Bio; 9:67-81, 1999. This article describes the CEA in technical terms.

224. Vander Heiden MG, Cantley LC, Thompson CB. Understanding the Warburg Effect: The Metabolic Requirements of Cell Proliferation. Science; 324(5390):1029-1033, 2009.

225. Vander Heiden MG, Cantley LC, Thompson CB. Understanding the Warburg Effect: The Metabolic Requirements of Cell Proliferation. Science; 324(5930):1029-1033, 2009.

THELMA LAMBROS: OVARIAN CANCER

226. Kauffman G, Pentimalli R, Doldi S et al. Michele Peyrone (1813–1883), Discoverer of Cisplatin. Platinum Metals Rev; 54(4): 250–256, 2010. This article provides the history of the discovery of cisplatin referred to later in the story.

227. Tobias JS, Griffiths CT. Management of Ovarian Carcinoma—Current Concepts and Future Prospects. N Engl J Med; 294:877-882, 1976.

228. "From Basic Research to Cancer Drug: The Story of Cisplatin," by Ricki Lewis in *The Scientist*, July 5, 1999.

229. Richardson GS, Scully RE, Najamosama N and Nelson JH. Common Epithelial Cancer of the Ovary. N Engl J Med; 312:474-448, 1985.

230. McGuire WP, Rowinsky EK, Rosenshein NB et al. Taxol: a unique antineoplastic agent with significant activity in advanced ovarian epithelial neoplasms. Ann Intern Med; 111(4):273-279, 1989.

231. Armstrong DK, Bundy B, Wenzel L et al. Intraperitoneal Cisplatin and Paclitaxel in Ovarian Cancer. N Engl J Med; 354:34-43, 2006.

232. Bryant HE1, Schultz N, Thomas HD et al. Specific killing of BRCA2-deficient tumours with inhibitors of poly(ADP-ribose) polymerase. Nature; 434(7035):913-917, 2005.

233. Fong PC, Boss DS, Yap TA et al. Inhibition of Poly(ADP-Ribose) Polymerase in Tumors from BRCA Mutation Carriers. N Engl J Med; 361:123-134, 2009.

ROBERT FENTON: PROSTATE CANCER

234. The PSA can also be broken down into "free PSA" and "total PSA." The free PSA is PSA which is inactivated in the prostate gland. As prostate cancers develop, the PSA can escape the gland and enter the blood before inactivation, thus the free PSA can be a lower percentage of the total in cancers. The use of this breakdown of the PSA is highly debated.

235. The website of Roswell Park has a brief history of Dr. Chu and the PSA. https://www.roswellpark.org/cancer/prostate/prevention-early-detection/screening/history-psa . Accessed 12/16.

236. Phillips, JL and Sinha A. Patterns, Art and Context: Donald Floyd Gleason and the Development of the Gleason Grading System. Urology; 74(3):497–503, 2009.

237. "Obituary for Dr. Donald Gleason" by Thomas Maugh II in *The Los Angeles Times* on January 19, 2009.

238. Chism DB, Hanlon AL, Troncoso P et al. The Gleason score shift: score four and seven years ago. Int J Radiat Oncol Biol Phys; 56(5):1241-1247, 2003.

239. Smith EB, Frierson HF, Mills SE et al. Gleason scores of prostate biopsy and radical prostatectomy specimens over the past 10 years. Cancer; 94: 2282–2287, 2002.

240. Bill-Axelson, A, Holmberg L, Garmo H et al. Radical Prostatectomy or Watchful Waiting in Early Prostate Cancer. N Engl J Med; 370:932-942, 2014.

241. Wilt TJ, Brawer MK, Jones KM et al. Radical Prostatectomy versus Observation for Localized Prostate Cancer. N Engl J Med; 367:203-213, 2012.

242. Widmark A, Klepp O, Solberg A et al. Endocrine treatment, with or without radiotherapy, in locally advanced prostate cancer (SPCG-7/SFUO-3): an open randomised phase III trial. Lancet; 373(9660):301-308, 2009.

243. Kantof PW, Higano CS, Shore ND et al. Sipuleucel-T Immunotherapy for Castration-Resistant Prostate Cancer. N Engl J Med; 363:411-422, 2010.

244. Longo D. New Therapies for Castration-Resistant Prostate Cancer. N Engl J Med; 363:479-481, 2010.

WILLIAM DENTON: MULTIPLE MYELOMA

245. Brown JR and Thornton JL. Percivall Pott (1714-1788) and Chimney Sweepers' Cancer of the Scrotum. Br J Ind Med; 14(1):68–70, 1957.

246. Principles & Practice of Lung Cancer: The Official Reference Text of the IASLC, 4e, by Harvey I. Pass, David P. Carbone, David H. Johnson, John D. Minna, Giorgio V. Scagliotti, Andrew T. Turrisi, III. Wolters Kluwer Health, 2010. Chapter 65.

247. McDonald JC and McDonald AD. The Epidemiology of mesothelioma in historical context. Eur Respir J; 9:1932-1942, 1996.

248. Veterans and Agent Orange: Health Effects of Herbicides Used in Vietnam http://www.nap.edu/catalog/2141.html. Accessed 12/16. This is the report of the National Academy of Sciences. It contains an excellent description of the soldiers who fought in the war beginning on page 75.

249. Veterans and Agent Orange: Health Effects of Herbicides Used in Vietnam http://www.nap.edu/catalog/2141.html. Accessed 12/16.

250. Institute of Medicine (US) Committee to Review the Health Effects in Vietnam Veterans of Exposure to Herbicides. Veterans and Agent Orange: Health Effects of Herbicides Used in Vietnam. Washington (DC): National Academies Press (US); 1994. 2, History of the Controversy Over the Use of Herbicides. Available from: https://www.ncbi.nlm.nih.gov/books/NBK236351/. Accessed 12/16.

251. <u>The Effects of Herbicides in South Viet Nam</u> by the Committee on the Effects of Herbicides in Viet Nam. National Academy of Sciences, Washington, DC, 1974. This report contains an interesting introduction about the challenges of forming the committee and reporting its results given the divisions over the war.

252. "For Maude DeVictor, Agent Orange Became an Obsession." By James Litke, Associated Press on Mar. 9, 1985.

253. Times Beach Site - Environmental Protection Agency. https://www.epa.gov/history/times-beach. Accessed 3/17.

254. Veterans and Agent Orange: Health Effects of Herbicides Used in Vietnam Committee to Review the Health Effects in Vietnam Veterans of Exposure to Herbicides, Institute of Medicine. ISBN:

0-309-55619-8, 832 pages, 6 x 9, (1994). This PDF is available from the National Academies Press at: http://www.nap.edu/catalog/2141.html. Accessed 12/16.

255. The opposite view from the IOM report can be found in <u>Politicizing Science: The Alchemy of Policymaking</u> edited by Michael Gough, The Hoover Institution Press, Stanford University, Stanford, California, 2003. Chapter 8 written by Gough is titled "The Political Science of Agent Orange and Dioxin."

256. Attal M, Harousseau JL, Stoppa AM et al. A Prospective, Randomized Trial of Autologous Bone Marrow Transplantation and Chemotherapy in Multiple Myeloma. N Engl J Med; 335:91-97, 1996.

257. A description of the program can be founded on the Institute's website.

258. Palumbo A, Cavallo F, Gay F et al. Autologous transplantation and maintenance therapy in multiple myeloma. N Engl J Med; 371:895-905, 2014.

259. This story was reported "Thalidomide Found to Slow a Bone Cancer" by Sheryl Gay Stolberg in *The New York Times* on November 18, 1999.

260. Singhal S, Mehta J, Desikan R et al. Antitumor activity of thalidomide in refractory multiple myeloma. N Engl J Med; 341:1565–1571, 1999.

261. Sanchez-Serrano I. Translational Research in the Development of Bortezomib: A Core Model. Disc Med; 5(30):527-533, 2005.

262. "Development of a Targeted Treatment for Cancer: The Example of C225 (Cetuximab)" by John Mendelsohn in <u>Molecular Targeting in Oncology</u> edited by Kaufam HL, Wadler S and Antman K. Humans Press, Totowa, NJ, 2008. See page 562.

263. De Weers M, Tai YT, van der Veer MS et al. Daratumumab, a novel therapeutic human CD38 monoclonal antibody, induces killing of multiple myeloma and other hematological tumors. J Immunol; 186:1840-48, 2011.

CAROL FEINMAN 4: BREAST CANCER

264. The Canadian Medical Hall of Fame website includes a description of Dr. Gold and a brief interview with him and his colleagues. http://cdnmedhall.org/inductees/dr-phil-gold. Accessed 3/17.

265. Hammarstrom S. The carcinoembryonic antigen (CEA) family: structures, suggested functions and expression in normal and malignant tissues. Sem Canc Bio; 9(2):67-81, 1999. This article describes the CEA in technical terms.

266. The website of Roswell Park has a brief history of Dr. Chu and the PSA. https://www.roswellpark.org/cancer/prostate/prevention-early-detection/screening/history-psa. Accessed 12/16.

JEFF STILLER: HEAD AND NECK CANCER

267. Volkow ND and McLellan AT. Opioid Abuse in Chronic Pain — Misconceptions and Mitigation Strategies. N Engl J Med; 374(13):1253-63, 2016.

268. Volkow ND and McLellan AT. Opioid Abuse in Chronic Pain — Misconceptions and Mitigation Strategies. N Engl J Med; 374(13):1253-63, 2016.

269. Volkow ND, Baler RD, Compton WM et al. Adverse Health Effects of Marijuana Use. N Engl J Med; 370:2219-2227, 2014.

270. Kandel ER and Kandel DB. A Molecular Basis for Nicotine as a Gateway Drug. N Engl J Med; 371:932-943, 2014.

271. Adolescent Substance Abuse: America's #1 Health Problem. A report by the National Center on Addiction and Substance Abuse at Columbia University. Available at www.centeronaddiction.org. Accessed 4/16.

272. Morpheus was one of the few Greek Gods who kept his or her name in Roman mythology, a fact noted in The Encyclopedia of Greco-Roman Mythology by Mike Davis-Kennedy, ABC-CLIO, Santa Barbara, CA, 1998.

273. Friedrich SR. Wilhelm Seturner and the Discovery of Morphine. Pharm Hist; 27(2): 61-74, 1985.

274. Forces of Habit: Drugs and the Making of the Modern World by David T. Courtwright, Harvard University Press, Cambridge, Massachusetts, 2001. See pages 31-34 for an overview of opium.

275. "As morphine turns 200, drug that blocks its side effects reveals new secrets." From the University of Chicago. Available at www.uchospitals.edu news from 05/19/2005, accessed 3/16.

276. Friedrich SR. Wilhelm Seturner and the Discovery of Morphine. Pharm Hist; 27(2): 61-74, 1985.

277. Ovid's *Metamorphoses Book XI.* ovid.lib.virginia.edu. Accessed 3/16.

278. Friedrich SR. Wilhelm Seturner and the Discovery of Morphine. Pharm Hist; 27(2): 61-74, 1985.

279. <u>Mythology</u> by Edith Hamilton, Little, Brown and Company, Boston, 1942. Page 43 and 334 describe the River of Lethe.

280. Ovid's *Metamorphoses Book XI (573-649)*. ovid.lib.virginia.edu. Accessed 3/16.

281. ancestry.com

282. "Opiate Addiction as a Consequence of the Civil War" by David T. Courtwright in <u>The Civil War Veteran: A Historical Reader</u>, edited by Larry M Logue and Michael Barton, New York University Press, New York and London, 2007. Courtwright provides a balanced discussion of both sides of this debate.

283. "Post-Traumatic Stress" by Eric T. Dean, Jr. in <u>The Civil War Veteran: A Historical Reader</u>, edited by Larry M Logue and Michael Barton, New York University Press, New York and London, 2007.

284. "Exempt from the Ordinary Rules of Life" by James Marten in <u>The Civil War Veteran: A Historical Reader</u>, edited by Larry M Logue and Michael Barton, New York University Press, New York and London, 2007.

285. "Opiate Addiction as a Consequence of the Civil War" by David T. Courtwright in <u>The Civil War Veteran: A Historical Reader</u>, edited by Larry M Logue and Michael Barton, New York University Press, New York and London, 2007.

286. Lewis DC and Zinberg NE. Narcotic Usage: II. A Historical Perspective on a Difficult Medical Problem. N Engl J Med; 270(20):1045-1050, 1964.

287. <u>An Anatomy of Addiction: Sigmund Freud, William Halsted and the Miracle Drug Cocaine</u> by Howard Markel. Pantheon Books,

New York, 2011. See pages 53-63 for the extraction and expansion of cocaine industry and page 93 for a discussion of the eye surgeries.

288. Sneader W. The Discovery of Heroin. Lancet; 352(9141):1697-1699, 1998. Heroin was removed from the history of Bayer.

289. Lewis DC and Zinberg NE. Narcotic Usage: II. A Historical Perspective on a Difficult Medical Problem. N Engl J Med; 270(20):1045-1050, 1964.

290. An Anatomy of Addiction: Sigmund Freud, William Halsted and the Miracle Drug Cocaine by Howard Markel, Pantheon Books, New York, 2011. This a fascinating book which juxtaposes the experiences of these two giants in medicine.

291. Halsted's radical surgery was based on the concept that the cancer spread through the lymph system, so removal of more lymph tissue would stop the spread. It was later understood that the cancers spread via the blood stream. The extensive surgery to remove more lymph and breast tissue was too late; the "horse was out of the barn." This led to the use of more a limited mastectomy and, with time, even lumpectomy and radiation in place of Halsted's surgery.

292. An Anatomy of Addiction: Sigmund Freud, William Halsted and the Miracle Drug Cocaine by Howard Markel, Pantheon Books, New York, 2011. Markel advances this idea on page 239.

293. "History of Drug Use and Drug Users in the United States" by Elaine Casey. From Facts about Drug Abuse-Participant Manual Publication, U.S. Government publications 79-FADA-041P, November 1978. Available from Schaffer Library of Drug Policy at www.druglibrary.org. Accessed 3/16.

294. Lewis DC and Zinberg NE. Narcotic Usage: II. A Historical Perspective on a Difficult Medical Problem. N Engl J Med; 270(20):1045-1050, 1964. The authors point out the difficulties outpatient programs faced both in terms of knowledge and the political and legal environment. They note the AMA resolution denouncing the outpatient treatment of addiction.

295. "New Anti-Drug Law is in Effect Today" in *The New York Times* on July 1, 1914.

296. Boylan credits Town in a letter to *The New York Times* published April 20, 1914.

297. The law provided for physicians to provide narcotics as part of their "professional practice." The practice was defined by the Court to exclude prescribing narcotics to addicts.

298. Lewis DC and Zinberg NE. Narcotic Usage: II. A Historical Perspective on a Difficult Medical Problem. N Engl J Med; 270(20):1045-1050, 1964.

299. Lewis DC and Zinberg NE. Narcotic Usage: II. A Historical Perspective on a Difficult Medical Problem. N Engl J Med; 270(20):1045-1050, 1964.

300. Lewis DC and Zinberg NE. Narcotic Usage: II. A Historical Perspective on a Difficult Medical Problem. N Engl J Med; 270(20):1045-1050, 1964.

301. Lewis DC and Zinberg NE. Narcotic Usage: II. A Historical Perspective on a Difficult Medical Problem. N Engl J Med; 270(20):1045-1050, 1964.

302. Courtwright DT. Preventing and Treating Narcotic Addiction — A Century of Federal Drug Control. N Engl J Med, 373:2095-2097, 2015.

303. *The Druggists Circular*, October 1922, page 392. A reproduction is available on Google Books. Several similar articles in the circular give the confusing history and debates about the narcotics laws of the time.

304. Brown LS. Substance Abuse and America: Historical Perspective on the Federal Response to a Social Phenomenon. J Natl Med Assoc; 73(6):497-506, 1981.

305. "History of Drug Use and Drug Users in the United States" by Elaine Casey. From Facts about Drug Abuse-Participant Manual Publication, U.S. Government publications 79-FADA-041P, November 1978. Available from Schaffer Library of Drug Policy at www.druglibrary.org. Accessed 3/16.

306. "History of Drug Use and Drug Users in the United States" by Elaine Casey. From Facts about Drug Abuse-Participant Manual Publication, U.S. Government publications 79-FADA-041P, November 1978. Available from Schaffer Library of Drug Policy at www.druglibrary.org. Accessed 3/16.

307. Kolodny A, Courtwright DT, Hwang CS et al. The Prescription Opioid and Heroin Crisis: A Public Health Approach to an Epidemic of Addiction. Ann Rev Pub Health; 36:559–574, 2015.

308. OxyContin Abuse and Diversion and Efforts to Address the Problem. United States General Accounting Office Report GAO- 04-110. December 2003. http://www.gao.gov/new.items/d04110.pdf. Accessed 4/16.

309. Kolodny A, Courtwright DT, Hwang CS et al. The Prescription Opioid and Heroin Crisis: A Public Health Approach to an Epidemic of Addiction. Ann Rev Pub Health; 36:559–574, 2015.

310. OxyContin Abuse and Diversion and Efforts to Address the Problem. United States General Accounting Office Report GAO- 04-110. December 2003. http://www.gao.gov/new.items/d04110.pdf. Accessed 4/16.

311. Kolodny A, Courtwright DT, Hwang CS et al. The Prescription Opioid and Heroin Crisis: A Public Health Approach to an Epidemic of Addiction. Ann Rev Pub Health; 36:559–574, 2015.

312. "In Guilty Plea, OxyContin Maker to Pay $600 Million," by Barry Meier in *The New York Times* on May 10, 2007.

313. Nelson LS, Juurlink DN, Perrone J. Addressing the Opioid Epidemic. JAMA; 314(14):1453-1454, 2015.

314. "Development of a Targeted Treatment for Cancer: The Example of C225 (Cetuximab)" by John Mendelsohn in Molecular Targeting in Oncology edited by HL Kaufam, S Wadler, and K Antman, Humans Press, Totowa, NJ, 2008.

DENISE FLINT: KIDNEY CANCER

315. Paget S. The Distribution of Secondary Growths in Cancer of the Breast. Lancet; 1:571-573, 1889.

316. Hart IR and Fidler IJ. Role of Organ Selectivity in Determination of Metastatic Patterns of B16 Melanoma. Can Res; 40:2281-2287, 1980.

317. Sonnenschein C and Soto A. Cancer Metastases: So close and so far. JNCI; 107(11): dvj236, 2015.

318. From "Milestones in Cancer: Observations from a ploughman" by Helen Dell in *Nature* April 1, 2006 | doi:10.1038/nrc1843.

319. Maher ER, Neumann HPH, Richard S. von Hippel-Lindau disease: A clinical and scientific review. Eur J Hum Gen; 19:617-623, 2011.

320. Cohen AJ, Li FP, Berg S et al. Hereditary Renal-Cell Carcinoma Associated with a Chromosomal Translocation. N Engl J Med 301:592-595, 1972.

321. In addition to the obvious fact they involve different genes, an important difference between the VHL translocation and the Philadelphia chromosome translocation is that the VHL translocation is inherited and all the cells in the person carry the defect. The Philadelphia chromosome translocation develops in the stem cells of the bone marrow during life but is not present at birth.

322. Clark PE and Cookson MS. The von Hippel-Lindau Gene: Turning Discovery into Therapy. Cancer; 113(7 suppl):1768-78, 2008.

323. "Prolonging the Life of Cancer Patients" gives a brief history of the development of sunitinib and is available at http://www.astp-proton.eu/prolonging-life-cancer-patients/. Accessed 5/16.

324. Fairlamb DJ. Spontaneous Regression of Metastasis of Renal Cancer: A report of two cases including the first recorded regression following irradiation of a dominant metastasis and review of the world literature. Cancer; 47:2102-2106, 1981.

325. Bukowski RM. Natural history and therapy of metastatic renal cell carcinoma. The role of IL-2. Cancer; 80:1198-1220, 1997.

326. Flanigan RC, Salmon SE, Blumenstein BA et al. Nephrectomy followed by interferon alfa-2b compared with interferon alfa-2b alone for metastatic renal-cell cancer. N Engl J Med; 345:1655-1659, 2001.

327. Weinstock M and McDermott DF. Emerging Role for Novel Immunotherapy Agents in Metastatic Renal Cell Carcinoma: From Bench to Bedside. 2015 ASCO Educational Book. e291. asco.org/edbook.

RACHAEL SIMON: BREAST CANCER

328. Selye H. A syndrome produced by diverse nocuous agents. Nature; 138(3479):32, 1936.

329. The Stress of Life (revised edition) by Hans Selye, McGraw-Hill Book Co, New York, 1976.

330. Bodily Changes in Pain, Hunger, Fear and Rage by Walter B. Cannon, D. Appleton and Company, New York and London, 1915.

331. The Stress of Life (revised edition) by Hans Selye, McGraw-Hill Book Co, New York, 1976. Page 174 to 177 describes the components of a panic attack.

332. The Stress of Life (revised edition) by Hans Selye, McGraw-Hill Book Co, New York, 1976. Page 1 starts a nice summary of the G.A.S.

333. The Stress of Life (revised edition) by Hans Selye, McGraw-Hill Book Co, New York, 1976. Page 375.

334. Smith MT, Guyton KZ, Gibbons CF et al. Key Characteristics of Carcinogens as a Basis for Organizing Data on Mechanisms

of Carcinogenesis. Environmental Health Perspectives, 2016. Online at http://dx.doi.org/10.1289/ehp.1509912. Accessed 3/17.

335. Hanoun M, Maryanovich M, Arnal-Estape, et al. Neural regulation of hematopoiesis, inflammation and cancer. Neuron; 86(2): 360–373, 2015.

336. Genentech: The Beginnings of Biotech by Sally Smith Hughes, The University of Chicago Press, Chicago, 2011. This book details the rise of the company.

337. From The Truth About the Drug Companies by Marcia Angell, Random House, New York, 2004.

338. Ullrich shares the credit with Robert Weinberg, a well-known scientist at MIT who found the Her-2-neu protein years earlier but whose work took him in other directions.

339. "Development of a Targeted Treatment for Cancer: The Example of C225 (Cetuximab)" by John Mendelsohn in Molecular Targeting in Oncology edited by Kaufman HL, Wadler S and Antman K. Humans Press, Totowa, NJ, 2008. See page 562.

340. Interferon: The science and selling of a miracle drug by Toine Pieters, Routledge, London and New York, 2005. This is a complete history of interferon.

Pieters, T. Interferon and its first clinical trial: looking behind the scenes. Med Hist 37(3):270-95, 1993. This article preceded the book and gives more detail into the initial discovery phase of interferon.

341. Her 2: The Making of Herceptin, a Revolutionary Treatment for Breast Cancer by Robert Bazell, Random House, New York,

1998. This is a very personally written book about the figures involved and chapter 5 details this story.

342. Her 2: The Making of Herceptin, a Revolutionary Treatment for Breast Cancer by Robert Bazell, Random House, New York, 1998. Page 50.

343. "Genentech-Roche Deal May Spur Similar Ties," by Andrew Pollack, Special to *The New York Times*, February 5, 1990.

344. Pegram M, Hsu S, Lewis G et al. Inhibitory effects of combinations of her-2/neu antibody and chemotherapeutic agents used for treatment of human breast cancers. Oncogene; 18(13):2241-2251, 1999.

345. Her 2: The Making of Herceptin, a Revolutionary Treatment for Breast Cancer by Robert Bazell, Random House, New York, 1998. Brazell covers these events in his book in pages 113-132.

346. The Emperor of All Maladies by Siddhartha Mukherjee, Scribner, New York, 2010. The description of this struggle is well told on beginning on page 423.

347. Slamon DJ, Leyland-Jones B, Shak S et al. Use of Chemotherapy plus a Monoclonal Antibody against HER2 for Metastatic Breast Cancer That Overexpresses HER2. N Engl J Med; 344:783-792, 2001.

348. Romond EH, Perez EA, Bryant J et al. Trastuzumab plus Adjuvant Chemotherapy for Operable HER2-Positive Breast Cancer. N Engl J Med; 353:1673-1684, 2005.

349. President Reagan honored Williams at a 1993 Commencement address at the Citadel. A nice report of this comes from "Lessons

from '82 Disaster Aided Hudson River Crash Pilots" by Josh Katz's article found on "finding Dulcinea, Librarian of the Internet" dated January 15, 2010.

350. The issues are well summarized in "A Crash's Improbable Impact" by Del Quentin Wilber in *The Washington Post*, January 12, 2007.

351. <u>To Err is Human: Building a Safer Health System</u> by the Institute of Medicine, November 1999 is available on the website of the National Academy of Science (www.nationalacademies.org).

352. The original studies used by the Institute of Medicine were:

Brennan TA, Leape LL Laird NM at al. Incidence of Adverse Events and Negligence in Hospitalized Patients — Results of the Harvard Medical Practice Study I. N Engl J Med; 324:370-376, 1991.

Leape LL, Brennan TA, Laird N et al. The Nature of Adverse Events in Hospitalized Patients. Results of the Harvard Medical Practice Study II. N Engl J Med; 324:377-84, 1991.

Thomas EJ, Studdert DM, Burstin HR et al. Incidence and Types of Adverse Events and Negligent Care in Utah and Colorado. Med Care; 38(3):261-71, 2000.

Two letters responding to the Harvard study were noteworthy:

Incidence of Adverse Events and Negligence in Hospitalized Patients. N Engl J Med; 325:210, 1991.

353. The Office of Inspector General report released in November 2010 called "Adverse Events in Hospitals: National Incidence among Medicare Beneficiaries," Daniel R. Levinson Inspector

General. It is available on the oig.hhs.gov website. This report includes a history of the issues, a review of Medicare charts, and proposals regarding hospital safety.

354. "Big Doses of Chemotherapy Drug Killed Patient, Hurt 2d" by Lawrence Altman in *The New York Times*, March 24, 1995.

355. Makary M and Daniel M. Medical error—the third leading cause of death in the US. BMJ; 2139:353-358, 2016.

356. Maizlin ZV1, Vos PM. Do we really need to thank the Beatles for the financing of the development of the computed tomography scanner? J Comput Assist Tomogr; 36(2):161-164, 2012.

CAROL FEINMAN 5: BREAST CANCER

357. Wachter RM. AIDS, Activism, and the Politics of Health. N Engl J Med; 326(2):128-133, 1992.

358. Kokler ES. Framing as a cultural resource in health social movements: funding activism and the breast cancer movement in the US 1990-1993. Soci Health Ill; 26(6): 820-844, 2004.

359. Wachter RM. AIDS, Activism, and the Politics of Health. N Engl J Med; 326(2):128-133, 1992.

360. Wachter RM. AIDS, Activism, and the Politics of Health. N Engl J Med; 326(2):128-133, 1992.

361. Wachter RM. AIDS, Activism, and the Politics of Health. N Engl J Med; 326(2):128-133, 1992.

362. Osuch JR, Silk K, Price C et al. A Historical Perspective on Breast Cancer Activism in the United States: From Education and

Support to Partnership in Scientific Research. J Women Health; 21(3):355-362, 2012.

363. Lerner BH. No shrinking violet: Rush Kushner and the rise of American breast cancer activism. West J Med; 174:362-365, 2001.

364. Osuch JR, Silk K, Price C et al. A Historical Perspective on Breast Cancer Activism in the United States: From Education and Support to Partnership in Scientific Research. J Women Health; 21(3):355-362, 2012.

365. King S. Pink Ribbons Inc: breast cancer activism and the politics of philanthropy. Int J Qual Stud Ed; 17(4):473-492, 2004.

366. Healy B. The Yentl Syndrome. N Engl J Med; 325(4):274-276, 1991.

367. Osuch JR, Silk K, Price C et al. A Historical Perspective on Breast Cancer Activism in the United States: From Education and Support to Partnership in Scientific Research. J Women Health; 21(3):355-362, 2012.

368. http://www.beautyoutofdamage.com/Aboutphoto.html. Accessed 3/17.

369. Turning Disease Into Political Cause: First AIDS, and Now Breast Cancer by Jane Gross, *The New York Times*, January 7, 1991.

370. Turning Disease Into Political Cause: First AIDS, and Now Breast Cancer by Jane Gross, *The New York Times*, January 7, 1991.

371. https://www.visualaids.org/projects/detail/the-red-ribbon-project. Accessed 3/17.

372. Wright PW. Red Ribbon. Texas Heart Inst; 40(4):384, 2013.

373. Through a City Archway: The Story of Allen and Hanburys, 1715-1954, by Desmond Chapman-Huston and Ernest C. Cripps, John Murray, London, 1954. Reviewed by Cope Z. Brit Med J; 1(4909):337, 1955.

374. Through a City Archway: The Story of Allen and Hanburys, 1715-1954, by Desmond Chapman-Huston and Ernest C. Cripps, John Murray, London, 1954. Reviewed by Cope Z. Brit Med J; 1(4909):337, 1955.

375. Perfecting the World: The Life and Times of Dr. Thomas Hodgkin 1789-1866 by Amalia and Edward Kass, Harcourt Brace Jovanovich, Orlando, 1988. Pages 17-27.

376. Page C and Humphrey P. Sir David Jack; an extraordinary drug discoverer and developer. Br J Clin Pharm; 75(5):1213-1218, 2013.

377. Dale DC. The Discovery, Development and Clinical Applications of Granulocyte Colony Stimulating Factor. Transactions of the American and Climatological Association. Volume 109, pages 27-38, 1988.

378. Gabrilove J. The Development of Granulocyte Colony-Stimulating Factor in its Various Clinical Applications. Blood; 80(6):1382-1385, 1992.

379. www.amegenhistory.com accessed 7/16.

380. The Crimean War: A History by Orlando Figes, Metropolitan Books, Henry Holt and Company, New York, 2010.

381. Heart and Soul. The Story of Florence Nightingale by Gena K. Gorrell, Tundra Books, Toronto, 2000.

382. <u>Heart and Soul. The Story of Florence Nightingale</u> by Gena K. Gorrell, Tundra Books, Toronto, 2000. See page 124.

383. <u>Clara Barton, Founder, American Red Cross</u> in American Women of Achievement Series by Leni Hamilton, Chelsea House Publishers, New York and Philadelphia, 1988.

384. <u>Clara Barton, Founder, American Red Cross</u> in American Women of Achievement Series by Leni Hamilton, Chelsea House Publishers, New York and Philadelphia, 1988.

385. RedCross.org accessed 7/16.

386. ons.org accessed 7/16.

DEBRA PACKARD: BREAST CANCER

387. Germain RN. Maintaining system homeostasis - the third law of Newtonian immunology. Nat immun; 13(10):902-906, 2012.

388. Eisenberg DM, Davis RB, Ettner SL et al. Trends in Alternative Medicine Use in the United States, 1990-1997. JAMA; 280:1569-1575, 1998.

389. <u>Richard Bright 1789-1858, Physician in an Age of Revolution and Reform</u> by Diana Berry and Campbell Mackenzie, Royal Society of Medicine Services Limited, London, 1992. Page 32.

390. <u>Richard Bright 1789-1858, Physician in an Age of Revolution and Reform</u> by Diana Berry and Campbell Mackenzie, Royal Society of Medicine Services Limited, London, 1992. Page 34.

391. <u>Richard Bright 1789-1858, Physician in an Age of Revolution and Reform</u> by Diana Berry and Campbell Mackenzie, Royal Society of Medicine Services Limited, London, 1992. Page 59.

392. Nagy J and Sonkodi S. Richard Bright in Hungary: A Reevaluation. Am J Nephrol; 17:387-391, 1997.

393. Richard Bright 1789-1858, Physician in an Age of Revolution and Reform by Diana Berry and Campbell Mackenzie, Royal Society of Medicine Services Limited, London, 1992. Pages 62 and 120.

394. Slater EAW. Bright and Bright's Disease. Res Medica; 2(2):43-46, 1960.

395. Thayer WS. Richard Bright: The Man and the Physician. Br Med J; 2(3471):87–93, 1927.

396. Barlow GH as quoted in Richard Bright 1789-1858, Physician in an Age of Revolution and Reform by Diana Berry and Campbell Mackenzie, Royal Society of Medicine Services Limited, London, 1992. Page 236.

397. Richard Bright 1789-1858, Physician in an Age of Revolution and Reform by Diana Berry and Campbell Mackenzie, Royal Society of Medicine Services Limited, London, 1992. Page 131.

398. Richard Bright 1789-1858, Physician in an Age of Revolution and Reform by Diana Berry and Campbell Mackenzie, Royal Society of Medicine Services Limited, London, 1992. Page 68 and 113.

399. New Guide to Health or Botanic Family Physician by Samuel Thomson. Printed for the Author, and sold by his General Agent, at the Office of the Boston Investigator. J. Q. ADAMS, Printer. 1835. www.swsbm.com/ManualsOther/Samuel_Thomson-Lloyd.pdf.

400. New Guide to Health or Botanic Family Physician by Samuel Thomson. Printed for the Author, and sold by his General Agent, at the Office of the Boston Investigator. J. Q. ADAMS, Printer. 1835.

www.swsbm.com/ManualsOther/Samuel_Thomson-Lloyd.pdf.
Page 25.

401. <u>New Guide to Health or Botanic Family Physician</u> by Samuel
Thomson. Printed for the Author, and sold by his General Agent, at
the Office of the Boston Investigator. J. Q. ADAMS, Printer. 1835.
www.swsbm.com/ManualsOther/Samuel_Thomson-Lloyd.pdf.
Page 26.

402. <u>Nature Cures: The History of Alternative Medicine in America</u>
by James C. Whorton, Oxford University Press, Oxford, 2002.
Pages 28 to 32 provide a very nice description of Thompson's
system and marketing.

403. <u>Nature Cures: The History of Alternative Medicine in America</u>
by James C. Whorton, Oxford University Press, Oxford, 2002.
This is nicely discussed beginning on page 33 and in the article
by Flannery below.

404. <u>Nature Cures: The History of Alternative Medicine in America</u>
by James C. Whorton, Oxford University Press, Oxford, 2002.
Page 39-40.

405. Flannery, MA. The early botanical medical movement as a reflection of life, liberty, and literacy in Jacksonian America. J Med Libr
Assoc; 90(4):442–454, 2002.

406. <u>Clara Barton, Founder, American Red Cross</u> in American Women
of Achievement Series by Leni Hamilton, Chelsea House
Publishers, New York and Philadelphia, 1988. Page 21.

407. Flannery, MA. The early botanical medical movement as a reflection of life, liberty, and literacy in Jacksonian America. J Med Libr
Assoc; 90(4):442–454, 2002.

408. Immediately after his U.S. report, Flexner wrote a similar, although less detailed description of medical education in Europe which was also clearly pro-German.

409. Ludmerer KM. Commentary: Understanding the Flexner Report. Acad Med; 85:193–196, 2010.

410. Duffy TP. The Flexner Report — 100 Years Later. Yale J Biol Med; 84(3):269–276, 2011.

411. Medical Education in the United States and Canada: A Report to the Carnegie Foundation For Teaching by Abraham Flexner, The Carnegie Foundation, New York, 1910. Reproduced by D.B. Updike, The Merrymount Press, Boston, 1960 and 1972.

412. Medical Education in the United States and Canada: A Report to the Carnegie Foundation For Teaching by Abraham Flexner, The Carnegie Foundation, New York, 1910. Reproduced by D.B. Updike, The Merrymount Press, Boston, 1960 and 1972. Page 179 and 180.

413. Barkin SL, Fuentes-Afflick E, Brosco JP et al. Unintended Consequences of the Flexner Report: Women in Pediatrics. Pediatrics; 126(6):1055-1057, 2010.

414. Medical Education in the United States and Canada: A Report to the Carnegie Foundation For Teaching by Abraham Flexner, The Carnegie Foundation, New York, 1910. Reproduced by D.B. Updike, The Merrymount Press, Boston, 1960 and 1972. Pages 155.

415. Medical Education in the United States and Canada: A Report to the Carnegie Foundation For Teaching by Abraham Flexner, The Carnegie Foundation, New York, 1910. Reproduced by D.B. Updike, The Merrymount Press, Boston, 1960 and 1972. Page 154.

416. Medical Education in the United States and Canada: A Report to the Carnegie Foundation For Teaching by Abraham Flexner, The Carnegie Foundation, New York, 1910. Reproduced by D.B. Updike, The Merrymount Press, Boston, 1960 and 1972. Page 64.

417. Medical Education in the United States and Canada: A Report to the Carnegie Foundation For Teaching by Abraham Flexner, The Carnegie Foundation, New York, 1910. Reproduced by D.B. Updike, The Merrymount Press, Boston, 1960 and 1972. Page 155.

418. Ludmerer KM. Commentary: Understanding the Flexner Report. Acad Med; 85:193–196, 2010.

419. Duffy TP. The Flexner Report — 100 Years Later. Yale J Biol Med; 84(3):269–276, 2011.

420. Medical Education in the United States and Canada: A Report to the Carnegie Foundation For Teaching by Abraham Flexner, The Carnegie Foundation, New York, 1910. Reproduced by D.B. Updike, The Merrymount Press, Boston, 1960 and 1972. Page 161.

421. Medical Education in the United States and Canada: A Report to the Carnegie Foundation For Teaching by Abraham Flexner, The Carnegie Foundation, New York, 1910. Reproduced by D.B. Updike, The Merrymount Press, Boston, 1960 and 1972. Page 162.

422. Nature Cures: The History of Alternative Medicine in America by James C. Whorton, The Oxford University Press, New York, 2002. Whorton's fascinating book covers each of these movements in detail in separate chapters.

423. Nature Cures: The History of Alternative Medicine in America by James C. Whorton, The Oxford University Press, New York, 2002. Page 18.

424. Nature Cures: The History of Alternative Medicine in America by James C. Whorton, The Oxford University Press, New York, 2002. Chapter 7. Page 141.

425. Autobiography of Andrew Still with a History of the Discovery and Development of the Science of Osteopathy by Andrew Still. 1897. Accessed in 1/16 on https://archive.org/details/autobiographyand00stiliala.

426. Autobiography of Andrew Still with a History of the Discovery and Development of the Science of Osteopathy by Andrew Still. 1897. Accessed in 1/16 on https://archive.org/details/autobiographyand00stiliala. Page 276.

427. Autobiography of Andrew Still with a History of the Discovery and Development of the Science of Osteopathy by Andrew Still. 1897. Accessed in 1/16 on https://archive.org/details/autobiographyand00stiliala. Page 63.

428. Autobiography of Andrew Still with a History of the Discovery and Development of the Science of Osteopathy by Andrew Still. 1897. Accessed in 1/16 on https://archive.org/details/autobiographyand00stiliala. Page 98-99.

429. Nature Cures: The History of Alternative Medicine in America by James C. Whorton. The Oxford University Press, New York, 2002. Page 145. Dr. Whorton's description and Still's own autobiography convey this sense.

430. Nature Cures: The History of Alternative Medicine in America by James C. Whorton, The Oxford University Press, New York, 2002. Chapter 8. Page 165.

431. The Chiropractor by D.D. Palmer, Beacon Light Printing Company, Los Angeles, 1914. Page 3.

432. Nature Cures: The History of Alternative Medicine in America by James C. Whorton, The Oxford University Press, New York, 2002. Page 233.

433. Carey TS, Garrett J, Jackman A et al. The Outcomes and Costs of Care for Acute Low Back Pain among Patients Seen by Primary Care Practitioners, Chiropractors, and Orthopedic Surgeons. N Engl J Med; 333:913-917, 1995.

434. *Hamlet* (1.5.167-8), Hamlet to Horatio

435. Podolsky SH and Kessselheim AS. Regulating Homeopathic Products—A Century of Dilute Interest. N Engl J Med; 374: 201-203, 2016.

436. Nature Cures: The History of Alternative Medicine in America by James C. Whorton. The Oxford University Press, New York, 2002. Chapter 9 is devoted to Naturopathy and much of this description comes from that work.

437. Whorton J. Benedict Lust, Naturopathy, and the Theory of Therapeutic Universalism. Iron Game Hist; 8:22-29, 2003.

438. Interferon: The science and selling of a miracle drug by Toine Pieters, Routledge, London and New York, 2005. Page 40. The cartoon is reproduced here.

439. Interferon: The science and selling of a miracle drug by Toine Pieters, Routledge, London and New York, 2005. Page 74.

440. Nature Cures: The History of Alternative Medicine in America by James C. Whorton, The Oxford University Press, New York, 2002. Chapter 11, page 248. This section of Dr. Whorton's book nicely expands on these concepts.

441. Steve Jobs by Walter Isaacson, Simon and Schuster, New York, 2011. Page 58.

442. Nature Cures: The History of Alternative Medicine in America by James C. Whorton, The Oxford University Press, New York, 2002. Pages 277 and 279.

443. Representative Thomas Harkin was critical to this effort and his interest had been spurred on the experiences of two of his sister who had breast cancer.

444. Nature Cures: The History of Alternative Medicine in America by James C. Whorton, The Oxford University Press, New York, 2002. Page 18.

445. Eisenberg DM, Davis RB, Ettner SL et al. Trends in Alternative Medicine Use in the United States, 1990-1997. JAMA; 280:1569-1575, 1998.

446. Angell M and Kassirer J. Alternative Medicine—The Risks of Untested and Unregulated Remedies. N Engl J Med; 339: 839-841, 1998.

447. Abrams DI and Weil AT. What's the Alternative? (letter to the editor). N Engl J Med; 366:2232-3, 2012.

448. The American College of Surgeons Cancer Program Standards website at https://www.facs.org/quality%20programs. Accessed 2/16.

449. From Oliver Wendell Holmes and quoted by A Yankauer in a review of <u>Nature Cures: The History of Alternative Medicine in America</u> by James Whorton, The Oxford University Press, New York, 2002. The review appeared in N Engl J Med 348; 2165-6, 2003.

450. Fisher B, Dignam J, Emir A et al. Tamoxifen and Chemotherapy for Lymph Node-Negative, Estrogen Receptor-Positive Breast Cancer. J Natl Cancer Inst; 89(22):1673-1682, 1997.

451. Mamounas EP. NSABP Breast Cancer Clinical Trials: Recent Results and Future Directions. Clin Med Res; 1(4):309–326, 2003.

452. Fisher B, Dignam J, Emir A et al. Tamoxifen and Chemotherapy for Lymph Node-Negative, Estrogen Receptor-Positive Breast Cancer. J Natl Cancer Inst; 89(22):1673-1682, 1997.

453. www.nsabp.pitt.edu/NSABP_Pathology.asp.

BILLY JACKSON: ESOPHAGEAL CANCER

454. Torek F. The First Successful Resection of the Thoracic Portion of the Esophagus for Cancer: A Preliminary Report. JAMA; 60(20):1533, 1913.

455. Eggers C. Franz JA Torek 1861-1938. Ann Surg; 110(4):797-799, 1939.

456. Brodsky JB, Lemmens JM. The history of anesthesia for thoracic surgery. Mierva Anestesiol; 73(10):513-24, 2007.

457. OD. Obituary I Lewis. Brit Med J; 285(2):982,1982.

SARAH TAYLOR: CERVICAL CANCER

458. Tan SY and Tatsumura Y. George Papanicolaou (1883-1962): Discoverer of the Pap smear. Singapore Med J; 56(10):586-587, 2015.

459. <u>Practical Treatise on The Diseases of the Lungs and Heart</u> by Walter Hayle Walshe, Taylor, Walton, & Maberly, London, 1851. Page 413.

460. <u>Practical Treatise on The Diseases of the Lungs and Heart</u> by Walter Hayle Walshe, Taylor, Walton, & Maberly, London, 1851. Page viii.

461. <u>The Anatomy, Physiology, Pathology and Treatment of Cancer</u> by Walter Hayle Walsh, William D. Ticknor and Company, Boston, 1844.

462. Hajdu SI and Ehya H. A note from History: Foundation of Diagnostic Cytology. Annal Clin Lab Science; 38(3):296-299, 2008.

463. Tan SY and Tatsumura. George Papanicolaou (1883-1962): Discoverer of the Pap smear. Singapore Med J; 56(10):586-587, 2015.

464. Traut HF and Papanicolaou. Cancer of the Uterus: The Vaginal Smear in Diagnosis. Cal West Med; 59(2):121-122, 1943.

465. Vilos GA. The History of the Papanicolaou Smear and the Odyssey of George and Andromache Papanicolaou. Obstect Gynecol; 91(3):479-483, 1998.

466. Meigs JV. Gynecology: Carcinoma of the Cervix. N Engl J Med; 230(19):577-582, 1944.

467. Beral V. Cancer of the cervix: a sexually transmitted infection? Lancet; 1(7865):1037-40, 1974.

468. Munoz N, Bosch S, and Kaldor JM. Does human papillomavirus cause cervical cancer? The state of epidemiological evidence. Br. J Cancer; 57:1-5, 1987.

469. Koss LG. Cytologic and Histologic Manifestations of Human Papillomavirus Infection of the Female Genital Tract and Their Clinical Significance. Cancer; 60:1942-1950, 1987.

470. Durst M, Gissman L, Ikenberg H et al. A papillomavirus DNA from a cervical carcinoma and its prevalence in cancer biopsy samples from different geographic regions. Proc Natl Acad Sci; 80:8212-3815, 1983.

471. Muller M, Zhou J, Reed TD et al. Chimeric Papillomavirus-like Particles. Virology; 234:93-111, 1997.

472. "HPV: the whole story, wart and all" by Emma Smith writing in the Science Blog of Cancer Research UK. September 16, 2014. Http://scienceblog.cancerresearchuk.org/2014/09/16/hpv-the-whole-story-warts-and-all/ accessed 10/24/16.

473. Koutsky LA, Ault KA, Wheeler CM et al. A controlled trial of a human papillomavirus type 16 vaccine. N Engl J Med; 347(21):1645-1651, 2002.

474. The HPV Vaccine: Access and Use in the U.S. The Henry J. Kaiser Family Foundation, September 2015 Fact Sheet. www.kff. org. Accessed 11/16.

475. Baily HH, Chuang LT, DuPont NC et al. American Society of Clinical Oncology Statement: Human Papillomavirus Vaccination for Cancer Prevention. J Clin Oncol; 34(15):1803-1812, 2016.

476. Tannock IF and Hickman JA. Limits to Personalized Cancer Medicine. N Engl J Med; 375(13):1289-1294, 2016.

CAROL FEINMAN 7: BREAST CANCER

477. McGuire WP, Rowinsky EK, Rosenshein NB et al. Taxol: a unique antineoplastic agent with significant activity in advanced ovarian epithelial neoplasms. Ann Intern Med; 111(4):273-9, 1989.

478. Abrams JB, Vena DA, Baltz J et al. Paclitaxel Activity in Heavily Pretreated Breast Cancer: A National Cancer Institute Treatment Referral Center Trial. J Clin Oncol; 13:2056-2065, 1995.

JOSEPH LAWRENCE: GLIOBLASTOMA

479. Ferguson S, Lesniak MS. Percival Bailey and the classification of brain tumors. Neurosurg Focus; 18(4):1-6, 2005.

480. Harvey Cushing: A Life in Surgery by Michael Biss, Oxford University Press, Oxford, 2005. This is a comprehensive biography of this remarkable man. The book is reviewed in Clarfield AM. Harvey Cushing: A Life in Surgery by Michael Biss (Review). N Engl J Med; 354: 534-535, 2006.

481. Harvey Cushing: A Life in Surgery by Michael Biss, Oxford University Press, Oxford, 2005. Page 164.

482. Harvey Cushing: A Life in Surgery by Michael Biss, Oxford University Press, Oxford, 2005. Page 228.

483. Harvey Cushing: A Life in Surgery by Michael Biss, Oxford University Press, Oxford, 2005. The biography covers this complexity beautifully.

484. Percival Bailey (1892-1973). A Biographical Memoir by Paul Mitchell. Bucy, National Academy of Sciences, Washington, D.C. 1989. Available at http://www.nasonline.org/publications/biographical-memoirs/memoir-pdfs/bailey-per.pdf. Accessed 1/17.

485. Percival Bailey (1892-1973). A Biographical Memoir by Paul Mitchell. Bucy, National Academy of Sciences, Washington, D.C. 1989. Available at http://www.nasonline.org/publications/biographical-memoirs/memoir-pdfs/bailey-per.pdf. Accessed 1/17.

486. Ferguson S, Lesniak MS. Percival Bailey and the classification of brain tumors. Neurosurg Focus; 18(4):1-6, 2005.

487. Rycaj K and Tang DG. Cancer Stem Cells and Radioresistance. Int J Radiat Biol; 90(8):615-621, 2014.

488. Lathia JD, Mack SC, Mulkearns-Hubert EE et al. Cancer stem cells in glioblastoma. Genes Dev; 29:1203-1217, 2015.

489. Newlands ES, Stevens MFG, Wedge SR et al. Temozolomide: a review of its discovery, chemical properties, pre-clinical development and clinical trials. Canc Treat Rev; 23:35-61, 1997.

490. Stupp R, Mason WP, van den Bent MJ et al. Radiotherapy plus concomitant and adjuvant temozolomide for glioblastoma. N Engl J Med; 352(10):987-996, 2005.

491. https://www.cancer.gov/about-cancer/treatment/drugs/fda-temozolomide. Accessed 1/17.

492. Adams and Victor's Principles of Neurology (Tenth Edition) by Allen Ropper, Martin A. Samuels, and Joshua P Klein, McGraw-Hill Education, 2014.

493. Paul Broca: Founder of French Anthropology, Explorer of the Brain by Francis Schiller, Oxford University Press, New York, 1992. First published by University of California Press, Berkley, 1979. This is a detailed biography of Broca and provides a discussion of these events as well as photographs of Tan's brain in the section "A Manner of Not Speaking." Slightly different perspectives of the debated are offered in the articles cited later.

494. Berker EA, Berker AH, Smith A. Translation of Broca's 1865 Report. Localization of Speech in the Third Left Frontal Convolution. Arch Neurol; 43:1065-1072, 1986.

495. Broca PP. Loss of Speech, Chronic Softening and Partial Destruction of the Anterior Left Lobe of the Brain. Bulletin de la Societe Anthropologique; 2:235-238, 1861. A translation by CD Green is found at psychclassics.yorku.ca/Broca/perte-e.htm. Accessed 1/17.

496. Berker EA, Berker AH, Smith A. Translation of Broca's 1865 Report. Localization of Speech in the Third Left Frontal Convolution. Arch Neurol; 43:1065-1072, 1986.

497. Harlow JM. Passage of An Iron Rod Through the Head. Boston Medical and Surgical Journal; 39(20):389-393, 1848.

498. Harlow JM. Recovery from the Passage of an Iron Bar through the Head. Read before the Massachusetts Medical Society, June 3, 1868. David Clapp & Son, Boston, 1869. https://en.wikisource.org/wiki/Author:John_Martyn_Harlow. Accessed 1/17.

499. Ratiu P, Talos IF. The Tale of Phineas Gage, Digitally Remastered. N Engl J Med; 351:e21, 2004.

500. The Man Who Mistook His Wife For a Hat by Oliver Sacks, Summit Books, New York, 1985. Page 154.

501. Thiebaut de Schotten M, Dell'Acqua, Ratiul et al. From Phineas Gage and Monsieur Leborgne to H.M.: Revisiting Disconnection Syndromes. Cerebral Cortex; 25:4812–4827, 2015.

502. "Soul has Weight, Physician Thinks." Special to The New York Times, March 11, 1907.

503. Carelli Frank. The book of death: weighing your heart. London J Prim Care; 4:86-87, 2011.

504. In Search of the Soul and the Mechanism of Thought, Emotion, and Conduct by Bernard Hollander.\, EP Dutton and Company, New York, 1920. Page 12. Available at https://archive.org/details/insearchofsoulme01holl.

505. Leonardo Da Vinci and the Search for the Soul by Rolando Frank Del Maestro. American Osler Society John P. McGovern Award Lectureship. Delivered April 27th, 2015 at the 45th Meeting of the American Osler Society Baltimore, Maryland.

506. Leonardo Da Vinci and the Search for the Soul by Rolando Frank Del Maestro. American Osler Society John P. McGovern Award Lectureship. Delivered April 27th, 2015 at the 45th Meeting of the American Osler Society Baltimore, Maryland.

507. Lokhorst, Gert-Jan, "Descartes and the Pineal Gland," The Stanford Encyclopedia of Philosophy (Summer 2016 Edition),

Edward N. Zalta (ed.), URL = <https://plato.stanford.edu/archives/sum2016/entries/pineal-gland/>. Accessed 3/17.

508. Fine HA. New Strategies in Glioblastoma: Exploiting the New Biology. Clin Cancer Res; 21(9):1984-1988, 2015.

509. Kirson ED, Daly V, Tovarys F et al. Alternating electric fields arrest cell proliferation in animal tumor models and human brain tumors. PNAS; 104(24):10152-10157, 2007.

510. Stupp R, Tallibert S, Kanner AA et al. Maintenance Therapy With Tumor-Treating Fields Plus Temozolomide vs Temozolomide Alone for Glioblastoma. JAMA; 314(23):2535-2543, 2015.

511. Sampson JH. Alternating Electric Fields for the Treatment of Glioblastoma (Editorial). JAMA; 314(23):2511-2513, 2015.

512. www.fda.gov/NewsEvents/Newsroom/PressAnnouncements/ucm465744.htm. Accessed 1/17.

513. Richmond M. Dame Cicely Saunders, founder of the modern hospice movement, dies. BMJ; 331(7510):238, 2005.

514. Baines M. From pioneer days to implementation: lessons to be learnt. Euro J Pall Care; 18(5): 223-227, 2011.

Provides perspective on this early period. Twycross RG. Choice of strong analgesic in terminal cancer: diamorphine or morphine? Pain; 3(2):93-104, 1977.

515. http://www.stchristophers.org.uk/about/damecicelysaunders/tributes. Accessed 1/17.

516. History of Hospice. National Hospice and Palliative Care Organization. http://www.nhpco.org/history-hospice-care. Accessed 1/17.

517. Friedrich MJ. Hospice care in the United States: A Conversation with Florence S. Wald. JAMA; 281(18):1683-5, 1999.

518. National Hospice and Palliative Care Organization Facts and Figures, 2015 Edition. http://www.nhpco.org/about-hospice-and-palliative-care/hospice-faqs. Accessed 1/17.

519. Kubler-Ross E. The Family Physician and the Dying Patient. Can Fam Physician; 18(10):79-83, 1972.

520. Friedrich MJ. Hospice care in the United States: A Conversation with Florence S. Wald. JAMA; 281(18):1683-1685, 1999.

521. Buck S. Policy and the Re-Formulation of Hospice: Lessons from the Past and Future of Palliative Care. J Hosp Palliat Nurs; 13(6):S35-S43, 2011.

522. Friedrich MJ. Hospice care in the United States: A Conversation with Florence S. Wald. JAMA; 281(18):1683-1685, 1999.

523. Buck S. Policy and the Re-Formulation of Hospice: Lessons from the Past and Future of Palliative Care. J Hosp Palliat Nurs; 13(6):S35-S43, 2011.

524. http://www.stchristophers.org.uk/about/damecicelysaunders/tributes. Accessed 1/17.

525. http://www.stchristophers.org.uk/about/damecicelysaunders/tributes. Accessed 1/17.

GLEN WATERS: LYMPHOMA

526. Hodgkin, T. On some marked appearances of absorbent glands and spleen. Medico-Chirurg. Tr. London; 17:68-114, 1832.

527. A very nice biography of Dr. Dorothy Reed Mendenhall appears at https://www.nlm.nih.gov/changingthefaceofmedicine/physicians/biography_221.html. Accessed 6/16.

528. Haggard HW, Smith GM. Johannes Müller and the Modern Conception of Cancer. The Yale Journal of Biology and Medicine; 10(5):419-436, 1938.

529. Degos L. John Hughes Bennett, Rudolph Virchow ... and Alfred Donne: the first description of leukemia. Hem J; 2:1, 2001.

530. Piller GJ. Leukaemia—A brief historical review from ancient times to 1950. Brit J Heam; 112:282-292, 2001.

531. Haggard HW and Smith GM. Johannes Muller and the Modern Conception of Cancer. Yale J of Biol and Med; 10(5):419-436, 1938.

532. The Non-Hodgkin's Lymphoma Pathologic Classification Project. Cancer 49:2112-2135, 1982.

533. Nadler LM, Stashenko P, Hardy R et al. Serotherapy of a Patient with a Mono-clonal Antibody Directed against a Human Lymphoma-associated Antigen. Cancer Res; 40:3147-3154, 1980.

534. Reff M, Carner K, Chambers KS et al. Depletion of B Cells In Vivo by a Chimeric Mouse Human Monoclonal Antibody to CD20. Blood; 83(4):435-445, 1994.

535. IDEC would go on to merge with Biogen in 2002.

536. Ecker DM, Jones SD, Levine H. The therapeutic monoclonal antibody market. mAbs; 7(1):9-14, 2015.

537. Jackson H. The Diagnosis and Treatment of Malignant Lymphoma. New Engl J Med; 201(26):1284-1285, 1929.

538. This description comes from <u>Blood</u> by James H. Jandl, Little, Brown and Company, Boston, 1987. Page 945.

539. <u>Blood</u> by James H. Jandl, Little, Brown and Company, Boston, 1987. Page 946.

540. Fisher RI, Gaynor ER, Dahlberg S et al. Comparison of a Standard Regimen (CHOP) with Three Intensive Chemotherapy Regimens for Advanced Non-Hodgkin's Lymphoma. N Engl J Med; 328:1002-6, 1993.

541. A picture of father and son appear in the history of Walter Reed at http://documentslide.com/documents/the-patient-is-first-and-lastalways-a-history-of-the-dept.html Accessed 12/16.

542. Bruton OC. Agammaglobulinemia. Pediatrics; 9:722-728, 1952.

543. Buckley RH. Commentary Agammaglobulinemia, by Col. Ogden C. Bruton, MC, USA, Pediatrics, 1952;9:722-8. Pediatrics; 102:213-215, 1998.

544. Byrd JC, Furman RR, Coutre SE et al. Targeting BTK with Ibrutinib in Relapsed Chronic Lymphocytic Leukemia. N Engl J Med; 369:32-42, 2013.

545. Foa R and Guarini A. A Mechanism-Driven Treatment for Chronic Lymphocytic Leukemia. N Engl J Med; 369:85-87, 2013.

546. Brody J, Kohrt H, Marabelle A et al. Active and Passive Immunotherapy for Lymphoma: Proving Principles and Improving Results. J Clin Oncol; 29:1864-1875, 2011.

547. Palanca-Wessels MC and Press OW. Advances in the treatment of hematologic malignancies using immunoconjugates. Blood; 123(15):2293-2301, 2014.

548. Topp MS, Gokburger N, Zugmaier G et al. Phase II Trial of the Anti-CD 19 Bispecific T Cell-Engager Blinatumomab Shows Hematologic and Molecular Remission in Patients With Relapsed or Refractory B-Precursor Acute Lymphoblastic Leukemia. J Clin Oncol; 32:4134-4140, 2014.

549. Maude SL, Frey N, Shaw P et al. Chimeric Antigen Receptor T Cells for Sustained Remission in Leukemia. N Engl J Med; 371(16):1507-1717, 2014.

550. Hoban MD and Bauer DE. A genome editing primer for the hematologist. Blood; 127:2525-2535, 2016.

ALISA COHEN: GENETIC TESTING

551. Hall JM, Lee MK, Newman B et al. Linkage of Early-Onset Familial Breast Cancer to Chromosome 17q21. Science; 250:1684-89, 1990.

552. "Breast Cancer Gene Offers Surprises," by Racheal Nowak in the News Section of Science; 265: 1796-1799, 1994.

553. Miki Y, Swensen J, Shattuck-Eidens D et al. A Strong Candidate Gene for the Breast and Ovarian Cancer Susceptibility Gene BRCA1. Science; 266:66-71, 1994.

554. https://ghr.nlm.nih.gov/gene/BRCA1#conditions. Accessed 11/16.

555. Weber BL. Susceptibility Genes for Breast Cancer. N Engl J Med; 331(22):1523-4, 1994.

556. The nomenclature used here was replaced by a more complex but scientifically more accurate system. These common mutations are often still referred to by their earlier designations.

557. www.knowbrca.org gives a comprehensive review. Accessed 11/16.

558. Neuhausen SL, Mazoyer S, Friedman L et al. Haplotype and Phenotype Analysis of Six Recurrent BRCA1 Mutations in 61 Families: results of an International Study. Am J Hum Genet 58:271-280, 1996.

559. Bar-Sade RB, Kruglikova A, Modan B et al. The del185AG BRCA1 Mutation Originated before the Dispersion of Jews in the Diaspora and Is Not Limited to Ashkenazim. Hum Molec Genet; 7(5):810-5, 1996.

560. Hamel N, Feng BJ, Foretova L et al. On the origin and diffusion of BRCA1 c.5526dupC (5382insC) in European populations. Eur J Hum Gen; 19:300-306, 2011.

561. "The Spanish Expulsion" from jewishvirtuallibrary.org. Accessed 11/16.

562. The Secret Jews of San Luis Valley by Jeff Wheelwright in *Smithsonian Magazine*, October 2008 at smithsonian.com. Accessed 11/16.

563. Collins FS. BRCA1- Lots of Mutations, Lots of Dilemmas. N Engl J Med; 334(3):186-188, 1996.

564. Semple J, Metcalfe KA, Lynch HT et al. International rates of breast reconstruction after prophylactic mastectomy in BRCA1 and BRCA2 mutation carriers. Ann Surg Oncol; 20(12): 3817-3822, 2013.

565. "My Medical Choice" by Angelina Jolie in *The New York Times*, May 14, 2014.

566. Finch AP, Lubinski J, Moller P et al. Impact of oophorectomy on cancer incidence and mortality in women with a BRCA1 or BRCA2 mutation. J Clin Oncol; 32(15):1547-1554, 2014.

567. Cannon-Albright LA, Thomas A, Goldgar DE, et al. Familiality of Cancer in Utah. Cancer Res; 54(9):2378-85, 1994.

568. Gold ER and Carbone J. Myriad Genetics: In the eye of the policy storm. Genet Med; 12(4 Suppl):S39–S70, 2010. This comprehensive article reviews the issues prior to the Supreme Court case.

569. Personal communication and author's observations.

570. Gold ER and Carbone J. Myriad Genetics: In the eye of the policy storm. Genet Med; 12(4 Suppl): S39–S70, 2010.

571. <u>Genetic Susceptibility to Breast and Ovarian Cancer: Assessment, Counseling and Testing Guidelines</u>. Published by the American

College of Medical Genetics, Bethesda, MD, 1999. Sponsored by New York State Department of Health.

572. Personal communication and author's observations.

573. Personal communication and author's observations.

574. "How a Breast Cancer Pioneer Finally Turned a Profit," by JJ Colao in *Forbes*, November 5, 2112.

575. Supreme Court of the United States *Association for Molecular Pathology et al. v. Myriad Genetics, Inc et al.* Certiorari to the United States Court of Appeals for the Federal Circuit. No. 12–398. Argued April 15, 2013—Decided June 13, 2013.

Index

Made in the USA
Middletown, DE
14 November 2017